How Medicines Work

Illustrated

How Medicines Work

Illustrated

William S. Hancock
Northeastern University, USA

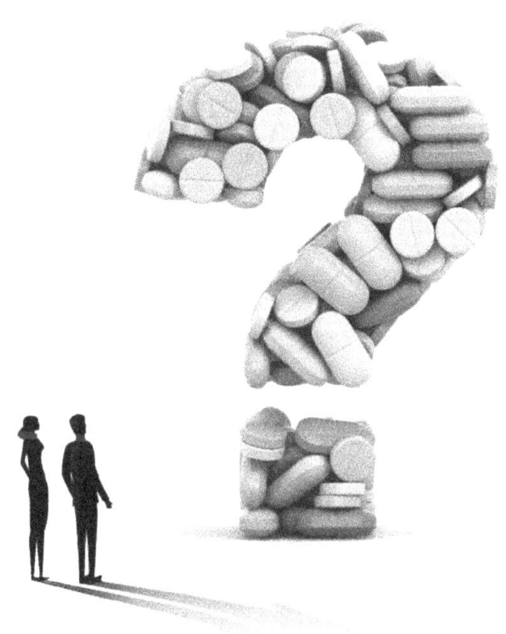

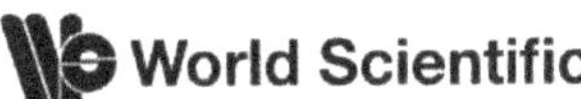

World Scientific

NEW JERSEY • LONDON • SINGAPORE • BEIJING • SHANGHAI • HONG KONG • TAIPEI • CHENNAI • TOKYO

Published by

World Scientific Publishing Co. Pte. Ltd.
5 Toh Tuck Link, Singapore 596224
USA office: 27 Warren Street, Suite 401-402, Hackensack, NJ 07601
UK office: 57 Shelton Street, Covent Garden, London WC2H 9HE

Library of Congress Cataloging-in-Publication Data
Names: Hancock, William S., author.
Title: How medicines work : illustrated / William S. Hancock.
Description: New Jersey : World Scientific, [2022]
Identifiers: LCCN 2022013265 | ISBN 9789811248191 (hardcover) | ISBN 9789811248207 (ebook) |
ISBN 9789811248214 (ebook other)
Subjects: MESH: Pharmacological Phenomena | Pharmacokinetics | Drug Therapy | Handbook | Pictorial Work
Classification: LCC RM300 | NLM QV 39 | DDC 615.1--dc23/eng/20220525
LC record available at https://lccn.loc.gov/2022013265

British Library Cataloguing-in-Publication Data
A catalogue record for this book is available from the British Library.

For any available supplementary material, please visit
https://www.worldscientific.com/worldscibooks/10.1142/12582#t=suppl

Table of contents

Table of contents ctd.

FOREWORD

By Stephen Wasserman, MD
Professor and Chairman, Emeritus
Department of Medicine
UC San Diego

William Hancock brings his more than 50 years of experience and expertise in analytic biochemistry and drug development to this book. He has deftly integrated and characterized classical and newly approved pharmaceutical and biologic agents by presenting their chemistry, biological mode of action, and relevance to medical disorders in clear prose and brilliantly explanatory figures and diagrams to enable the reader to understand the drug, its chemistry, and its mode of action. The book is especially timely as medical therapy moves from treating populations to individualized personalized medicine. As one with more than 50 years of experience in medical education and training and clinical practice, I can see the utility of this material to a broad variety of learners and caregivers. For the beginner in biomedical therapeutics, the material provides concise and clear descriptions of drugs and their role in various pathobiological processes. For the more seasoned learner such as advanced medical students and residents in training, it provides important material at one's fingertips without fighting through algorhythmic thickets presented on frequently accessed electronic data bases. For the practitioner, this book enables important discussions with patients by providing the physician with simple to describe figures explaining the most advanced new therapeutics for disorders commonly seen in clinical practice. By focusing only on approved therapeutics, the contents of this book eliminate the potential confusion of the learner and the educator so often engendered when agents studied in animal or cellular model systems but not yet studied in human disease are added into the mix. I anticipate wide use of this book in medical schools and physician's offices.

FOREWORD

By Kathryn C. Zoon, PhD
Scientist Emerita, NIH
Former Scientific Director, NIAID, NIH
Former Director, CBER, FDA

William Hancock has over 50 years of experience in chemistry and has been involved in the analytical characterization of biopharmaceuticals since the mid-1980s. He is a recognized leader in both industry and academic institutions for developing methods to characterize proteins and glycoproteins. He was one of the driving forces for the first Well Characterized biotechnological Product (WCBP) symposium in the mid-1990s. These symposia still occur on an annual basis. Bill along with his colleagues were instrumental in engaging industry, regulatory and academic scientists to focus on the establishment of tests and criteria for biopharmaceuticals that could facilitate their development, production, and quality. At that time, I was then Director of the Food and Drug Administration's Center for Biologics Evaluation and Research (CBER). My colleagues at CBER and I led the development of regulatory guidance for biotechnology products since the early 1980s and these activities continued throughout my tenure at FDA. It was a natural partnership of regulators, academics, and industry to facilitate the advancement of biotechnology-derived medicines. Together, scientists shared their successes and challenges, which was especially important to the moving the field of biopharmaceuticals forward and to the rapid advances in medical treatments.

This book provides examples of important medicines that have been approved by regulatory authorities to prevent or treat a variety of diseases. FDA was at the forefront of approving many of these new medicines such as monoclonal antibodies, mRNA vaccines for COVID-19, growth factors and cytokines, and targeted cancer therapies. The development and application of innovative technologies and the collaborative efforts of scientists and physicians at government and private institutions have contributed and will continue to advance the availability of new medicines to the public.

FOREWORD

By Kenneth R. Miller, PhD
Director, Biologics Operation, AstraZeneca

"A picture is worth a thousand words" is an often-used phrase meaning a complex concept can be described through the use of one image. In the case of "How Medicines Work: Illustrated," this phrase is quite appropriate. As a biochemist by training and someone who has been in the biopharmaceutical industry for more than 15 years, I am always looking for effective ways to teach undergraduate and graduate students what can be a complicated subject, how medicines work. William Hancock, in this highly illustrated book that you are about to read, has done a masterful job of using visuals to explain the cellular biochemistry of diseases and how medicines are used to treat those diseases. Perfect examples of this are the easy-to-understand explanations in Chapter 6 of Hemophilia A and the bispecific antibody that was approved by the US FDA under breakthrough therapy designation for its treatment and in Chapter 7 of human papillomavirus (HPV) and a vaccine that prevents its infection.

I first met William ("Bill") Hancock at a well-characterized biotechnology products symposium a few years ago and have had the great pleasure to get know him better since then. I had the opportunity over the past year to work closely with Bill to organize a kickoff session during the 25th anniversary celebration of the CASSS-sponsored WCBP meetings. During this session, Bill was joined by other pioneers in the development and regulation of well-characterized biotechnology products for a fireside chat that I moderated. I am particularly impressed by the broad experience that Bill has, and the ease with which he shares his extensive knowledge. Bill's career has spanned across the biopharmaceutical industry, scientific instrumentation suppliers, academia, and for a brief time as a visiting scientist at the FDA, where he established a high-performance liquid chromatography (HPLC) assay for the activity of recombinant-DNA-derived human insulin.

Bill is highly recognized in the field of analytical chemistry, including his pioneering work in the area of separation and characterization of biomolecules. He has served as an Associate Editor for *Analytical Chemistry* and as the founding Editor-in-Chief of the *Journal of Proteome Research*. With his extensive experience in individual drug approvals, he has given testimony before the Senate Judiciary Committee on the topic of review and approval of off-patent biological products. CASSS, which is a not-for-profit professional scientific society, has recognized the significant contributions of Bill over the years by establishing the William S. Hancock Award for Outstanding Achievements in CMC Regulatory Science. This award is given on an annual basis to someone who has significantly contributed to the advancement of scientific principles, applied technologies, and/or science-based regulations in the areas of manufacturing process, technology development, characterization, analysis, and quality of biotechnology-derived pharmaceuticals.

Besides being a valuable resource for the education of undergraduate and graduate students, "How Medicines Work: Illustrated" is also valuable for anyone in the pharmaceutical industry to have. With its clear and concise descriptions, it is the perfect reference to have close at hand when discussing diseases and medicines with those in the general public, who do not have formal scientific training. I look forward to referencing "How Medicines Work: Illustrated" when I have conversations with family and friends about diseases and medicines, and will be recommending for them to add it to their personal library so that they can have informed discussions with their healthcare providers.

FOREWORD

By Jeffrey C. Travis, PhD, FAACC

Biomedical technology continues to expand exponentially and once unapproachable new drug targets, as well as well-established ones, are now able to be exploited with breakthrough FDA-approved pharmaceuticals, from small molecules to biologics, cell and gene therapies, across the whole disease spectrum. Using novel mechanisms of action, it can be increasingly more difficult to recall the rapidly expanding number of trade and generic names for drugs and match them to very specific functions in pathology.

Professor Hancock's new book (How Medicines Work: An Illustrated View*)* provides a unique medical resource and quick reference for established and recently approved new drugs and their essential mechanisms of action for specifically targeted diseases. In one or two pages for each drug, he concisely reviews the disease, the medicine (including when approved by FDA), and the essential mechanism of action on the cell and disease biology. Using a skillful combination of technical jargon and easy-to-read text, combined with associated highly colorful and descriptive diagrams, this book provides a quick reference suitable across a wide range of readers. I believe those of us in the clinical pathology profession; from clinical pathologists to clinical chemists, clinical microbiologists, medical technologists, physicians, nurses, lab assistants, and technicians, can find this a very useful resource for quick review or to learn specific drug mechanisms, as well as trade-generic name associations. There is no question patients also can benefit from this book as its reading style and concise descriptions can help them better understand why their medical provider has prescribed a specific drug and how they can benefit from it.

Preface

The rapid advance in medical knowledge based on the sequencing of the human genome, with the associated fields of epigenomics, transcriptomics, proteomics, and metabolomics, has resulted in a significant increase in knowledge of the cause of a wide range of diseases and potential therapies. In addition, the areas of drug research have experienced a parallel evolution in both the design of small molecule, antibody, and peptide drugs as well as the new DNA, RNA, and cell therapies.

The explosion in knowledge presents challenges across the field of medicine ranging from faculty and student educational practices, to patient–doctor interactions, to regulatory bodies, and pharmaceutical research programs. In each area of biological research, the amount of detailed knowledge has become overwhelming to all except specialized research practitioners and is accompanied by extensive use of acronyms, which hinders understanding. The positive side of this increase in biological research has been the approval of valuable new medicines for the treatment of both rare and chronic diseases (50+ approved by the FDA each year).

With the well-known aphorism "A picture is worth a thousand words" this book provides an illustrated view of how a broad range of approved medicines work for the major disease classes. The different chapters will include viral and bacterial infections, cancer, high blood pressure, diabetes, autoimmune and neurological disorders, as well as recent FDA approvals of medicines for rare diseases. The individual descriptions will be based on normal and disease biology resulting from a fusion of different areas, such as the physiological biochemistry of organs, endocrinology, clinical chemistry, pharmacology, and organic chemistry. By the study of the organ, we can describe the disease process as well as understanding how each medicine will interact with carrier proteins, transporters, metabolizing enzymes, and multiple receptors. Such insights will aid understanding of how the medicine works.

The book structure will progress from a description of the digestive organs and processing the molecules of life, the body's protective systems, the maintenance of physiological homeostasis, brain function and disorders, to breakthrough therapies, with the final chapter on the properties of viruses, diseases, and medicines.

It is the author's hope that this book shows readers the power of illustrations to convey a global view of disease processes and the diversity of modern medicines. The book has been prepared with the goal that it will be a valuable tool for medical education, as well as the development and regulation of powerful new medicines.

Biographical Information

Areas of technology development during my career:

The broad scope of this book on the spectrum of medicines for human diseases originated from the different aspects of my long career in education, government service, and analytical biotechnology.

The understanding of the role of proteins in biological systems was promoted by three significant developments that were a focus of my research. Firstly, the ability to synthesize proteins by chemical and then recombinant DNA procedures enabled the genesis of the biotechnology industry. The products of these syntheses created the need for a high-efficiency analytical method for purity analysis and structure-function studies. The development of reversed-phase high-performance liquid chromatography (HPLC) coupled with mass spectrometry provided a premier tool for intact protein analysis and peptide mapping for the identification of amino acid substitutions. This technology has become an integral part of manufacturing and quality control in the biotechnology industry. Subsequently, success in sequencing the human genome, coupled with protein and peptide analysis by mass spectrometry and HPLC, created the new field of proteomics which enable the global study and understanding of the role proteins play in disease biology.

Cumulated experience in medical research

(Location and calendar year given below)

The chemical synthesis of acyl carrier protein and studies of fatty acid biosynthesis (1971) **//** Identification of proteins involved in thyroid function (thyroid-stimulating hormone [TSH] and parathyroid hormone [PTH]) **//** Chemical synthesis of apolipoprotein C-I and study of lipid transport and heart disease **//** Developed a new analytical technique, reversed-phase HPLC for analysis of proteins and peptide mapping to characterize protein variants, as there was a need to analyze proteins in biological samples. The broad impact of this new analytical method was described in two CRC Handbooks, “HPLC for the Separation of Amino Acids, Peptides and Proteins.” **//** Measurement of plasma amino acids, enkephalins, and rotavirus envelope proteins (1972–1984)

// HPLC for the study of apolipoproteins and variants in the transport of cholesterol and lipids in the blood and role in hyperlipoproteinemias (1980) // Keynote presentation on the HPLC technique at the first FDA Consensus Forming Meeting for the regulation of biotechnology drugs (1983) // Development of an HPLC assay of insulins at the FDA (1984) // Application of HPLC to recombinant DNA products and monitoring of protein pharmaceuticals for a range of diseases, for example, diabetes, hormonal insufficiencies, asthma, blood disorders, multiple cancers, and infectious diseases (1985) // Development of mass spectrometry methods in the analysis of blood biomarkers for disease diagnosis and the characterization of adenovirus vectors used in gene therapy. Later, ion trap mass spectrometry enabled the development of proteomic analysis of blood, cerebrospinal fluid, and cancer cell lines (1994–2002) // Proteomic analysis was applied to a wide range of diseases: 1) Cancer, ranging from breast, pancreas, stomach, colon, brain, head and neck, and renal 2) Infectious disease—AIDS 3) Cardiovascular diseases, diabetes, metabolic syndrome, and gastric bypass 4) Polycystic kidney disease 5) Glycoproteomics measured the changing glycans in cancer and infectious diseases and was also applied to the characterization of biosimilar antibody therapeutics (2002–2018) // Review of drug approvals for small molecules, biotechnology, and cell therapy medicines (2019).

History

1968—1970 in Organic Chemistry, University of Adelaide
1971—Post doctorate with Professor P.R. Vagelos, School of Medicine, Washington University, St. Louis
1972—Professor in Biochemistry, Massey University, New Zealand
1980—Sabbatical, Department of Internal Medicine at Baylor College of Medicine, Houston
1984—Visiting Scientist at Bureau of Drugs, FDA, Washington, D.C.
1985—Staff Scientist, Director of Analytical Chemistry, Acting Director of Pharmacology, Genentech California
1994—Principal Scientist, HP Laboratories
1996—Adjunct Professor of Chemical Engineering, Yale University, New Haven, Connecticut
2000—Vice President, Proteomics Development, Thermo Finnigan, San Jose, California
2001—Founding Editor-in-Chief, Journal of Proteomic Research, American Chemical Society
2002—Brad Street Chair, Barnett Institute, Northeastern University, Boston, Massachusetts
2007—Cochair National Cancer Institute Alliance of Glycobiologists for Detection of Cancer
2008—Visiting Professor, Yonsei University, Seoul, Korea
2009—Adjunct Professor of Clinical Proteomics, Macquarie University, Australia
2015—Member of FDA Advisory Committee
2018—Adjunct Professor—Department of Medicine, University of California, San Diego
2018—Research affiliate—MIT, Boston, Massachusetts
2019—Senior Regulatory Consultant—Health Science Authority, Singapore

Acknowledgments

*At the beginning of gathering ideas of writing this book, my wife was my sounding board. After listening to my general idea of this book, my wife Agnes suggested this book is better illustrated; quoting her "A picture is worth a thousand words." I owe her a thousand thanks in words.

*Steve Wasserman and Jess Mandel, colleagues in the Department of Medicine at UCSD, offered their critiques in a significant way, along with encouragements to the concept of an illustrated book. Additionally, I also received helpful inputs from Nai-Wen Chi, Nick Webster, Sven Heinz, and Brian Hinds.

*Tony Chen provided reviews of each of the summaries on medicines.

*Jeff Travis reviewed the clinical chemistry aspects of the book contents.

*Kathy Zoon offered valuable insights into medicines for viral diseases, with further detail provided by Jim Tartaglia.

*Di Wu helped with creating chemical structures., Manveen Sethi on glycobiology, Francisca Gbormittah on additional disease topics, and John de la Parra on natural products.

*Cheng Leng and Agnes Chan, colleagues at Health Science Authorities in Singapore exposed me to the regulatory world in SE Asia, as well as the broad range of medicines that are impacting health in this diverse region. Freddie Foo, to whom I give my special thanks, for highlighting the importance of biochemical knowledge in the world's regulatory process.

*Barry Karger, George O'Doherty, Sunny Zhao, and Alex Makriyannis, my colleagues at Northeastern University, have given advice regarding analytical, organic chemistry, and cannabinoid development.

*Stacy Springs, Donovan Guttieres, and Jim Leung, my colleagues at MIT, offered insightful input in the area of noncommunicable diseases.

*Additionally, John Frenz, Erno Pungor, Arne Staby, and Ralph Riggin had provided valuable input.

*Steve Kent has a special mention for having introduced me to my publisher, World Scientific Press (WSP).

I acknowledge and express gratitude to the creators of SMART_PPT for the extensive set of medical illustrations some of which I have used in the book. https://smart.servier.com

Valuable sources of information included
https://www.fda.gov/drugs/new-drugs-fda-cders-new-molecular-entities-and-new-therapeutic-biological-products/novel-drug-approvals-2021
https://www.drugs.com/top200/ and
https://www.mayoclinic.org/diseases-conditions
https://www.rxlist.com/drugs
https://clincalc.com/DrugStats/Top200Drugs.aspx
The vector used to illustrate cultural diversity was obtained at pic3 https://www.freepik.com/free-vector/cultural-diversity_4589959.htm

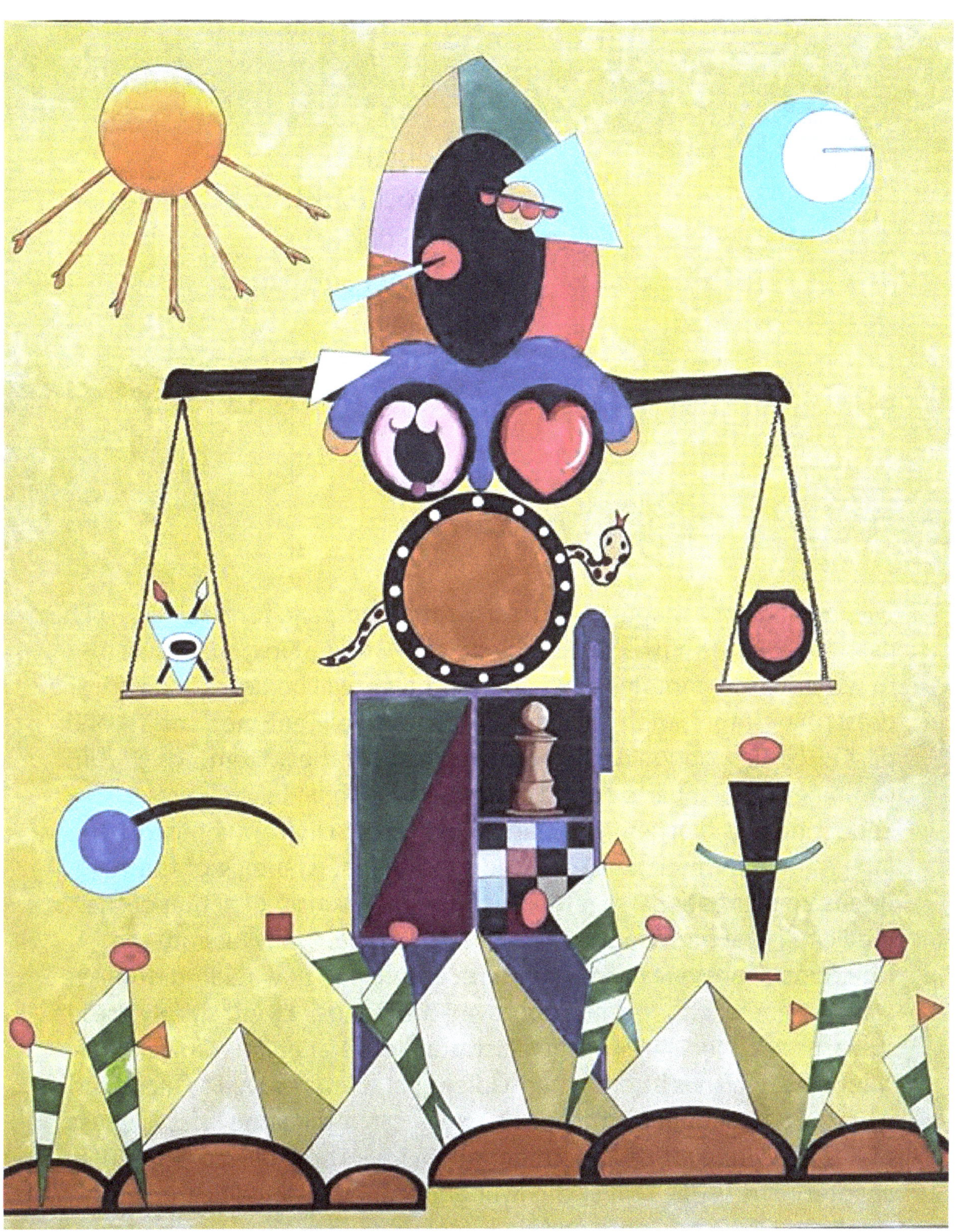

“The ancient art of medicine”. Painting by William Hancock.

Chapter 1 The chemistry of life

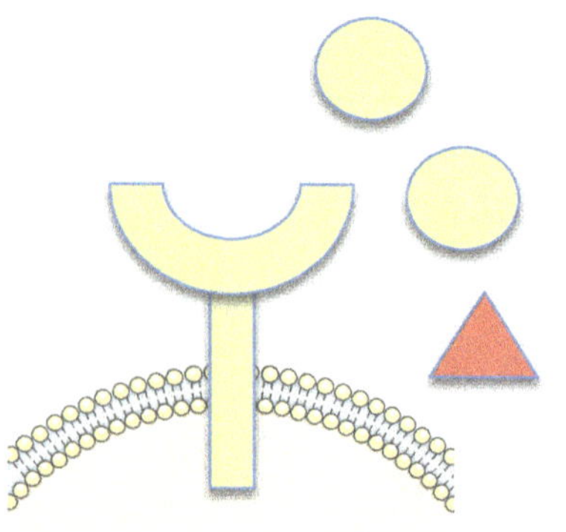

Introduction
The biochemistry of enzymes and related diseases
Receptors and actions of medicines
Detoxification pathways

Overview

The introductory chapter will describe the **two-page format** that will be used to illustrate how a selected medicine works. First, the disease, together with symptoms and patient profiles, will be described with the prescribing information and composition of the medicine. The second part is the description of the normal biology of the system, which will combine relevant parts of organic chemistry, organ biochemistry, endocrinology, biochemical pharmacology, and clinical chemistry. The integrated information will be used to gain understanding of the disease perturbations, together with the mechanism of action of the medicine. The medicines selected in this chapter will illustrate the **functions of enzymes and protein receptors** and how related diseases can be treated with recently approved medicines. **Ethnic differences** in diseases and medicines will be illustrated with variabilities in l**actose tolerance**, which is a common excipient in tablets, as well as a common variant of **alcohol dehydrogenase**, which can reduce the effectiveness of nitroglycerine for the treatment of angina. The final section of the chapter reviews the role of the liver and kidney in detoxification of small molecule medicines and their metabolites.

How to develop a broad understanding of how different therapies work in the context of modern medicine?

We define "medicine" as a substance that provides favorable therapeutic benefits in a patient. Examples of common medicines include analgesics (paracetamol), antibiotics (penicillin), hormones (insulin), and vaccines (polio).

1 The goal of this text is to provide an account of how a medicine works by focusing on the **biochemistry of the body's organs** and describing the **metabolism of the biological macromolecules**, that is DNA, RNA, proteins, polysaccharides, and lipids in **the context of the major organs of the body**.

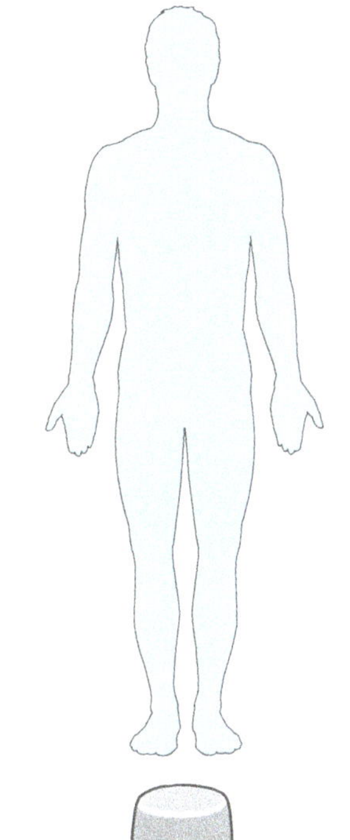

3 Medical research studies the extensive detail about a selected biological process, but such detail does not inform the nonexpert as to the immediate question of **how does the medicine work**. To avoid this problem, this book will **describe** with extensive illustrations **an important pathway** that the medicine acts on.

2 By the study of the organ, we can understand how each medicine will **interact with carrier proteins, transporters, metabolizing enzymes, and multiple receptors**. Such insights will aid **understanding of how the medicine works**.

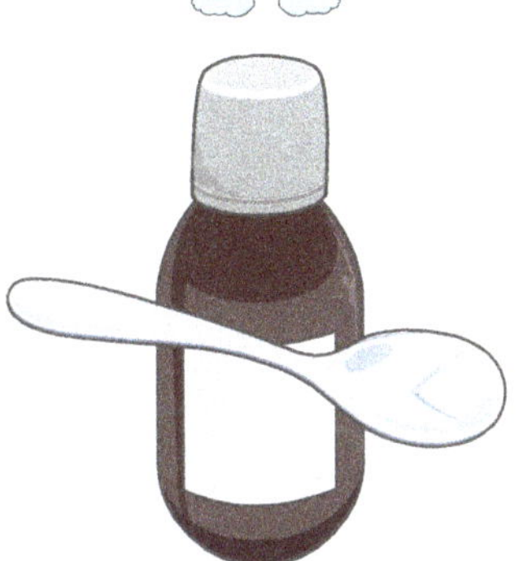

4 Now, we have set the stage. We will **study how the approved medicines work for the major classes of diseases,** such as viral and bacterial infections, cancer, high blood pressure, diabetes, autoimmune, and neurological disorders.

5 We will then use this approach to gain insights into **recent FDA approvals** of novel medicines as well as some of the **most prescribed** in the United States. Each description will include the biochemistry of the disease and the therapeutic mechanism.

Selected drugs approved by the FDA ✓ = Drugs approved recently (2017–2020)
Examples listed in Chapter 1 (Brand name)

Invasive breast cancer (Raloxifene)
Adenosine deaminase (Revcovi ✓)

Phenylketonuria (Palynziq✓)
Angina (Nitrostat)

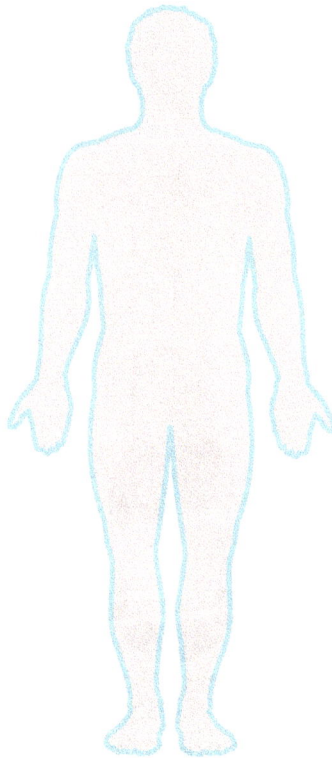

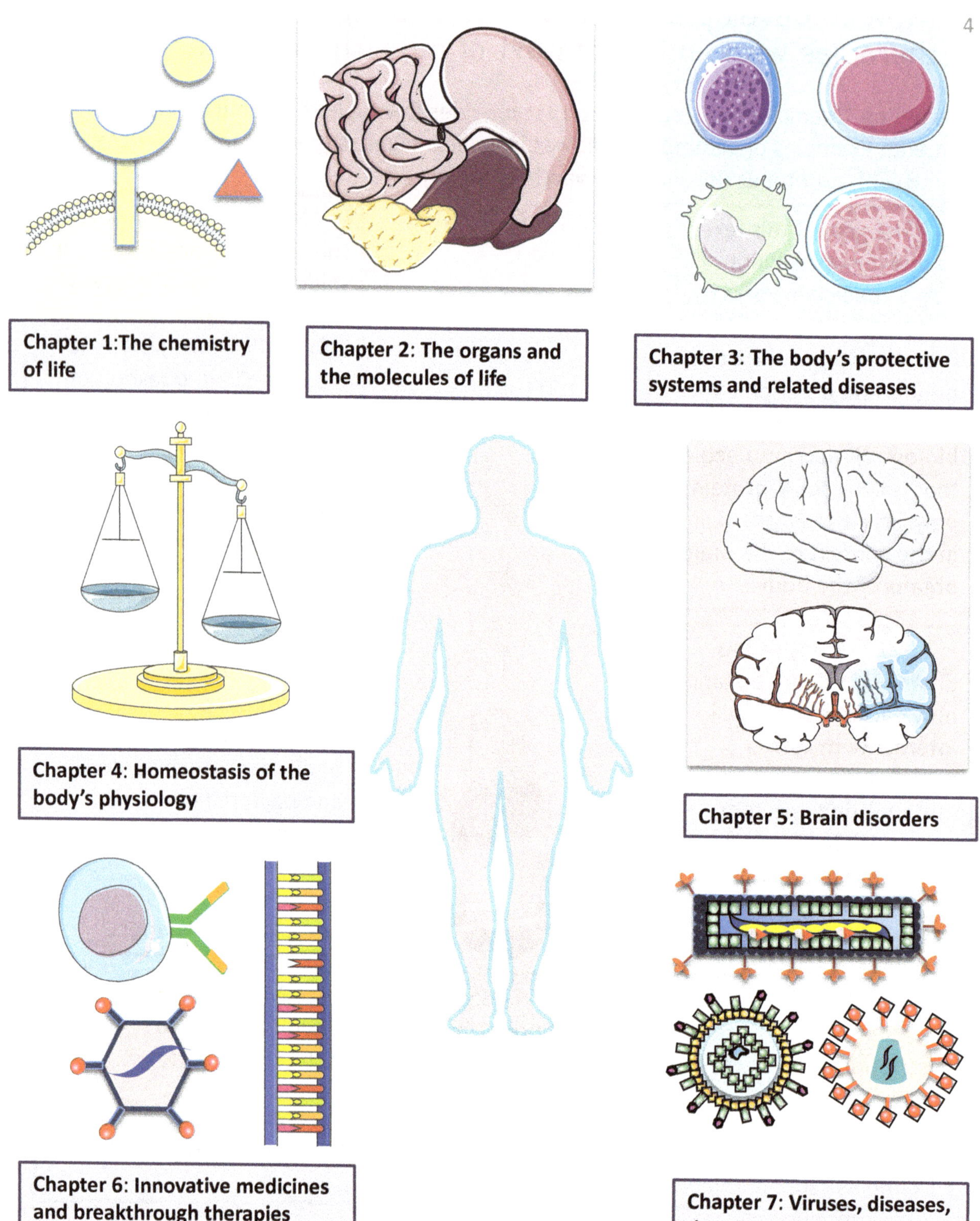
Chapter 1:The chemistry of life
Chapter 2: The organs and the molecules of life
Chapter 3: The body's protective systems and related diseases
Chapter 4: Homeostasis of the body's physiology
Chapter 5: Brain disorders
Chapter 6: Innovative medicines and breakthrough therapies
Chapter 7: Viruses, diseases, drugs, and vaccines

Introduction: Chapter outlines

The science behind understanding drug action

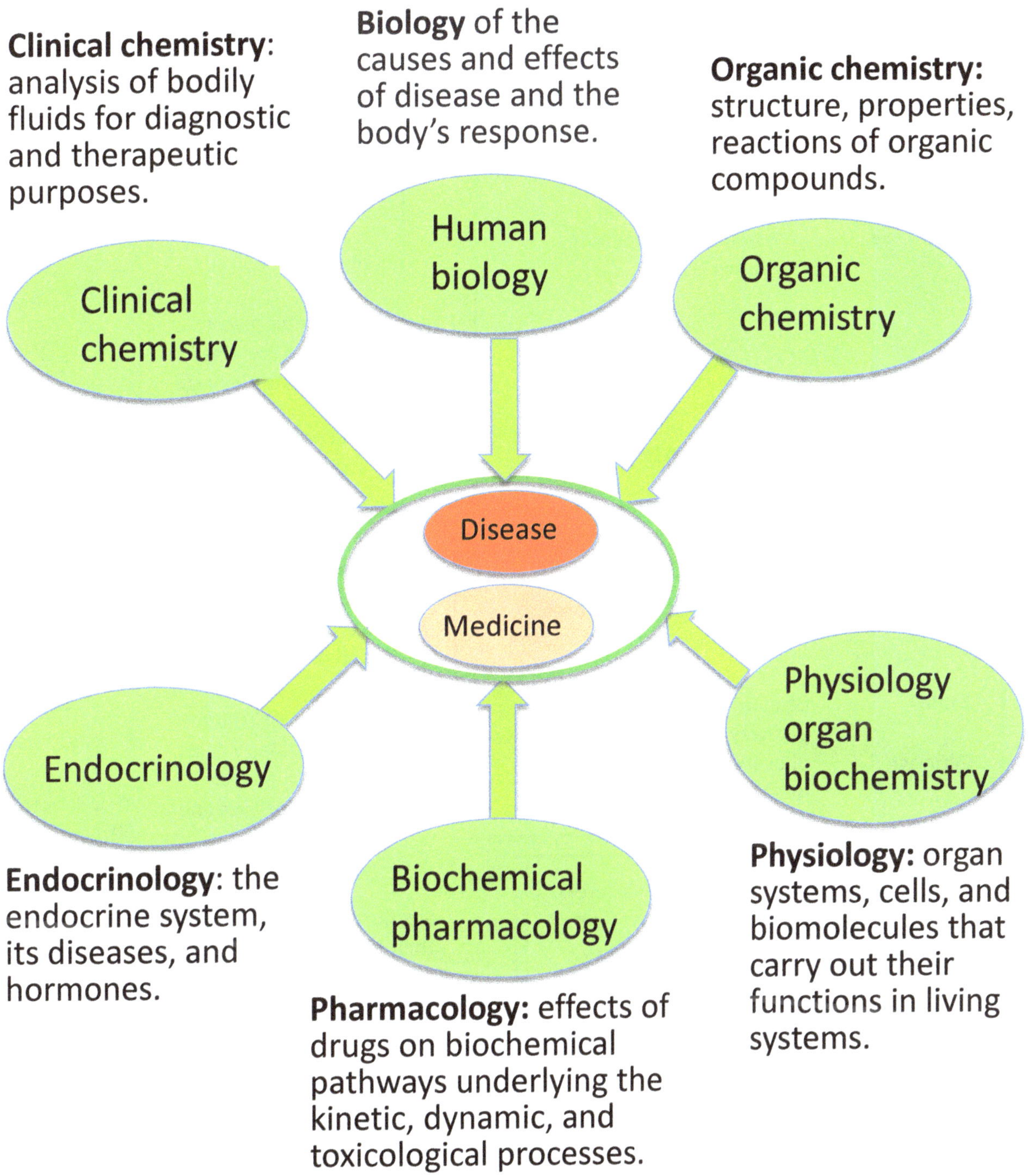
Clinical chemistry: analysis of bodily fluids for diagnostic and therapeutic purposes.
Biology of the causes and effects of disease and the body's response.
Organic chemistry: structure, properties, reactions of organic compounds.
Human biology
Clinical chemistry
Organic chemistry
Disease
Medicine
Endocrinology
Physiology organ biochemistry
Biochemical pharmacology
Endocrinology: the endocrine system, its diseases, and hormones.
Physiology: organ systems, cells, and biomolecules that carry out their functions in living systems.
Pharmacology: effects of drugs on biochemical pathways underlying the kinetic, dynamic, and toxicological processes.

Introduction: The sciences behind understanding of medicines

Organ biochemistry

Each organ has a unique metabolic profile with biochemical processes that are regulated by the physiological actions of specific hormone systems.

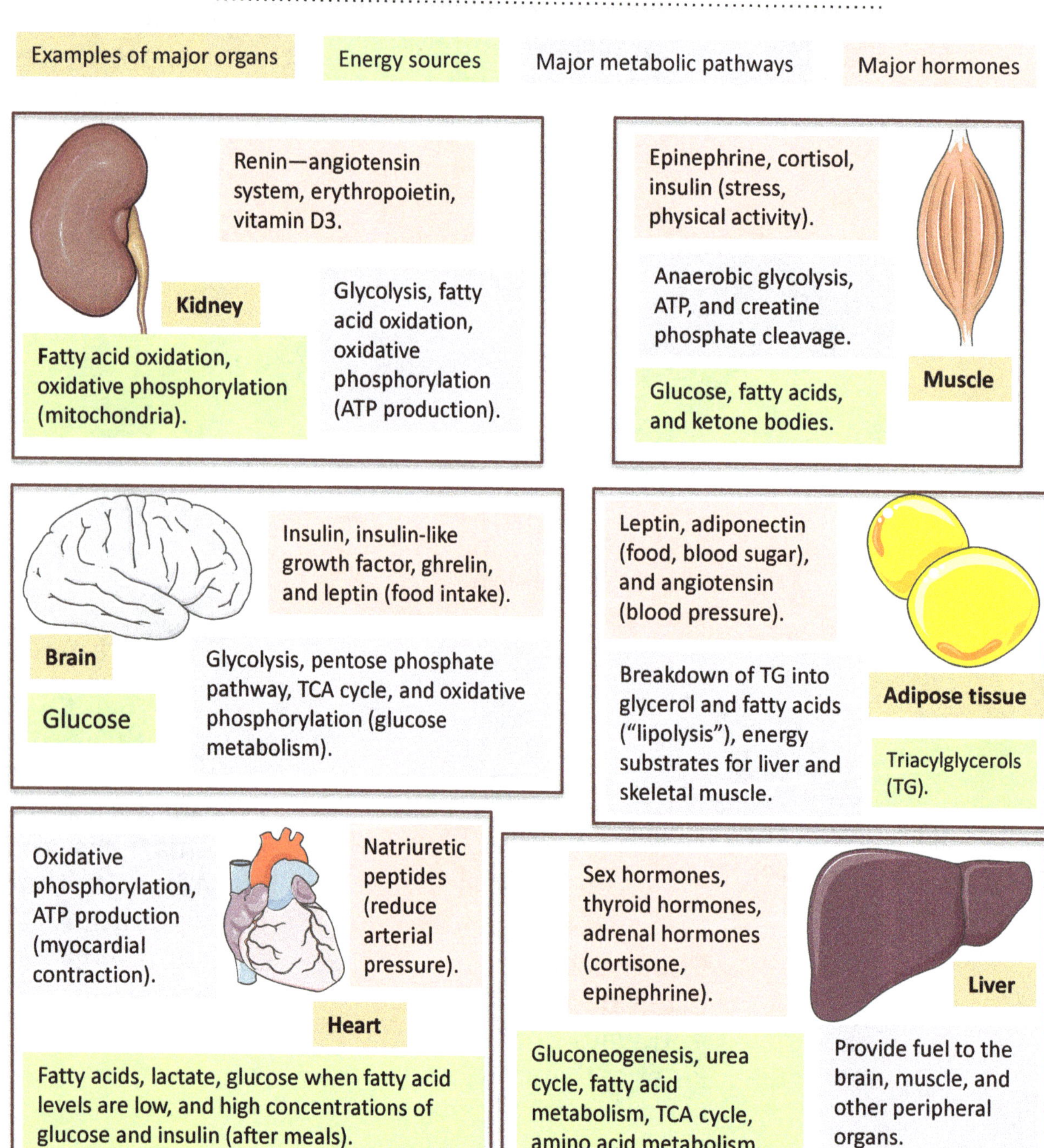

Examples of major organs
Energy sources
Major metabolic pathways
Major hormones
Renin—angiotensin system, erythropoietin, vitamin D3.
Kidney
Glycolysis, fatty acid oxidation, oxidative phosphorylation (ATP production).
Fatty acid oxidation, oxidative phosphorylation (mitochondria).
Epinephrine, cortisol, insulin (stress, physical activity).
Anaerobic glycolysis, ATP, and creatine phosphate cleavage.
Muscle
Glucose, fatty acids, and ketone bodies.
Insulin, insulin-like growth factor, ghrelin, and leptin (food intake).
Brain
Glucose
Glycolysis, pentose phosphate pathway, TCA cycle, and oxidative phosphorylation (glucose metabolism).
Leptin, adiponectin (food, blood sugar), and angiotensin (blood pressure).
Breakdown of TG into glycerol and fatty acids ("lipolysis"), energy substrates for liver and skeletal muscle.
Adipose tissue
Triacylglycerols (TG).
Oxidative phosphorylation, ATP production (myocardial contraction).
Natriuretic peptides (reduce arterial pressure).
Heart
Fatty acids, lactate, glucose when fatty acid levels are low, and high concentrations of glucose and insulin (after meals).
Sex hormones, thyroid hormones, adrenal hormones (cortisone, epinephrine).
Liver
Gluconeogenesis, urea cycle, fatty acid metabolism, TCA cycle, amino acid metabolism.
Provide fuel to the brain, muscle, and other peripheral organs.

Introduction: Metabolic profiles of major organs

How the medicine summaries are organized in a two-page report

Page 1

The disease — Disease symptoms — Incidence by gender and ethnicity

The medicine

Generic name — Brand name — FDA, year of approval

Medicine information — Structure of medicine

Page 2

Action of medicine on cell and disease biology

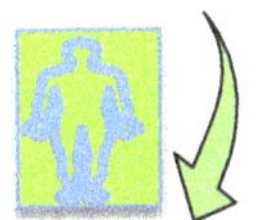
Biology pathways

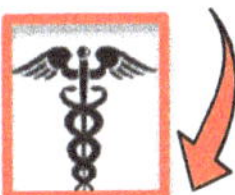
Disease pathways

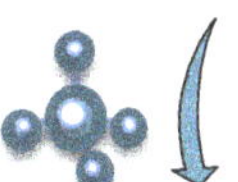
Medicine pathways

Names of medicines

Generic and brand names must be unique to prevent drug mix-ups.

① **Generic name**

- Name based on physiological function or chemical structure.
- Approved by WHO
- Name is a collection of short name fragments (stems), e.g., -mab, monoclonal antibody or –nib, inhibitor

Example

① Lanadelumab

② Takhzyro

② **Brand name**

- Exclusive company name with patent protection that is generated on FDA approval .
- Marketing name is often used by doctors on prescriptions.
- Follow on companies use the same generic name with new brand name.

Simplified terminology used in medicine summaries

Book describes a wide range of drugs, organs, mechanisms, and thus terminology.

Students who started medical school in 2010 will master only 6% of the knowledge available in 2020. Today?

Doubling time of medical knowledge in 1950 (50 years); 1980 (7 years); 2010 (3.5 years); and in 2020s projected to be 0.2 years.

Specialist literature is full of technical terms, acronyms, and other abbreviations.

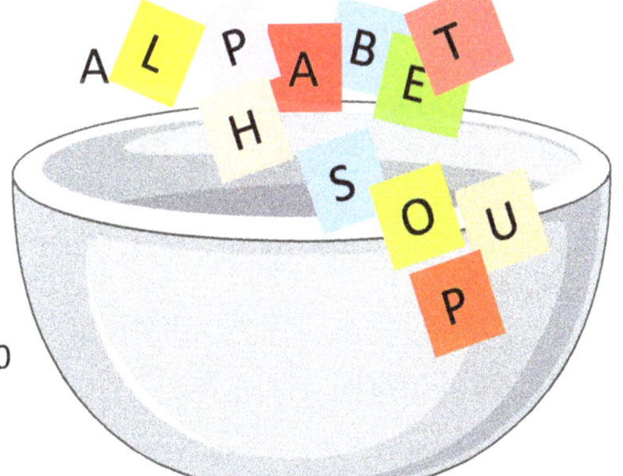

Example 1—NHP
Nonhuman primate
Nonhemoglobin protein.

Example 2—ACHE
Acetyl choline esterase
ACE—Angiotensin-converting enzyme.

Example 3—Receptor blocker or inhibitor
Pharmacology terms
Agonists, antagonists, inverse agonist.

Introduction: The structure of summaries for medicines

How do enzymes work?

Enzymes are true catalysts as they speed up reactions but are not consumed and do not become part of the products.

(1) Active site

Binding site	**Catalytic site**
Forms temporary bonds with the substrate (reactants).	Catalyzes a specific reaction with the substrate.

In an active site, the side chains of specific amino acids are located in a 3D environment favorable for catalyzing the reaction to generate products.

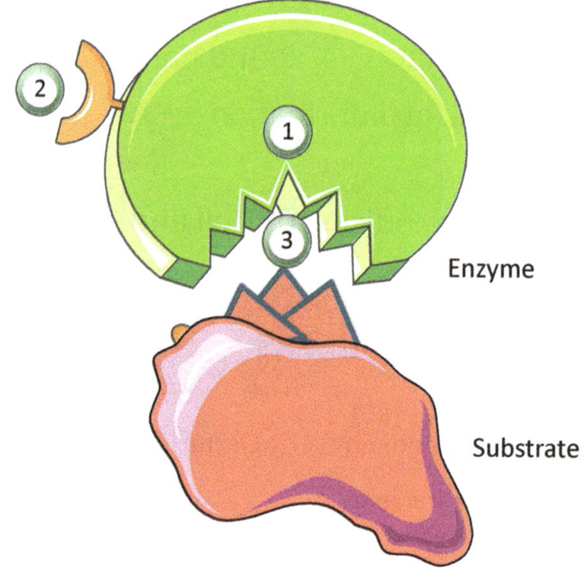

(2) **Enzyme activators** are ions, small organic molecules, peptides, proteins, and lipids that increase the velocity of enzymatic reaction. Their actions are opposite to the effect of enzyme inhibitors.

(3) An **enzyme inhibitor** binds to an enzyme and reduces activity, either blocking the entry of a substrate to the active site or hindering the catalytic reaction.
Inhibition can either be reversible or irreversible (binding noncovalently or forming a covalent bond with the catalytic site).

Specificity
Each enzyme **catalyzes specific biochemical reactions**, e.g.,
Amylase (mouth, carbohydrate)
Pepsin (stomach, protein)
Lipase (small intestine, lipid)
Trypsin (small intestine, protein)
Lactase (small intestine, carbohydrate)

Most enzymes have a characteristic optimum pH where the enzyme shows maximum catalytic activity, e.g., the optimum pH for salivary amylase, pepsin, lysosomal enzymes, acid phosphatase, and alkaline phosphatase are 6.8, 1–2, 5.0, 4–5, and 9–10, respectively.

For body fluids (blood), the **pH is normally 7.35–7.45**.
- < 7.35, > 7.45, promotes illness
- < pH's depress brain function
- > pH's cause neuronal irritability
- Severe diabetic ketoacidosis pH < 7.0

Lactose as an excipient: Lactase deficiencies

Lactose is commonly used as a **filler for solid dosage forms** to produce tablets of sufficient hardness and with good disintegration properties.

An **excipient** is an inert substance formulated alongside the active ingredient of a medication for the purpose of

- Long-term stabilization
- Bulking up solid formulations with potent active ingredients
- Facilitate drug absorption or enhancing solubility
- Inert, no effect of action of the drug ingredients

Lactose is widely available with a bland taste, excellent physical and chemical stability, and water solubility.

Lactose is a component of about **20% of prescriptions** and 6% of over-the-counter medications.

Lactase is located in the brush border of the small intestine and is essential to the complete **digestion of whole milk** by breaking down lactose.

Lactose intolerance is a digestive disorder caused by the **inability to digest lactose** (main diary component).

Ingestion of medications with a lactose excipient a patient may consume over **10 g of lactose a day**, in addition dietary lactose.

In highly sensitive individuals, symptoms may occur after ingestion of as little as 200 mg of lactose.

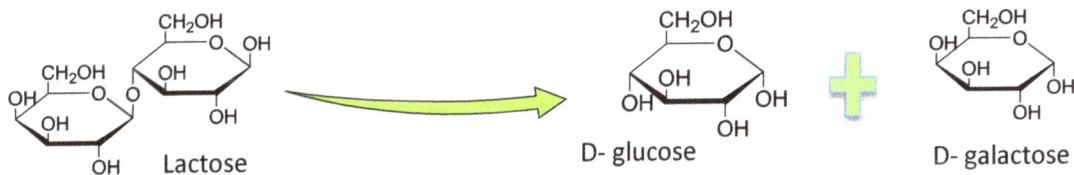

Lactose → D- glucose + D- galactose

Some 65% of the global population is lactose intolerant but with large variation from under 10% in Northern Europe but up to 95% in parts of Asia and Africa.

(1) **Lactose is broken down in the small intestine by lactase** to glucose and galactose, then absorbed by the small intestine and little lactose enters the large intestine (colon).

Ingested lactose is not completely hydrolyzed within the small intestine in individuals with low lactase levels.

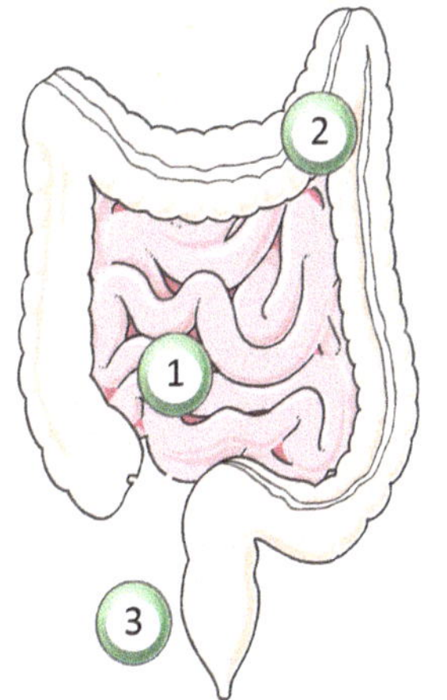

(2) When lactose is metabolized in the large intestine (colon) by bacteria, **gases such as hydrogen and methane** will be produced as well as small peptides and toxins.

These products cause symptoms of **stomach cramps**, bloating, flatulence, diarrhea, muscle cramps, and headache.

(3) Unabsorbed lactose raises the osmotic pressure **in the colon**, preventing water reabsorption and causing a **laxative effect.**

The biochemistry of enzymes: Lactose metabolism in the small intestine

The disease: Adenosine deaminase deficiency (ADA)

Adenosine deaminase deficiency (ADA) and severe combined immunodeficiency (SCID) is due to mutations in the adenosine deaminase (ADA) gene, which results in **elevated levels of adenosine and deoxyadenosine** in the blood and urine. Patients are unable to fight off infections, such as bacterial, viral, and fungal infections due to **low levels of lymphocytes.**

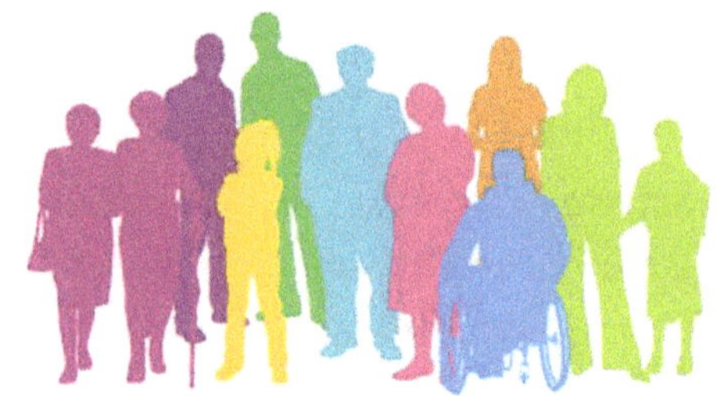

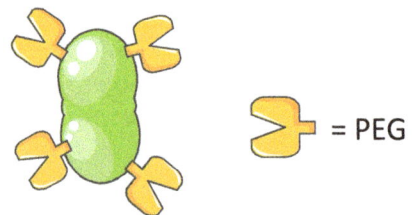

Incidence by gender and ethnicity

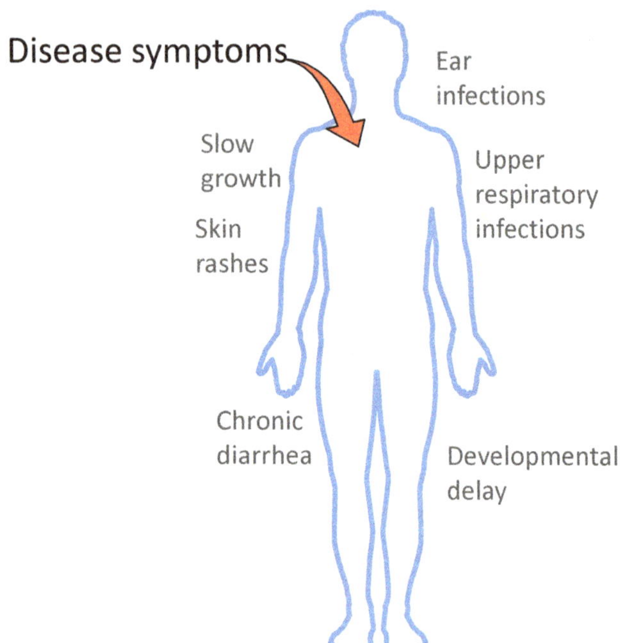

SCID is diagnosed by 3 months of age and the most common form is X-linked in males but other forms can present in males and females equally. Greater risk of ADA occurs in ethnic groups such as Finnish, North Africans, Italians, Navajos, and Apaches.

The medicine

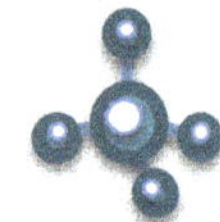

Elapegademase; Revcovi, FDA Approval 2018

Administered by intramuscular injection

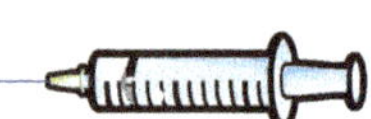

Elapegademase is a modified form of **bovine adenosine deaminase** (rADA) made in ***Escherichia coli*** and **conjugated** with 13 **PEG groups** to increase the circulating half-life and minimize immunogenicity.

PEGylation (pegylation) is the process of attachment of polyethylene glycol (PEG) polymer chains.

Action of Elapegademase on cell and disease biology

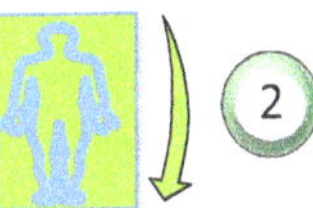

1. **Deoxyadenosine (dAdo)** is the DNA nucleoside that pairs with deoxythymidine (T) in double-stranded DNA.
2. **Ribonucleotide reductase (RNR)** catalyzes formation of **deoxyribonucleotides** (loss of 2'-hydroxyl group of ribose) and **regulates DNA synthesis rate** (constant ratio of DNA to cell mass) during cell division and DNA repair .
3. In lymphocytes, **adenosine deaminase eliminates dAdo** from degraded DNA.

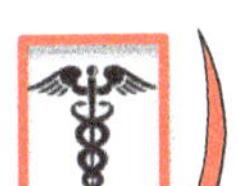

4. **T cells** undergo proliferation and **development in the thymus** and ADA-SCID patients typically have a small, underdeveloped thymus.
5. **dAdo** blocks cell division by **inhibiting enzyme RNR** and DNA synthesis and kills immature T lymphocytes, which results in ADA-SCID.

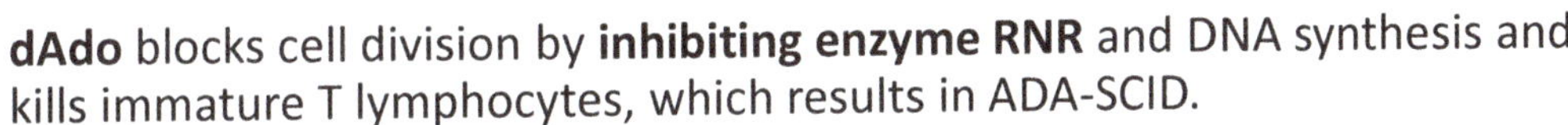

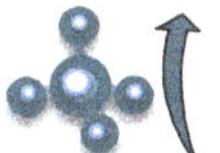

6. **Elapegademase replaces** mutated and **inactive Adenosine deaminase.**

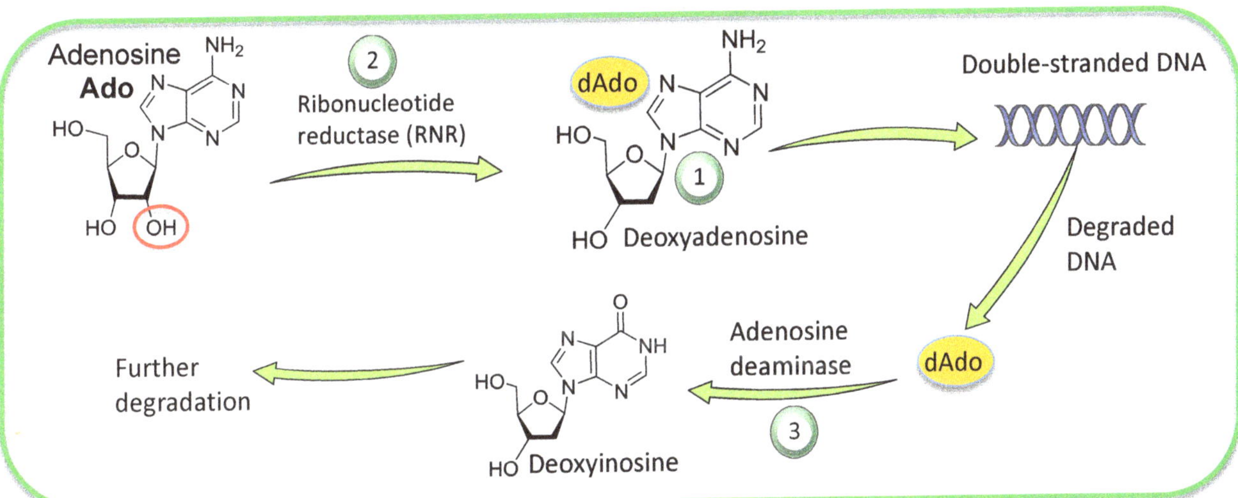

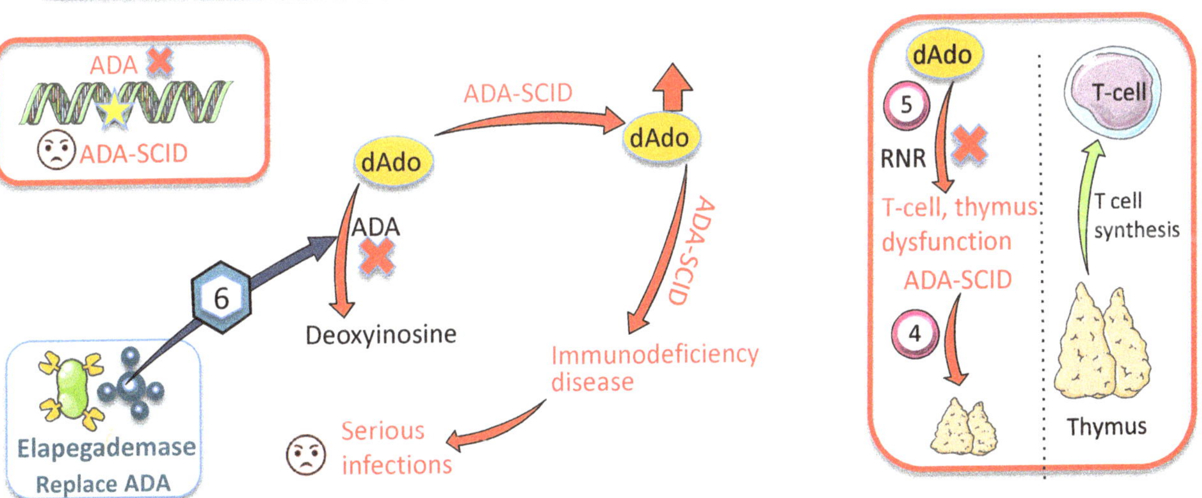

The disease: Phenylketonuria

Phenylketonuria (PKU) is an inherited disease caused by **mutations** in both alleles of the gene for **phenylalanine hydroxylase (PAH)**, which results in a liver enzyme deficiency. PAH catalyzes the conversion of phenylalanine to tyrosine. High phenylalanine levels during childhood cause profound cognitive, developmental, and learning defects.

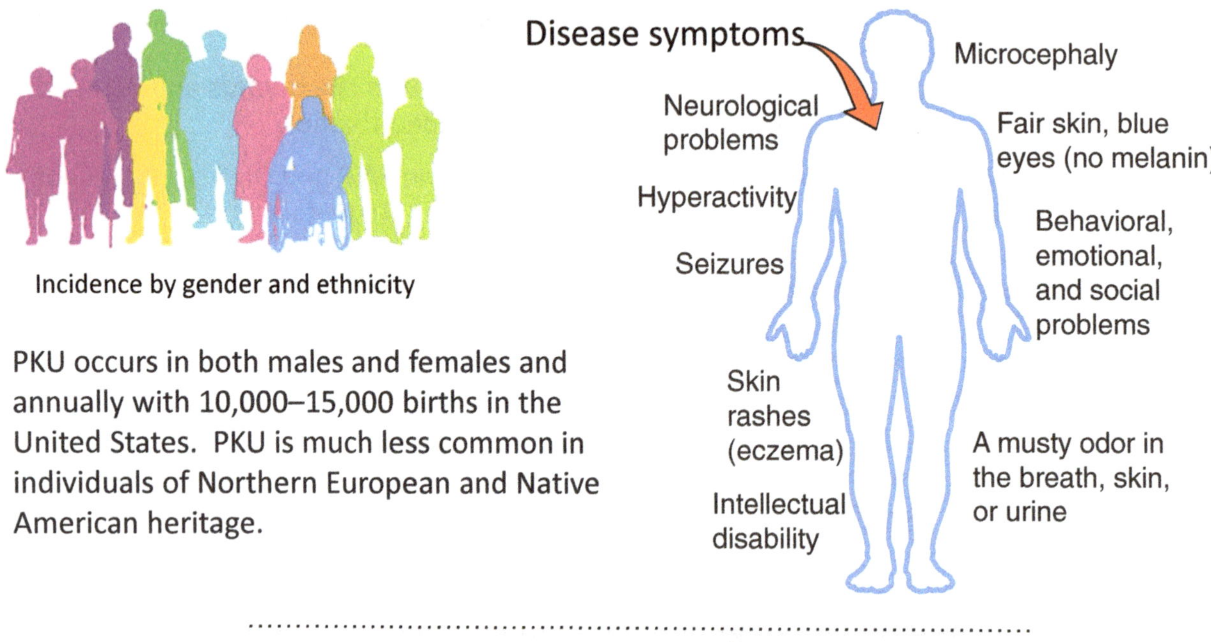

Incidence by gender and ethnicity

PKU occurs in both males and females and annually with 10,000–15,000 births in the United States. PKU is much less common in individuals of Northern European and Native American heritage.

The medicine

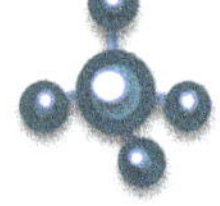

Pegvaliase; Palynziq, FDA Approval 2018

Administered by subcutaneous injection

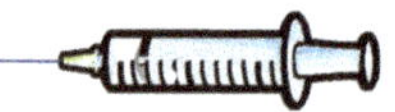

Pegvaliase is a recombinant phenylalanine ammonia lyase (PAL) enzyme derived from a cyanobacterium and expressed in *E. coli* with the addition of polyethylene glycol (PEG) groups to reduce immune recognition of the bacterial protein and also to increase the half-life.

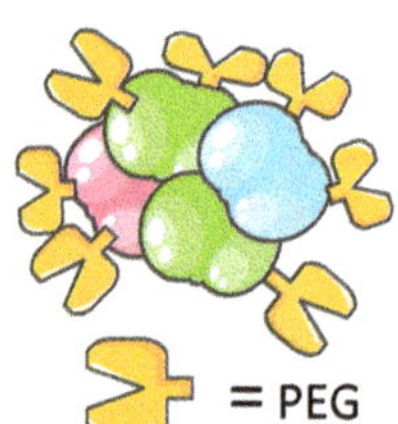

PEGylation (pegylation) is the process of attachment of polyethylene glycol (PEG) polymer chains.

Action of Pegvaliase on cell and disease biology

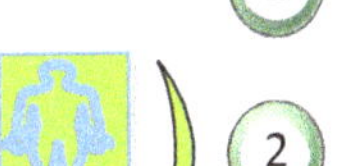

1 **Phenylalanine** is an essential amino acid for the **synthesis of tyrosine,** proteins, catecholamine neurotransmitters, and melanin.

2 **Phenylalanine hydroxylase (PAH)** catalyzes the hydroxylation of phenylalanine to tyrosine in the liver.

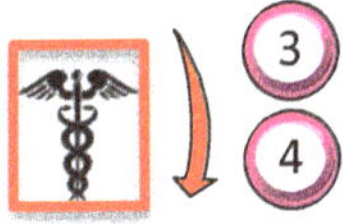

3 **Mutated**, inactive **PAH** results in **phenylalanine accumulation** in the body.

4 In the **brain, excess phenylalanine** reduces glutamate synapse transmission with myelin damage, **toxicity** to the hypothalamic-pituitary-adrenal axis .

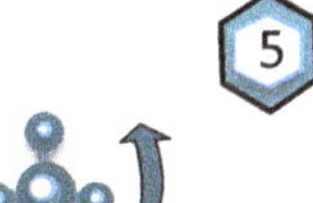

5 **Palynziq** (phenylalanine ammonia lyase [PAL]) **substitutes** for the **deficient PAH enzyme** and **converts phenylalanine to trans-cinnamic acid,** which is excreted in the urine.

6 Palynziq **reduces blood phenylalanine levels** both in the blood and brain tissue.

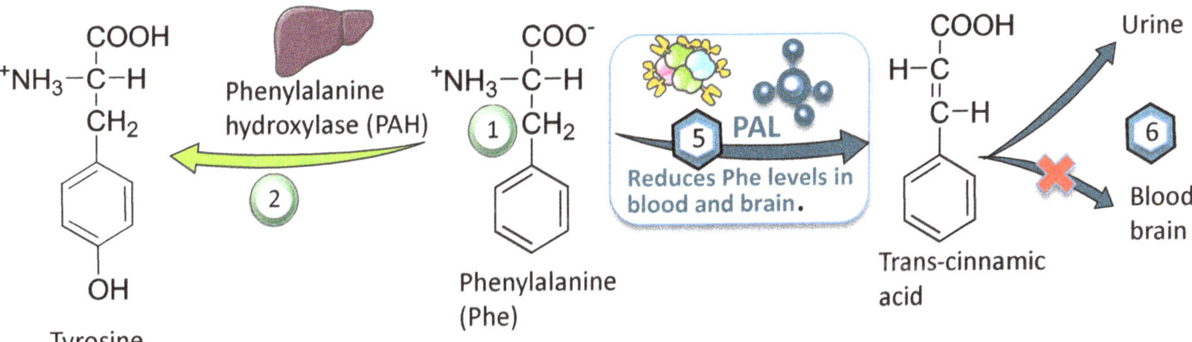

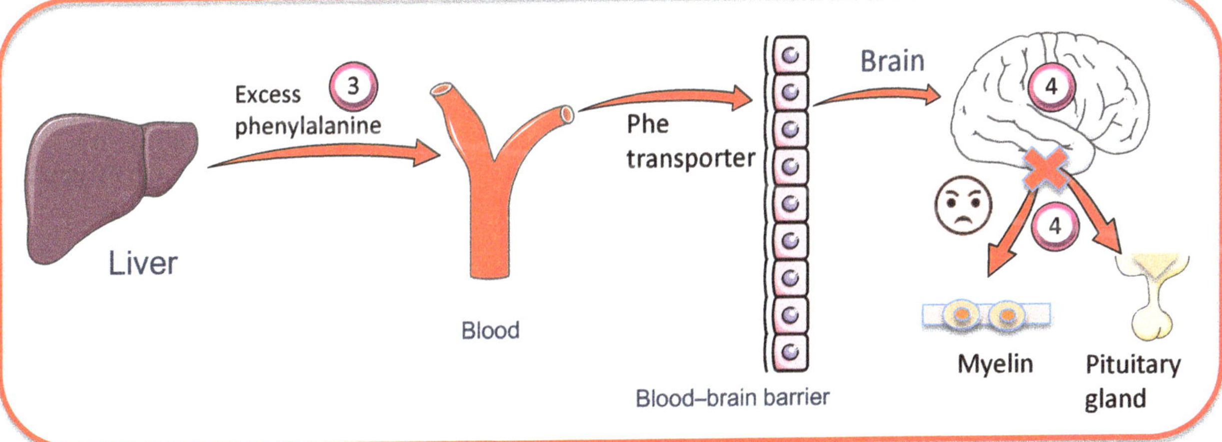

Protein targets for actions of medicines

The main classes of protein targets are receptors, ion channels, enzymes, and transporters (carrier molecules).

1 **Receptors** (protein or glycoprotein) are located both on the cell surface or within the cell such as the nuclear membrane.

Receptors **initiate a chemical response** (signaling cascade) that induces cell growth, division, death, or opens membrane channels.

Receptor families are targeted by **medicines** that produce specific biochemical **alterations in receptors.**

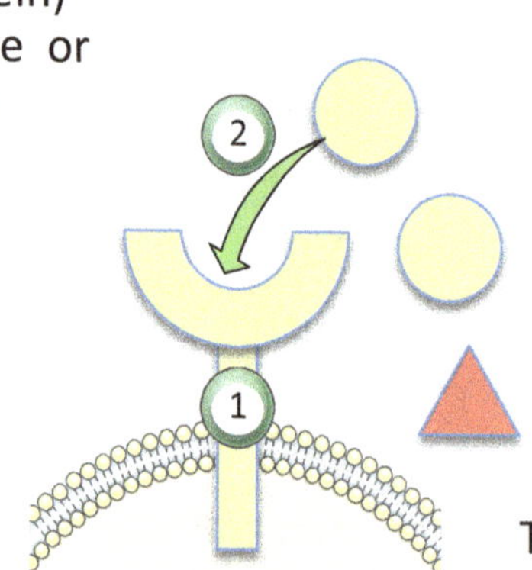

2 The function of a receptor is to receive a signal by the **binding of a signaling molecu**le such as insulin or dopamine.

The signaling molecule can effect cell function without entering the cell.

There are **three main classes** of receptors: ion channel-linked, G protein-coupled, and enzyme-linked receptors.

Ion channel receptors

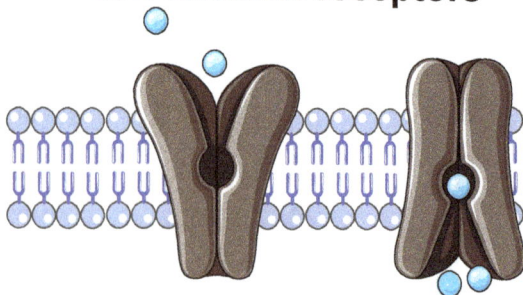

Ion channel receptors are multimeric proteins in the plasma membrane and form a passageway for ions.

A chemical signal allows the channel to open and close to regulate the flux of ions in and out of the cell.

Ion channels were targets for the first synthesized drugs, local anaesthetic agents, which are sodium channel blockers and bind to an intracellular portion of the channels and thus block movement of ions.

Transporters

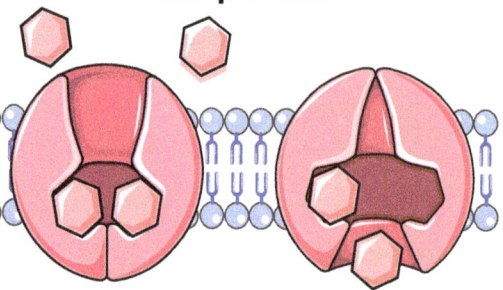

Transporters accumulate high concentrations of required molecules, such as glucose or amino acids.

Regulate the movement of a substance across a membrane against its concentration gradient.

The carrier proteins have specific receptors to bind and transport required molecules.

Transporters are important in the effectiveness and safety of drugs.

Receptors and actions of medicines

G protein-coupled receptors (GPCRs)

GPCRs account for ~4% of the total protein coding sequences in humans and are the most important druggable targets in medicine. These receptors activate a G-protein that will in turn activate secondary messengers such as cyclic AMP and Protein kinase A.

G proteins (guanine nucleotide-binding proteins) act as molecular switches inside cells to transmit signals from a variety of stimuli outside a cell to the interior.

Binding of a signaling molecule to a **G-protein-coupled receptors** (GPCR) activates G protein to GTP, which then triggers adenyl cyclase to **produce cyclic AMP (cAMP).**

Protein kinase A (PKA) promotes a cascade of **signaling reactions involved in the family of enzymes** which regulate glycogen, sugar, and lipid metabolism.

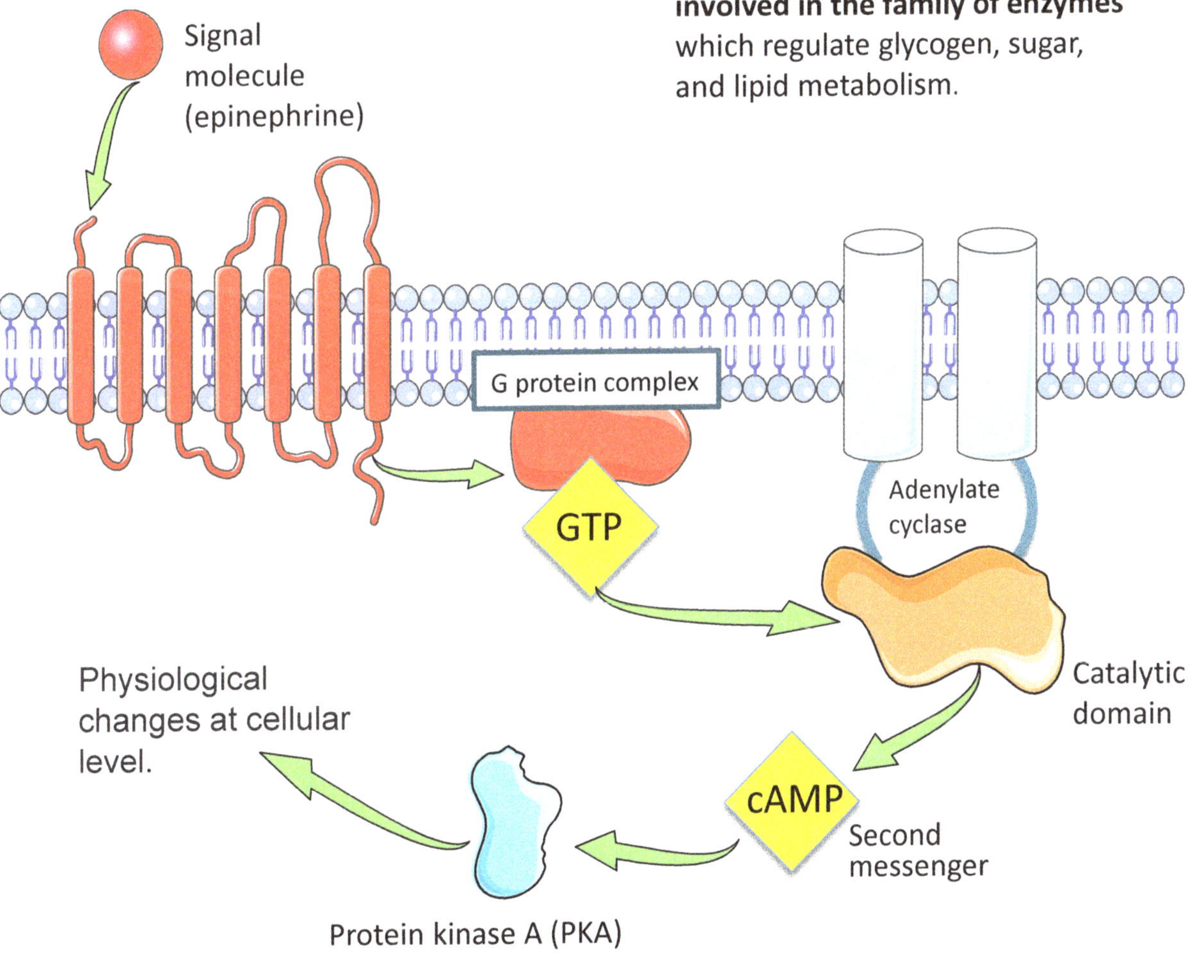

The disease: Angina

Angina is a type of chest pain caused by reduced blood flow to the heart muscle and is a symptom of coronary artery disease. Angina (angina pectoris) is described as squeezing, pressure, heaviness, and chest tightness.

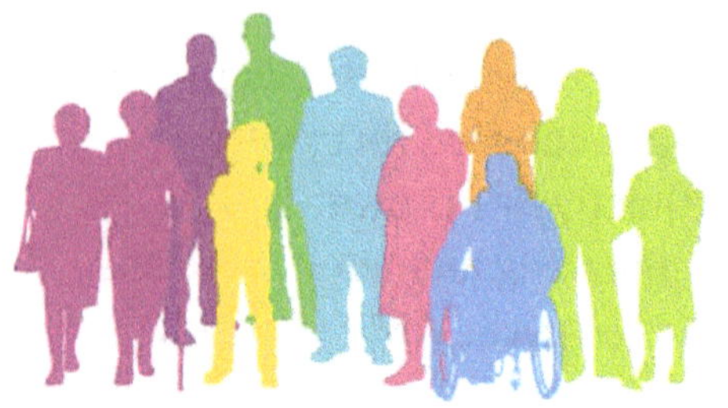

Incidence by gender and ethnicity

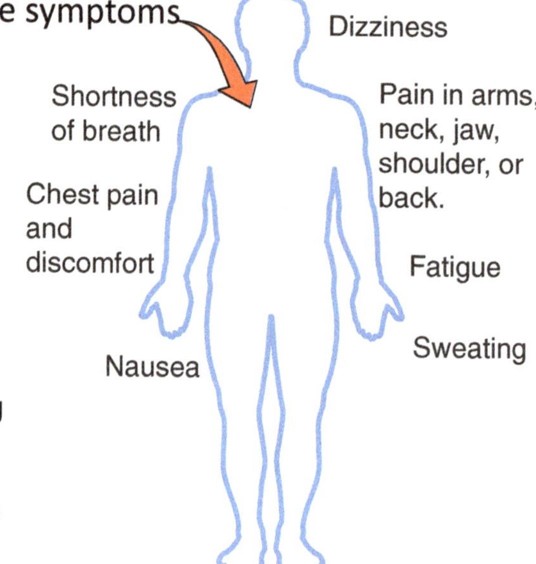

In stable angina, the risk for significant coronary artery disease was 0.34 for women compared with men, with black women having the lowest risk-adjusted odds compared with other females. Among Asian groups, heart disease rates vary widely. South Asians tend to have higher rates of coronary artery disease.

The medicine

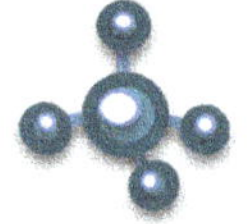

Nitroglycerin; Nitrostat, FDA Approval 1982

184th most US prescribed drug, (2019), 3.2 million prescriptions

Nitrostat (nitroglycerin) prevents chest pain (angina) in people with coronary artery disease. The drug works by relaxing vascular smooth muscle and widening blood vessels, so blood can flow more easily to the heart. **Nitroglycerin also produces relaxation of small blood vessels**, reducing peripheral resistance to blood flow as well promoting pooling in the venous system and reducing cardiac work.

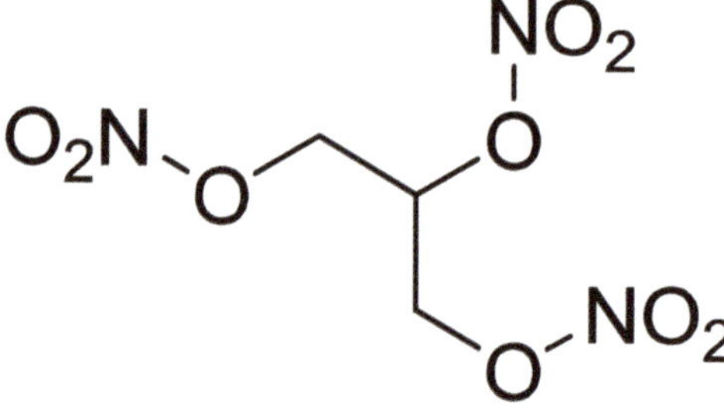

Receptors: Angina, relaxation of smooth muscle cells, Nitroglycerin

Action of Nitroglycerin on cell and disease biology

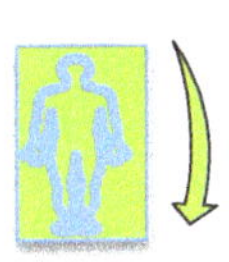

1. **Mitochondrial aldehyde dehydrogenase (ALDH2)** catalyzes the **reduction of nitroglycerin** to 1,2-glyceryl dinitrate and nitrite, which is metabolized in the mitochondria to nitric oxide.

2. **ALDH2** plays a role in the **bioactivation of NTG** in humans.

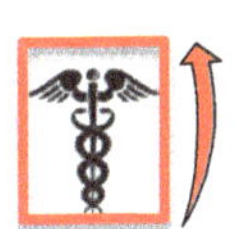
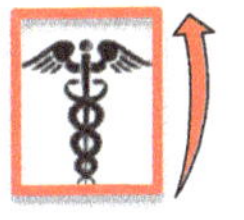

3. **ALDH2 variant** contains a mutation (glutamate to lysine at position 487) with a **loss of ALDH2 activity** in both heterozygotes and homozygotes.

4. 50% of the East Asian population have an **inactive variant of ALDH2, impaired alcohol metabolism**, and variable therapeutic efficacy for NTG.

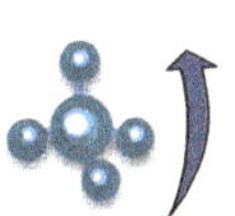

5. **Nitroglycerin** production of NO relaxes small blood vessels by **activating** the **cyclic GMP signaling pathway** in smooth muscle.

6. NO-mediated signals induce **dephosphorylation of myosin light chains** that regulate the contractile state of smooth muscle, which results in a **widening of blood vessels**.

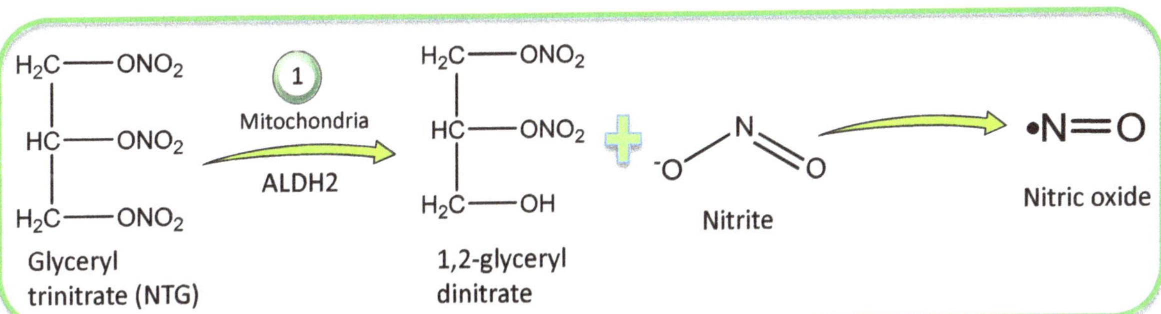

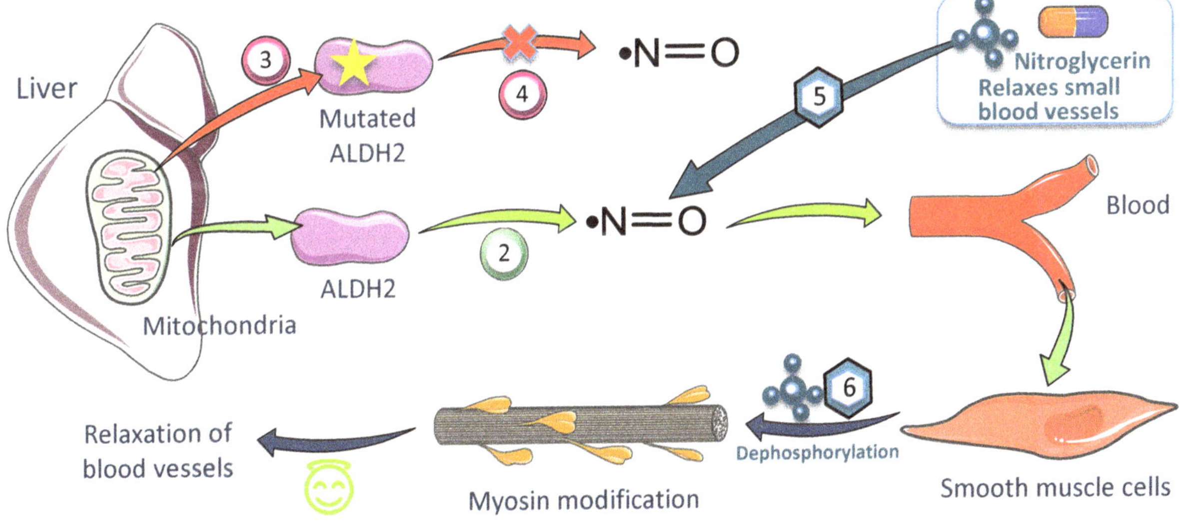

Receptors: Angina, relaxation of smooth muscle cells, Nitroglycerin

The disease: Invasive breast cancer

Invasive breast cancer involves spreading of cancer into surrounding breast tissue. Most breast cancers are invasive and the two most common are **invasive ductal carcinoma and invasive lobular carcinoma**. Women who have had breast cancer and chemotherapy have a higher risk for osteoporosis.

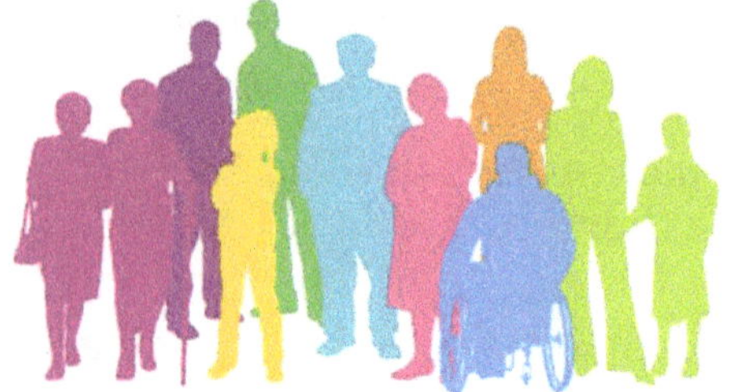

Incidence by gender and ethnicity

Disease symptoms

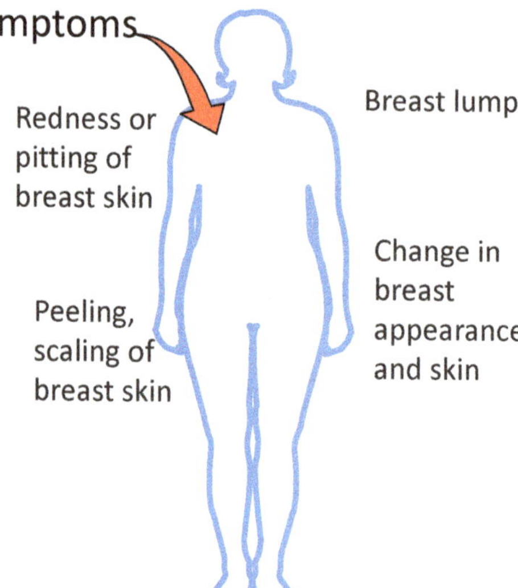

The majority of breast cancers occur in women 50 years or older. Among women aged 40 – 50, African American women have a higher incidence of breast cancer than white women and the highest death rate from breast cancer. Asian American women have the lowest death rate.

The medicine

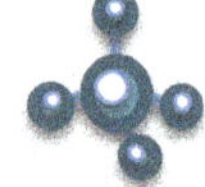

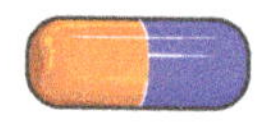

273rd most US prescribed drug, (2019), 1.5 million prescriptions

Raloxifene; Evista, FDA Approval 1999

Raloxifene is approved for the prevention of **osteoporosis in postmenopausal women**. Raloxifene significantly reduces the risk for invasive breast in postmenopausal women at high risk of the disease. Also raloxifene is used to **reduce the risk of invasive breast cancer** in postmenopausal women with osteoporosis.

HO S OH O N O

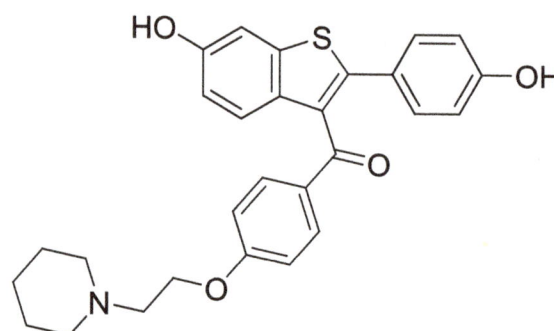

Receptors: Invasive breast cancer, Raloxifene

Action of Raloxifene on cell and disease biology

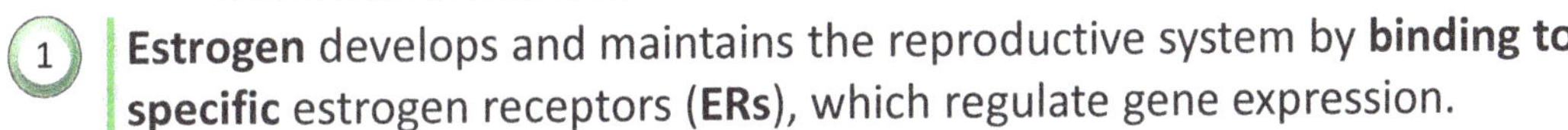

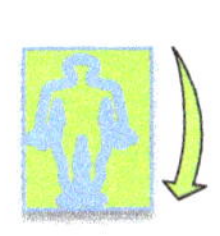

1 **Estrogen** develops and maintains the reproductive system by **binding to specific** estrogen receptors (**ERs**), which regulate gene expression.

2 The **G-protein-coupled estrogen receptor-1** (GPER-1) is expressed on the endoplasmic reticulum and mediates **estrogen receptor signaling**.

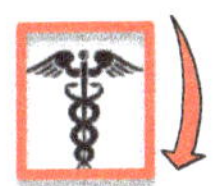

3 **Estrogen effects tumors** via genotoxic effects of **estrogen metabolites** and as a promoter of premalignant cancer cell proliferation.

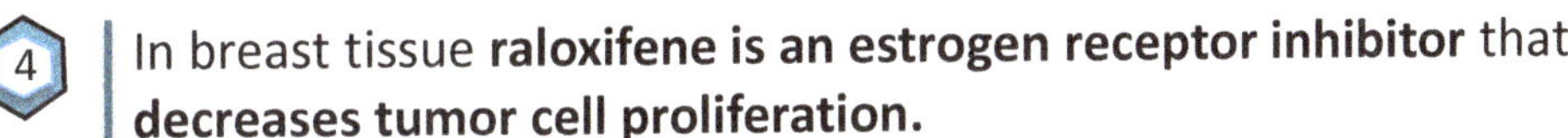

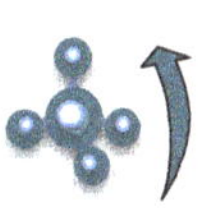

4 In breast tissue **raloxifene is an estrogen receptor inhibitor** that **decreases tumor cell proliferation.**

5 Raloxifene **activates** the G protein-coupled estrogen receptor 1 (**GPER1**), which may have **antiproliferative effect** in breast cancer cells.

6 **Raloxifene reduces** epidermal growth factor receptor (**EGFR**) **expression**, which increases apoptosis of cancer cells.

7 **Raloxifene reduces** breast cancer **tumor growth,** prevents cytokine production, recruitment of macrophages, and lymphocytes into the tumor.

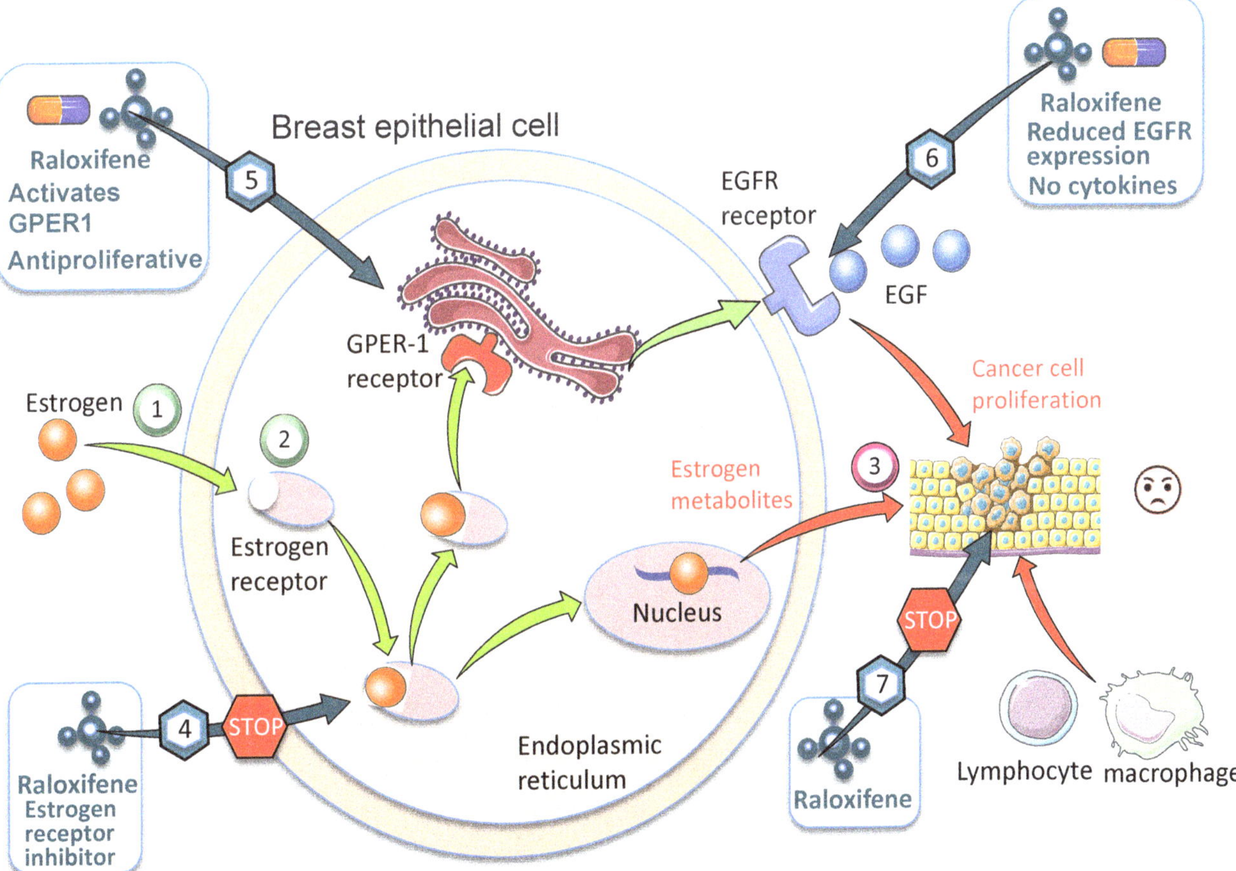

Receptors: Invasive breast cancer, Raloxifene

Detoxification pathways

The liver plays an important role in protecting the body from potentially toxic drugs by their conversion into more water-soluble metabolites, which can be efficiently eliminated from the body via the urine.

1 Protection of the liver stems from the expression of a wide variety of enzymes, which can transform foreign compounds and drugs (xenobiotics).

2 The enzymes have broad substrate specificity that allows the processing of the vast array of different chemical structures of drugs. Enzymes either catalyze oxidation, reduction, and hydrolysis reactions (Phase I) and/or conjugation (Phase II) of functional groups on the drug.

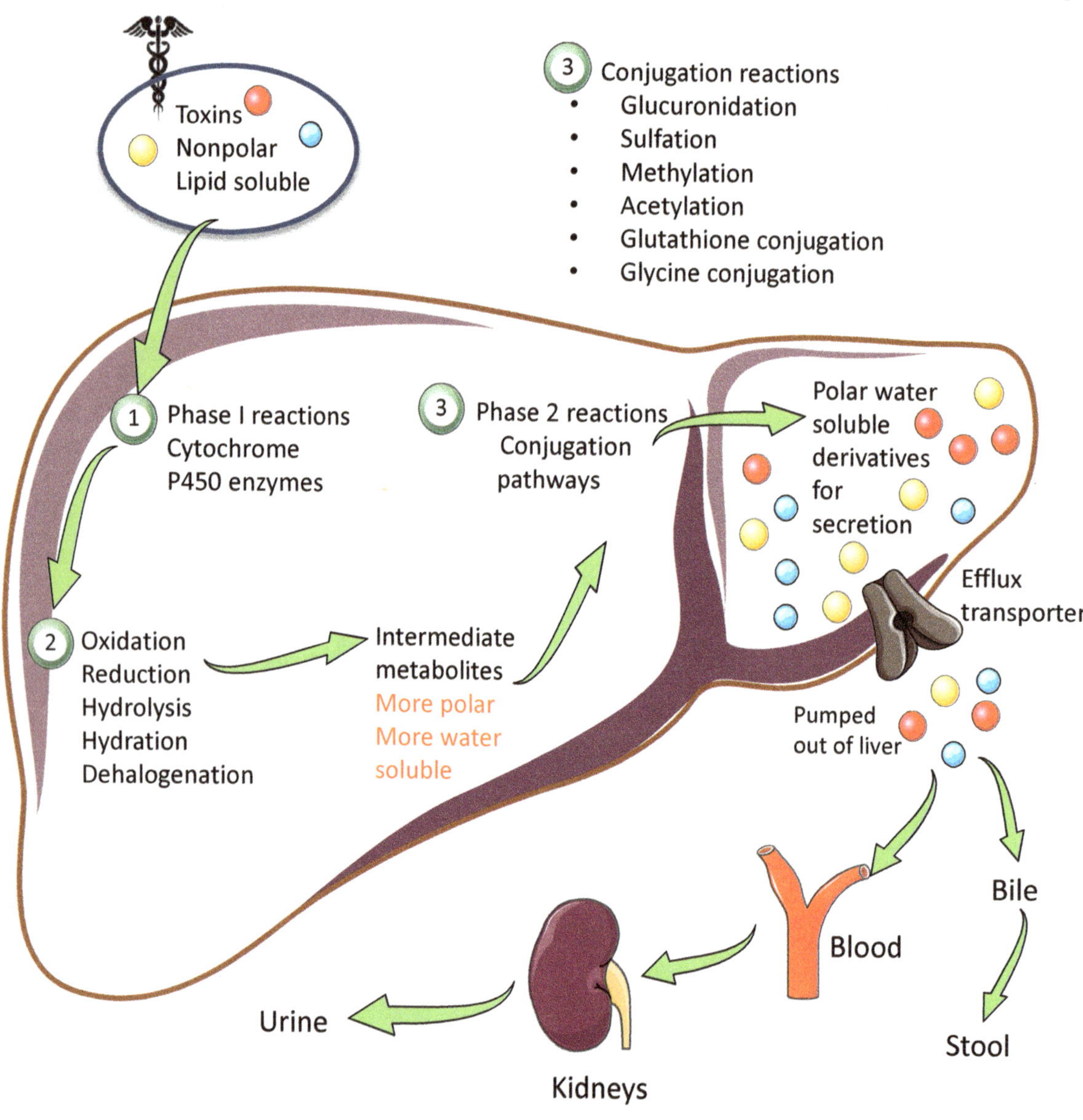

Detoxification pathways: Liver function in elimination of drugs

Examples of enzymatic biotransformation

Hydrolysis

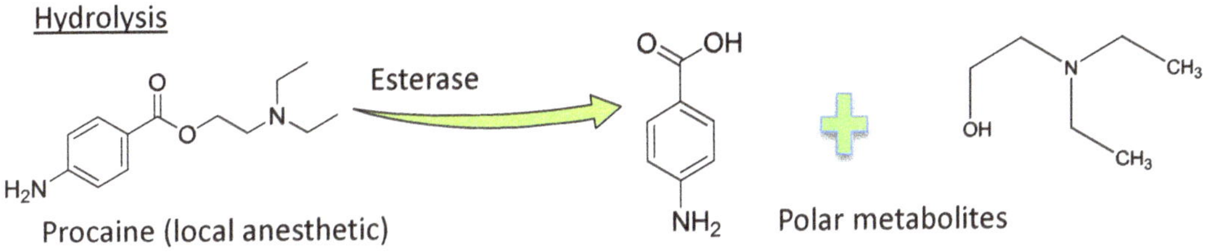

Esterase

Procaine (local anesthetic)

Polar metabolites

Reduction

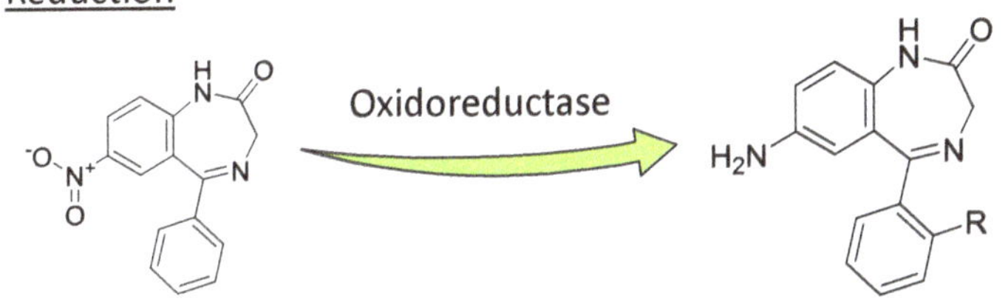

Oxidoreductase

Nitrazepam (hypnotic)

Polar metabolite

Glucuronidation

Glucuronosyl transferase

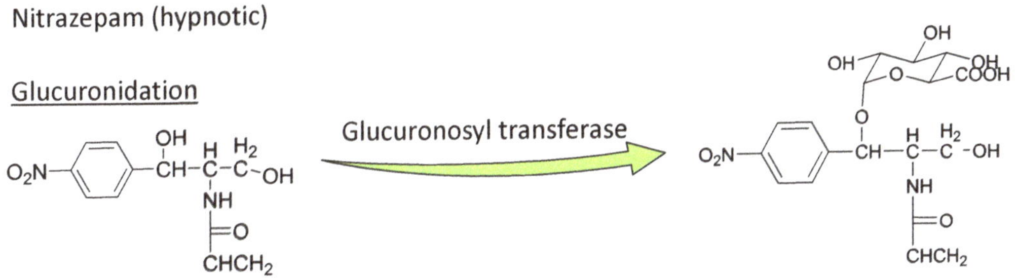

Chloramphenicol (antibiotic)

Polar metabolite

Kidney function

The function of the kidney is to maintain the **overall fluid balance** and returning vital substances such as vitamins, amino acids, glucose, hormones into the bloodstream, and filtering out waste materials such as urea and creatinine and toxic substances. The **kidneys are the primary excretory organs** for xenobiotics and their polar metabolites.

Substances with a low molecular weight, low lipophilicity, charged at pH 7.4, are eliminated effectively via the kidney.

Renal excretion does not occur for drugs with a molecular weight above 45kDa, strong protein binding, or high lipophilicity.

The kidney possesses most of the common xenobiotic metabolizing enzymes (with lower activity than the liver) with important contributions to the body's metabolism of drugs.

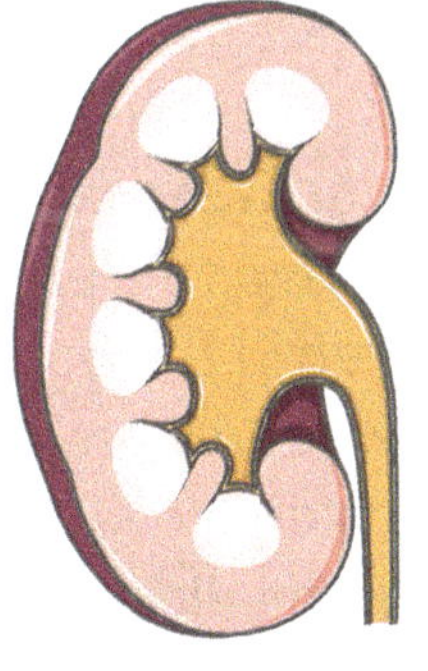

Relation between kidney and liver in the excretion of drugs depends on the physicochemical properties of each substance.

Xenobiotic metabolism converts nonpolar drugs to polar products that will not be reabsorbed from urine or bile.

Xenobiotic metabolism in the kidney by certain metabolizing enzymes may **result in the production of potent toxicants** (nephrotoxicity).

Detoxification pathways: Kidney function in elimination of drugs

Chapter 2 The organs and molecules of life

How the body digests food and provides the building blocks for life.

The gastrointestinal tract.

The pancreas gland with secretions of enzymes and hormones.

The role of the liver in protein, nucleic acid, polysaccharide, and lipid metabolism.

Selected medicines approved by the FDA.
✓ = Drugs approved recently (2017-2020)

GI system
Gastroesophageal reflux disease
- Prilosec

Gastrointestinal stromal tumor
- Ayvakit ✓

Liver
Transplant rejection
- Myfortic

Gout
- Zyloprim

Diabetes
- Amaryl

Elevated cholesterol
- Nexletol ✓
- Lipitor
- Colcrys

Overview

The ingestion of food provides the building blocks of life, which include the macromolecules, nucleic acids, proteins, polysaccharides, and lipids. This chapter will describe the organ biochemistry of the mouth, stomach, small and large intestine, as well as the pancreas and liver. The biochemistry provides an understanding of the diseases that occur in the digestive systems and the mechanism of action of the medicines used to treat these diseases.
Although many of the medicines covered in the book involve recent approvals from the FDA, this chapter will include heavily prescribed medicines such as statins for treatment of elevated cholesterol levels and a drug to stimulate insulin secretion in diabetes. The use of medicines to regulate nucleic acid metabolism in the liver can interfere in the supply of nucleotides required for lymphocyte proliferation and offer therapeutic options for diseases ranging from cancer, viral infections, and autoimmune disorders.

How the body digests food and provides the building blocks for life

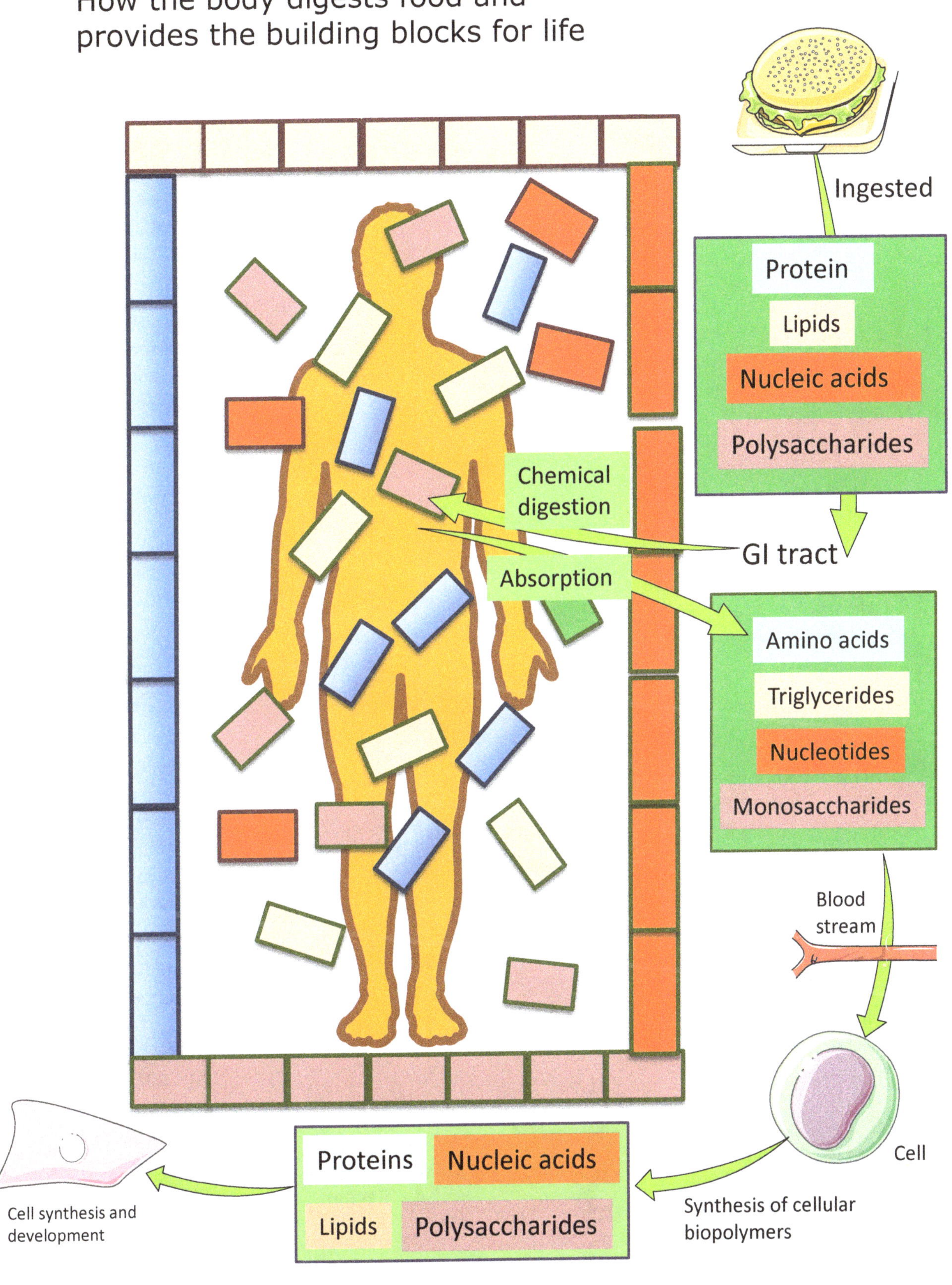

The digestive system: Gastrointestinal (GI) tract

GI tract is made up of a series of hollow organs, the mouth, esophagus, stomach, small and large intestine, and anus.

pH varies in the human digestive tract.

1 **Saliva of pH** is between 6.5 and 7.5. After chewing and swallowing, food enters the **upper portion** of the **stomach** with pH 4.0–6.5.

2 **Lower portion of the stomach** secretes HCl and pepsin to a pH 1.5–4.0.

3 **pH gradually increases in the small intestine** from 6 to 7.4 in the final part of small intestine.

4 **Rectum has a pH 6.7** with the passage of waste products.

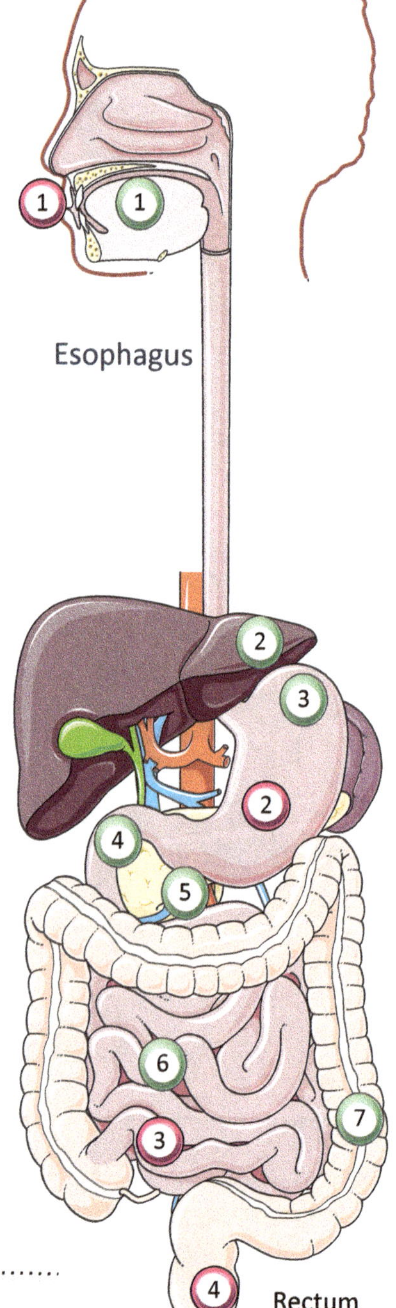

1 **Digestion begins in the mouth** with mechanical digestion (chewing and swallowing) and chemical digestion of carbohydrates and fats.

2 **Liver metabolizes ingested compounds** and produces bile to help break down fats and remove waste products.

3 **Stomach performs mechanical digestion** of food.

4 **Duodenum (digestion of food)**, both mechanical digestion and chemical digestion of proteins and fats.

5 **Pancreatic secretion (enzymes, hormones)** to the intestine for the digestion of proteins, carbohydrates, lipids, and nucleic acids.

6 **Small intestine** (responsible for most of the absorption of nutrients).

7 **Large intestine** (colon) mechanical digestion and mixing of food.

The mouth—the start of the digestive tract

Food consists of proteins, nucleic acids, lipids, and polysaccharides, which must be broken in the GI system into low-molecular weight fragments such as peptides, nucleotides, fatty acids, and simple sugars before absorption into the blood stream.

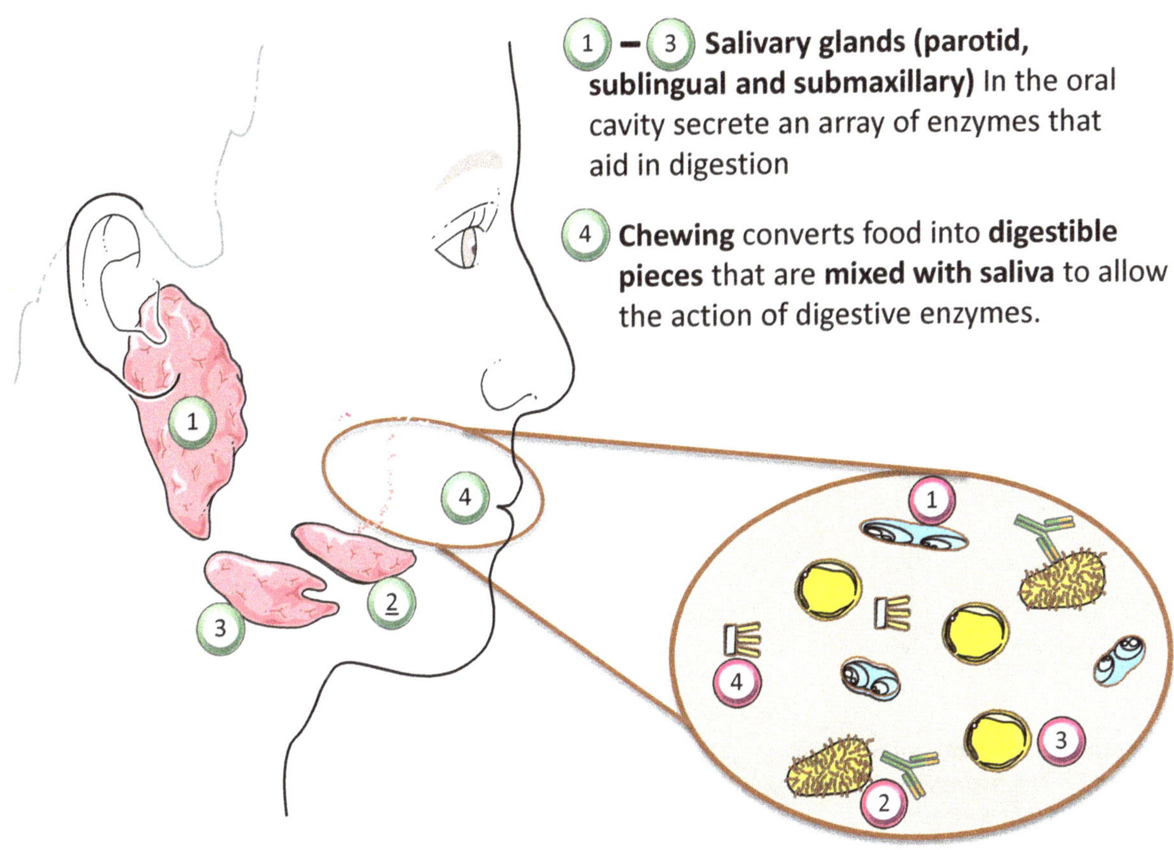

(1) – (3) **Salivary glands (parotid, sublingual and submaxillary)** In the oral cavity secrete an array of enzymes that aid in digestion

(4) **Chewing** converts food into **digestible pieces** that are **mixed with saliva** to allow the action of digestive enzymes.

(4) **Lingual lipase** hydrolyzes **triglycerides** into glycerides and free fatty acids for absorption by the small intestine.

(4) **30% of fat** is hydrolyzed by lingual lipase in 1–20 minutes of ingestion.

(1) **White blood and epithelial cells.**

(2) **IgA and lysozyme** offer a defense against bacteria, viruses, microorganisms.

(3) **Alpha-amylase** breaks down starch and glycogen into maltose and glucose.

(3) **About 5% of starches are digested in saliva that** minimize tooth decay.

The stomach

The stomach plays a major role in digestion both in a mechanical sense by mixing and crushing the food and by **digestion of proteins** with the enzyme **pepsin** (unlike carbohydrate and lipids where the mouth provides initial digestion). The amino acids that are released by protein digestion are absorbed across the intestinal wall into the circulatory system, where they can be used for protein synthesis.

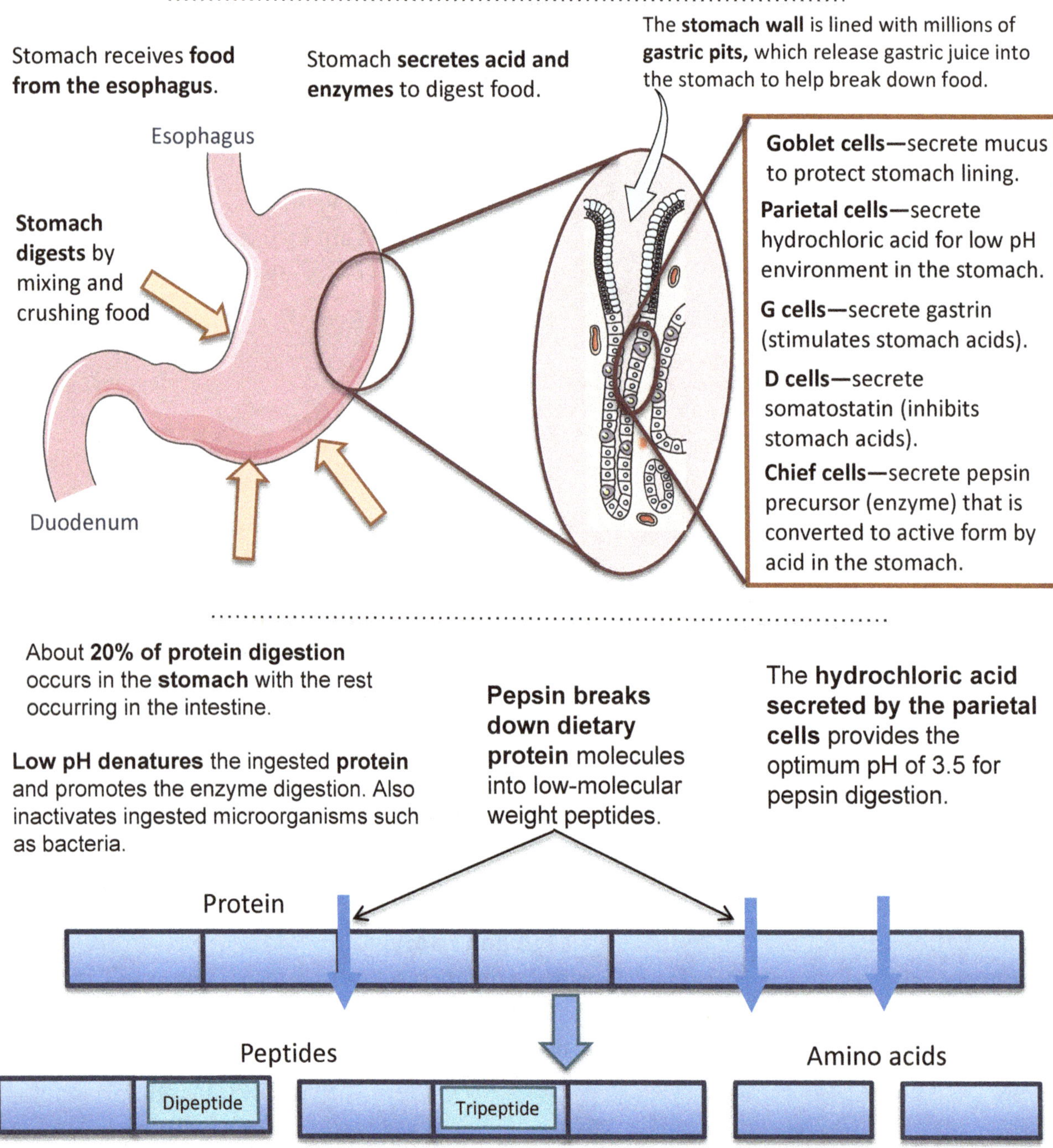

Stomach receives **food from the esophagus.**
Stomach **secretes acid and enzymes** to digest food.
The **stomach wall** is lined with millions of **gastric pits,** which release gastric juice into the stomach to help break down food.
Esophagus
Stomach digests by mixing and crushing food
Duodenum
Goblet cells—secrete mucus to protect stomach lining.
Parietal cells—secrete hydrochloric acid for low pH environment in the stomach.
G cells—secrete gastrin (stimulates stomach acids).
D cells—secrete somatostatin (inhibits stomach acids).
Chief cells—secrete pepsin precursor (enzyme) that is converted to active form by acid in the stomach.
About **20% of protein digestion** occurs in the **stomach** with the rest occurring in the intestine.
Low pH denatures the ingested **protein** and promotes the enzyme digestion. Also inactivates ingested microorganisms such as bacteria.
Pepsin breaks down dietary protein molecules into low-molecular weight peptides.
The **hydrochloric acid secreted by the parietal cells** provides the optimum pH of 3.5 for pepsin digestion.
Protein
Peptides
Dipeptide
Tripeptide
Amino acids

Molecules of life: The stomach, digestion of dietary proteins

Small intestine

1 **The duodenum** is largely responsible for the **digestion of food**. The later stages of the small intestine (jejunum and ileum) absorb nutrients into the bloodstream.

2 The small intestine breaks down food using **enzymes released** by the **pancreas** and **bile from the liver**.

3 **Contents** of the small intestine start out semi-solid but are **liquefied** by adding water, bile, enzymes, and mucous.

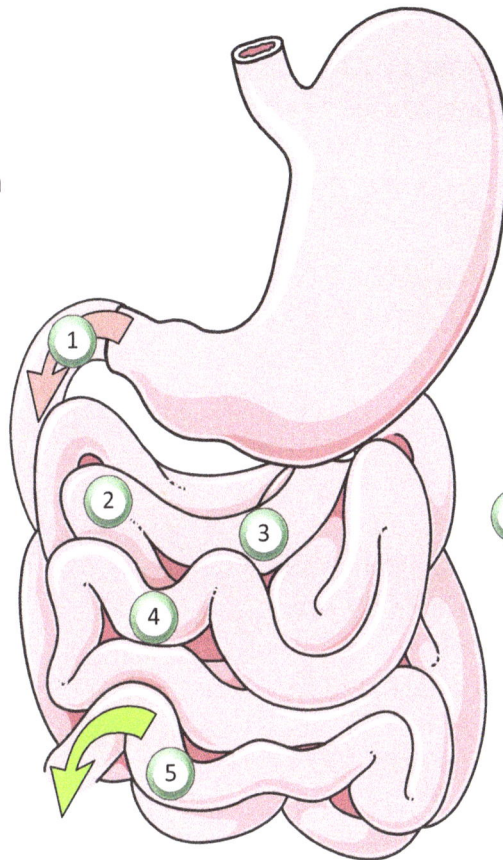

4 As the food moves through the 22-foot long muscular tube, it mixes with **digestive secretions** from the **pancreas and liver**.

5 Once the nutrients have been absorbed in the small intestine, the **residual food and liquid moves on to the** large intestine **(colon)**.

Nucleosidases and nucleases for the **digestion of DNA and RNA** are produced in the pancreas and secreted in the small intestine.

Bile acids and **pancreatic lipase** are added to **chyme** (gastric juices) to allow lipids to be absorbed (triglyceride, cholesterol) from the stomach.

Triglyceride molecules are enzymatically **digested** to yield **monoglycerides** and fatty acids, which can be transported to the inner surface of the small intestine.

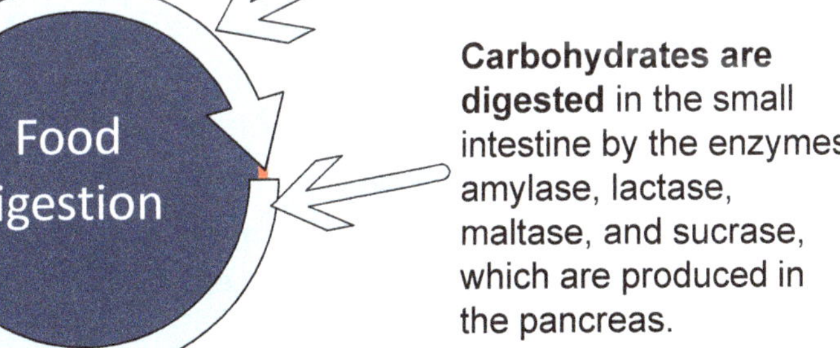

The **diversity of dietary proteins** with variable amino acid sequences requires that digestion in the intestine occurs with a **network of proteases** with different specificities.

Carbohydrates are digested in the small intestine by the enzymes amylase, lactase, maltase, and sucrase, which are produced in the pancreas.

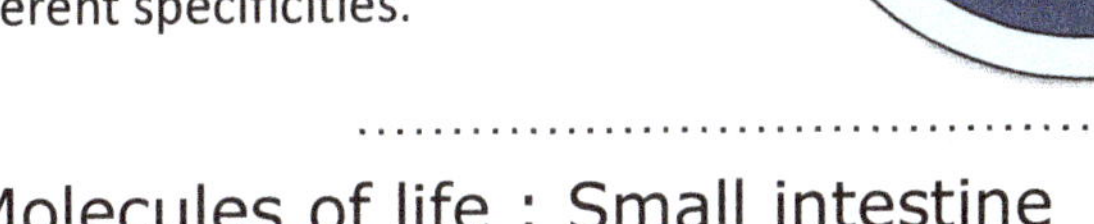

Gastroesophageal reflux disease (GERD)

Gastroesophageal reflux disease (GERD) occurs when **acid and food in the stomach back up** into the esophagus. It causes heartburn and other symptoms.

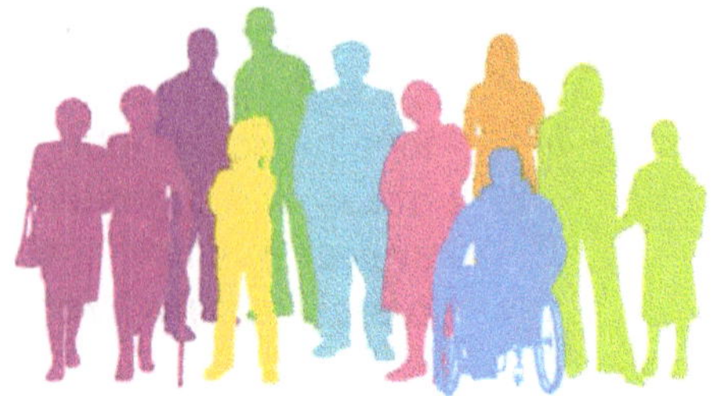

Incidence by gender and ethnicity

GERD occurs more in females than in males (ratio 1.6) and disease incidence increases in patients older than 50 years. Cuacasian individuals have a higher risk of complications such as esophagitis than African Americans and Asians.

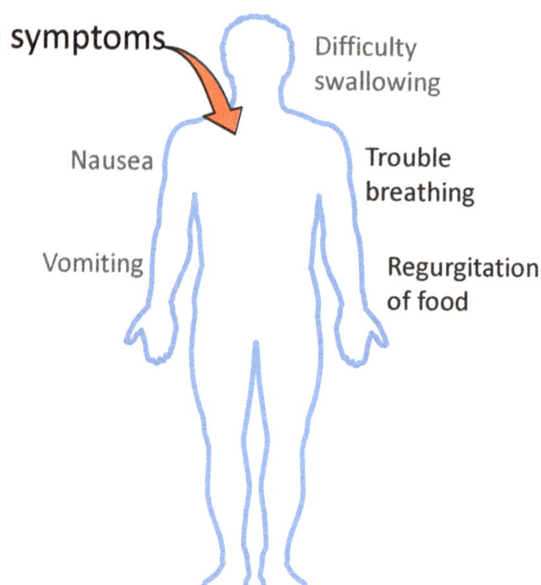

The medicine

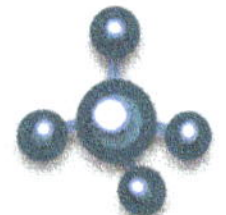

Omeprazol; Prilosec, FDA Approval 1989

Eighth Most US Prescribed Drug, (2019), 52.5 million prescriptions

Omeprazol is used when there is too much acid in the stomach and can result in gastric and duodenal ulcers, erosive esophagitis, and **gastroesophageal reflux disease** (GERD). Omeprazol promotes healing of peptic ulcers. **Omeprazole is absorbed in the small intestine** and diffuses into the parietal cells of the stomach. It is a prodrug that **activates in an acidic environment.**

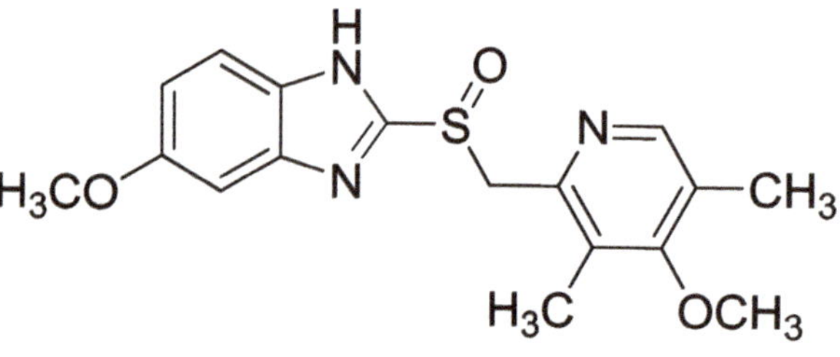

The stomach: Gastroesophageal reflux disease, Omeprazol

Action of Omeprazol on cell and disease biology

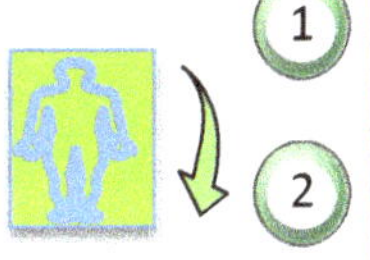

1 **Parietal cells** are epithelial cells in the lining of the pits of the stomach and **secrete H^+ into the stomach** in exchange for potassium ions (K^+).

2 The ATPase enzyme (**H^+/K^+) proton pump) is** located on the stomach inner cell lining. **Gastric acid is formed** when chloride ions (Cl^-) flow out.

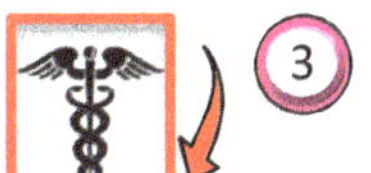

3 **GERD** occurs when the lower muscle of the esophagus does not close properly, allowing **stomach acid** and food back up (reflux) **into the esophagus.**

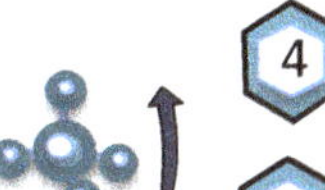

4 **Omeprazole is absorbed** in the **small intestine,** accumulates in the stomach parietal cells, activated in the secretory lining.

5 **Omeprazole** reduces gastric acid production by irreversibly **inhibiting** the **proton pump** in the parietal cells and **acid secretion is suppressed** until new proton pump molecules have been synthesized (24–48 hours).

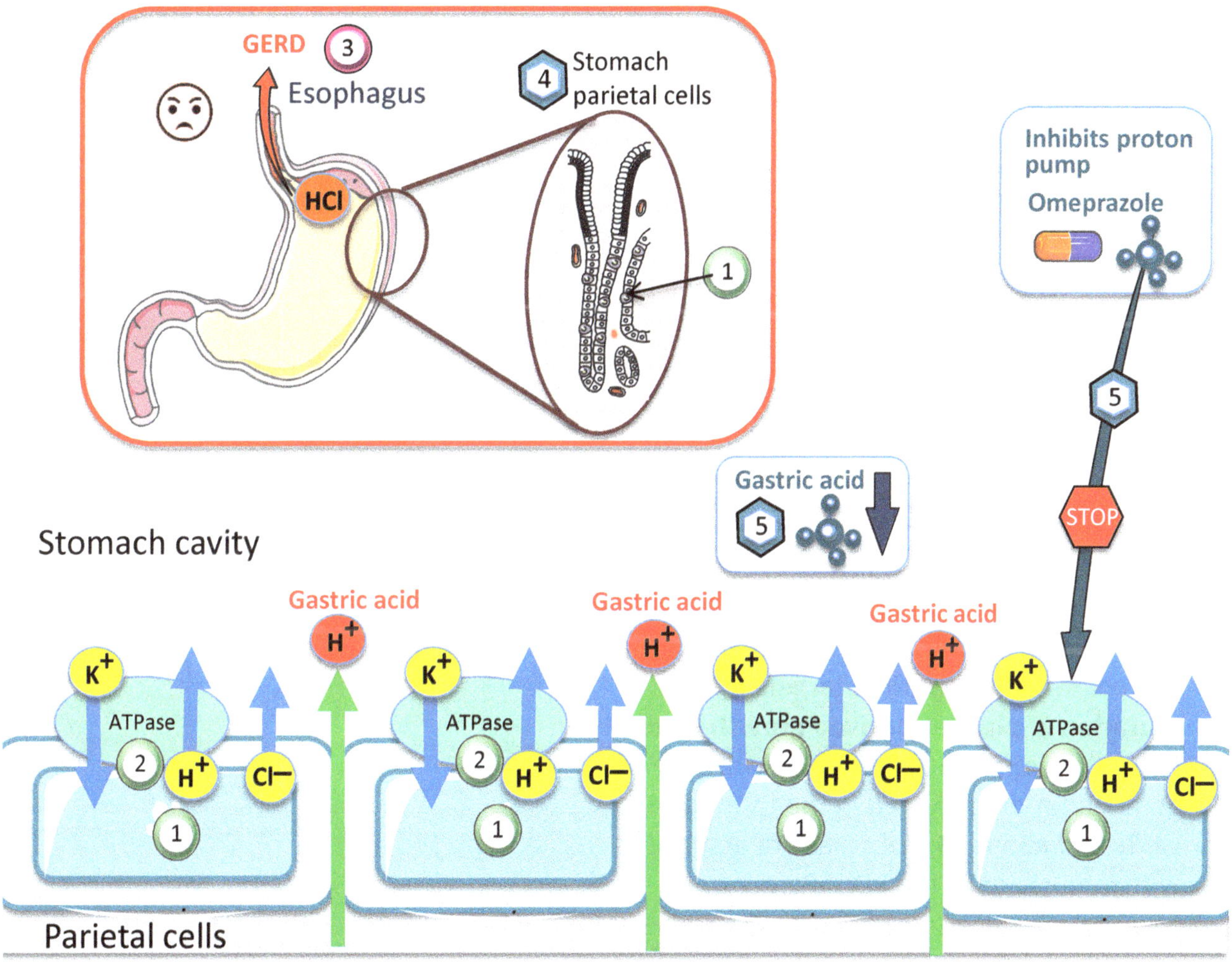

The stomach: Gastroesophageal reflux disease, Omeprazol

The disease: Gastrointestinal stromal tumors (GISTs) 30

Gastrointestinal stromal tumors (GISTs) are rare connective tissue malignancies in the gastrointestinal tract, most often in the stomach or small intestine, which is caused by **abnormal platelet-derived growth factor receptor alpha (PDGFRα) gene** and has spread throughout the body (metastatic GIST).

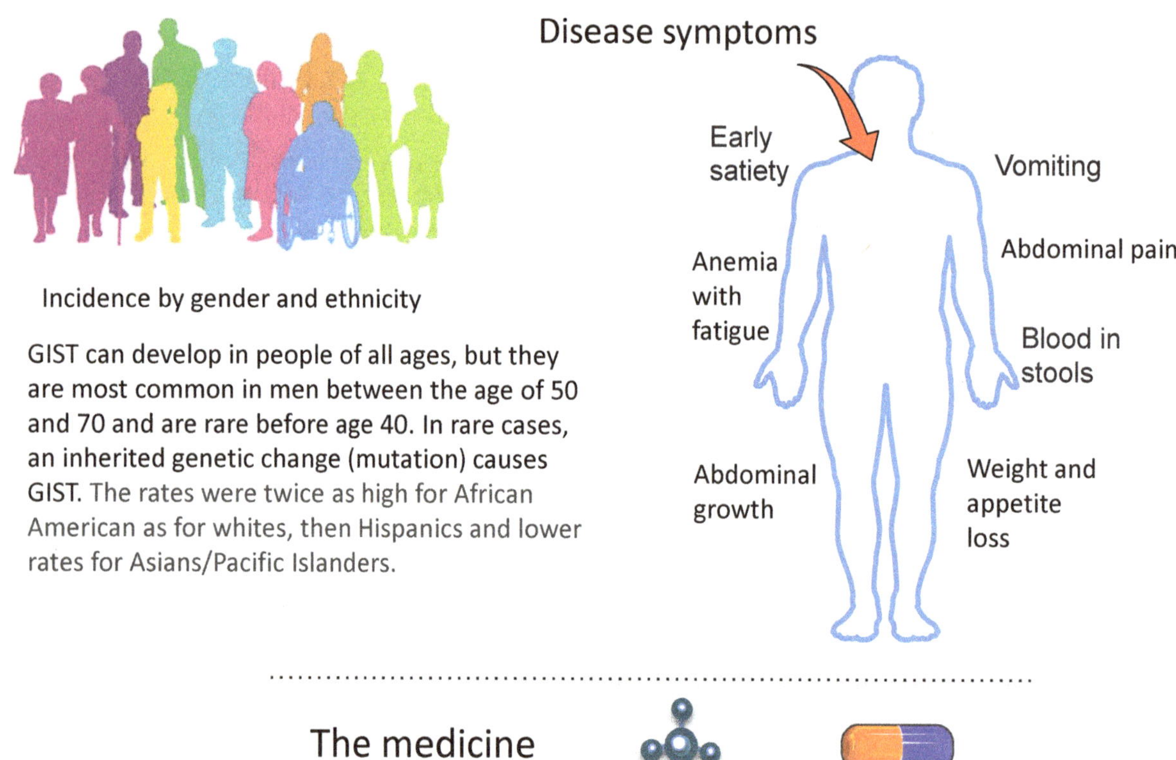

Incidence by gender and ethnicity

GIST can develop in people of all ages, but they are most common in men between the age of 50 and 70 and are rare before age 40. In rare cases, an inherited genetic change (mutation) causes GIST. The rates were twice as high for African American as for whites, then Hispanics and lower rates for Asians/Pacific Islanders.

The medicine

Avapritinib; Ayvakit, FDA Approval 2021

Avapritinib is the first tyrosine kinase inhibitor for the treatment of gastrointestinal stromal tumors (GIST). Avapritinib targets a rare **mutation in platelet-derived growth factor receptor alpha (PDGFRα)**. There are several gene mutations involved in the formation of GISTs and about 10% of cases are associated with a mutation in the PDGFRα gene.

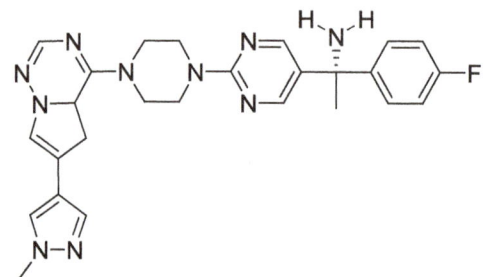

Action of Avapritinib on cell and disease biology

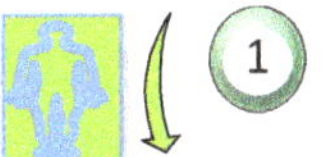

1 **Interstitial cells of Cajal (ICC) in the muscle layers** of the GI tract mediate communications (autonomic nervous system, smooth muscle).

2 A **gastrointestinal stromal tumor** (GIST) occurs in the ICC cells of the gastrointestinal tract with **mutations** in **platelet-derived growth factor receptor alpha** (PDGFRA), activation of the tyrosine kinase signaling pathways.

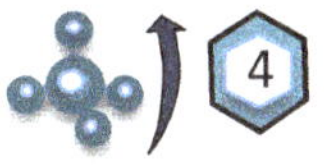

3 The constant activation of these cellular pathways results in uncontrolled cell growth and **proliferation of cancer cells** that leads to GIST formation.

4 **Ayvakit is a selective inhibitor of** PDGFRA that **blocks the mutated kinase** and the cancer cells from growing.

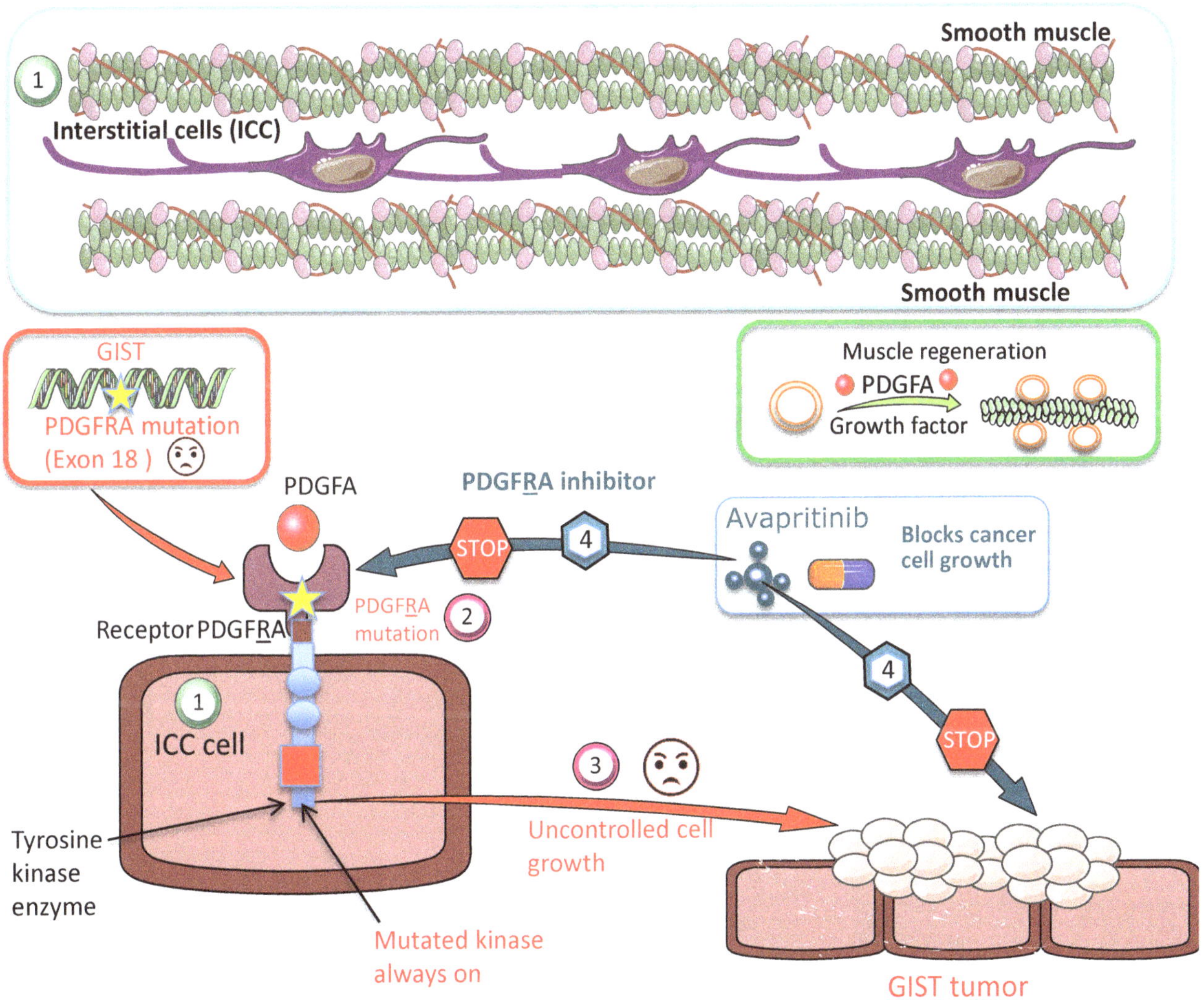

Small intestine: Gastrointestinal stromal tumors, Avapritinib

Pancreas

The exocrine pancreas is the organ with the **highest level of protein synthesis** producing enzymes for the breaking down of macromolecules in our diet. For homoeostasis, the pancreas must produce sufficient enzymes to **match the dietary intake** and digestion of proteins, fats, carbohydrates, and nucleic acids.

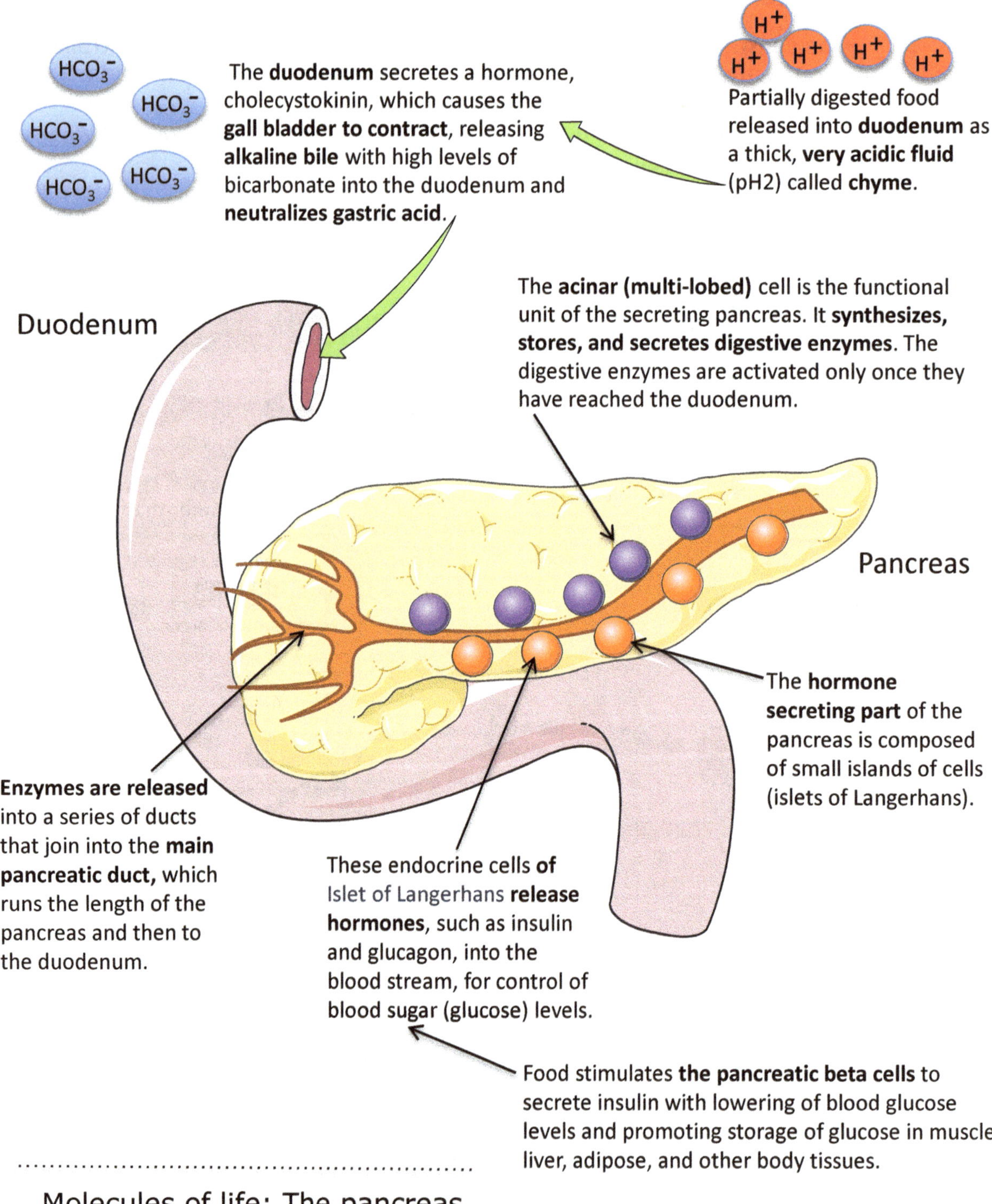

HCO_3^-
HCO_3^-
HCO_3^-
HCO_3^-
HCO_3^-
The **duodenum** secretes a hormone, cholecystokinin, which causes the **gall bladder to contract**, releasing **alkaline bile** with high levels of bicarbonate into the duodenum and **neutralizes gastric acid**.
H^+
H^+
H^+
H^+
H^+
Partially digested food released into **duodenum** as a thick, **very acidic fluid** (pH2) called **chyme**.
Duodenum
The **acinar (multi-lobed)** cell is the functional unit of the secreting pancreas. It **synthesizes, stores, and secretes digestive enzymes**. The digestive enzymes are activated only once they have reached the duodenum.
Pancreas
The **hormone secreting part** of the pancreas is composed of small islands of cells (islets of Langerhans).
Enzymes are released into a series of ducts that join into the **main pancreatic duct,** which runs the length of the pancreas and then to the duodenum.
These endocrine cells **of** Islet of Langerhans **release hormones**, such as insulin and glucagon, into the blood stream, for control of blood sugar (glucose) levels.
Food stimulates **the pancreatic beta cells** to secrete insulin with lowering of blood glucose levels and promoting storage of glucose in muscle, liver, adipose, and other body tissues.

Liver structure and function

The liver is the largest organ inside the body with many important metabolic functions such as the storage of some vitamins, minerals, and glucose, processing nutrients such as proteins, fats, and carbohydrates, as well as blood detoxification.

1 Hepatocyte (performs most of the liver's functions)

- **Synthesis** of nonessential **amino acids**, blood **proteins**, albumins, α- and β-globulins, blood clotting factors, fibrinogen, lipoproteins, and enzymes.
- **Nucleotides** (purines and pyrimidines) are primarily produced in the liver.
- Hepatocytes synthesize and store glucose based on needs.
- **Bile** production and excretion.

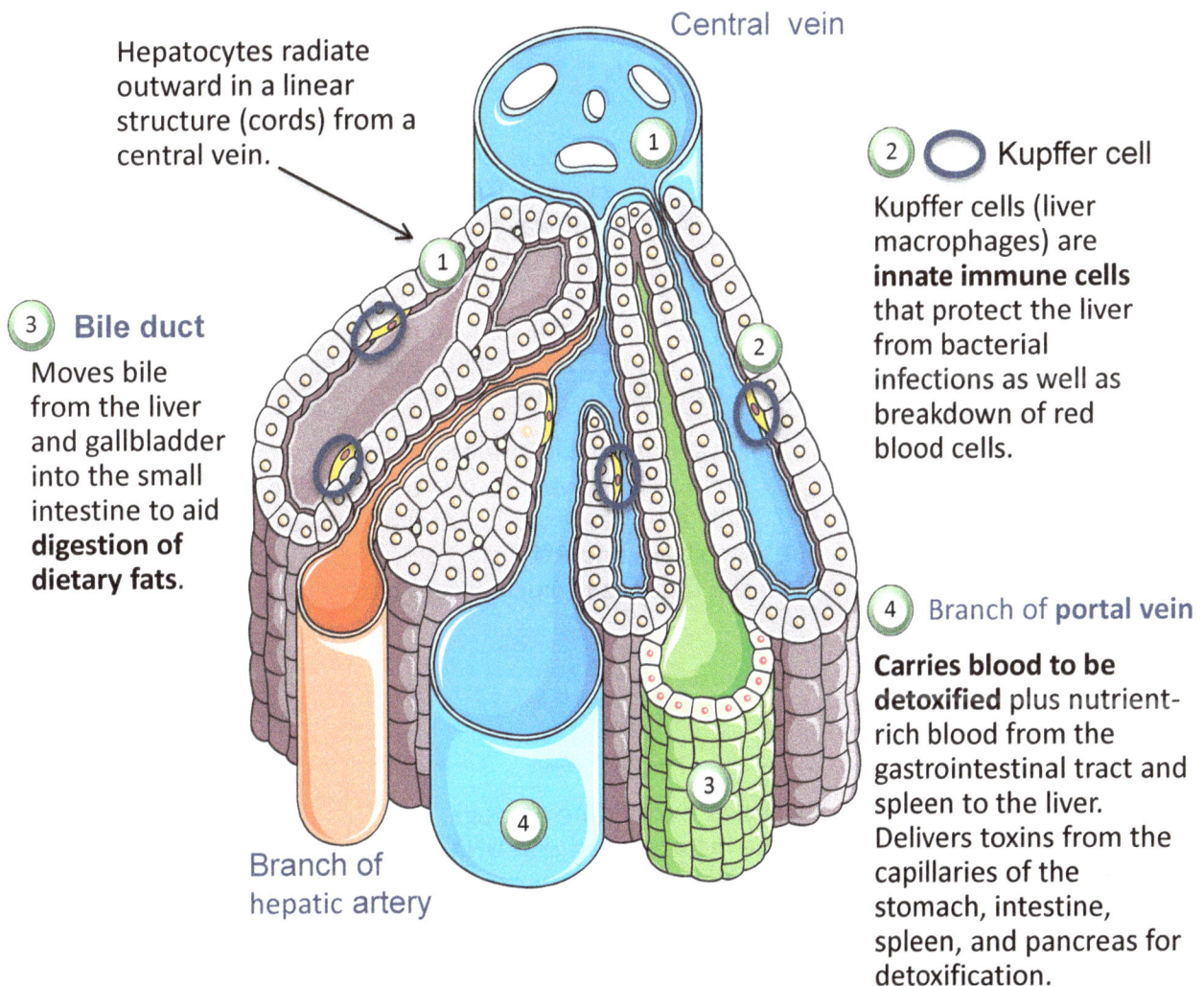

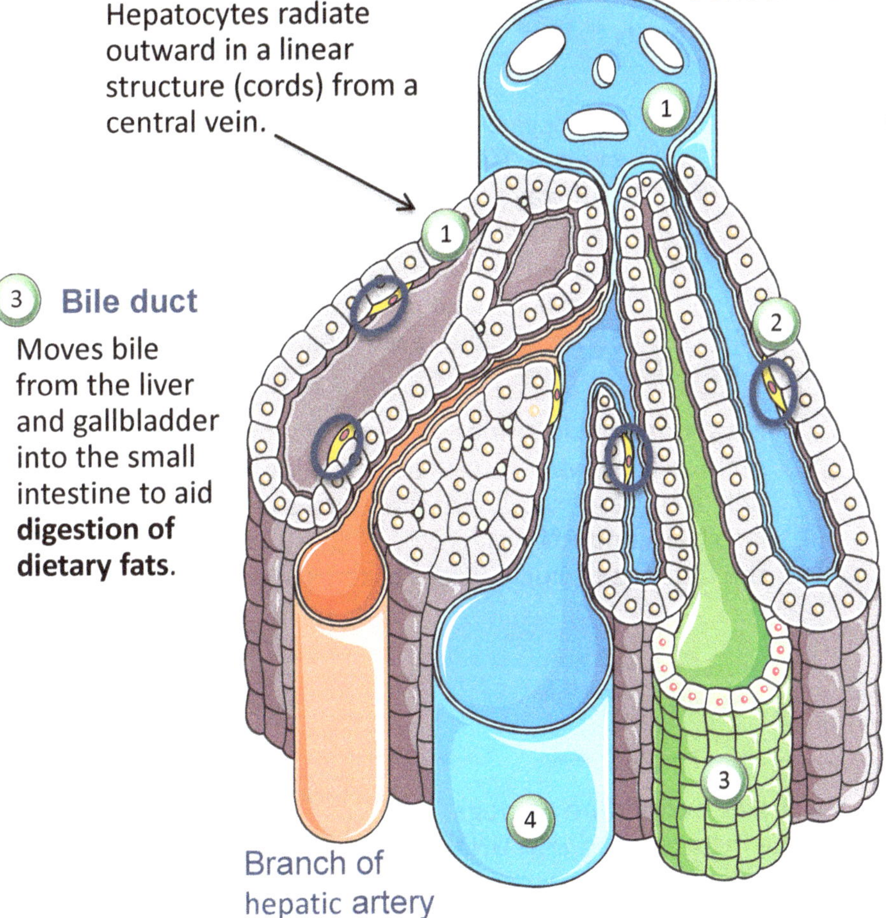

3 Bile duct

Moves bile from the liver and gallbladder into the small intestine to aid **digestion of dietary fats.**

2 Kupffer cell

Kupffer cells (liver macrophages) are **innate immune cells** that protect the liver from bacterial infections as well as breakdown of red blood cells.

4 Branch of **portal vein**

Carries blood to be detoxified plus nutrient-rich blood from the gastrointestinal tract and spleen to the liver. Delivers toxins from the capillaries of the stomach, intestine, spleen, and pancreas for detoxification.

Nucleic acid metabolism

The process by which nucleic acids (DNA and RNA) are synthesized and degraded.

1 **Nucleotides** and their constituent bases (purines and pyrimidines) are supplied by **dietary intake** but not incorporated directly into tissue nucleic acids. In what is called **salvage pathways**, the nucleic acids are **hydrolyzed** by a series of enzymes to yield **nucleotides**.

2 **Nucleotides** are supplied by **synthesis in tissues** from low-molecular weight precursors.

1 Salvage pathways

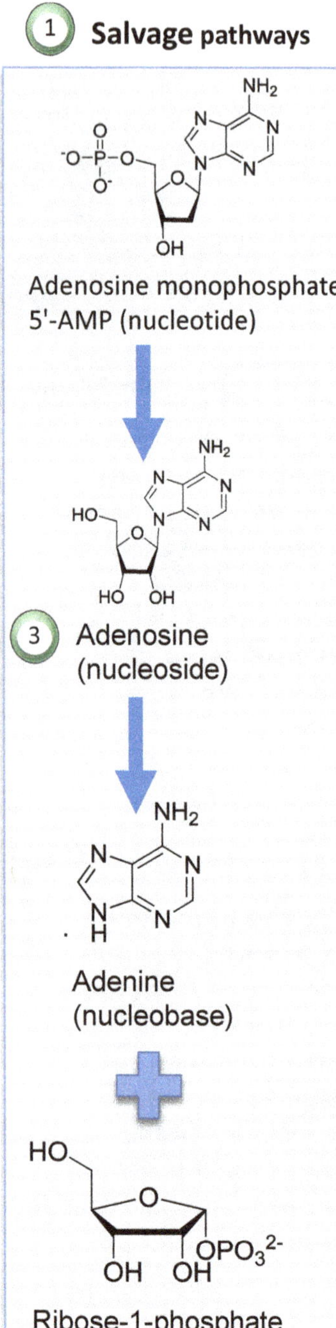

2 Nucleotide biosynthesis

The liver is the **major site** of de novo **nucleotide synthesis**, for the replenishment and maintenance of intracellular pools.

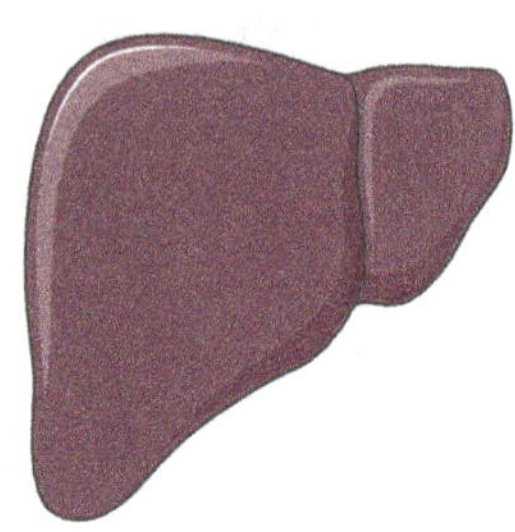

Chemical linkage of phosphate, pentose sugar, and either purines (adenine or guanine) or pyrimidines (cytosine, thymine, or uracil).

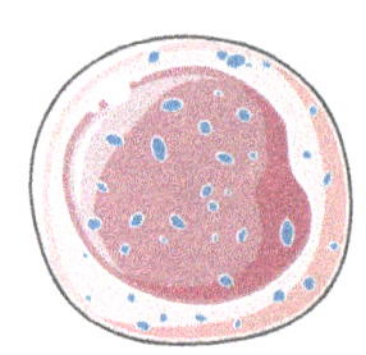

The cells of **immune system** use **salvage pathways** and dietary sources to fulfill their own **nucleotide needs** during periods of rapid proliferation during immune responses.

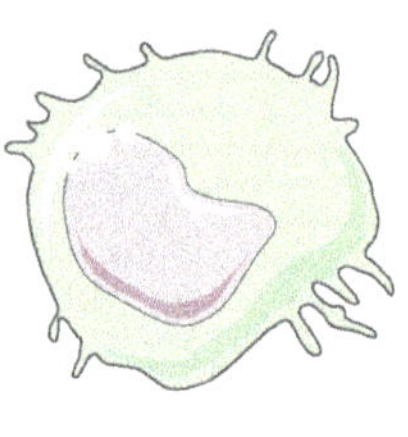

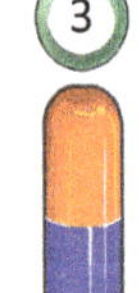

3 Most **nucleoside <u>analogs</u>** are active only after metabolic activation to the nucleotide form. Not only are these fraudulent nucleotides **incorporated into DNA and RNA** macromolecules but also **distort the balance of nucleic acid precursors.**

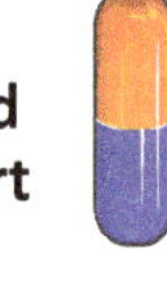

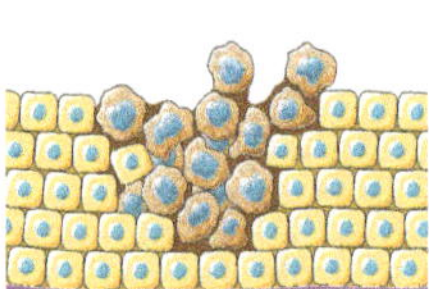

Purine or pyrimidine analogs can be incorporated into DNA and used as **anticancer drugs** as proliferating cells require de novo synthesis of nucleotides.

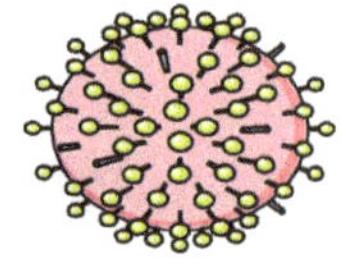

Nucleoside analogs with high antiviral potency treat acute infections caused by RNA and DNA viruses (HIV, hepatitis B or C viruses, and herpes viruses).

Nucleotide biosynthesis

Cells require a **balanced quantity of purines and pyrimidines** for growth, proliferation, survival.

Purine biosynthesis

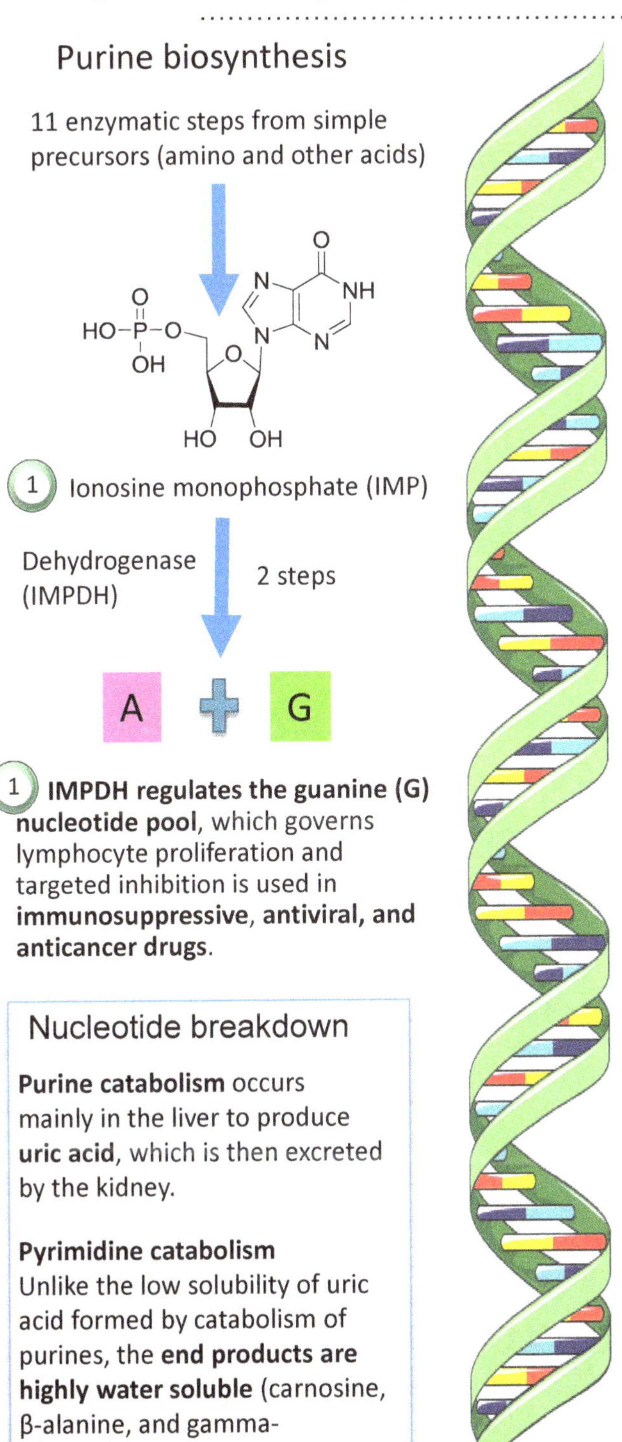

11 enzymatic steps from simple precursors (amino and other acids)

1 Ionosine monophosphate (IMP)

Dehydrogenase (IMPDH)

2 steps

A + G

1 **IMPDH regulates the guanine (G) nucleotide pool**, which governs lymphocyte proliferation and targeted inhibition is used in **immunosuppressive**, **antiviral, and anticancer drugs**.

Nucleotide breakdown

Purine catabolism occurs mainly in the liver to produce **uric acid**, which is then excreted by the kidney.

Pyrimidine catabolism
Unlike the low solubility of uric acid formed by catabolism of purines, the **end products are highly water soluble** (carnosine, β-alanine, and gamma-aminoisobutyrate).

Pyrimidine biosynthesis

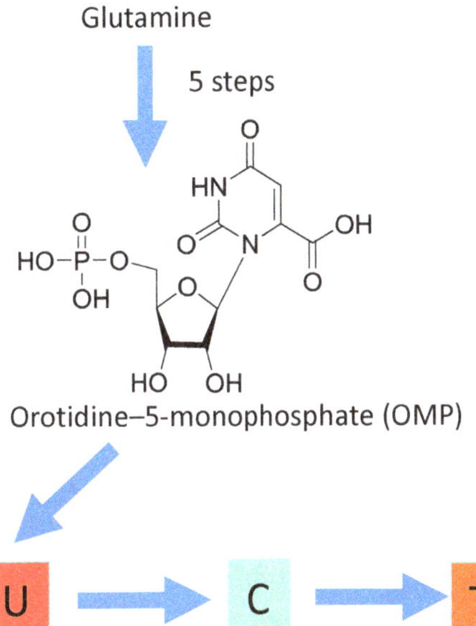

Glutamine

5 steps

Orotidine–5-monophosphate (OMP)

U → C → T

Purine or pyrimidine analogs
Antimetabolites, including potential anticancer drugs, are converted to analogues of cellular nucleotides by enzymes of the purine or pyrimidine metabolic pathway and then **interfere with DNA replication**.

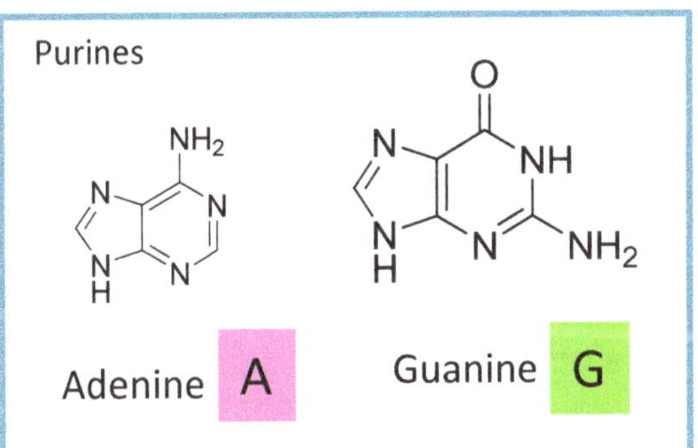

Pyrimidines

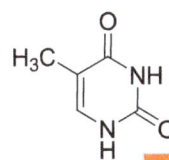

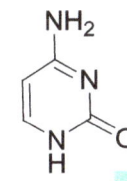

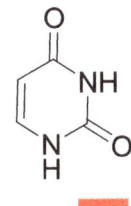

Thymine T   Cytosine C   Uracil U

The medical conditions include **immune system rejection** in allogenic renal, cardiac, or hepatic organ transplants as well as **inflammatory skin conditions**, psoriasis, and connective tissue disorders.

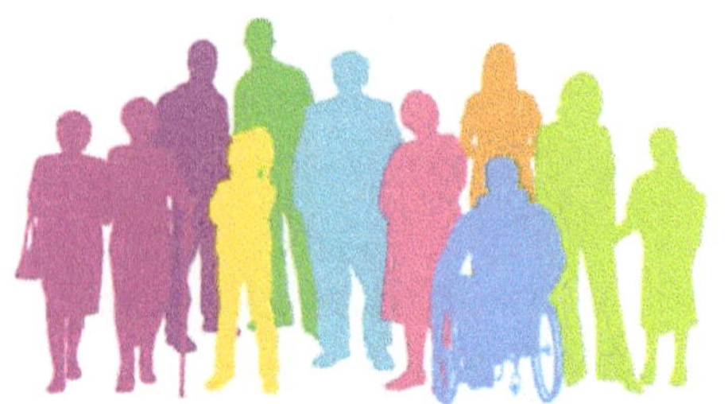

Incidence by gender and ethnicity

For skin disorders infectious diseases are more common in men, whereas autoimmune and allergic diseases are more common in women. For psoriasis, no age or gender differences in disease severity were observed.

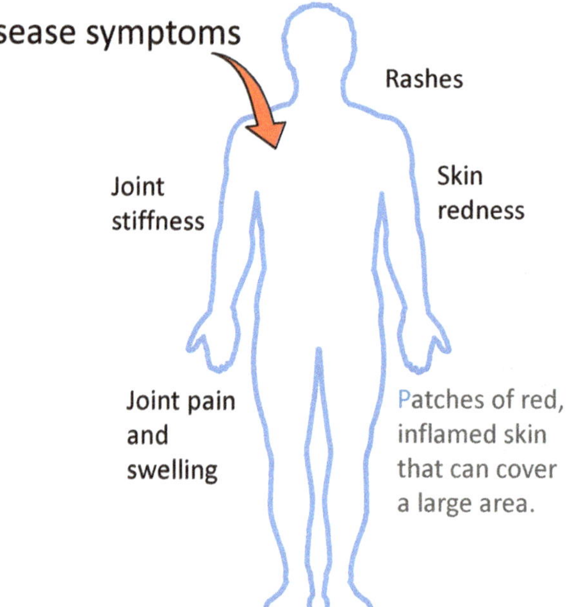

The medicine

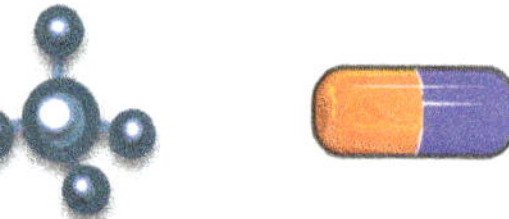

Mycophenolic acid; Myfortic , FDA Approval 2000

Mycophenolic acid is used for the prevention of acute allograft rejection. MPA is an **immunosuppressant** that is also effective in the treatment of inflammatory diseases, including systemic lupus erythematosus, and dermatology applications such as psoriasis.

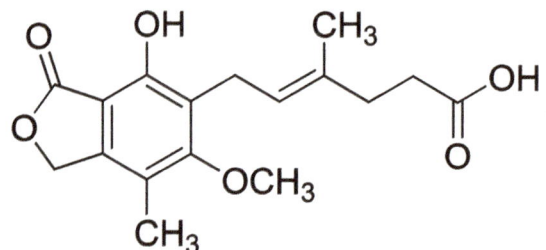

Action of Mycophenolic acid on cell and disease biology

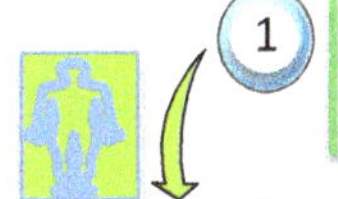

1 **Helper T cells** become **activated** by interacting with **dendritic cells**. Self-reactive T cells can cause pathological autoimmune disease**.**

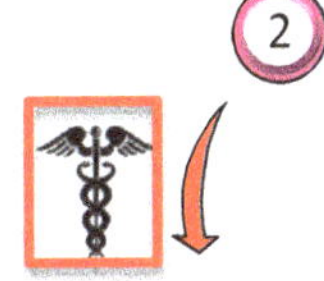

2 In **allograft rejection**, recipient T cells recognize donor-derived antigens, activated with clonal expansion, migrate to the graft with tissue destruction.

Psoriasis is mediated by T cells and dendritic cells, activate cytokine producing T cells that produce abundant psoriatic cytokines.

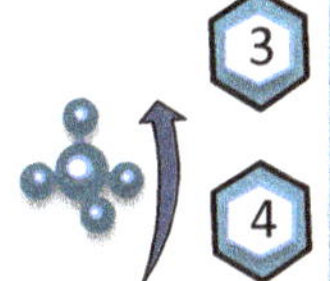

3 **Mycophenolic acid (MPA) inhibits IMP** and produces immunosuppression by inhibition of de-novo purine synthesis **(**DNA,RNA).

4 **MPA depletes guanosine nucleotides preferentially** in **T and B lymphocytes,** inhibits their proliferation, suppressing cell-mediated immune responses and antibody formation.

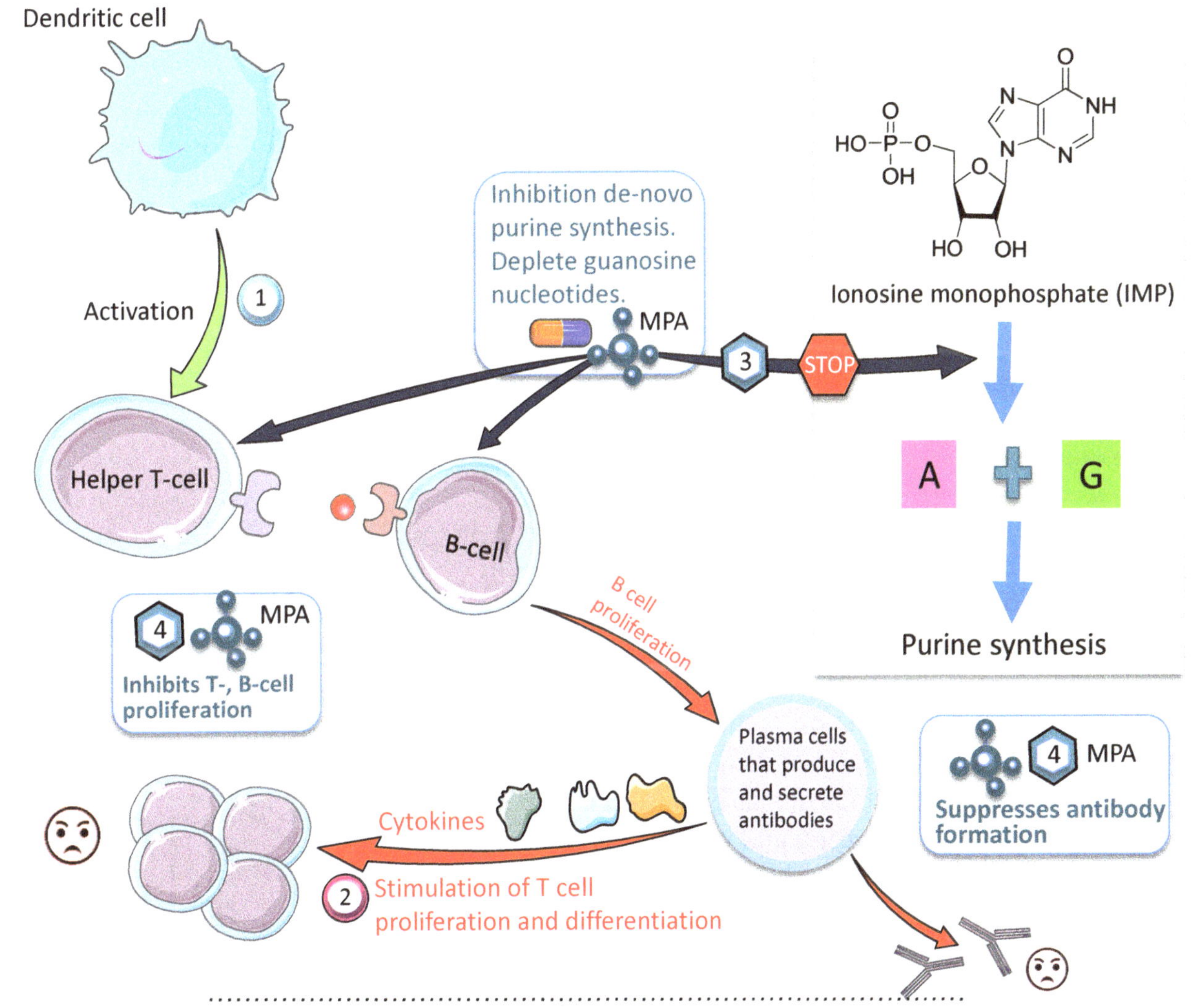

Nucleic acid metabolism : Immune system rejection, Mycophenolic acid

The disease: Gout

Gout refers to disease that occurs in response to the **presence of urate crystals in joints, bones, and soft tissues**. It may result in an acute arthritis (a gout flare) and chronic arthritis.

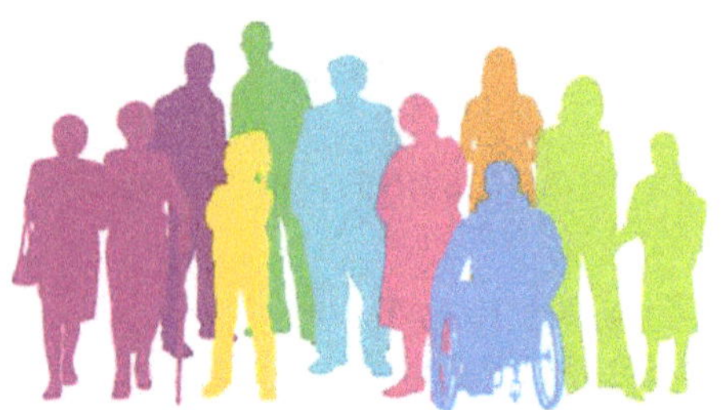

Incidence by gender and ethnicity

The prevalence of gout was higher in men than women (6 vs. 1 /1,000) but the gap narrowed with increasing age. Compared to whites, ethnic minorities, especially blacks, have higher prevalence of gout.

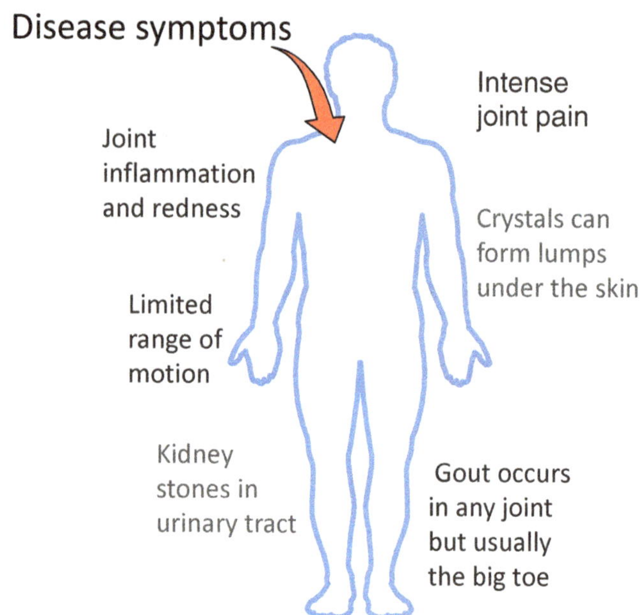

43rd Most US Prescribed Drug, (2019), 15.9 million prescriptions

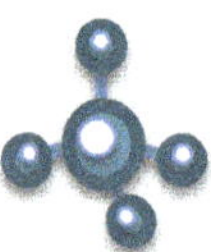

The medicine

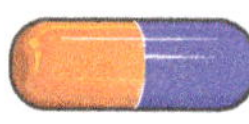

Allopurinol; Zyloprim, FDA Approval 1982

Allopurinol reduces the production of uric acid in the body. Uric acid buildup in the blood (hyperuricemia) can lead to **gout or kidney stones**. With cancer**,** chemotherapy treatment can generate a large increase in blood uric acid levels. Average levels of serum uric acid have also increased due to changes in diet and obesity and metabolic syndrome as well as medications that increase uric acid levels (low dose aspirin and diuretics).

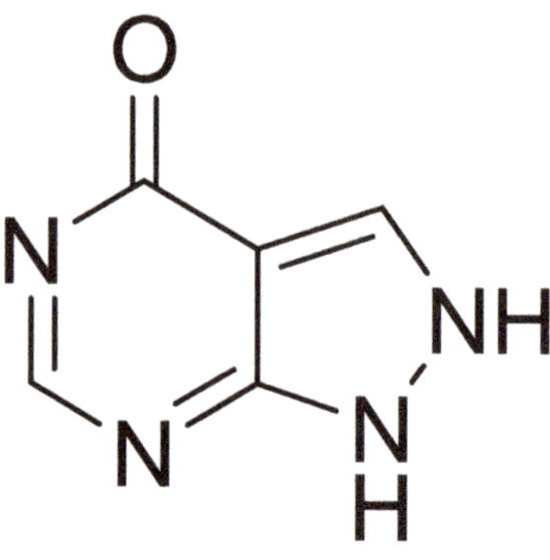

Nucleic acid metabolism: Gout, Allopurinol

Action of Allopurinol on cell and disease biology

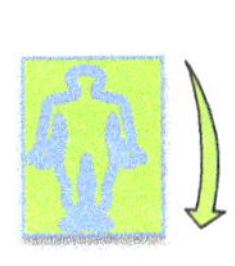

1 **Uric acid** is produced by **liver breakdown of purines** then transported to the blood and kidneys where it is excreted from the body in urine.

2 **Xanthine oxidase (XO)** catalyzes the **oxidation of hypoxanthine to xanthine** and then to **uric acid.**

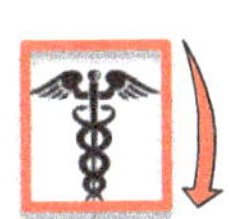

3 **Excess uric acid in the blood can form crystals** that results in gout, a type of arthritis that causes intense pain, swelling, and stiffness in a joint.

4 The acute symptoms of gout are triggered by the **inflammatory response to urate crystals**, mediated by macrophages and neutrophils.

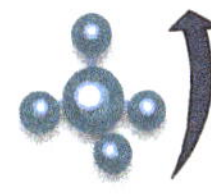

5 **Allopurinol** is an **inhibitor of xanthine oxidase.**

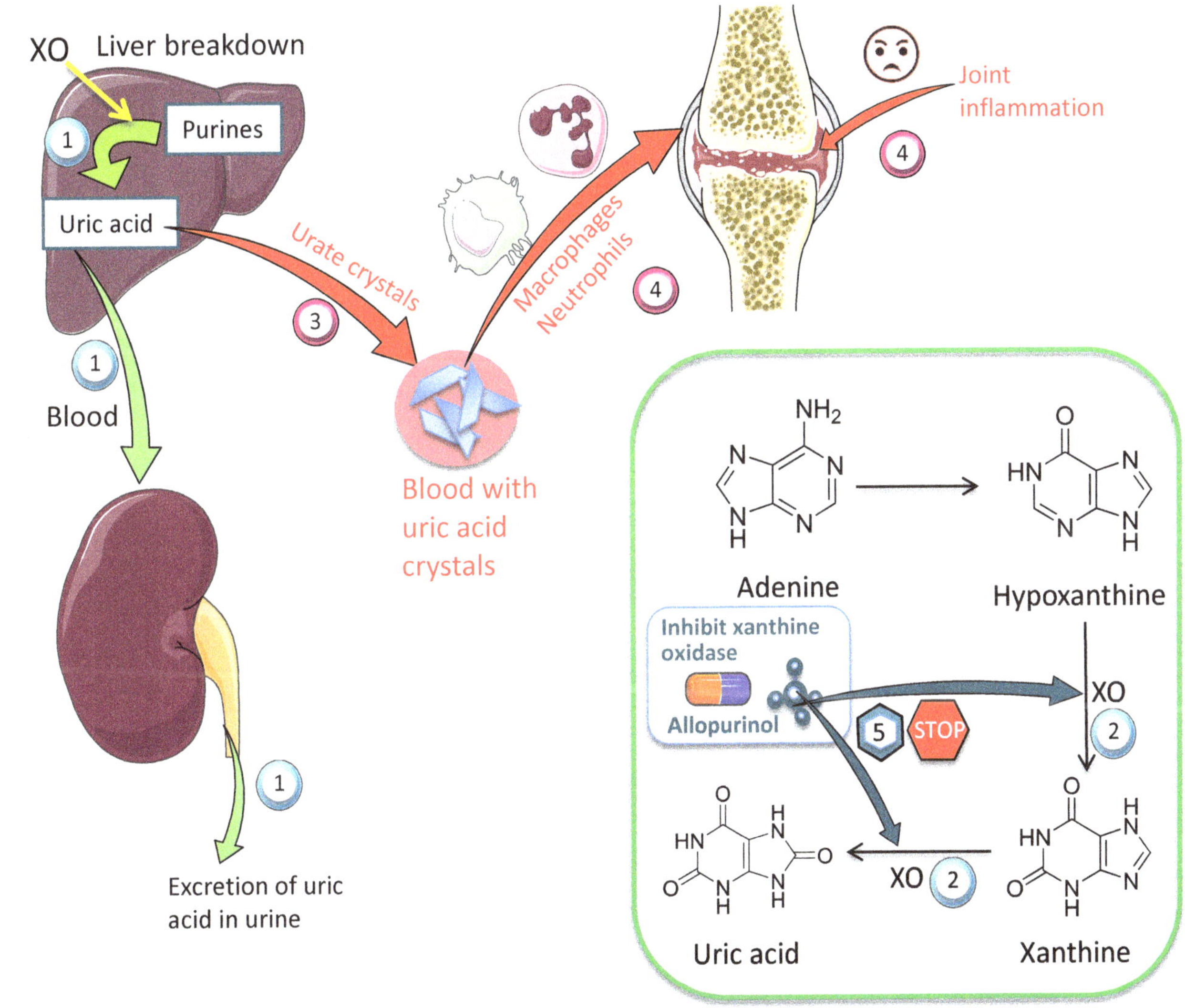

The role of the liver in carbohydrate metabolism

The liver plays a central role in balancing uptake and storage of glucose to regulate the body's energy needs.

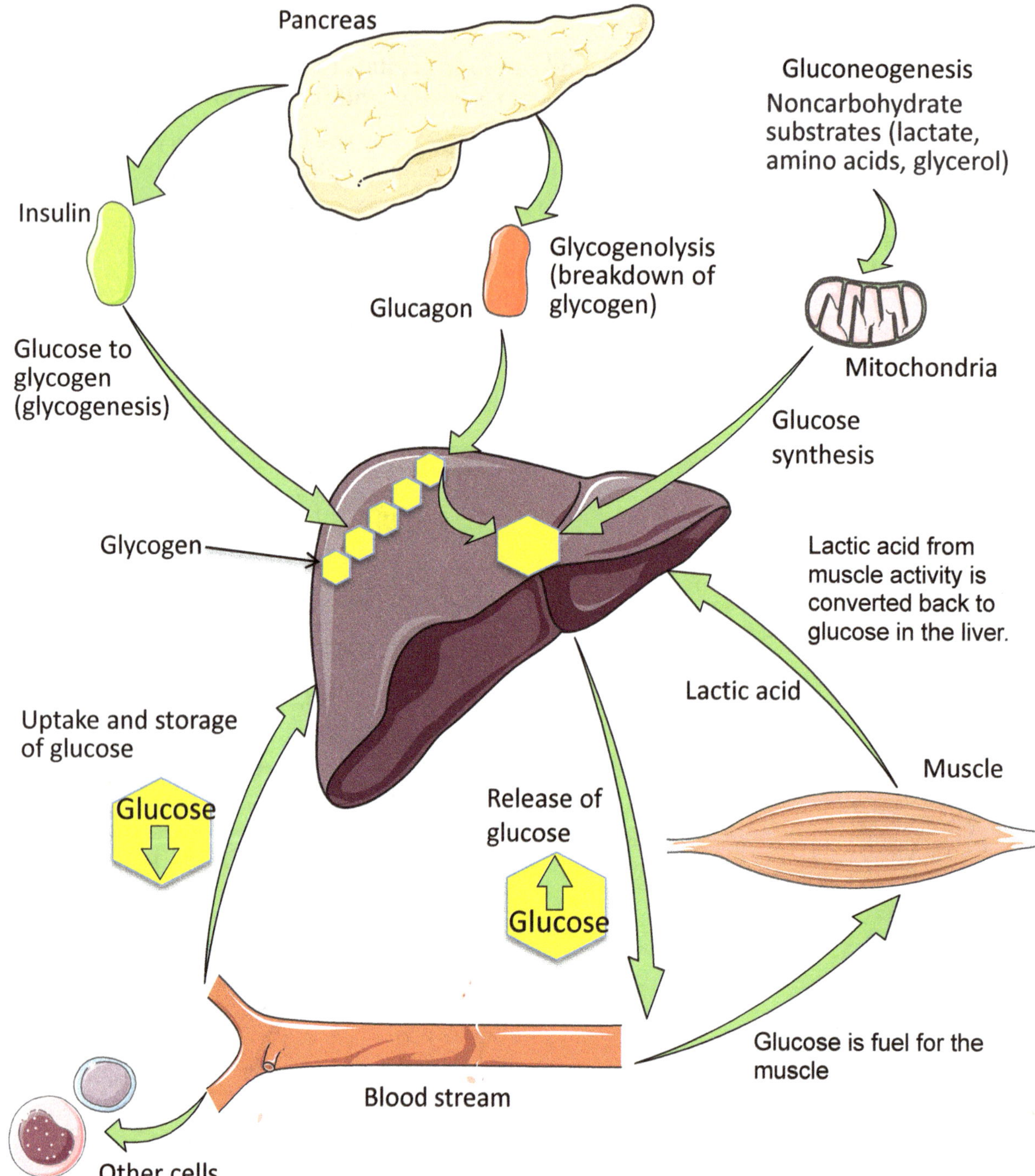

Lipid Metabolism in the liver

1. The major site for converting **excess carbohydrates, lipids, and proteins into fatty acids** and triglyceride, which are then exported and stored in adipose tissue.
2. **Triglycerides** are oxidized to produce **ketone bodies** (water-soluble molecules with ketone groups, e.g., acetoacetate), which are exported in large quantities into blood to be metabolized by other tissues.
3. **Lipoproteins** contain synthesized fatty acids, triglycerides, and cholesterol and are transported to the rest of the body.
4. Excess cholesterol and phospholipids are **excreted in bile** as cholesterol or bile acids.

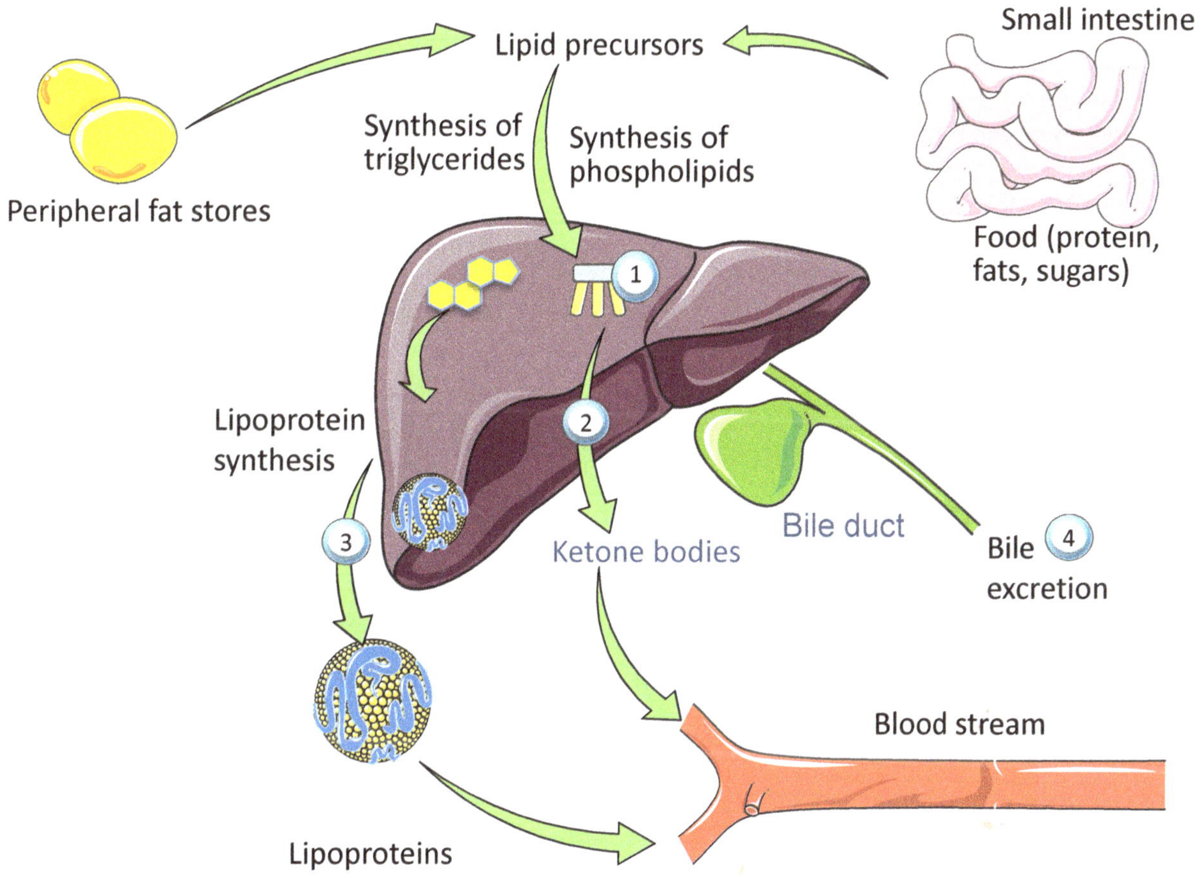

The disease: Type 2 diabetes

Type 2 diabetes (T2D) is characterized by **persistent hyperglycemia** as a result of β cell dysfunction coupled with **insulin resistance**.

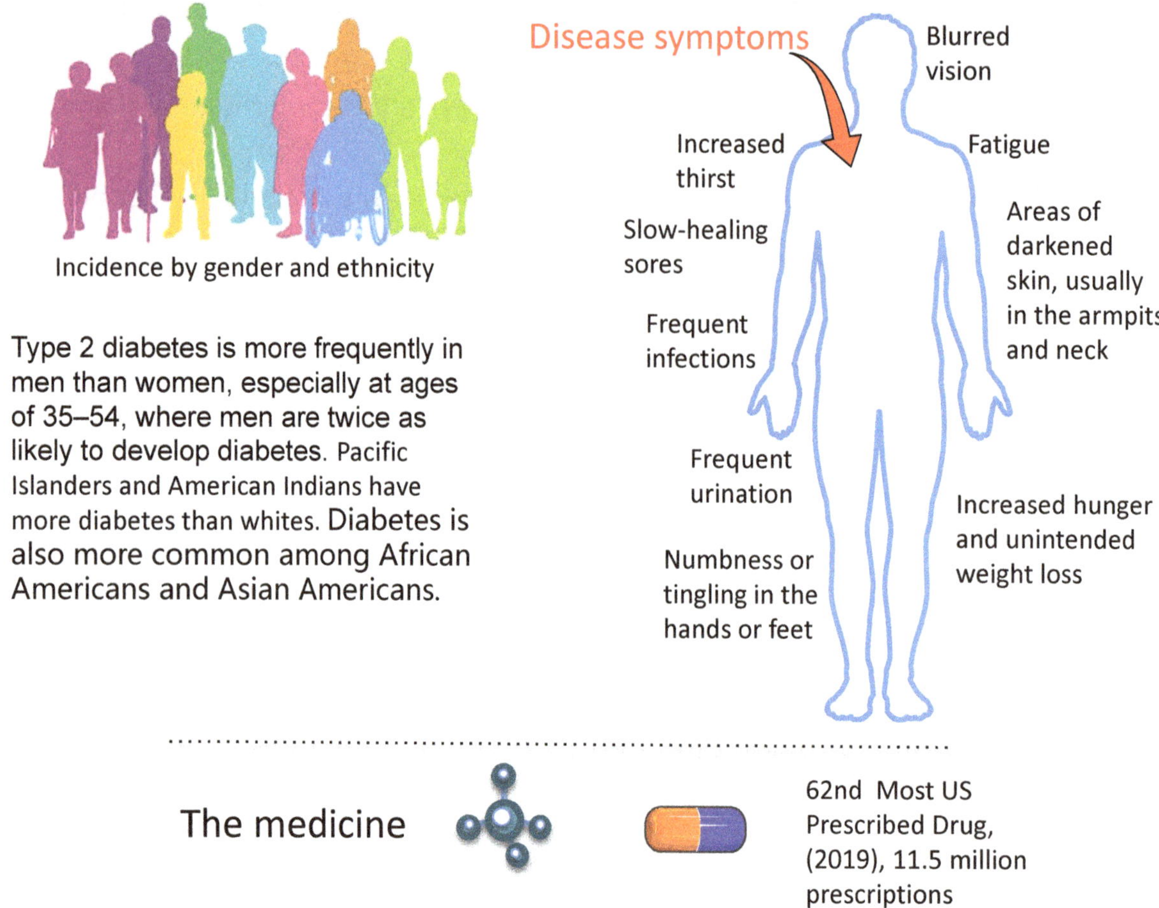

Incidence by gender and ethnicity

Type 2 diabetes is more frequently in men than women, especially at ages of 35–54, where men are twice as likely to develop diabetes. Pacific Islanders and American Indians have more diabetes than whites. Diabetes is also more common among African Americans and Asian Americans.

The medicine

62nd Most US Prescribed Drug, (2019), 11.5 million prescriptions

Glimepiride; Amaryl, FDA Approval 1995

Glimepiride improves glycemic control with type 2 diabetes and reduces the risk of cardiovascular death. **Glimepiride binds to sulfonylurea receptors (SUR-1)** on functioning pancreatic beta cells to acutely lower plasma glucose by stimulating the release of insulin.

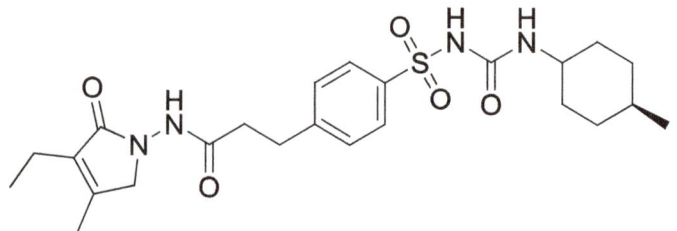

Carbohydrate metabolism: Type 2 diabetes, Glimepiride

Action of Glimepiride on cell and disease biology

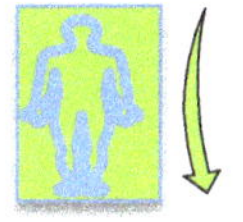

1. **Glucose transporter 2 (GLUT2)** is the primary glucose sensor and transporter in pancreatic beta cells.
2. The pancreatic **β-cell ATP channel** is composed of two subunits (channel and sulfonylurea receptor, SUR1) to link ATP generation to insulin secretion. When **ATP channels are open, insulin secretion is suppressed.**
3. **Closure of the ATP channel** results in membrane depolarization, voltage-dependent Ca^{2+} entry with a **rise in cytosolic Ca^{2+}**, which results in transport of secretory granules of insulin to the cell surface and **insulin secretion**.

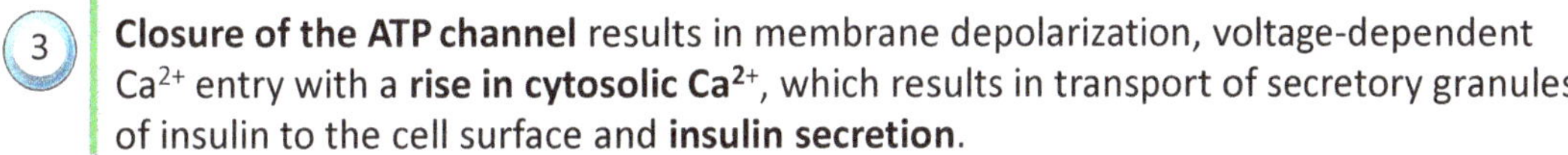

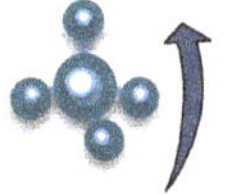

4. **Glimepiride** promotes insulin secretion by binding to the **regulatory sulfonylurea receptor-1 (SUR1) subunit** and **closes the ATP channels** with membrane depolarization.

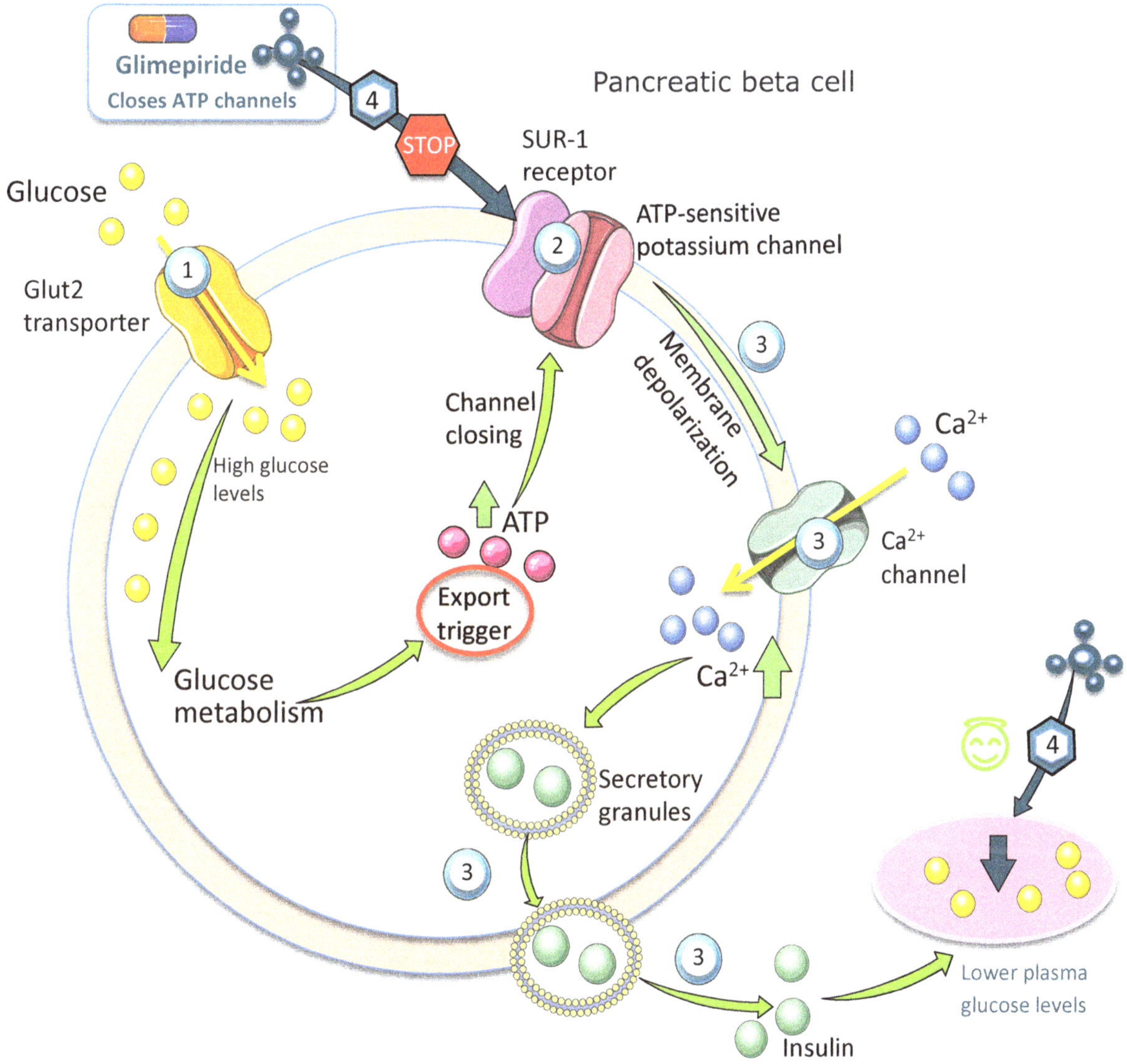

Cholesterol biosynthesis

Acetyl-CoA

↓

Acetoacetyl-CoA

↓

Hydroxymethylglutaryl (HMG)-CoA

HMGCR ↓

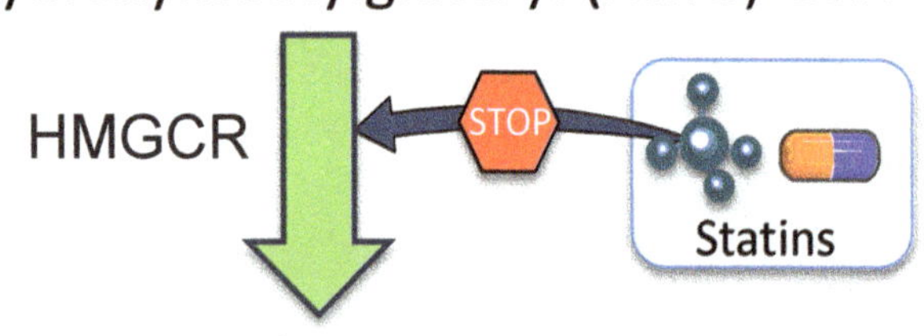

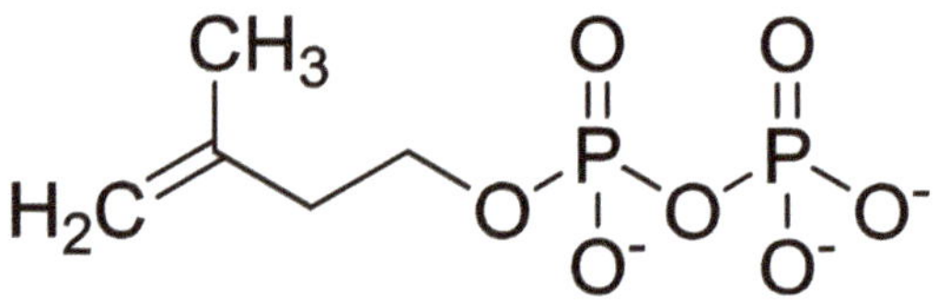

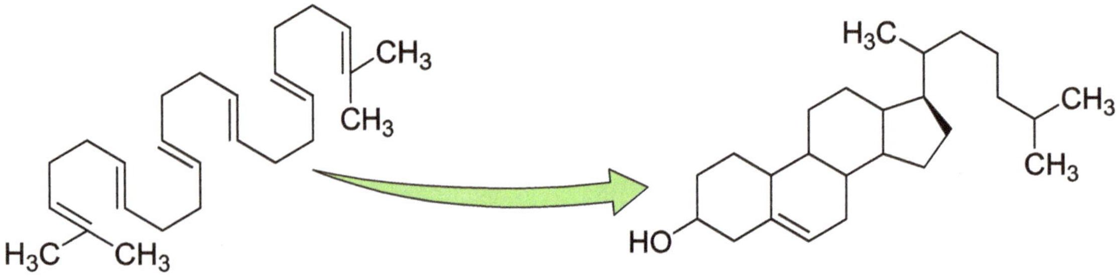

Mevalonate

Several steps ↓

Isopentenyl pyrophosphate (IPP)

Several steps ↓ Condense 6 molecules IPP

Cholesterol levels in the body come from either **dietary intake or biosynthesis**. In healthy adults, cholesterol is synthesized in the liver and intestine, producing ~80% of the total daily cholesterol requirement (~1 g).

HMG-CoA Reductase (HMGCR) is the **rate-controlling** enzyme of the metabolic pathway responsible for **cholesterol biosynthesis**.

Squalene

Cholesterol

Molecules of life: Cholesterol biosynthesis

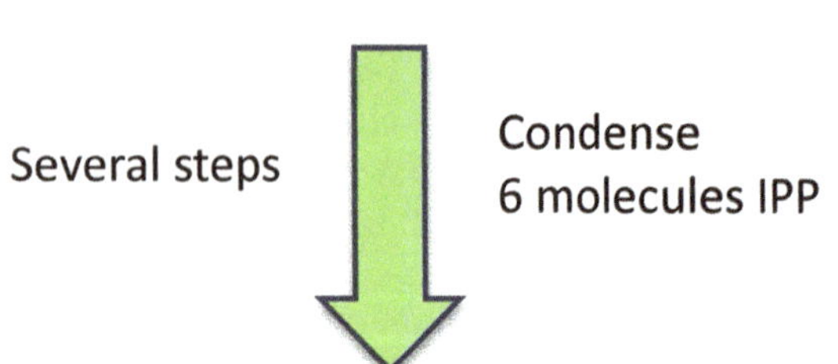

LDL and HDL and cholesterol metabolism

There are four major classes of circulating lipoproteins (**chylomicrons**, **very low-density lipoproteins** [**VLDL**], **low-density lipoproteins** [**LDL**], and **high-density lipoproteins** [**HDL**]), which transport hydrophobic lipid molecules in the blood or extracellular fluid.
LDL particle is 50% cholesterol by weight and 25% is protein.
HDL particles consist of 20% cholesterol by weight and 50% protein.

2. **Individuals with familial hypercholesterolemia** have high levels of circulating LDL due to **defective LDL receptors** with lack of clearance of LDL from the circulation.

3. **High levels of LDL cholesterol** greatly increase the risk for **atherosclerosis** because LDL particles contribute to the formation of atherosclerotic plaques.

4. **High levels of HDL cholesterol can be protective** as HDL transports cholesterol from cells back to the liver, which reduces plaque formation.

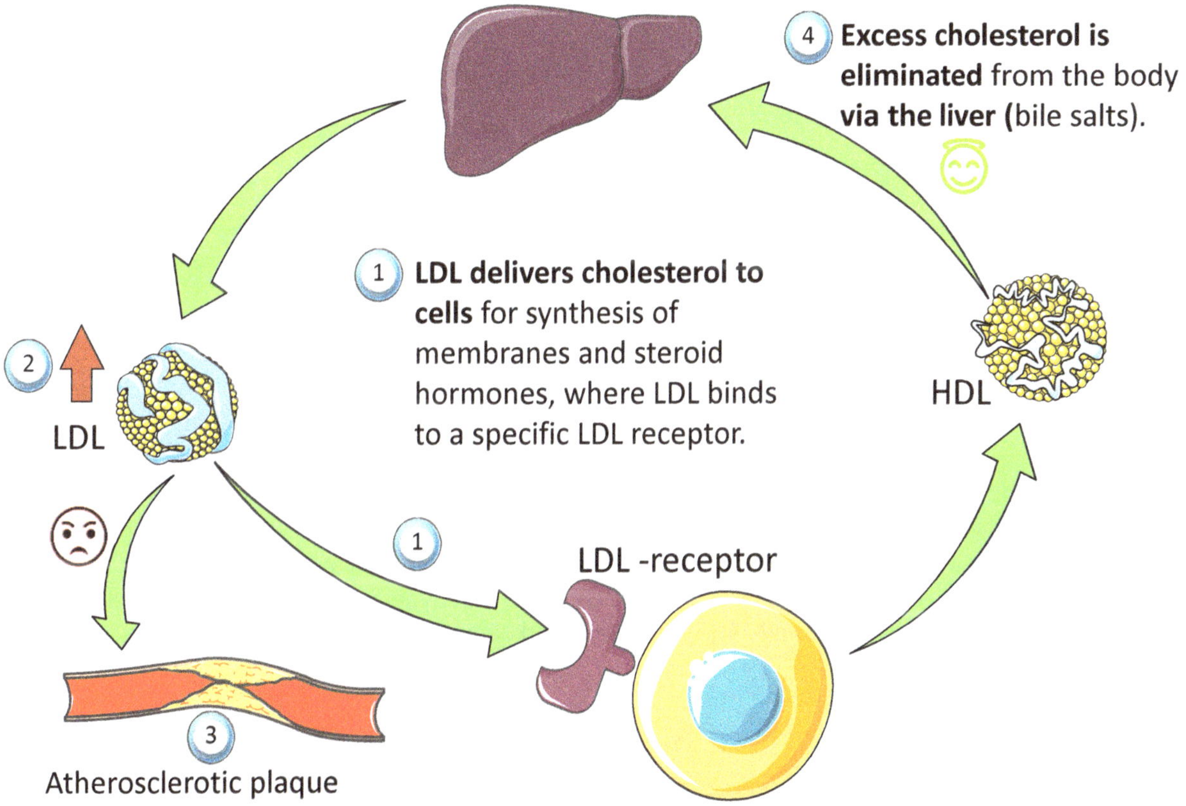

4 Excess cholesterol is eliminated from the body via the liver (bile salts).
1 LDL delivers cholesterol to cells for synthesis of membranes and steroid hormones, where LDL binds to a specific LDL receptor.
2
LDL
HDL
1
LDL -receptor
3
Atherosclerotic plaque

The disease: Heterozygous familial hypercholesterolemia

Heterozygous familial hypercholesterolemia (FH, high levels of LDL cholesterol) are caused by **genetic mutations** or lifestyle factors and can significantly increase the risk of mortality from cardiovascular disease. About 1 in 4 patients with elevated LDL-C are only partially managed by diet and maximum doses of statins and require additional treatment.

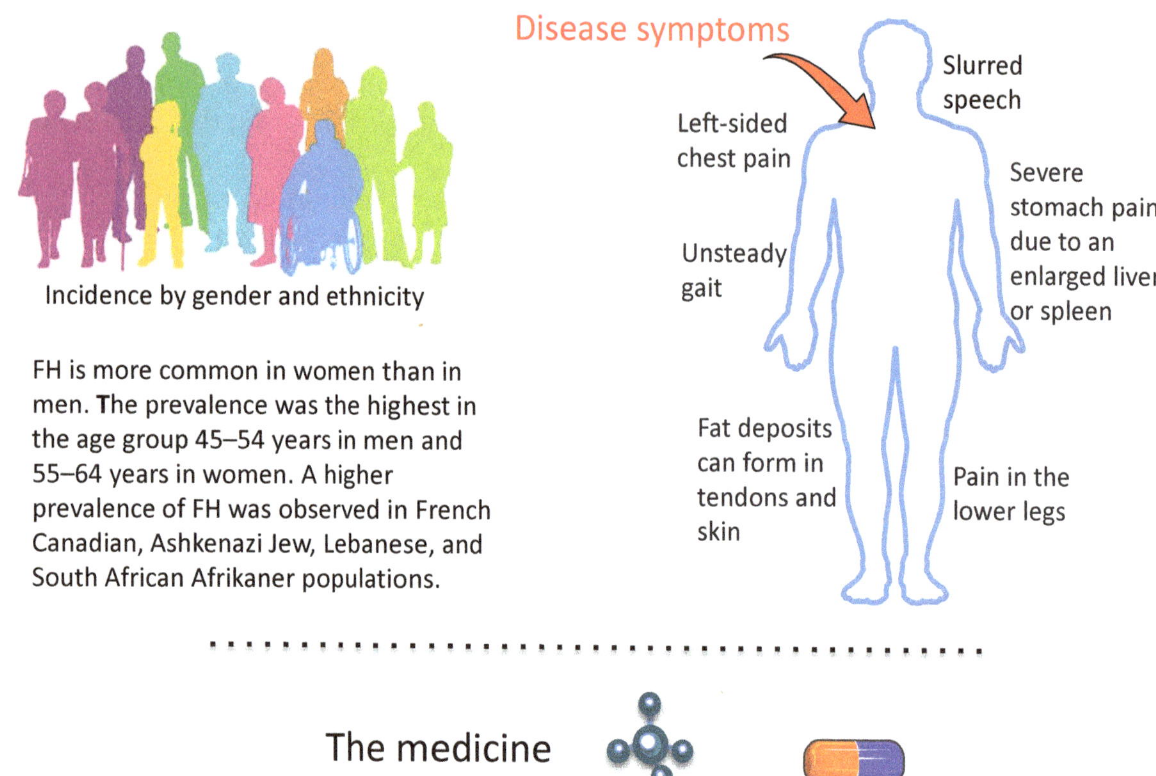

Incidence by gender and ethnicity

FH is more common in women than in men. The prevalence was the highest in the age group 45–54 years in men and 55–64 years in women. A higher prevalence of FH was observed in French Canadian, Ashkenazi Jew, Lebanese, and South African Afrikaner populations.

The medicine

Bempedoic acid ; Nexletol, FDA Approval 2020

Bempedoic acid is for the treatment of hypercholesterolemia in adults with heterozygous familial hypercholesterolemia, or with established atherosclerotic cardiovascular disease. The prodrug bempedoic acid is activated enzymatically to **inhibit** the **cytoplasmic enzyme ATP citrate lyase** (ACLY). Nexletol significantly lowers elevated levels of LDL cholesterol in hypercholesterolemic patients by 30% as a single therapy and an additional 24% when combined with statin therapy.

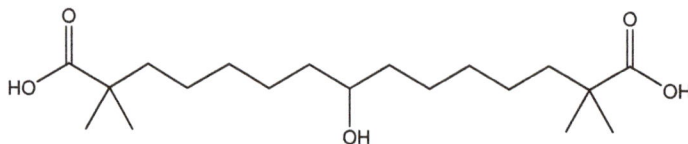

Cholesterol metabolism: Hypercholesterolemia, Bempedoic acid

Action of Bempedoic acid on cell and disease biology

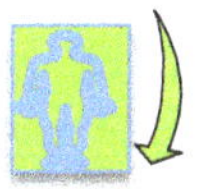

1 **Acetyl-CoA** in the cytosol is required for **cholesterol synthesis.**

2 Bempedoic acid (BemA) is **activated** to BemA-CoA in the liver by **addition of coenzyme A** (CoA).

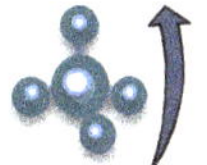

3 BemA **inhibits ATP citrate lyase** (ACLY) and cholesterol synthesis.

4 Bempedoic acid treatment **increases amount of the LDL receptor** and LDL uptake, with clearance of cholesterol in the liver as bile salts and a resulting decrease in levels of circulating LDL cholesterol.

2 Activation of bempedoic acid (BemA)

BemA + CoA + ATP → BemA-CoA (Very long-chain acyl-CoA synthetase)

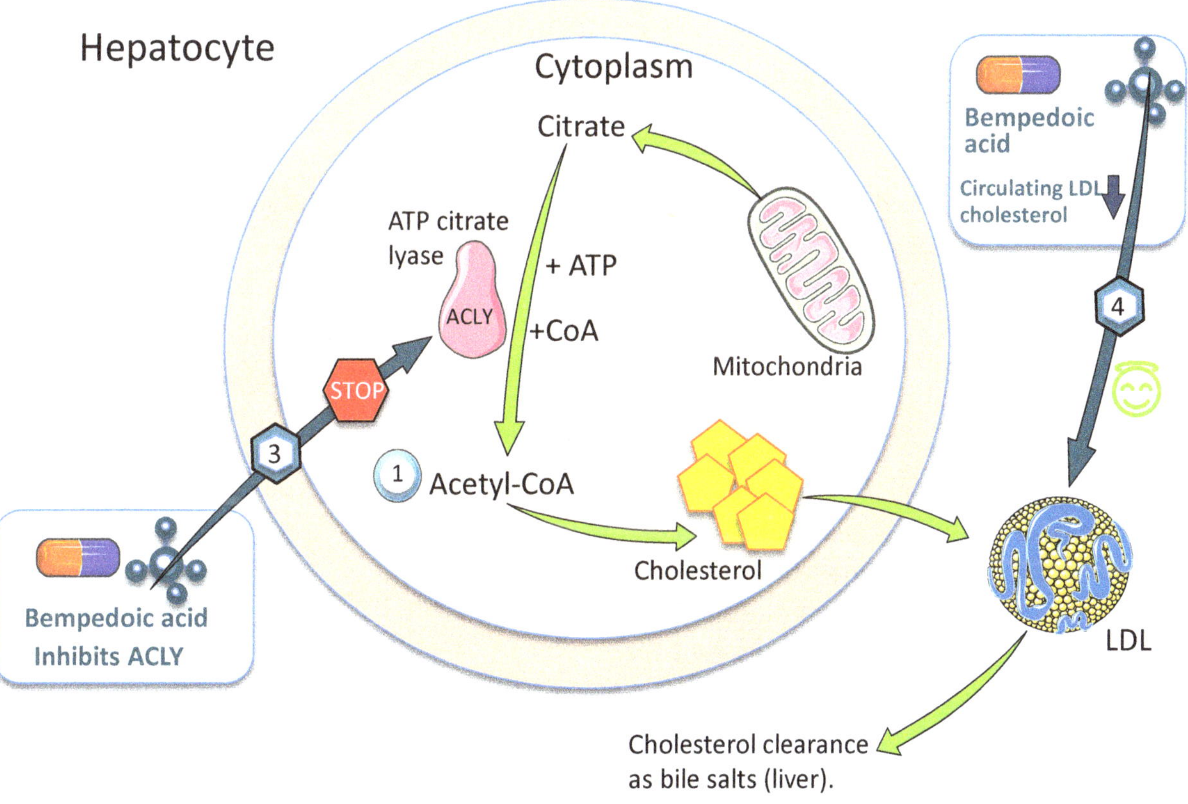

Cholesterol metabolism: Hypercholesterolemia, Bempedoic acid

The disease: Hypercholesterolemia

High cholesterol levels in the blood with increased risk of stroke, heart attack, or other heart complications especially in people with type 2 diabetes and coronary heart disease.

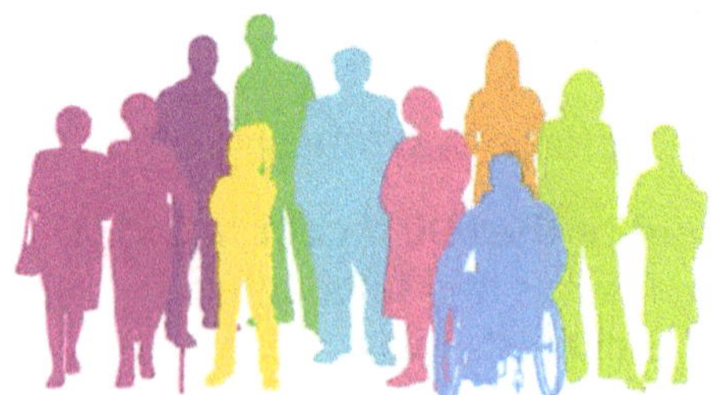

Incidence by gender and ethnicity

Western European countries have the highest and African countries have the lowest LDL cholesterol levels. In the United States, non-Hispanic white men have an incidence of high LDL cholesterol levels at 29.4%, non-Hispanic Black men at 30.7%, and Mexican American men at 38.8%. LDL was increased among Asian Americans compared with non-Hispanic whites. Non-Hispanic white and Mexican American women have rates of 32%, whereas LDL is higher in non-Hispanic Black women at 33.6%.

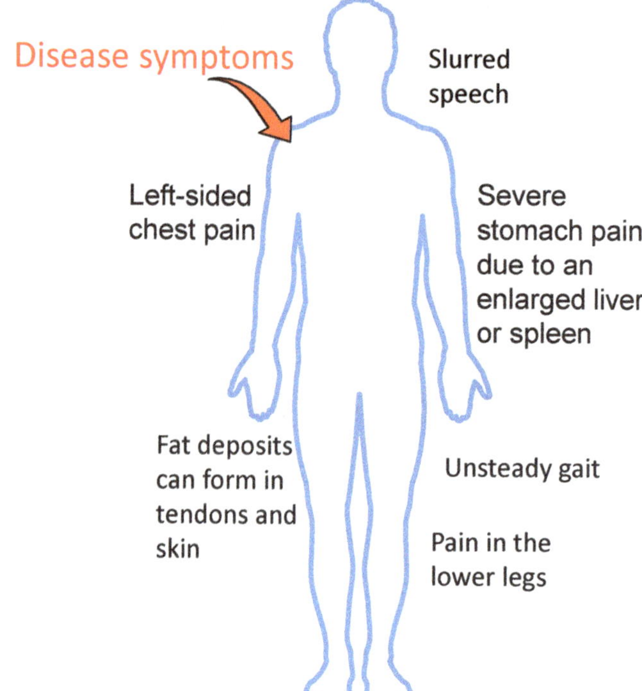

The medicine

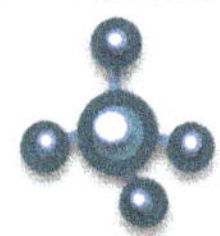

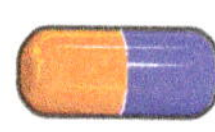

Atorvastatin; Lipitor, FDA Approval 1996

First Most US Prescribed Drug, (2019), 112 million prescriptions

Atorvastatin is used to reduce the risk of heart attack in people who have heart disease. Atorvastatin **blocks the synthesis of cholesterol** with lowering of plasma cholesterol and triglycerides levels and increasing the amount of high-density lipoprotein (HDL) cholesterol.

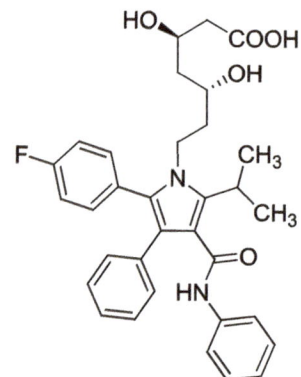

Cholesterol metabolism: Hypercholesterolemia, Atorvastatin

Action of Atorvastatin on the cell and disease biology

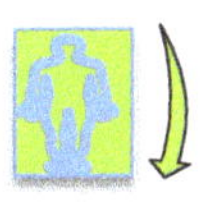

1 **LDL complex** consists mainly of cholesterol and is the vehicle for **delivering cholesterol** via the blood to body tissues.

2 In the early stages of atherosclerosis, **LDL that has entered the artery wall** attracts and is **engulfed by macrophages** that ingest LDL particles.

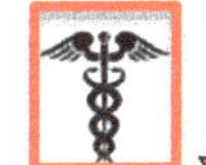

3 **LDL-laden macrophages become foam cells** that promote development of atherosclerotic plaques.

4 **Atorvastatin inhibits HMG-CoA (coenzyme A) reductase,** which is the rate-limiting step in cholesterol synthesis in the liver.

5 Molecular features of atorvastatin for recognition by HMG-CoA reductase.

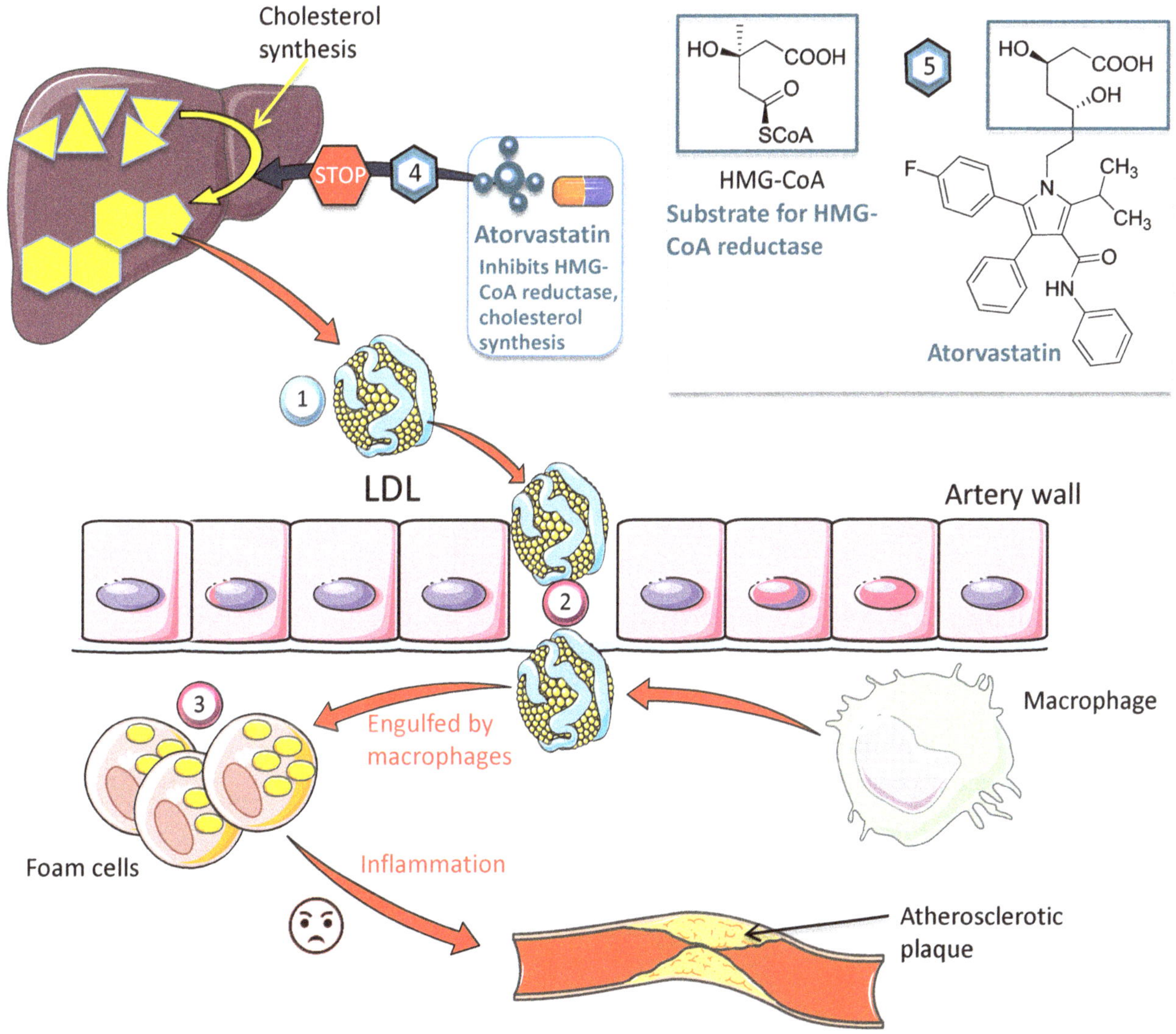

Cholesterol synthesis

STOP

4

Atorvastatin

Inhibits HMG-CoA reductase, cholesterol synthesis

HO COOH O SCoA

HMG-CoA

Substrate for HMG-CoA reductase

5

HO COOH OH F N CH_3 CH_3 O HN

Atorvastatin

1

LDL

Artery wall

2

3

Engulfed by macrophages

Macrophage

Foam cells

Inflammation

Atherosclerotic plaque

Cholesterol metabolism: Hypercholesterolemia, Atorvastatin

Chronic coronary artery disease

Chronic coronary artery disease occurs with a reduction of blood flow to the heart muscle due to **build-up of cholesterol-containing plaques** (atherosclerosis) in the coronary arteries with symptoms such as angina and shortness of breath with physical activity.

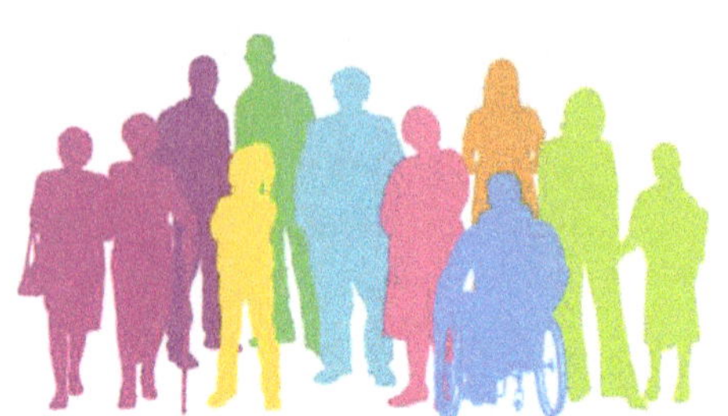

Incidence by gender and ethnicity

White men are about 6 times more likely to die of coronary heart disease than white women and develop disease at a younger age and at a greater rate. CHD prevalence is highest among blacks and Hispanics, and American Indian/Alaskan Natives have lower incidences of CHD. Asians or Pacific Islanders have significantly lower rates.

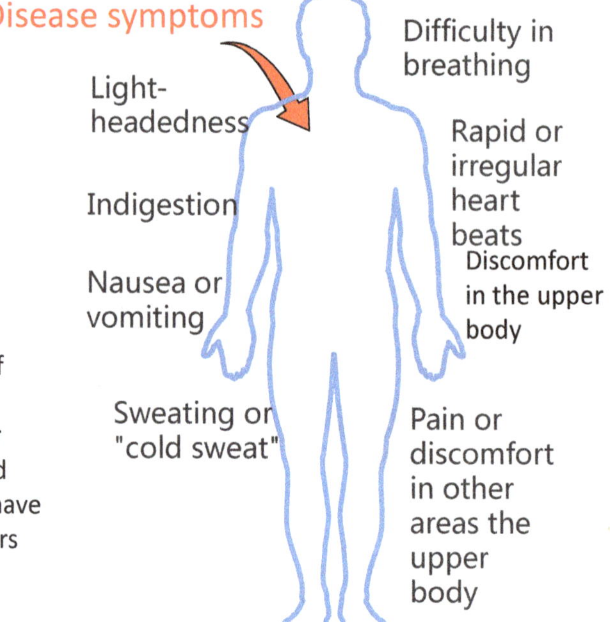

The medicine

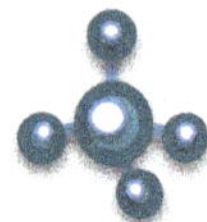

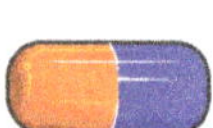

Colchicine; Colcrys, FDA Approval 2009

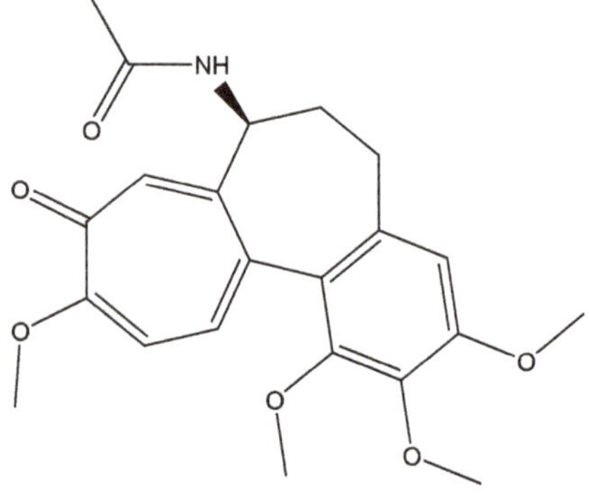

Colchicine is an **anti-inflammatory agent** that is used to reduce myocardial injury in an infarcted area. Colchicine **reduces** elevated levels of **Interleukin 1 beta** (IL-1β) and neutralizes inflammatory activity. Colchicine was approved by the FDA for the treatment of acute gout flares.

Action of Colchicine on cell and disease biology

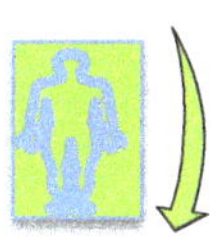

1 **Crystalized cholesterol** is highly immunogenic and activates the macrophage NLRP3 inflammasome, which is is a multimeric protein complex that **triggers** the release of **proinflammatory cytokine IL-1β.**

2 In the **inflammasome complex, the adaptor bridges** between recognition receptors for the **foreign body and enzyme caspase** that produces IL-1β.

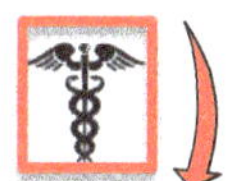

3 **Atherosclerosis** is a chronic inflammatory disease of the arterial wall with formation of **foam cells** (lipid-laden macrophages). **The inflammatory cascade** drives **plaque progression** and instability.

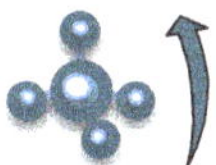

4 **Colchicine inhibits tubulin** polymerization, assembly, and activation of the macrophage NLRP3 inflammasome.

Activated macrophage cell

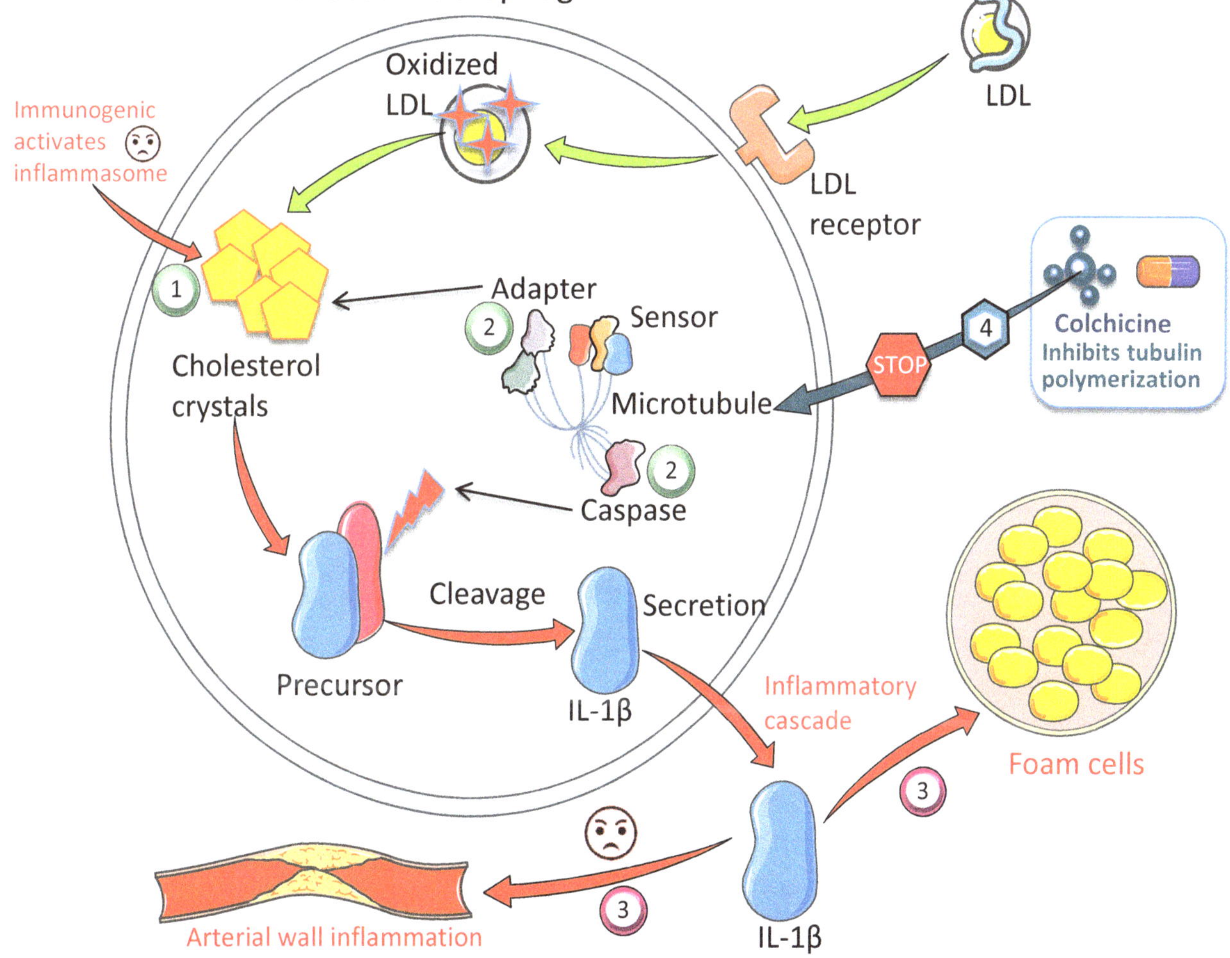

Oxidized LDL
LDL
LDL receptor
Immunogenic activates inflammasome
1
Cholesterol crystals
Adapter
2
Sensor
Microtubule
2
Caspase
Colchicine Inhibits tubulin polymerization
4
STOP
Cleavage
Secretion
Precursor
IL-1β
Inflammatory cascade
Foam cells
3
IL-1β
3
Arterial wall inflammation

Cholesterol metabolism: Coronary artery disease, Colchicine

Chapter 3 The body's protective systems and related diseases

How the body fights the hostile external environment through the protective systems of eyes, mouth, lungs, skin, the immune system, and related medicines.

The parts of the body's protective systems
The innate and adaptive immune system
Diseases of the eye and medicines
A medicine for lung cancer
Skin diseases and medicines
Blood cell disorders and medicines

Selected medicines approved by the FDA for the treatment of these diseases.
✓ = Drugs approved recently (2017–2020) (Brand name)

Eye diseases

- **Wet macular degeneration** (Beovu ✔)
- **Thyroid eye disease** (Tepezza ✔)
- **Neurotropic keratitis** (Oxervate ✔)
- **Optica spectrum disorder** (Enspryng ✔)

Lung disease

- **Nonsmall cell lung cancer** (Lorbrena ✔)

Skin diseases

- **Epithelioid sarcoma** (Tazverik ✔)
- **Psoriasis** (Skyrizi ✔)
- **Acne vulgaris (** Aklief ✔)
- **Erythropoietic protoporphyria** (Scenesse ✔)

Blood cells and related diseases

- **Platelet disorders** (Cablivi ✔, Mulpleta ✔, Doptelet ✔)
- **White blood cell disorders** (Oncovin, Polivy ✔, Xpovio ✔)

Overview

The survival of life in a hostile environment includes the hazards of intaking essential nutrients of oxygen, water, and food. Food provides the building blocks for the essential molecules of the body and energy needed for the required processes of biosynthesis, catabolism, movement, and transport within the body. The organs involved in nutrient intake and their primary defense systems are shown in the introduction. Although the impact of viruses on the lung and the defensive systems are listed here, the biology of viruses as well as related diseases and medicines are described in detail in Chapter 7. However, this chapter does list examples of standard and newly developed medicines to treat the diseases of the eye, lung, skin, and blood cells.

Diseases of the body's protective systems: Overview

The overlying mucus layer of the cornea consists of mucin (large heavily glycosylated proteins) to **create a physical barrier** against microbial invasion.

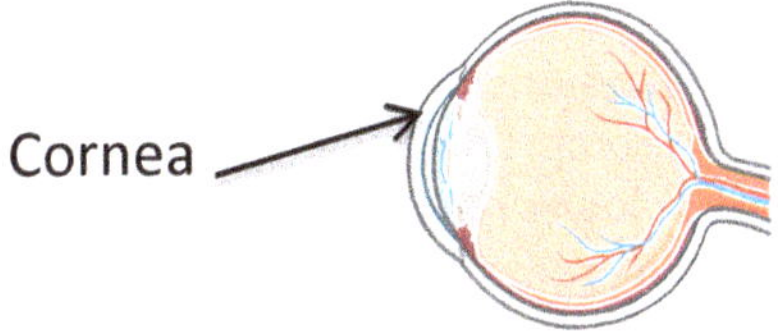

If a microbe penetrates the protective mucin layer a series of successive antimicrobial defenses can be recruited, antimicrobial peptides, e.g., β-defensin and enzymes (lysozyme).

Salivary defense proteins such as lysozyme, amylase, defensins, proline-rich proteins, and mucins generate innate immunity.

Removal of microorganisms by passage of air over **cilia in nasopharynx.** (1)

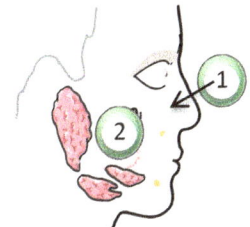

Salivary secretory immunoglobulins, heat shock proteins for **innate, and acquired immunity**.

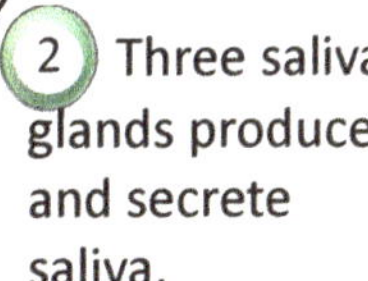

Saliva provides an immune defense of the oral and upper gastrointestinal mucosal surfaces.

(2) Three saliva glands produce and secrete saliva.

The lungs have their own large and layered antimicrobial defense system to protect against inhaled microorganisms.

Hair-like projections (cilia) lining the trachea move microorganisms out of the airway and from the lungs.

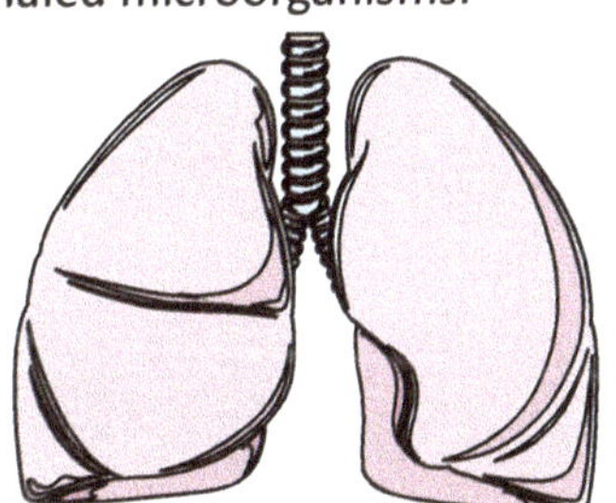

The barrier of the epithelium produces **mucus and surfactant proteins** to sweep away pathogens.

Epithelium releases **antimicrobial peptides** or stimulates cytokine release to maintain sterility of the lungs.

Low pH in stomach inhibits microbial growth.

Rapid pH increase in transition to intestine **blocks pathogen growth.**

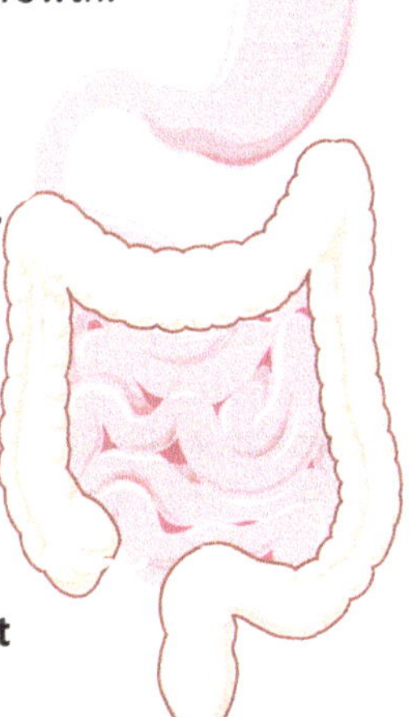

Normal bacterial colonies compete with pathogens for attachment sites and nutrients.

Flushing the urinary tract prevents colonization.

Skin is the largest organ of the body and continuously confronts the external environment.

Skin acts as a physical barrier and produces a number of antimicrobial peptides and **proteins (AMPs)** such as human defensins.

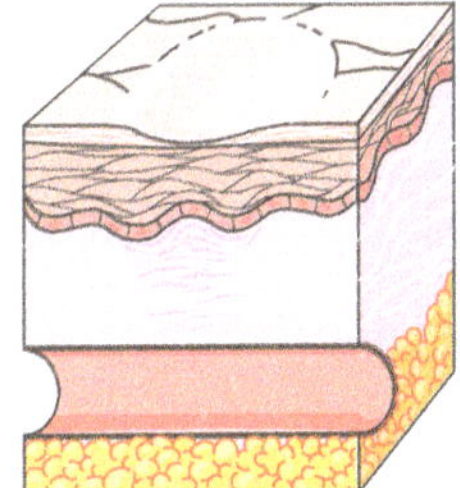

AMPs direct antimicrobial activities against various bacteria, viruses, and fungi and also activate cellular immune responses.

AMPs are mediators of inflammation with effects on epithelial and inflammatory cells, influencing cell proliferation, and **attracting macrophages and neutrophils to the site of infection.**

The parts of the body's protective systems

The lung and viral infections

Viral infections of the lungs represent a significant source of illness experienced by otherwise healthy adults and children. Lower respiratory tract infections and resulting infection-related mortality currently rank seventh among all causes of deaths in the United States.

Influenza virus

- **Types A and B** being clinically relevant for humans.
- Transmitted predominantly by **aerosol infection of mucous membranes** of the mouth, nose, eyelids, windpipe, and lungs.
- Most infections affect the **upper respiratory tract.**
- **Symptoms** include fever, chills, muscle aches, cough, congestion, headaches, and fatigue.

Herpes simplex virus type 1 (HSV-1)

- Transmitted by oral-to-oral contact in sores, saliva, and surfaces in or around the mouth.
- Associated with **pulmonary disease**, mostly in severely immunocompromised patients.
- Virus reaches the **lower respiratory tract** by aspiration and symptoms include, fever, cough, and bronchospasm **pneumonia**.

Coronaviruses

- Spreading via small droplets from coughing, sneezing, or touch.
- Affects the **upper respiratory system** with **flu-like symptoms.**
- Effects the **lower respiratory system** with cough, difficulty breathing.
- Severe cases with **acute respiratory distress syndrome**.

Adenovirus

- Spread through personal contact, droplet particles, or transmission via contaminated surfaces.
- Latent/persistent infection is **associated with chronic obstructive pulmonary disease (COPD)**.
- Infection of the **lower respiratory tract** causes clinical symptoms ranging from mild to acute respiratory disease.

Respiratory syncytial virus (RSV)

- Spread from coughs or sneezes from an infected person and by surface transmission.
- **Inflammation of the small airways** in the lung.
- **Pneumonia** in young children.
- Respiratory illness in older adults.
- Infection can **spread to the lower respiratory tract**, causing inflammation of the small airway passages and pneumonia.

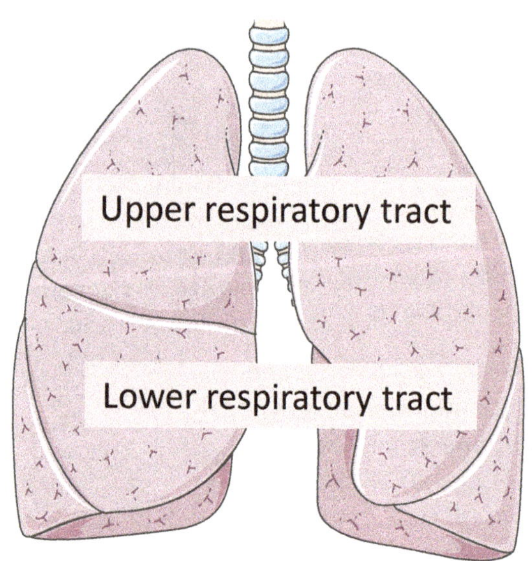

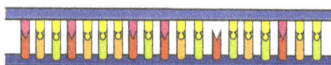

Enveloped viral genomes

- **Influenza** (negative-sense single-strand RNA)
- **Herpes** (double-stranded linear DNA)
- **Adenovirus** (double-stranded linear DNA)
- **Coronavirus** (positive-sense single-strand RNA)
- **RSV** (negative-sense single-strand RNA)

Positive-sense viral RNA can be translated by the host cell, whereas **negative-sense viral RNA** must first be converted to positive-sense RNA (RNA polymerase).

The innate and adaptive immune system

Peripheral blood mononuclear cells (PBMC) consists of any peripheral blood cell having a round nucleus that provide critical components of the **innate and adaptive immune system**, which defends the body against viral, bacterial, and parasitic infection and destroys tumor cells and foreign substances.

Percentage of total PBMC fraction

Innate Immunity (1–12 hours)

- Dendritic cells (1%–2%)
- Neutrophils
- Macrophage
- Natural Killer (NK) cells (5%–10%)
- Natural antibodies
- Complement

Innate lymphoid cells straddle these two arms, respond to infection quickly, and secrete a suite of inflammatory mediators.

Adaptive immunity (1–3 days)

- B lymphocytes (5%–15%)
- Helper and cytotoxic T lymphocytes (45%–70%)
- Cytokines
- High-affinity antibodies

Dendritic cells form an interface between the innate and adaptive immune system and act as sentinels that respond to a range of external cues re the bodily environment and allow the selection of rare, antigen-reactive T cell clones.

NK cells belong to the innate system that plays an important role in the **early phase of immune defense** against microbial infections, and tumor growth and dissemination with a population of highly specialized large **granular lymphocytes** with released cytokines and chemokines.

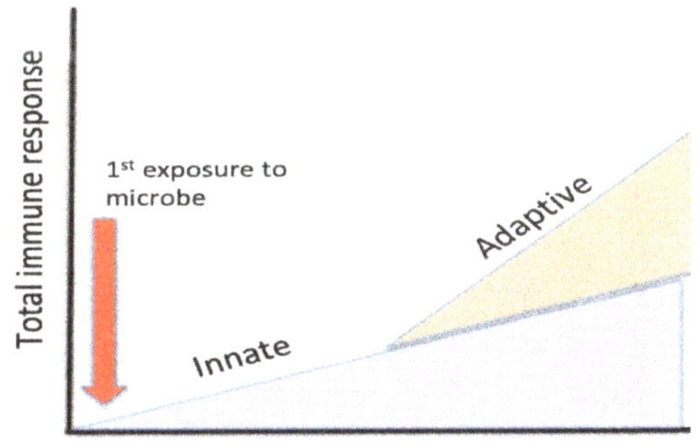

B lymphocytes (CD 19⁺), when activated, differentiates into plasma cells that secrete antibodies that target free antigens, which are specific to a pathogen.

T lymphocytes contain the CD3 (cluster of differentiation 3) receptor, which helps activate both **helper ($CD4^+$) and cytotoxic ($CD8^+$) T cells**

$CD4^+$ T cells have multiple functions: activation of the cells of the innate immune system, e.g., B-lymphocytes, cytotoxic T cells, and cytokine secretion. Also play critical role in the suppression of an uncontrolled immune reaction.

$CD8^+$ cytotoxic cells (or killer T cells) kill infected or malignant cells secretion of cytokines, primarily TNF-α and IFN-γ and cytotoxic granules. $CD8^+$ T cells contribute to excessive immune response (immunopathology).

Peripheral blood cells ⟶ Innate and adaptive immune system

1 Peripheral blood is the flowing, circulating blood of the body, through which the cells are circulated through the body.

Peripheral blood is an important component in the body's overall immunity, which is enhanced by the transport of defense mechanisms to sites of disease or infection.

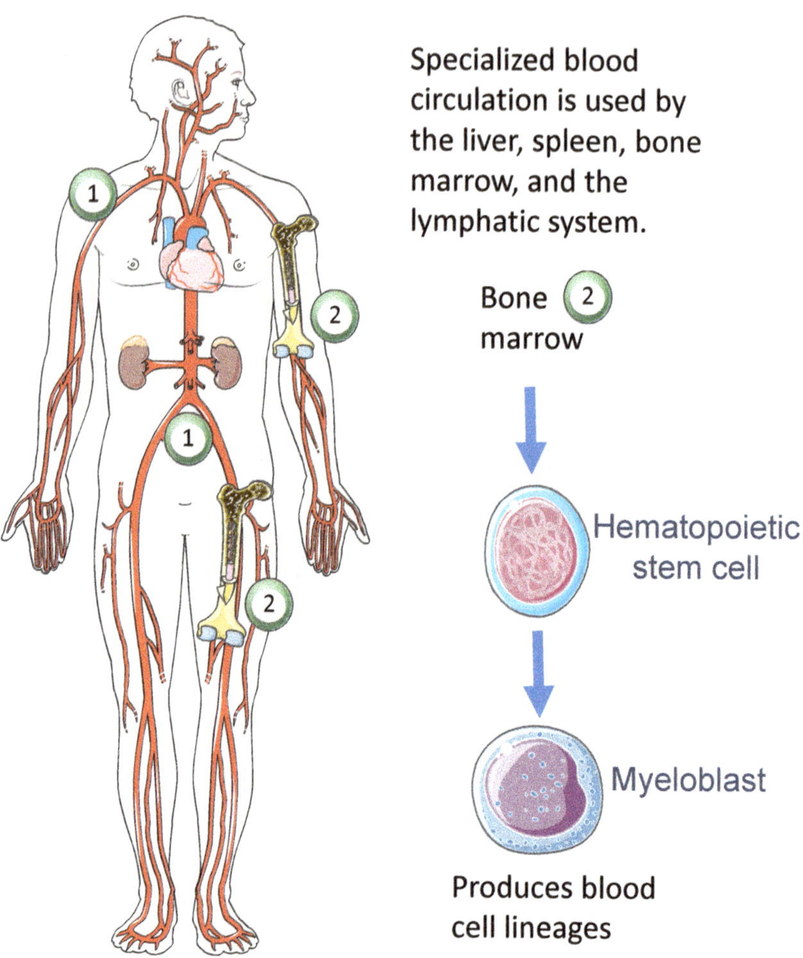

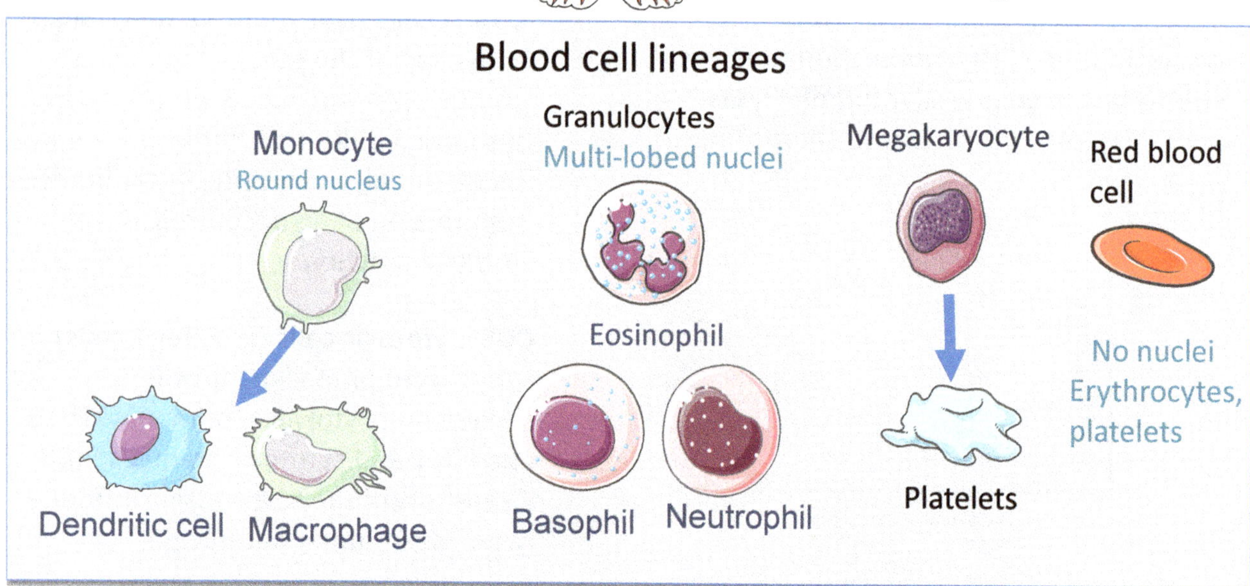

Diseases of the body's protective systems: Blood cell function

Production of plasma cells

A NK cell that has granules (small particles) with enzymes that can kill tumor cells or virally infected cells.

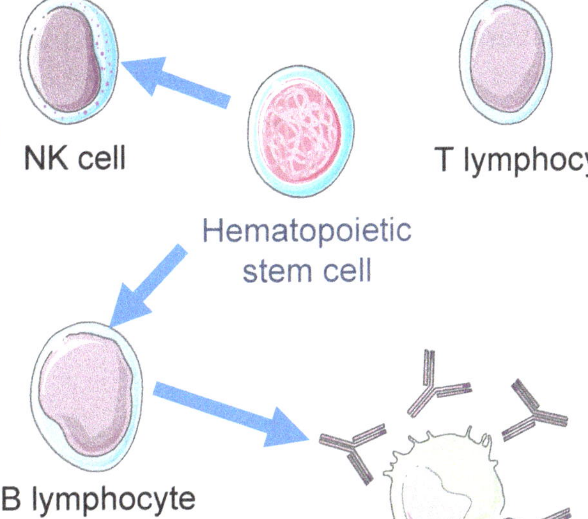

T cells multiply In the thymus and differentiate into helper, regulatory, or cytotoxic T cells or become memory T cells.

Activated B cells can begin secreting antibody as small lymphocytes, but mature to **large plasma cells**.

Every plasma cell divides repeatedly to form a clone that continuously secretes large amounts of only one specific type of antibody.

With the existence of a vast number of B-cell clones, the resulting **antibody repertoire** can respond to the numerous foreign substances to which the body is exposed.

Antibody production continues for several days or months, until the antigen has been overcome. The initial burst of antibody production gradually decreases as the stimulus is removed.

Many plasma cells die after several days, some survive in the bone marrow and lymph nodes, and continue to secrete antibodies into the blood.

The antibodies are transported from the plasma cells by the **blood and the lymphatic system** to the site containing the target antigen **and initiate destruction of the foreign substance.**

Plasma cell disorder

Normally, plasma cells make up less than 1% of the cells in the bone marrow. In multiple myeloma, typically **the majority of bone marrow cells are cancerous plasma cells.**

The overabundance of these cells suppresses the development of other normal bone marrow elements such as white blood cells and platelets.

Thus, people with plasma cell disorders are often at higher risk of infections. The large number of abnormal plasma cells can damage vital organs, especially the kidneys and bones.

The disease is accompanied by production of a large amount of a single type of antibody known as the M-protein at the expense of other types of normal antibodies.

The disease: Wet macular degeneration

Wet macular degeneration is a chronic eye disorder with blurred vision/blind spot and caused by **abnormal blood vessels leaking fluid** or blood into the macula with effects on central vision. Damaged blood vessels can occur in diabetic retinopathy, after eye surgery, age-related degeneration, or inflammatory diseases.

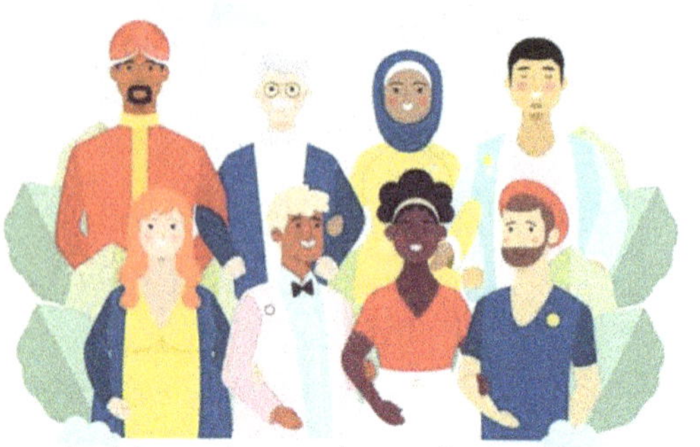

Incidence by gender and ethnicity

Macular degeneration increases with age and affects more than 14% of white Americans age 80 and older (female: male ratio is 2.3:1). Whites have the highest risk, followed by Chinese and Hispanic people and the African Americans with lowest risk. Whites are also more likely to go blind than African Americans.

Disease symptoms

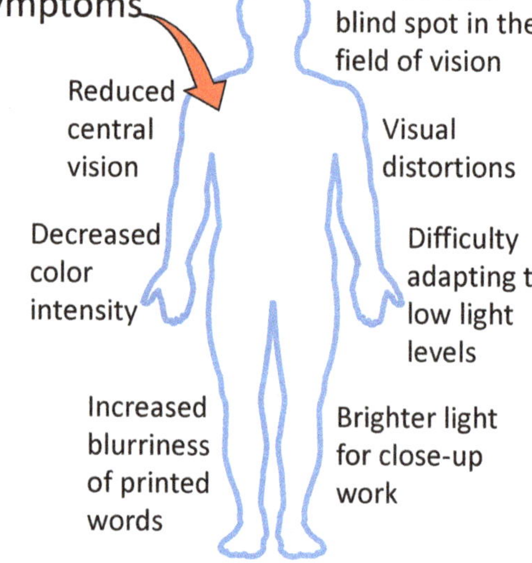

The medicine

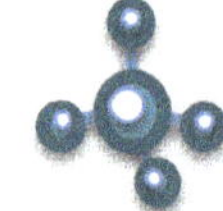

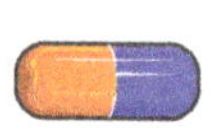

Brolucizumab; Beovu, FDA Approval 2019

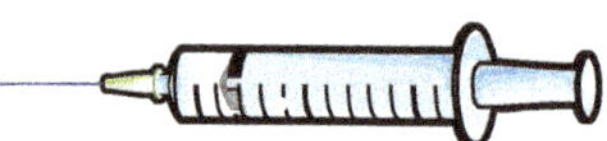

Direct injection into the vitreous humor of the eye (intravitreal).

Brolucizumab is a single-chain antibody fragment (scFv) against vascular endothelial growth factor (VEGF) designed to inhibit the activation of VEGF receptors by blocking interaction of VEGF with the receptor.

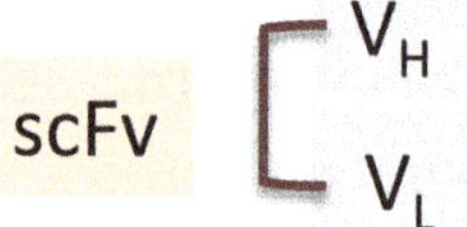

Fusion protein-variable regions of heavy and light antibody chains connected by a peptide.

Action of Brolucizumab on cell and disease biology

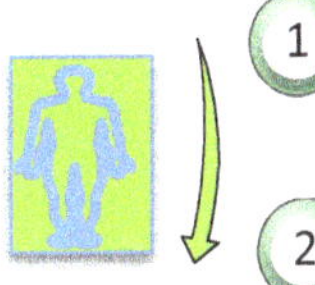
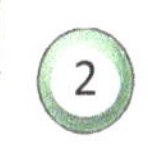

1 **The macula is part of the light-sensitive retina** at the inside back layer of the eye with a **high concentration of photoreceptor cells** and is responsible for sharp, detailed central vision.

2 **Fluid leaking from these abnormal blood vessels disrupts the normal structure of the retina** and ultimately destroys the macula.

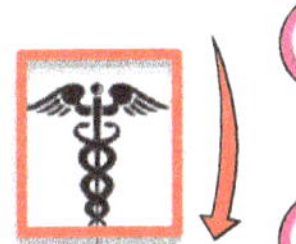
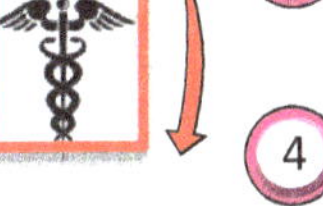

3 **Fluid build up in the macula** with increased leakage from abnormal retinal blood vessel **causes deterioration of the central portion of the retina** and loss of central vision.

4 **Increased signaling through the VEGF pathway** is associated with abnormal formation of new blood vessels, disruption of cell–cell gap junctions, and fluid accumulation in the deep retina that can destroy the macula.

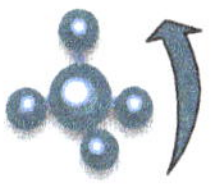

5 **Brolucizumab binds to VEGF,** blocks interaction with VEGF receptors, **suppresses endothelial cell proliferation**, blood vessels formation, and vascular permeability.

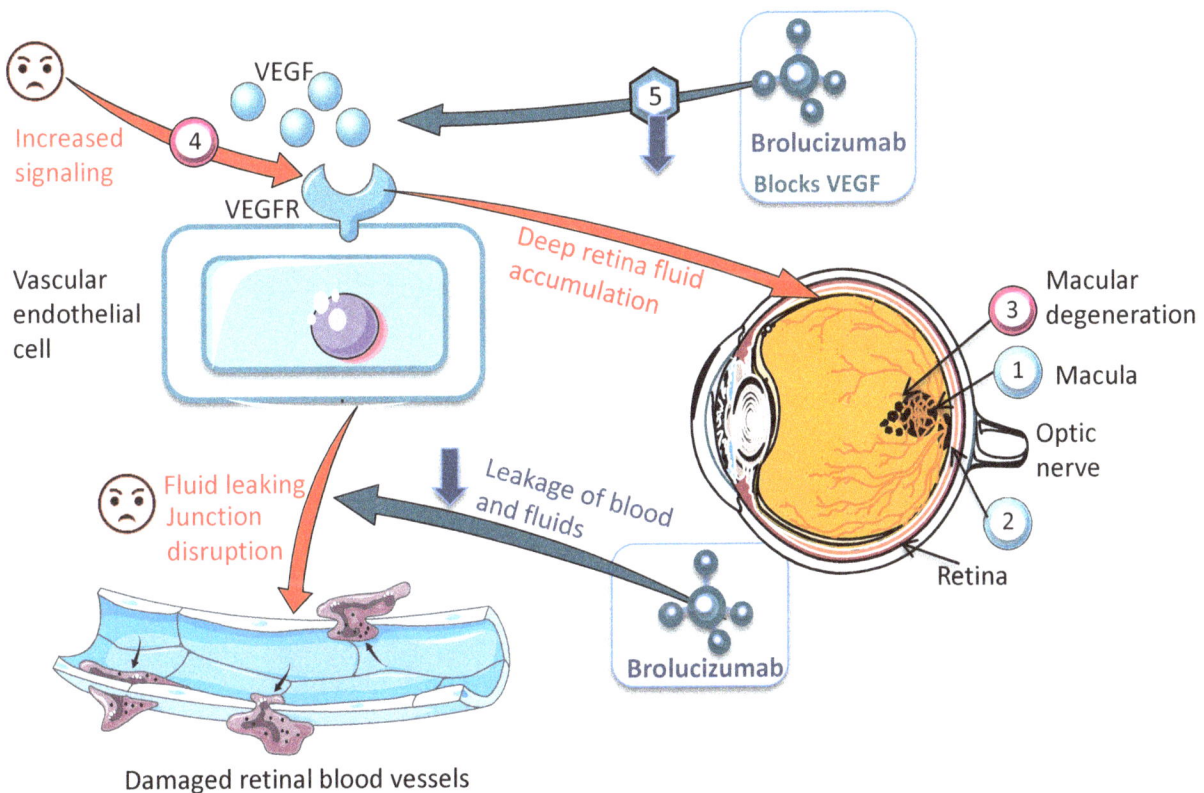

Thyroid eye disease (TED) is a rare condition associated with **Graves' disease** (**autoimmune** hyperthyroidism) with **inflammation** of the orbital tissues, causing eye pain, double vision, and light sensitivity.

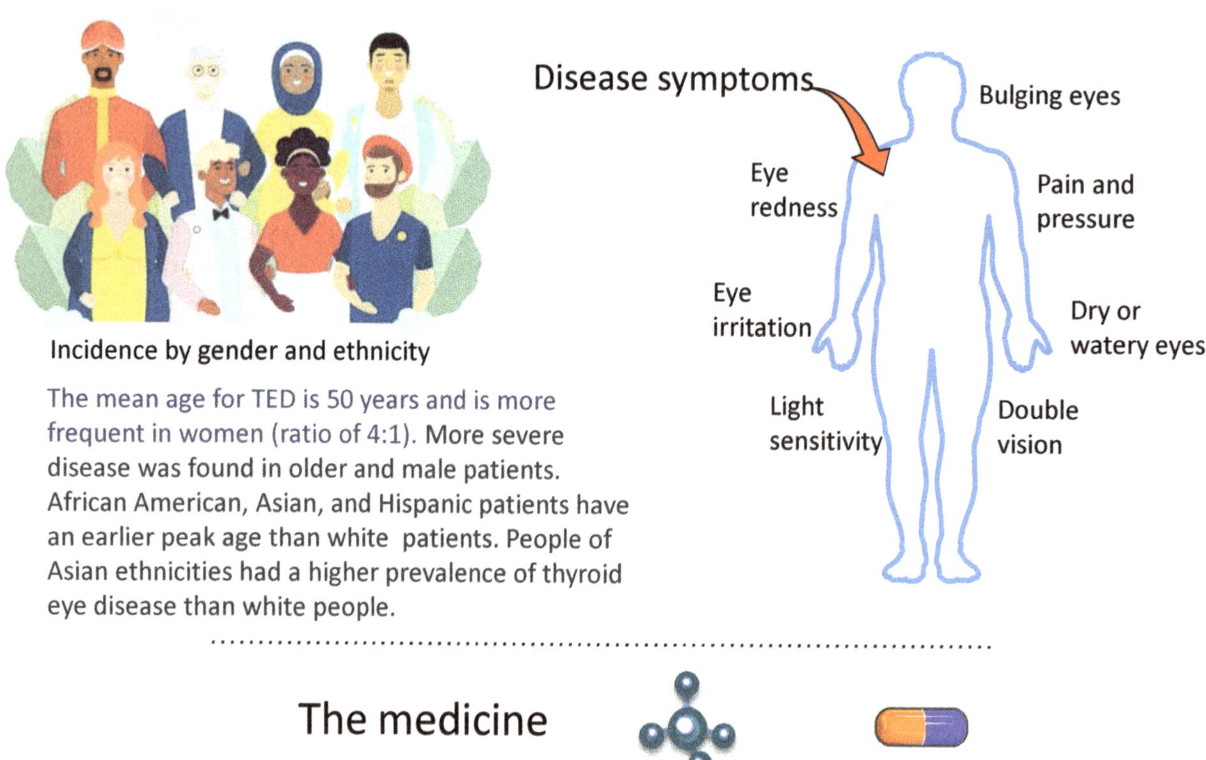

Incidence by gender and ethnicity

The mean age for TED is 50 years and is more frequent in women (ratio of 4:1). More severe disease was found in older and male patients. African American, Asian, and Hispanic patients have an earlier peak age than white patients. People of Asian ethnicities had a higher prevalence of thyroid eye disease than white people.

The medicine

Teprotumumab: Tepezza, FDA Approval 2020

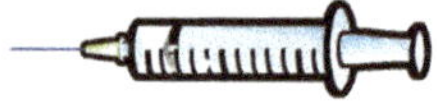

Delivery: 8 intravenous infusions over a period of 24 weeks.

Teprotumumab is a fully humanized monoclonal antibody (mAb), which is a **targeted inhibitor of the insulin-like growth factor-1 receptor** (IGF-1R).

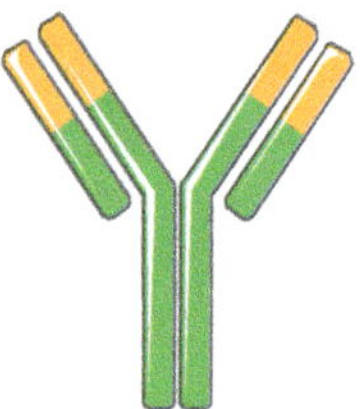

Action of Teprotumumab on cell and disease biology

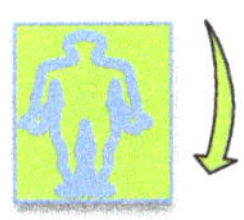

Orbital fibroblasts orchestrate tissue remodeling and recruitment of lymphocytes to sites of inflammation .

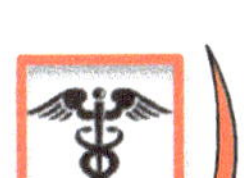

Graves' disease is an autoimmune disorder, **antibodies (TRAb)** binds and chronically **stimulates TSHr** (receptor for thyroid-stimulating hormone).

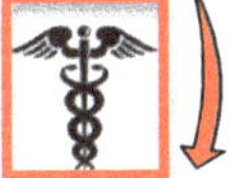

TED fibroblasts have higher **levels of** insulin-like growth factor 1 **(IGF-IR)** than normal fibroblasts.

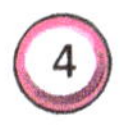
Pathogenic autoantibodies (TRAb) **stimulate the TSHr/IGF-1R complex** in orbital fibroblasts, produce hyaluronic acid, fat, muscle adjacent to the eye.

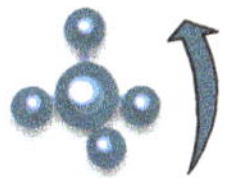

Teprotumumab binds to IGF-1R and inhibits IGF-1 function and blocks downstream TSH-R signaling, reducing pathogenic autoantibody stimulation.

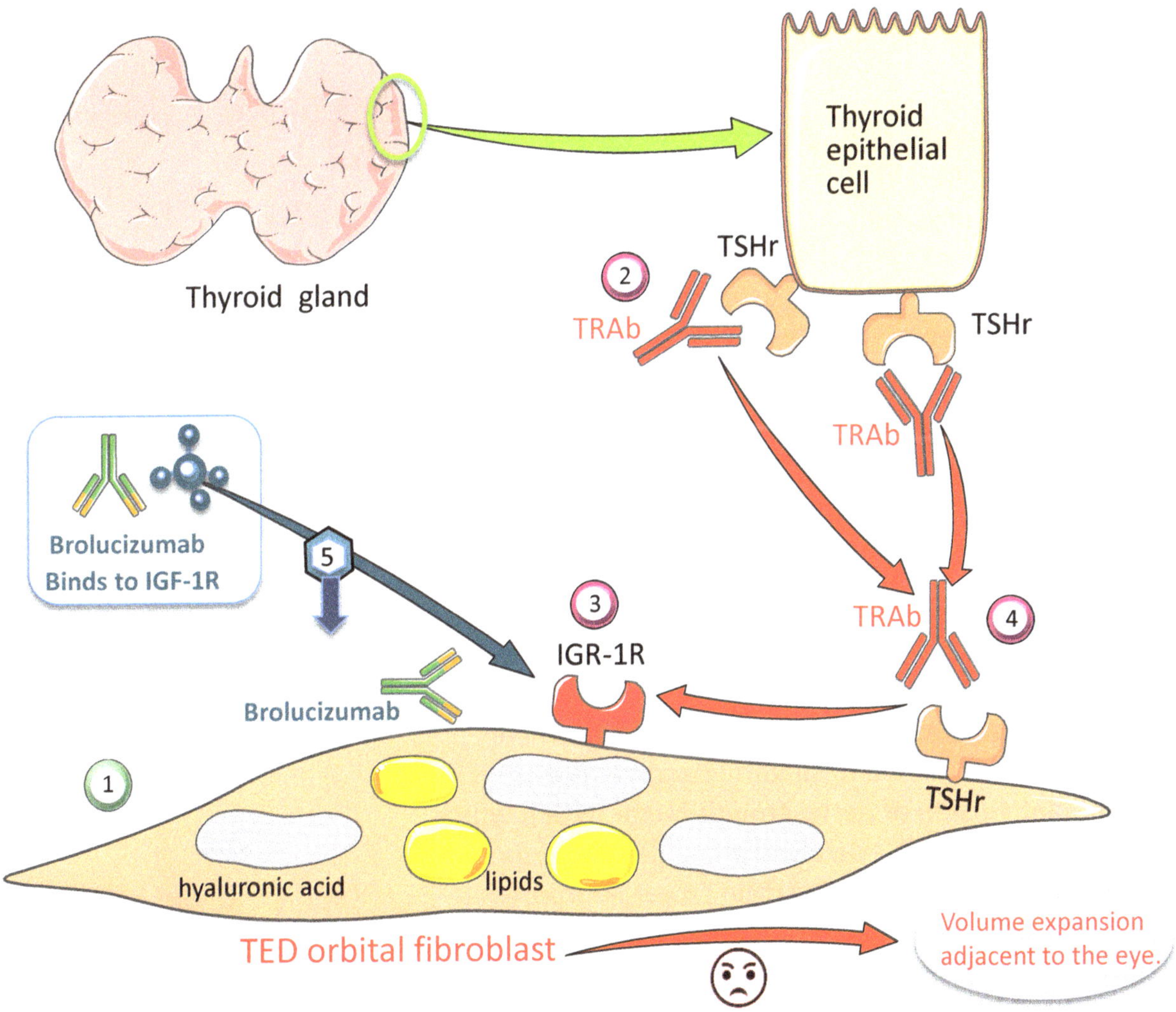

Thyroid gland

Thyroid epithelial cell

TSHr

2

TRAb

TSHr

TRAb

Brolucizumab Binds to IGF-1R

5

3

IGR-1R

TRAb

4

Brolucizumab

1

TSHr

hyaluronic acid

lipids

TED orbital fibroblast

Volume expansion adjacent to the eye.

Diseases of the eye: Thyroid eye disease, Teprotumumab

The disease: Neurotropic keratitis

Neurotropic keratitis is a rare and serious disease and commonly caused by **herpes simplex and zoster viral infections** or systemic conditions like diabetes, multiple sclerosis, and leprosy. It involves a loss of corneal sensation, spontaneous epithelium breakdown, and results in corneal thinning, ulceration, and perforation.

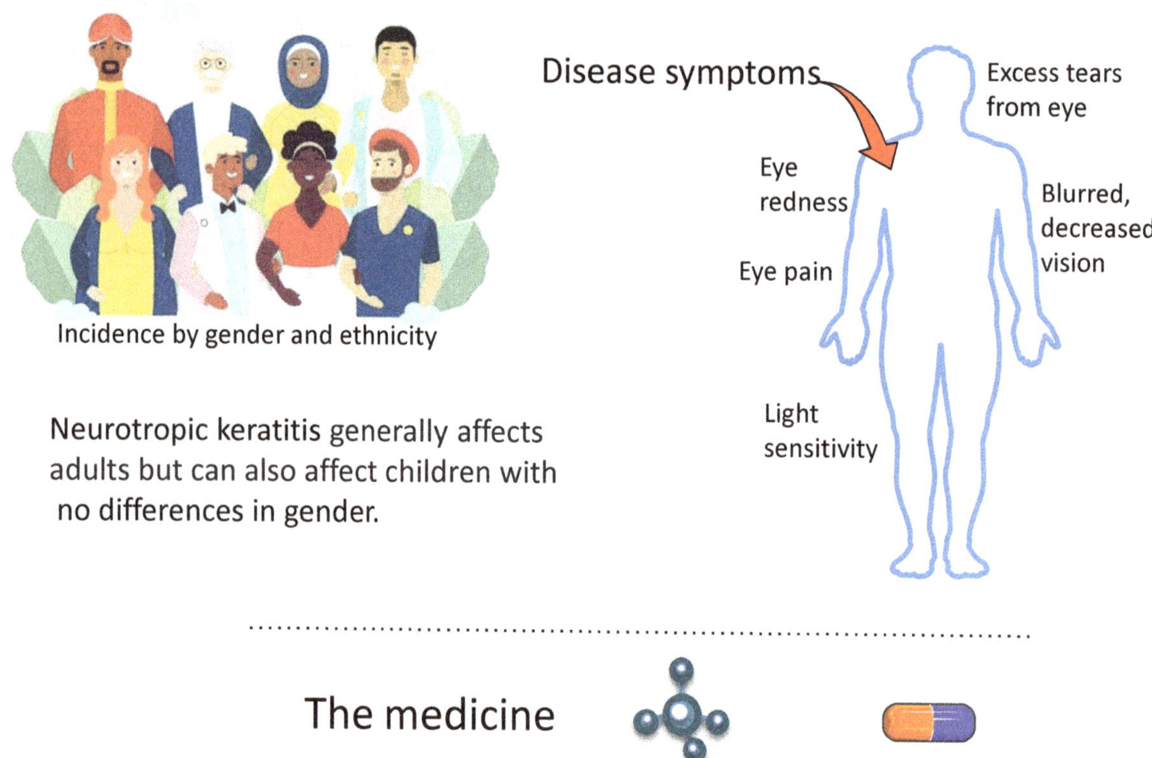

Neurotropic keratitis generally affects adults but can also affect children with no differences in gender.

The medicine

Cenegermin: Oxervate, FDA Approval 2018

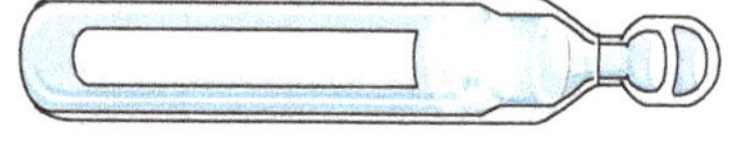

Delivered as eye drops

Cenegermin treats neurotrophic keratitis with corneal healing as an alternative to surgery. Oxervate is **a recombinant version of nerve growth factor (NGF), which is a neuropeptide** that is involved in maintenance, growth, proliferation, and **survival of certain target neurons, including those in the eye**. Oxervate is administered as eye drops to allow **restoration of corneal integrity**.

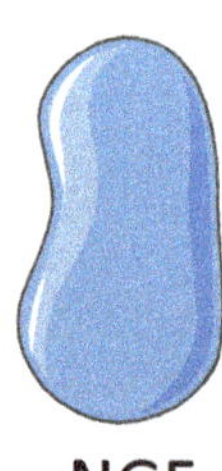

NGF

Action of Cenegermin on cell and disease biology

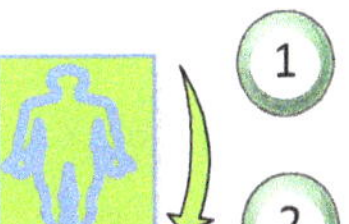

1 Nerve growth factor is a protein produced in the retina and is involved in the **differentiation and maintenance of neurons.**

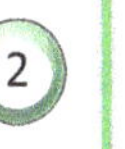

2 NGF binds to NGF receptors (NGFR) expressed on front-most region of the eye, on binding **NGF stimulates corneal healing** and sensitivity.

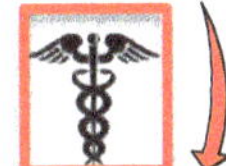

3 **Neurotropic keratopathy** results from **impaired corneal stimulation** and **NGF** production due to a lesion in the trigeminal nerve or its branches that can cause corneal anesthesia (loss of sensation).

4 **Cenegermin** promotes the differentiation and maintenance of neurons and acts through specific high-affinity **nerve growth factor receptors**.

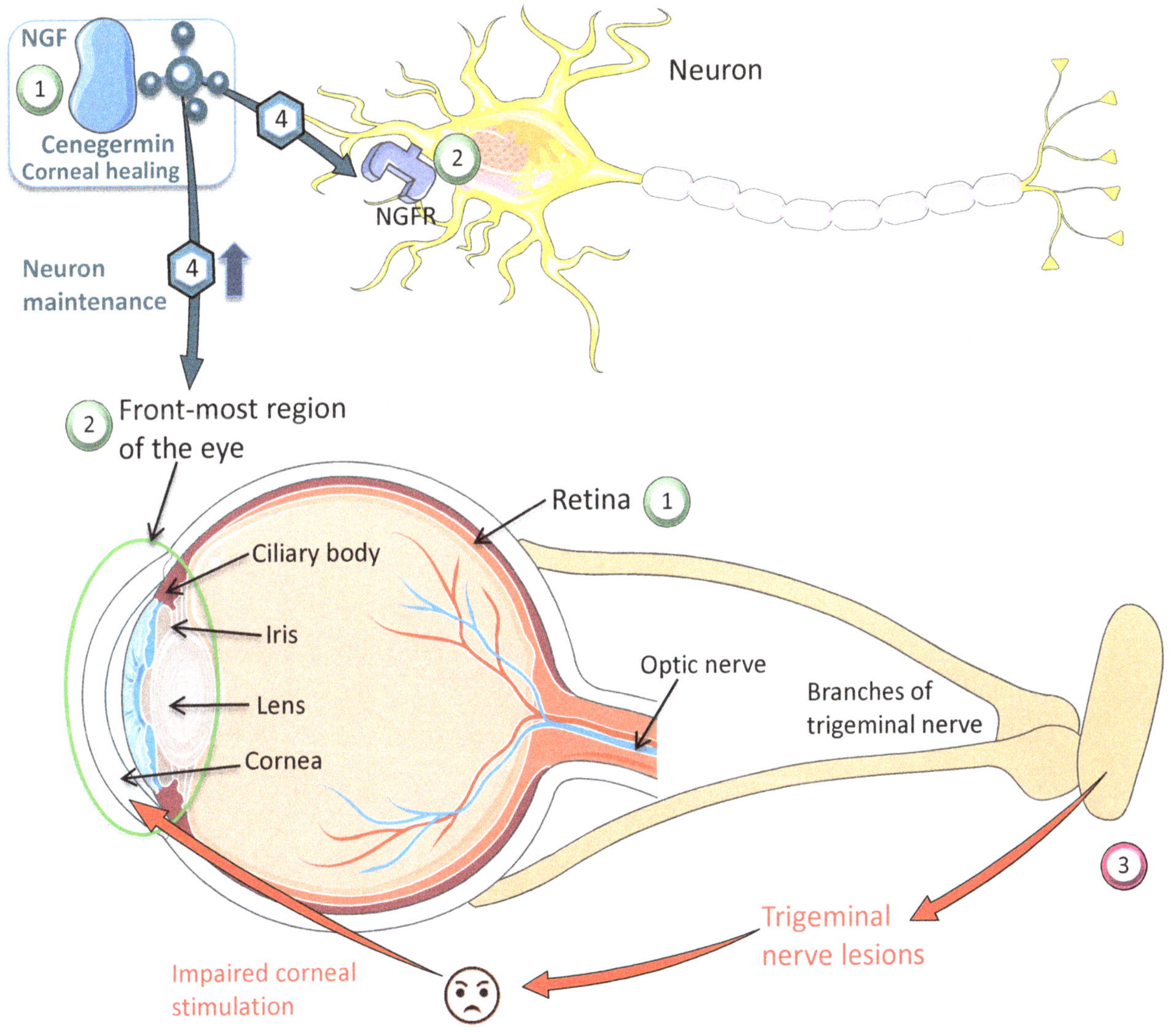

Diseases of the eye: Neurotropic keratitis, Cenegermin

The disease: Neuromyelitis optica spectrum disorder

Neuromyelitis optica spectrum disorder (NMOSD) is a rare chronic autoimmune disease that most commonly **affects the optic nerves and spinal cord with vision loss and serious disability**. NMOSD is characterized by **anti-aquaporin 4 (AQP4) antibody-mediated attack on astrocytes**, which results in inflammation of the optic nerve .

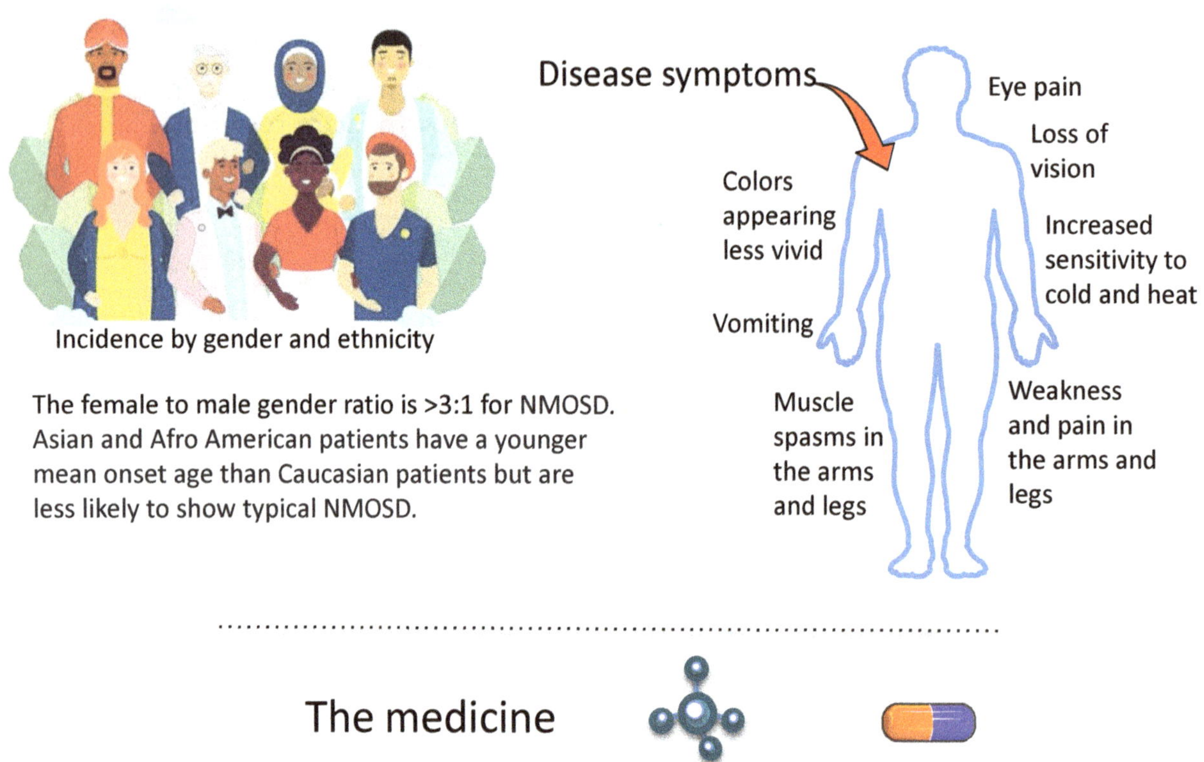

Incidence by gender and ethnicity
The female to male gender ratio is >3:1 for NMOSD. Asian and Afro American patients have a younger mean onset age than Caucasian patients but are less likely to show typical NMOSD.
Disease symptoms
Eye pain
Loss of vision
Colors appearing less vivid
Increased sensitivity to cold and heat
Vomiting
Muscle spasms in the arms and legs
Weakness and pain in the arms and legs

The medicine

Satralizumab; Enspryng, FDA Approval 2020

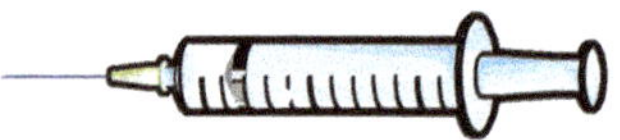

Delivered by subcutaneous injection

Satralizumab is for neuromyelitis optica spectrum disorder (NMOSD**)** patients who are positive for aquaporin-4 (AQP4) antibody**. Interleukin-6 (IL-6)** is involved in the production of **anti-AQP4 antibody and inflammation** in the central nervous system. **Satralizumab** is a long-acting humanized antibody that targets the IL-6 receptor with **inhibition of IL-6-mediated signaling.**

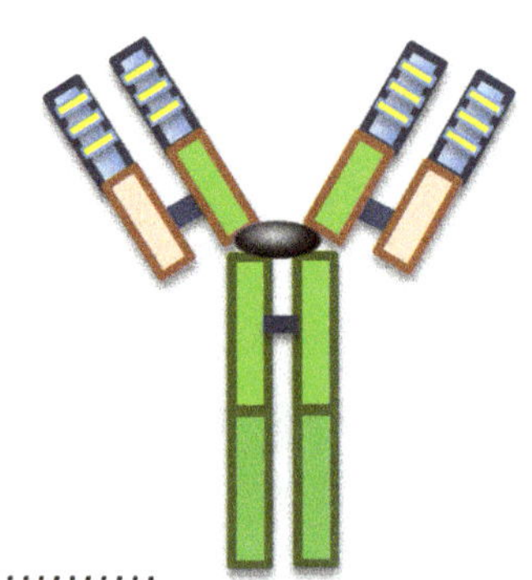

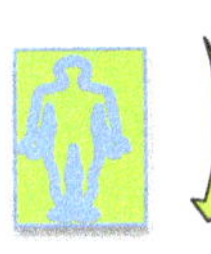
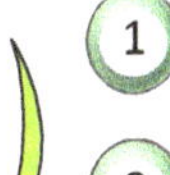

1. The blood–brain barrier is maintained by active interactions between astrocytes and endothelial cells.
2. Interleukin-6 (**IL-6**) regulates the transition from **neutrophils to macrophages** from acute to chronic **inflammation** as well as stimulating T- and B-cells .
3. Aquaporin-4 (**AQP4**) is the most abundant **water channel** in the optic nerves.

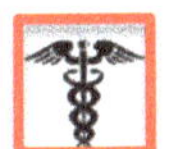
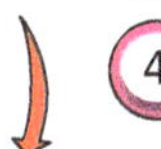

4. **Neutrophils** produce of **APQ4 antibodies**, blood–brain barrier disruption, activation of proinflammatory T-lymphocytes with inflammatory infiltrates.

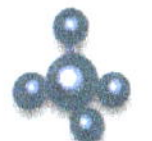

5. **Satralizumab** targets the **IL-6 receptor** and inhibits IL-6-involved pathways.

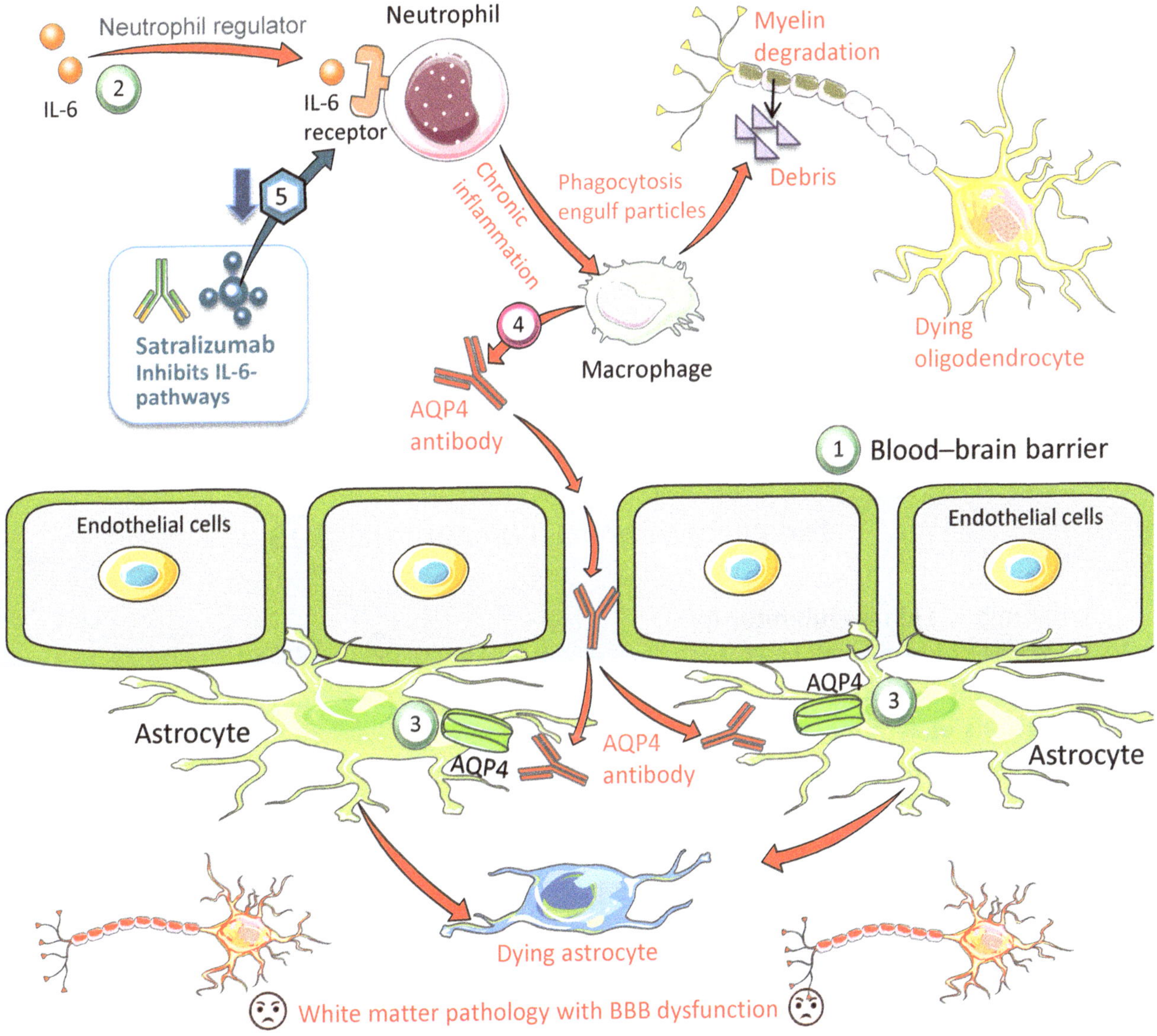

Neutrophil regulator
Neutrophil
IL-6
2
IL-6 receptor
Myelin degradation
Debris
5
Chronic inflammation
Phagocytosis engulf particles
Satralizumab Inhibits IL-6-pathways
4
Macrophage
Dying oligodendrocyte
AQP4 antibody
1 Blood–brain barrier
Endothelial cells
Endothelial cells
AQP4
3
Astrocyte
3
AQP4
AQP4 antibody
Astrocyte
Dying astrocyte
White matter pathology with BBB dysfunction

The disease: Non small cell lung cancer

Non small cell lung cancer (NSCLC) accounts for approximately 85% of all lung cancers and is divided into adenocarcinoma, squamous cell carcinoma, and large cell carcinoma. Some 3%–5% of NSCLC tumors are due to a rearrangement of the lymphoma kinase (ALK) gene.

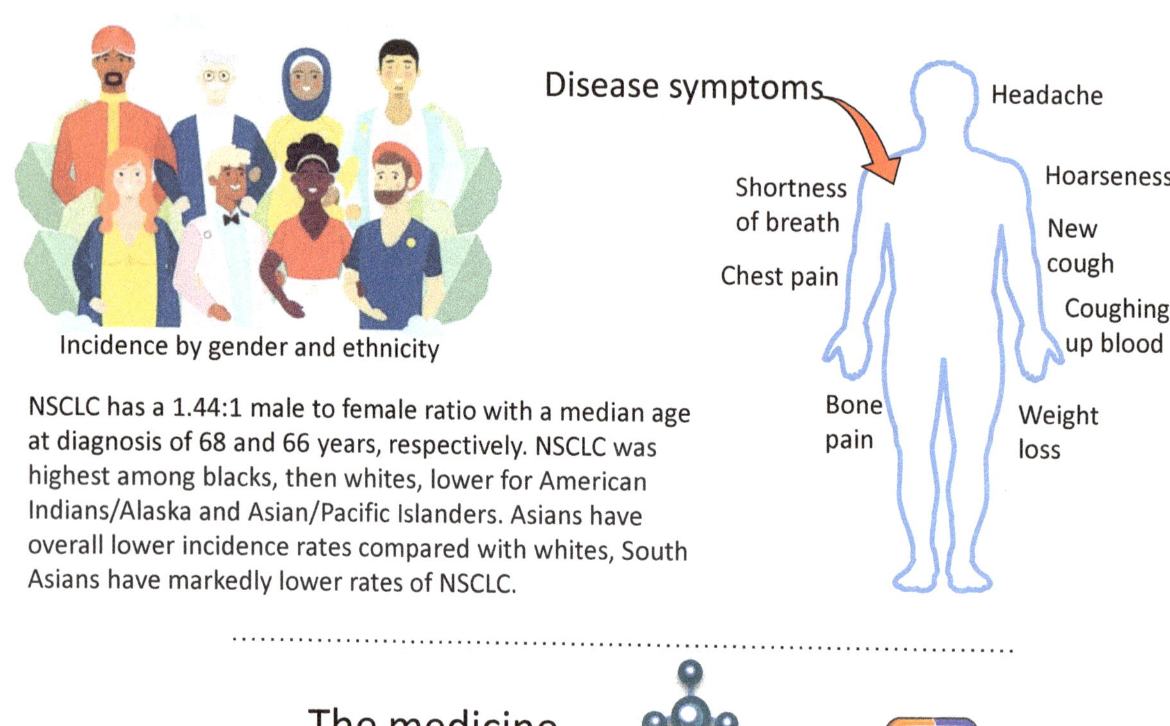

Incidence by gender and ethnicity

NSCLC has a 1.44:1 male to female ratio with a median age at diagnosis of 68 and 66 years, respectively. NSCLC was highest among blacks, then whites, lower for American Indians/Alaska and Asian/Pacific Islanders. Asians have overall lower incidence rates compared with whites, South Asians have markedly lower rates of NSCLC.

The medicine

Lorlatinib; Lorbrena, FDA Approval 2018

Lorlatinib is a **kinase inhibitor** for treatment of **non small cell lung cancer (NSCLC)** caused by **mutations of lymphoma kinase (ALK) gene**, which are resistant to other anti-cancer drugs and has metastasized to other regions including the brain. Lorlatinib can cross the blood–brain barrier to shrinks tumors in the brain.

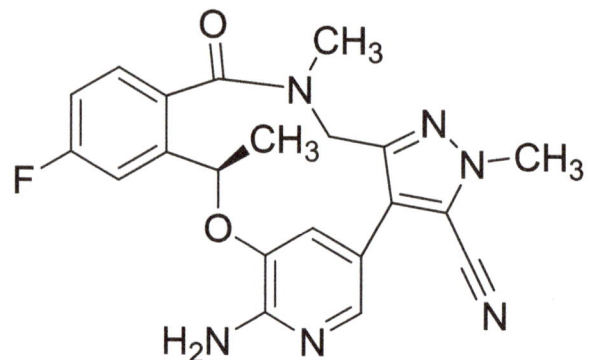

A medicine for lung cancer: Non small cell lung cancer, Lorlatinib

Action of Lorlatinib on cell and disease biology

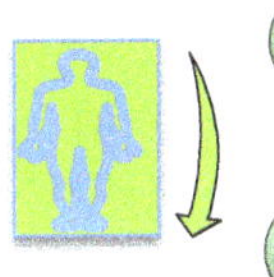

1 Anaplastic lymphoma receptor tyrosine kinase (**ALK**) is a **membrane-associated tyrosine kinase** primarily involved in the early developmental processes and regulates the proliferation of nerve cells.

2 ALK gene can form several fusion genes that become **oncogenic drivers**. The most common fusion occurs with EML4 gene (microtubule associated protein) and accounts for about 30% of ALK+ NSCLC.

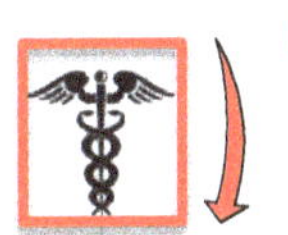

3 Oncogenic drivers generated by variants of the ALK gene result in **dysregulation of the cell cycle checkpoints**, proliferation, and promotion of the cancer process.

ALK-positive lung cancer starts as a single solid tumor, likely to spread quickly to other lung lobes and the other lung.

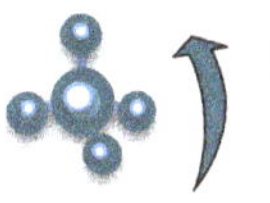

4 **Lorlatinib is a kinase inhibitor** with activity against the products from multiple rearrangements of the ALK gene as well as against multiple alterations of the ALK enzyme.

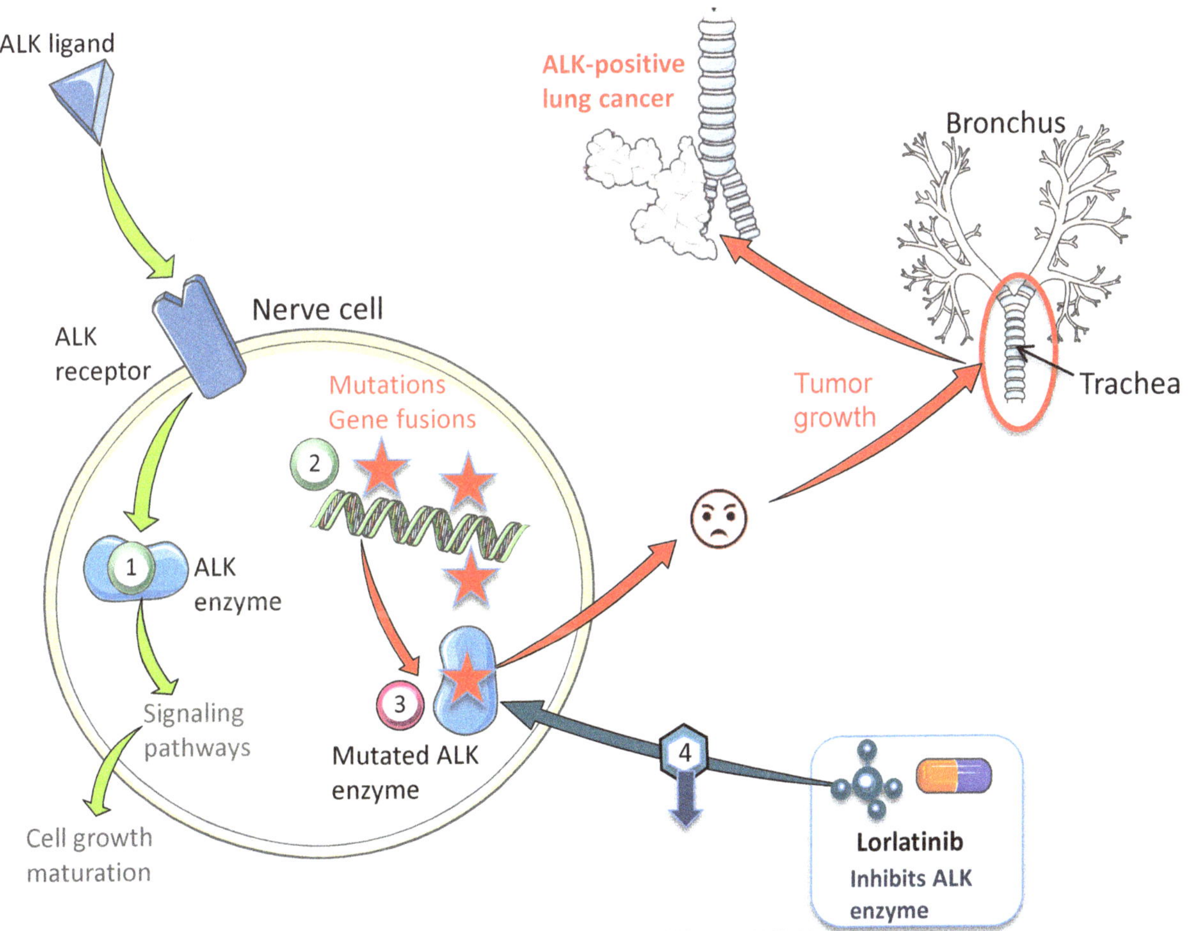

A medicine for lung cancer: Non small cell lung cancer, Lorlatinib

The disease: Epithelioid sarcoma

Epithelioid sarcoma is a rare subtype of **soft tissue sarcoma**, which commonly begins in the soft tissue under the skin of an extremity, such as a hand, forearm, and leg. Frequent causes are inherited syndromes, chemical exposures, and previous radiation treatment. Surgery, chemotherapy, or radiation are used for localized cancer, but 50% of patients have metastatic disease at the time of diagnosis.

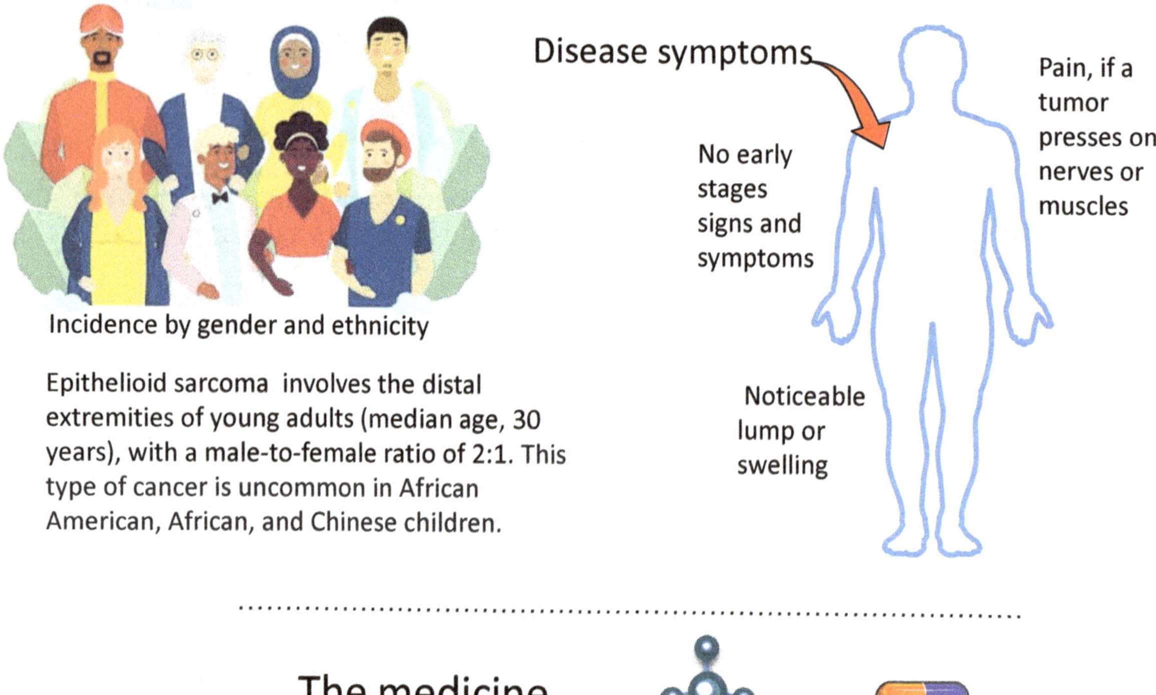

Incidence by gender and ethnicity

Epithelioid sarcoma involves the distal extremities of young adults (median age, 30 years), with a male-to-female ratio of 2:1. This type of cancer is uncommon in African American, African, and Chinese children.

The medicine

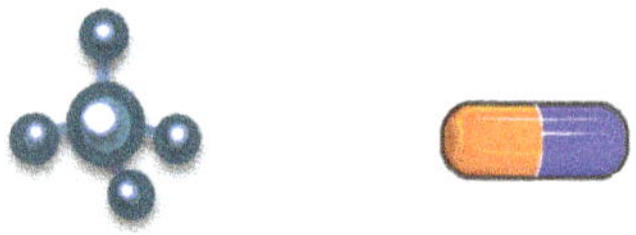

Tazemetostat: Tazverik, FDA Approval 2020

Tazemetostat is prescribed for metastatic or locally advanced **epithelioid sarcoma**. It is an oral small-molecule inhibitor that **blocks the activity of EZH2 methyltransferase**, which can play a key role in proliferation of the cancer cells.

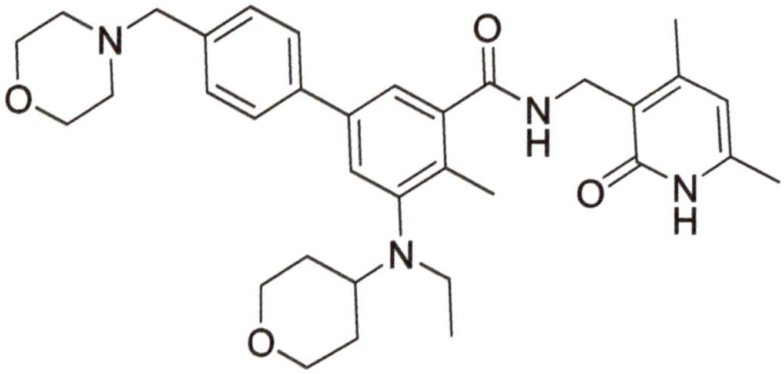

Action of Tazemetostat on cell and disease biology

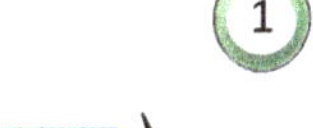

1 In the **chromatin complex, eight histone molecules** (H2A, H2B, H3, and H4) are organized into an octamer, which is wrapped by core DNA.

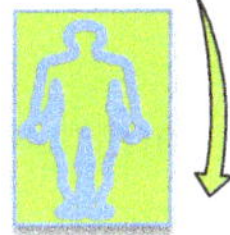

2 **Epigenetic modifications of histone proteins** occurs by **methylation** (Me) via the enzyme histone N-methyltransferase (gene **EZH2).**

3 **Histone H3** is involved in controlling **nucleosome structure** in chromatin.

4 **Repression of transcription** is achieved by altering the structure of chromatin to form large inaccessible DNA regions (heterochromatin).

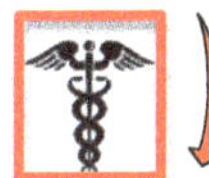

5 **EZH2** is a gene suppressor that is **mutated** and overexpressed in most solid tumors resulting in repressed heterochromatin with **inactivation** of many **tumor suppressor genes** and resulting tumor cell proliferation.

6 **Tazemetostat inhibits both mutated and normal EZH2.** Tazverik decreases histone methylation, alters gene expression associated with cancer pathways with decreased tumor cell proliferation.

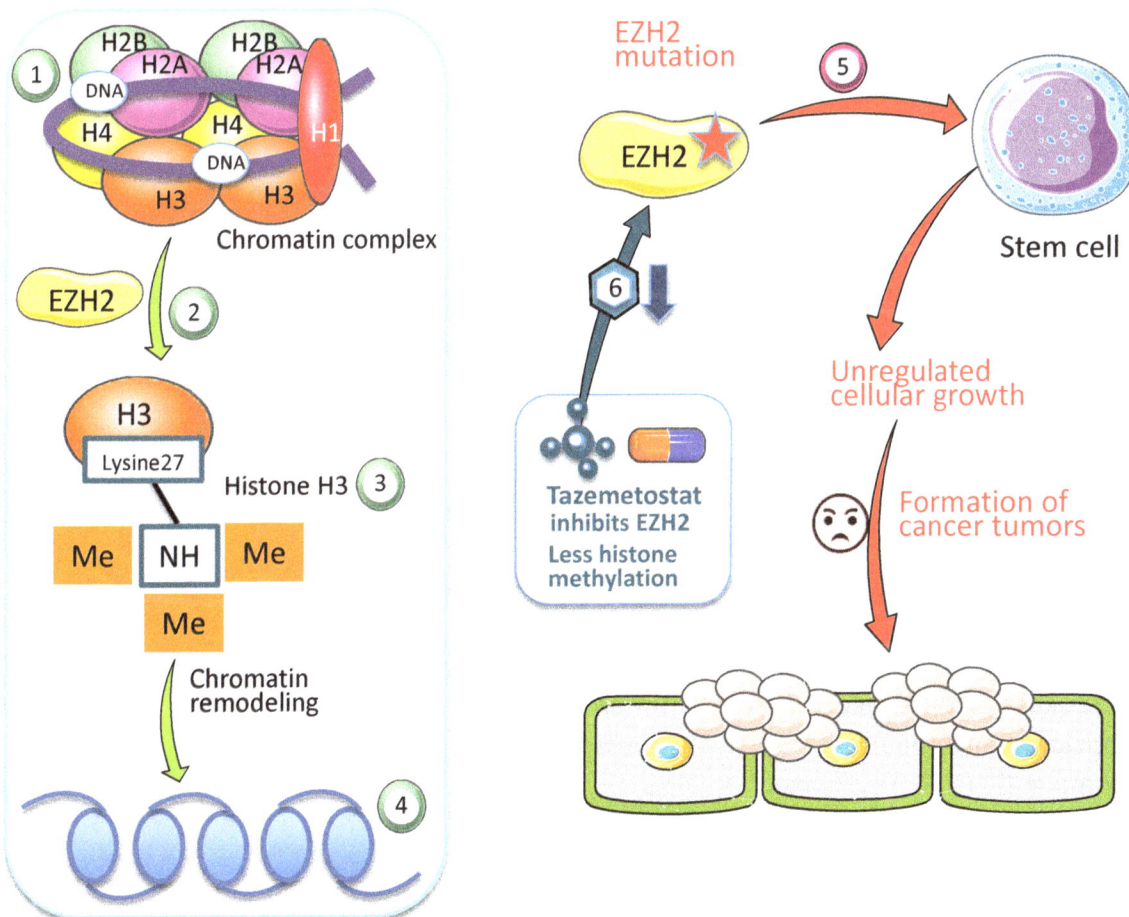

1 H2B H2A H2B H2A DNA H4 H4 DNA H1 H3 H3

Chromatin complex

EZH2 2

H3 Lysine27 Histone H3 3

Me NH Me Me

Chromatin remodeling

4

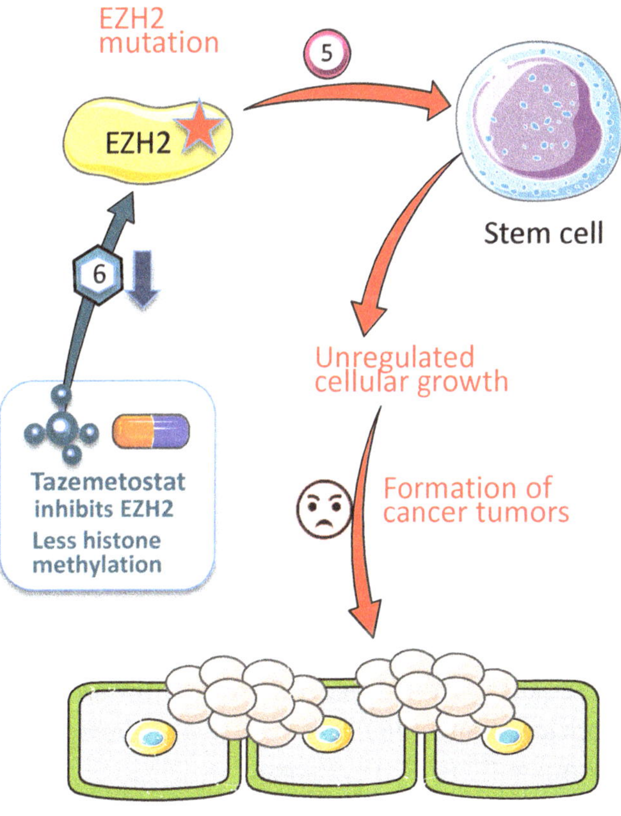

The disease: Psoriasis

Psoriasis is a chronic skin disease associated with overactive inflammatory and immune responses with hyper-proliferation of keratinocytes. In **plaque, psoriasis** 80%–90% of patients have **thick, raised patches (plaques) generated by this hyper-proliferation**, mostly on the knees, elbows, scalp, and is accompanied by severe itching, pain, and bleeding of psoriatic patches.

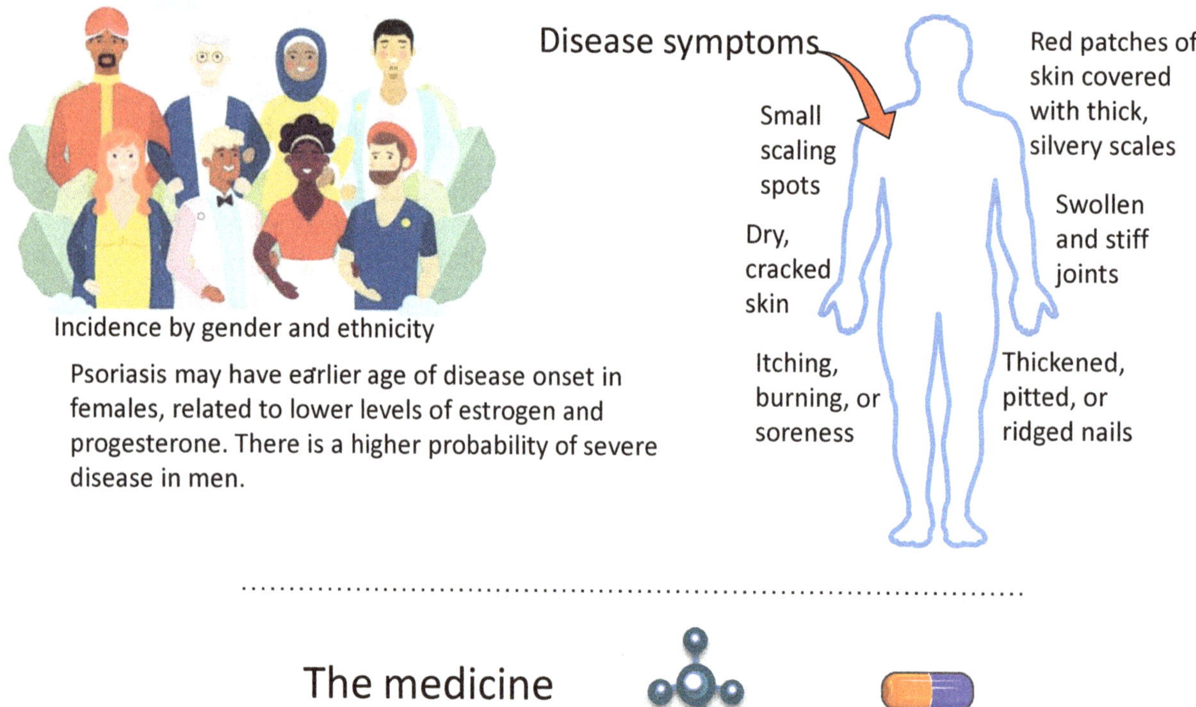

Incidence by gender and ethnicity

Psoriasis may have earlier age of disease onset in females, related to lower levels of estrogen and progesterone. There is a higher probability of severe disease in men.

The medicine

Risankizumab; Skyrizi, FDA Approval 2019

Risankizumab is prescribed for plaque psoriasis in adults who are candidates for systemic therapy. A broad immunosuppressant drug (methotrexate) is less safe/effective than **targeted inhibition of a cytokine Interleukin IL-23**. **Risankizumab is a humanized** IgG1 **monoclonal antibody** that selectively **binds to** interleukin 23 (IL-23) cytokine.

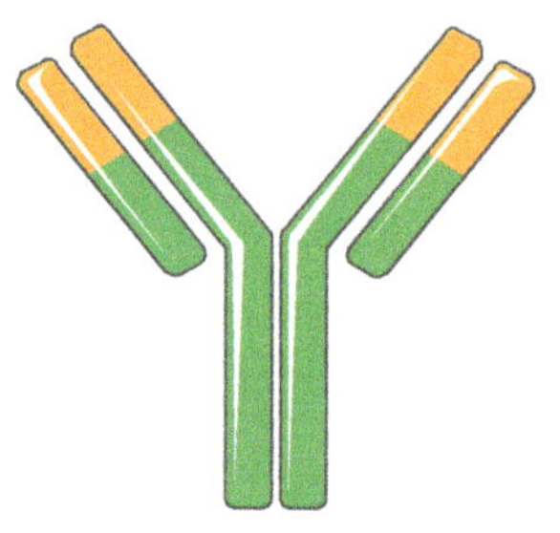

Skin diseases and medicines: Psoriasis, Risankizumab

Action of Risankizumab on cell and disease biology

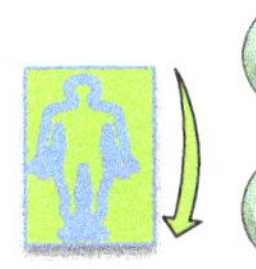

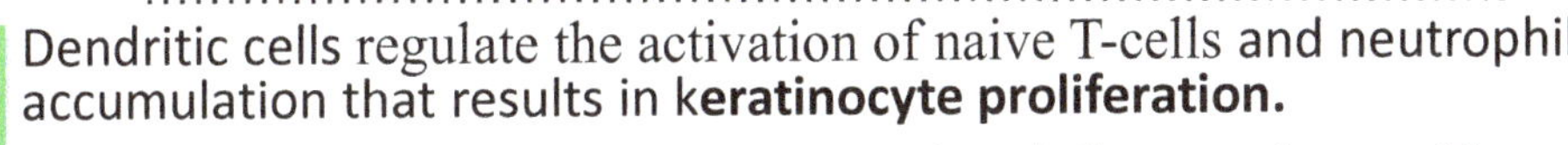

1 Dendritic cells regulate the activation of naive T-cells and neutrophil accumulation that results in **keratinocyte proliferation.**

2 **Interleukins (IL)** are cytokines that **regulate inflammation and immune cells** (activation, differentiation, proliferation, maturation, migration, adhesion).

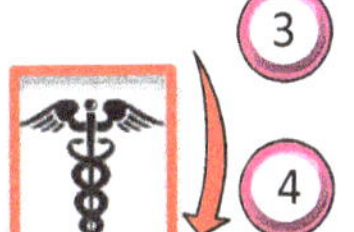

3 T-cells (**Th17**) are involved in **defense against external pathogens and** secrete IL-17 but also cause **chronic inflammation** and tissue destruction.

4 **Overproduction of IL-23 occurs in the upper dermis** with excessive Th17 cell accumulation and **excess IL-17, 22**.

5 **Activated neutrophils** travel to the skin lesion to undergo cell death and can contribute to ongoing inflammation and tissue destruction.

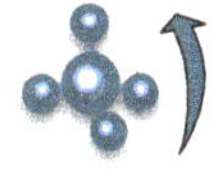

6 **Risankizumab antibody blocks IL-23 activity and prevents** release of pro-inflammatory **cytokines and chemokines.**

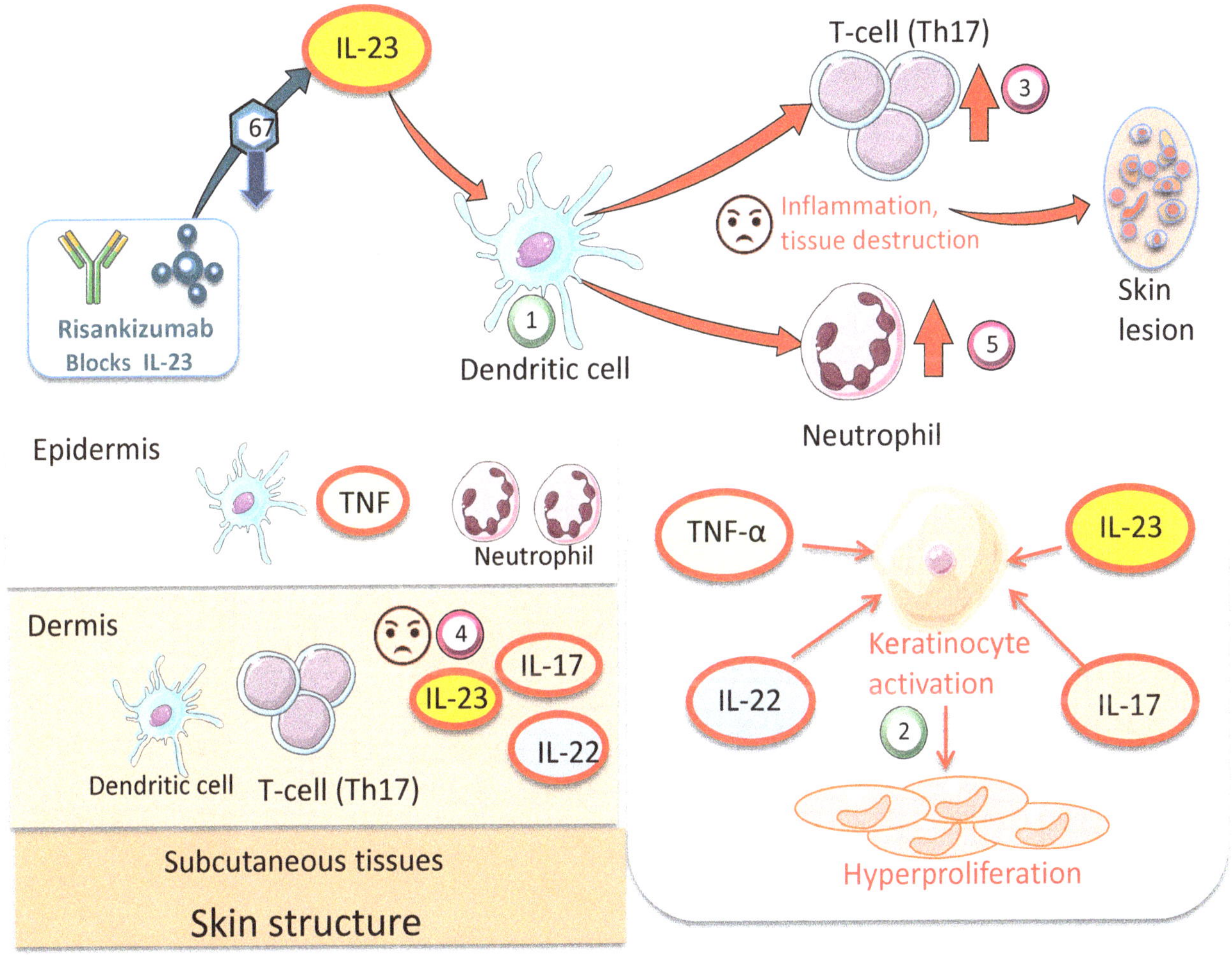

IL-23

67

T-cell (Th17)

3

Inflammation, tissue destruction

Skin lesion

Risankizumab Blocks IL-23

1

Dendritic cell

5

Neutrophil

Epidermis

TNF

Neutrophil

Dermis

4

IL-17

IL-23

IL-22

Dendritic cell

T-cell (Th17)

Subcutaneous tissues

Skin structure

TNF-α

IL-23

Keratinocyte activation

IL-22

IL-17

2

Hyperproliferation

The disease: Acne vulgaris

Acne vulgaris is a common chronic skin disease involving blockage and/or **inflammation of hair follicles** and **secretions of sebaceous gland (sebum)**. Acne can present as noninflammatory or inflammatory lesions, which affect the face, back, and chest.

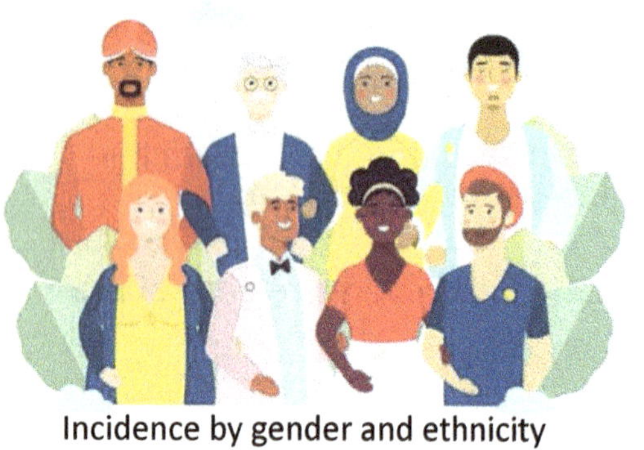

Incidence by gender and ethnicity

During adolescence, acne vulgaris is more common in males than in females, whereas in adulthood it is more common in women than in men. Clinical acne was more prevalent in African American and Hispanic women than in Continental Indian, Caucasian, and Asian women.

Disease symptoms

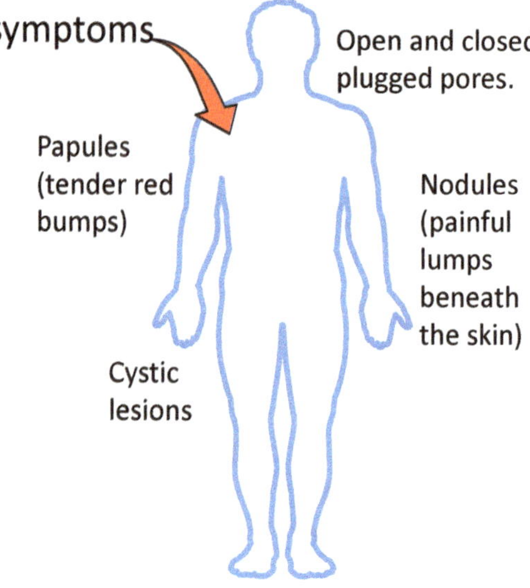

The medicine

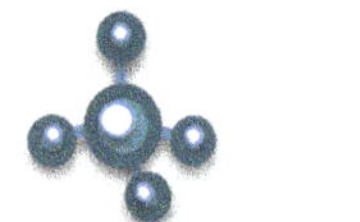
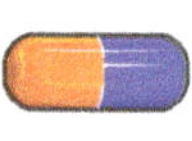

Trifarotene; Aklief, FDA Approval 2019

Trifarotene is an **agonist of retinoic acid receptors** (RAR), especially the **gamma subtype** of RAR. **Stimulation of RAR** and associated genes are associated with cell differentiation and **mediation of inflammation.**

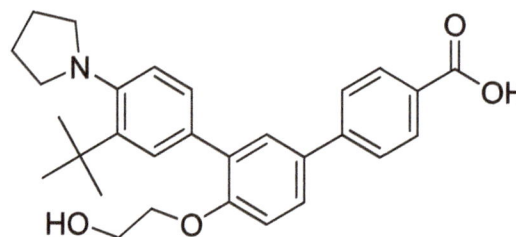

Action of Trifarotene on cell and disease biology

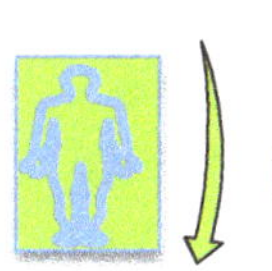

1 **Retinoic acid (RA) is the active metabolite of Vitamin A** and acts through **retinoic acid receptors (RARs) in the nucleus**. RARs regulate embryo development as well as adult tissue homeostasis.

2 **Sebaceous glands arise from keratinocytes** in the hair follicle and secrete sebum (oily, waxy matter) to lubricate the hair and skin.

3 **Retinoid receptor (RAR) and pathways are active in human sebocytes to regulate growth,** development, and lipid synthesis via gene activation/repression.

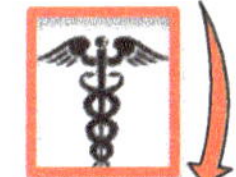

4 Acne develops from **proliferation of layers of epidermal cells** and causes excessive oil production and opportunistic bacterial infections.

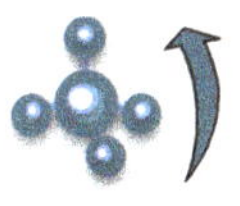

5 **Trifarotene stimulates retinoic acid receptors (RAR)** to modulate genes for cell differentiation and **inflammation with** significant **decreases** in numbers of **sebocyte cells** and **lipid-forming colonies.**

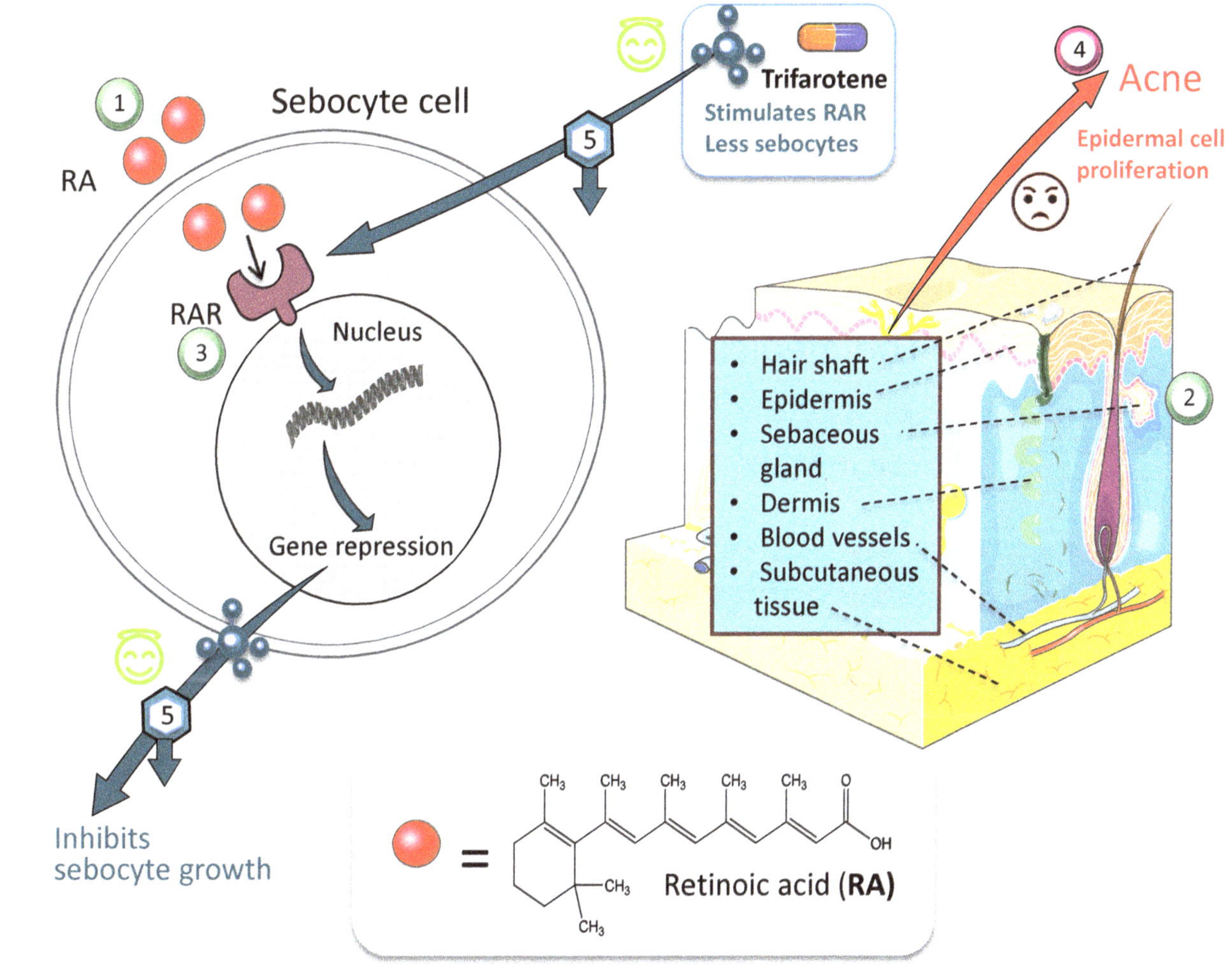

The disease: Erythropoietic protoporphyria

Erythropoietic protoporphyria (EPP) is a rare disorder caused by mutations with **impaired activity of ferrochelatase**, an enzyme involved in hemoglobin production. **Ferrochelatase catalyzes the final step in the biosynthesis of heme B** from protoporphyrin IX, which **leads to an accumulation of protoporphyrin IX (PpIX). Light reaching the skin can react with PPIX causing intense skin pain** skin, redness and thickening.

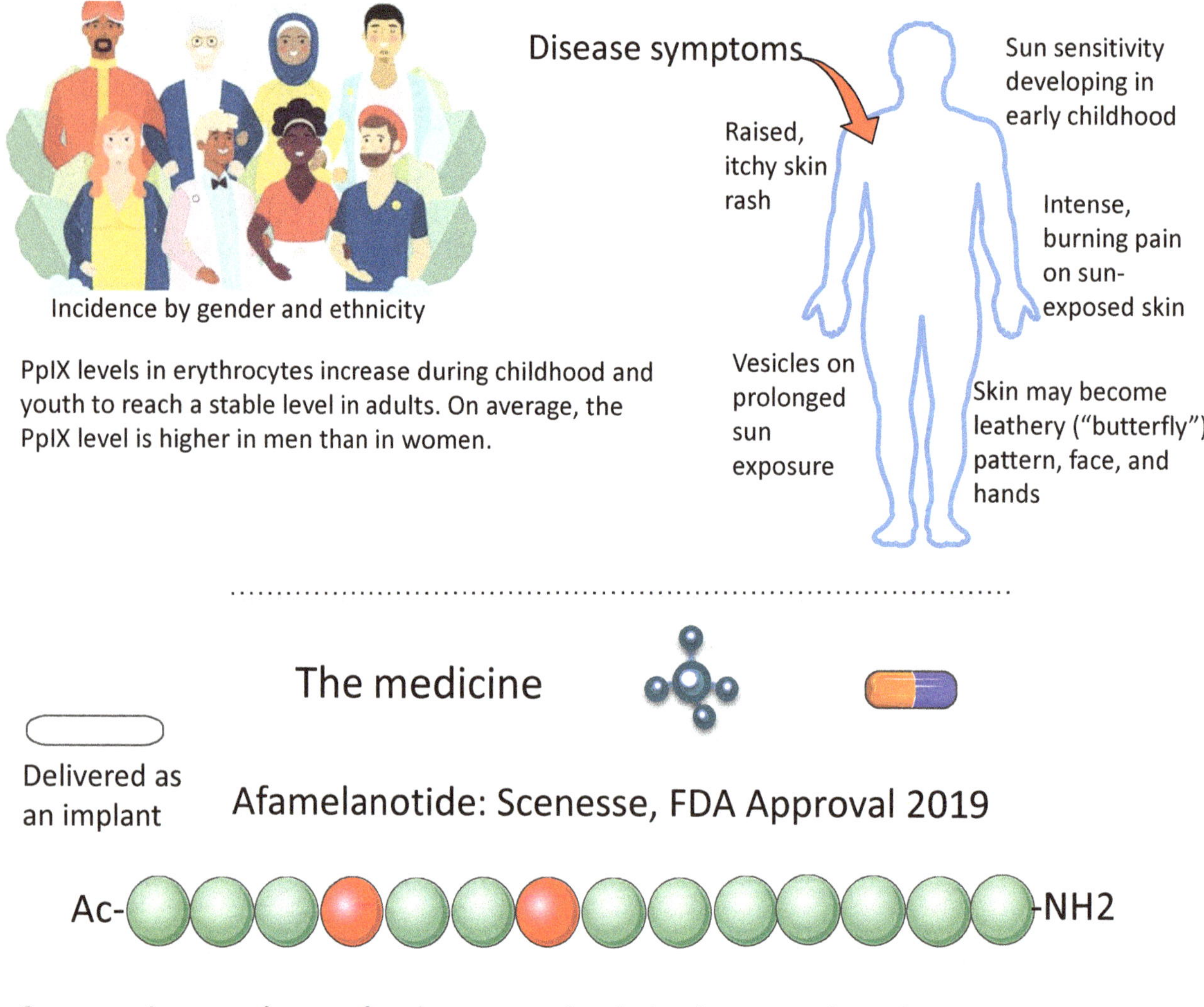
Incidence by gender and ethnicity
PpIX levels in erythrocytes increase during childhood and youth to reach a stable level in adults. On average, the PpIX level is higher in men than in women.
Disease symptoms
Raised, itchy skin rash
Sun sensitivity developing in early childhood
Intense, burning pain on sun-exposed skin
Vesicles on prolonged sun exposure
Skin may become leathery ("butterfly") pattern, face, and hands
The medicine
Delivered as an implant
Afamelanotide: Scenesse, FDA Approval 2019
Ac-
-NH2

Scenesse is an **analogue of melanocyte-stimulating hormone (MSH)** with two amino acid substituents (denoted in red), which significantly increases both the activity and stability of the peptide. It stimulates **alpha-MSH melanocortin-1 receptor (MC1R)** and increases the production of dark melanin pigments in the skin independent of exposure to sunlight or artificial light.

Action of Afamelanotide on cell and disease biology

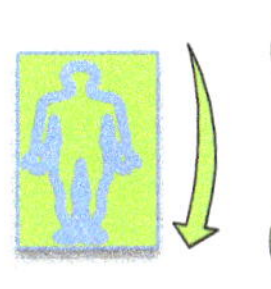

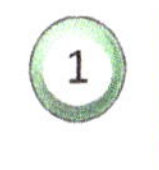

1 **α-Melanocyte-stimulating hormone** (α-MSH) on **binding** to melanocortin-1 receptor (MC1R) promotes **melanin synthesis.**

2 **Melanin** protects against melanoma by reducing exposure to UVB irradiation, scavenging oxygen free radicals and by stimulating DNA repair.

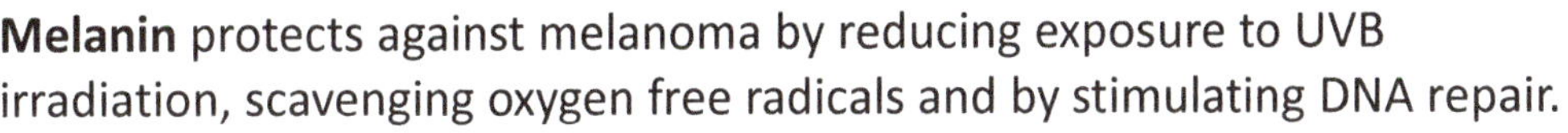

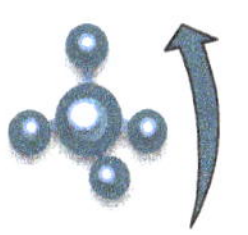

3 **Afamelanotide** has a skin protective effect through selective binding and **activation of the MC1R receptor** in melanocytes, which results in **melanin synthesis** and melanocyte proliferation.

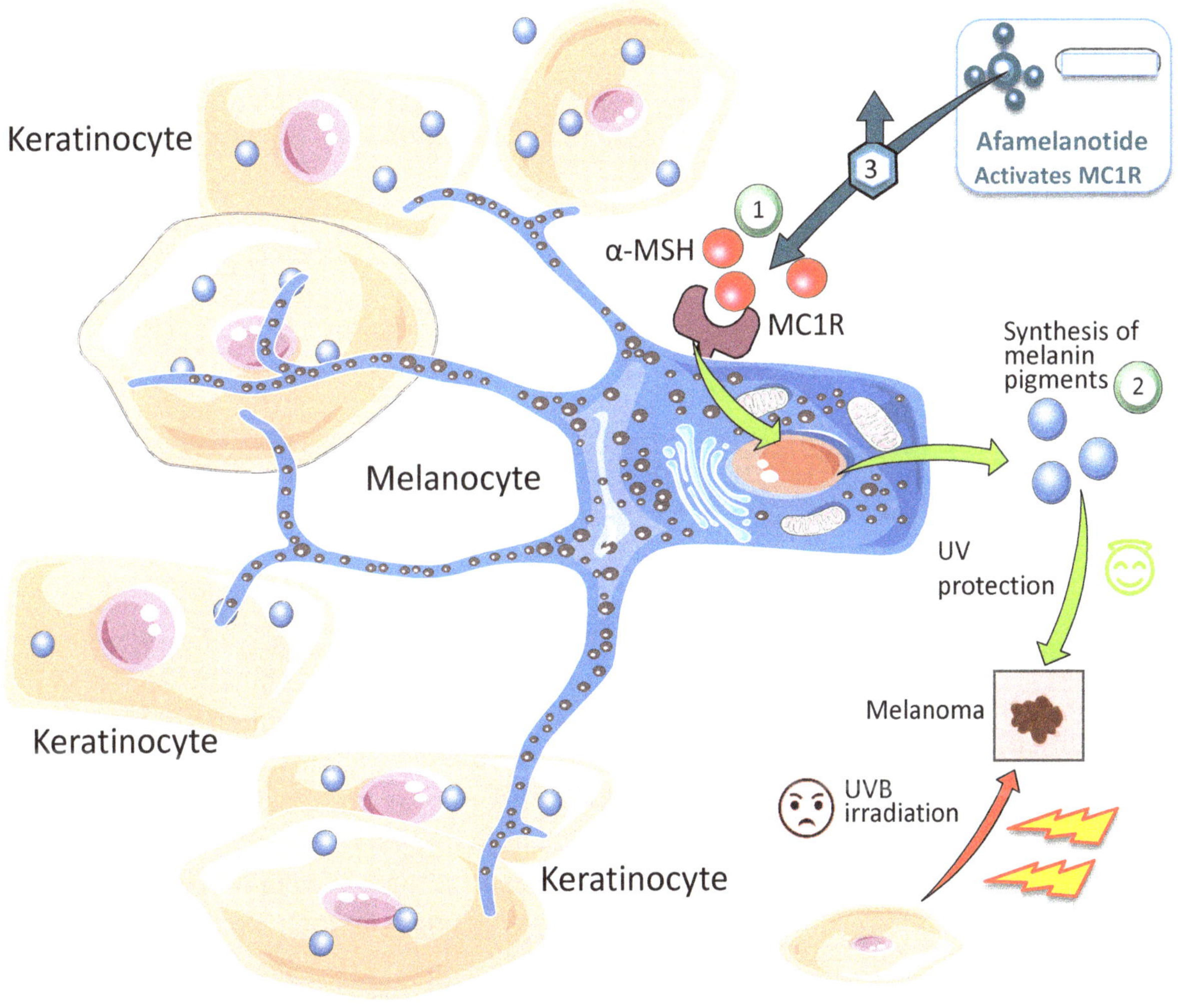

Keratinocyte

Afamelanotide
Activates MC1R

3

1

α-MSH

MC1R

Synthesis of melanin pigments 2

Melanocyte

UV protection

Keratinocyte

Melanoma

UVB irradiation

Keratinocyte

The disease: Acquired thrombotic thrombocytopenic purpura

Acquired thrombotic thrombocytopenic purpura (aTTP) is caused by unrestrained growth of microthrombi composed of von Willebrand factor and platelets (extensive blood clots in the small blood vessels) which cause thrombocytopenia.

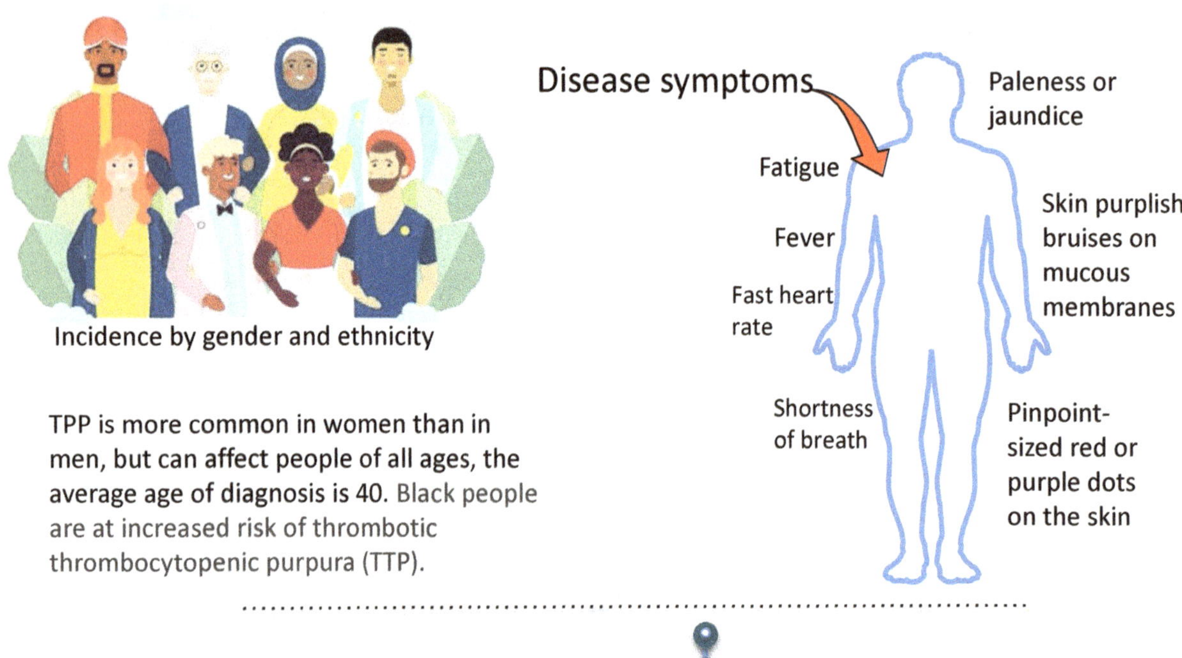

TPP is more common in women than in men, but can affect people of all ages, the average age of diagnosis is 40. Black people are at increased risk of thrombotic thrombocytopenic purpura (TTP).

The medicine

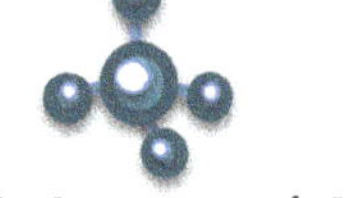

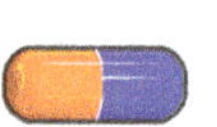

Caplacizumab; Cablivi, FDA Approval 2019

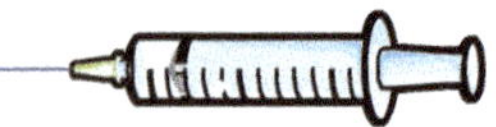

Bolus intravenous injection prior to plasma exchange followed by a subcutaneous injection.

Caplacizumab specifically blocks the interaction between von Willebrand factor (vWF) and platelets effecting platelet adhesion and consumption. The result is inhibition of the formation of micro-clots (microthrombi).

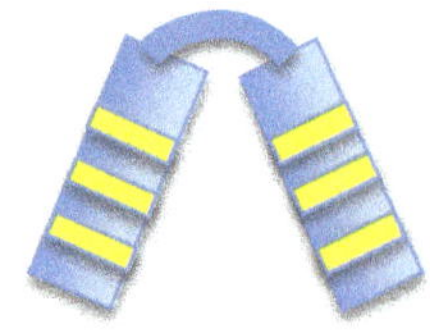

Caplacizumab consists of two identical nanobody building blocks connected by tri-alanine linker sequence. The nanobody contains single-domain heavy-chain antibody fragments each with three binding regions directed against the A1 domain of von Willebrand factor.

Action of Caplacizumab on cell and disease biology

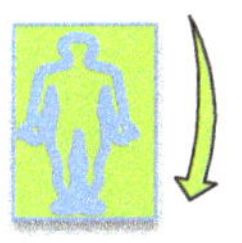

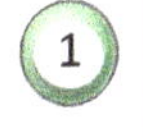

vWF is an **adhesive plasma glycoprotein**, which performs its hemostatic functions and binds to glycoproteins on platelets surface.

Glycoprotein (**GpIb**) functions as a **platelet receptor** for VWF.

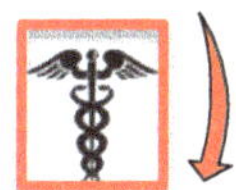

Microthrombi are composed of large complexes of **platelets and von Willebrand factor** and are associated with a higher death rate for patients with cardiovascular disease, especially for sudden deaths.

Caplacizumab binds to the A1 domain of vWF and **blocks** the **interaction** of ultra large von Willebrand Factor (**vWF**) multimers with **platelets**.

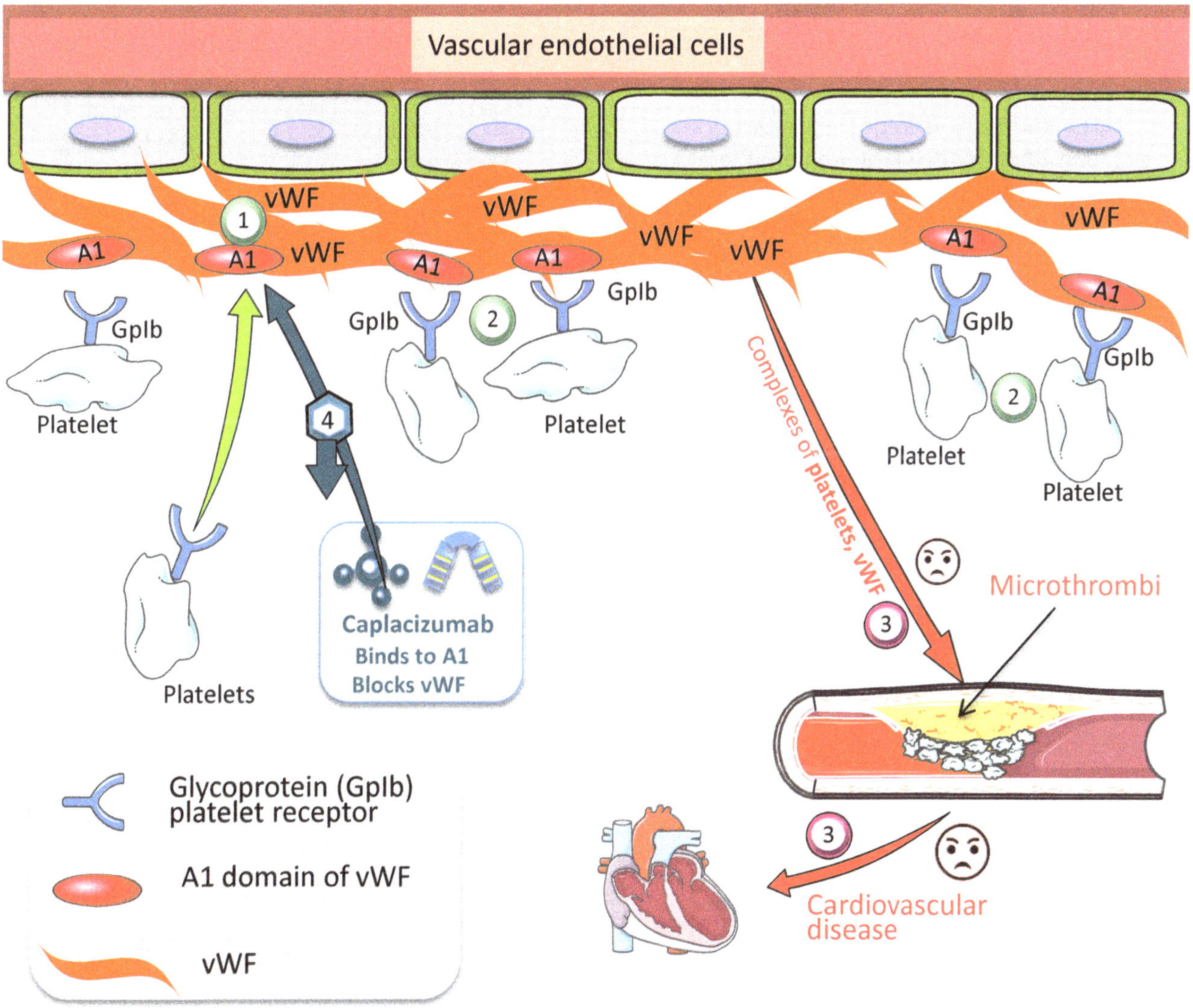

Vascular endothelial cells

vWF

vWF

vWF

vWF

vWF

vWF

1

A1

A1

A1

A1

A1

A1

GpIb

GpIb

GpIb

GpIb

GpIb

2

2

Platelet

Platelet

Platelet

Platelet

4

Complexes of **platelets, vWF**

3

Microthrombi

Platelets

Caplacizumab
Binds to A1
Blocks vWF

Glycoprotein (GpIb) platelet receptor

A1 domain of vWF

vWF

3

Cardiovascular disease

The disease: Thrombocytopenia

Thrombocytopenia has a low platelet count with a resulting deficiency in blood clotting. Autoimmune diseases, certain cancers, resulting medications, and treatments can cause thrombocytopenia. Surgical procedure preparation for adults with chronic liver disease drug treatment is proscribed to boost platelet levels.

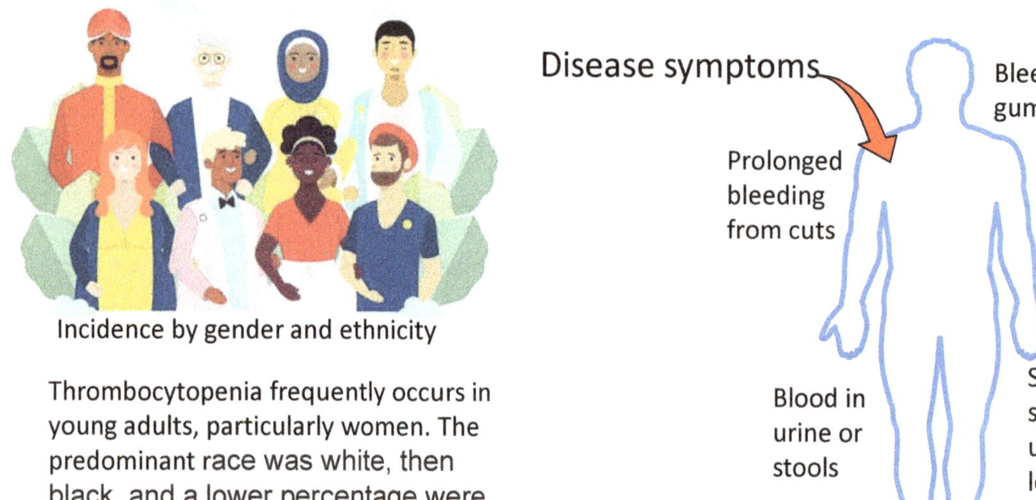

Incidence by gender and ethnicity

Thrombocytopenia frequently occurs in young adults, particularly women. The predominant race was white, then black, and a lower percentage were classified as other (Asian, mixed race, native American, and Hispanic).

The medicine

Lusutrombopag, Mulpleta, FDA Approval 2018

Avatrombopag, Doptelet, FDA Approval 2018

Lusutrombopag and Avatrombopag are **thrombopoietin (TPO) mimetics** that can bind to and activate TPO receptors and increase platelet production.

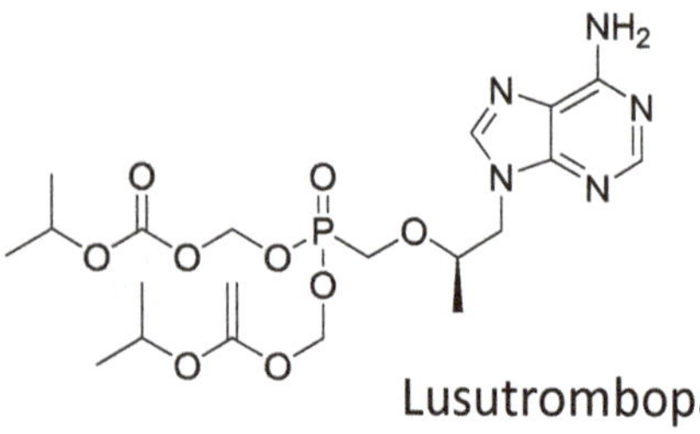

Lusutrombopag

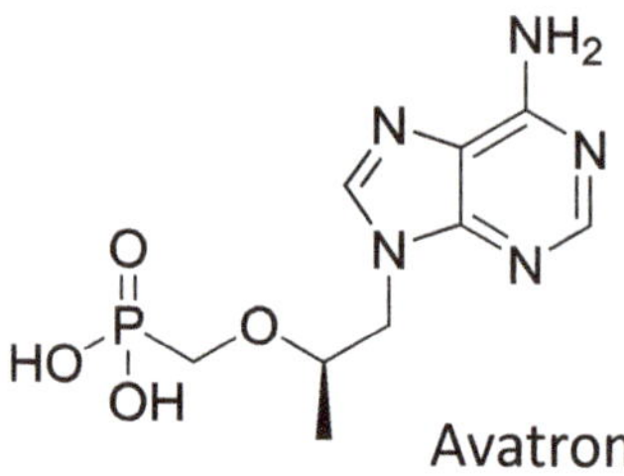

Avatrombopag

Blood cell disorders and medicines: Thrombocytopenia, Lusutrombopag, Avatrombopag,

Action of Lusutrombopag, Avatrombopag on cell and disease biology

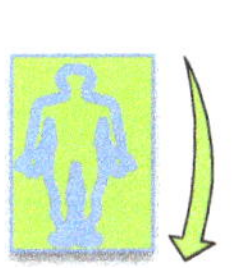
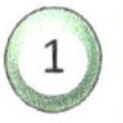

1 **Thrombopoietin (TPO) is a glycoprotein hormone** produced by the liver.

2 **TPO** binds to its receptor and **stimulates the production and differentiation of megakaryocytes** and platelet synthesis.

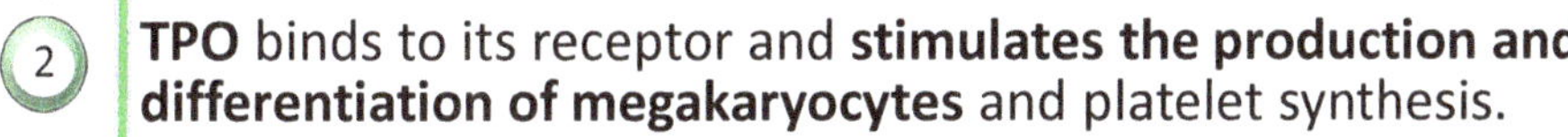

3 **Megakaryocytes** are bone marrow cells that **bud off large numbers of platelets**.

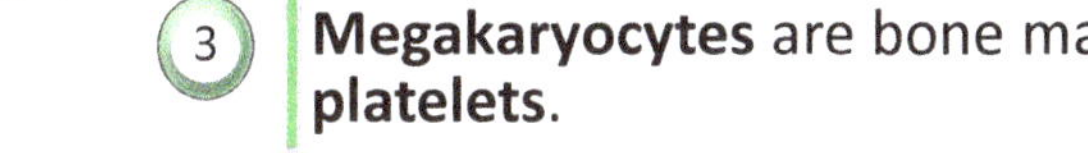

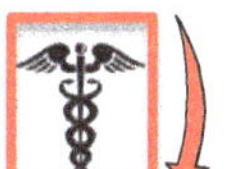

4 People with **thrombocytopenia** have **low platelet levels** and typically receive platelet transfusions immediately prior to a medical procedure. Platelets help form blood clots in the vascular system and prevent bleeding.

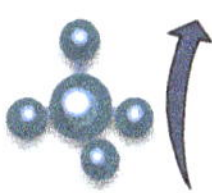

5 **Lusutrombopag, Avatrombopag activate thrombopoietin receptors (TPO-R)** on **megakaryocytes** in the bone marrow to produce more platelets.

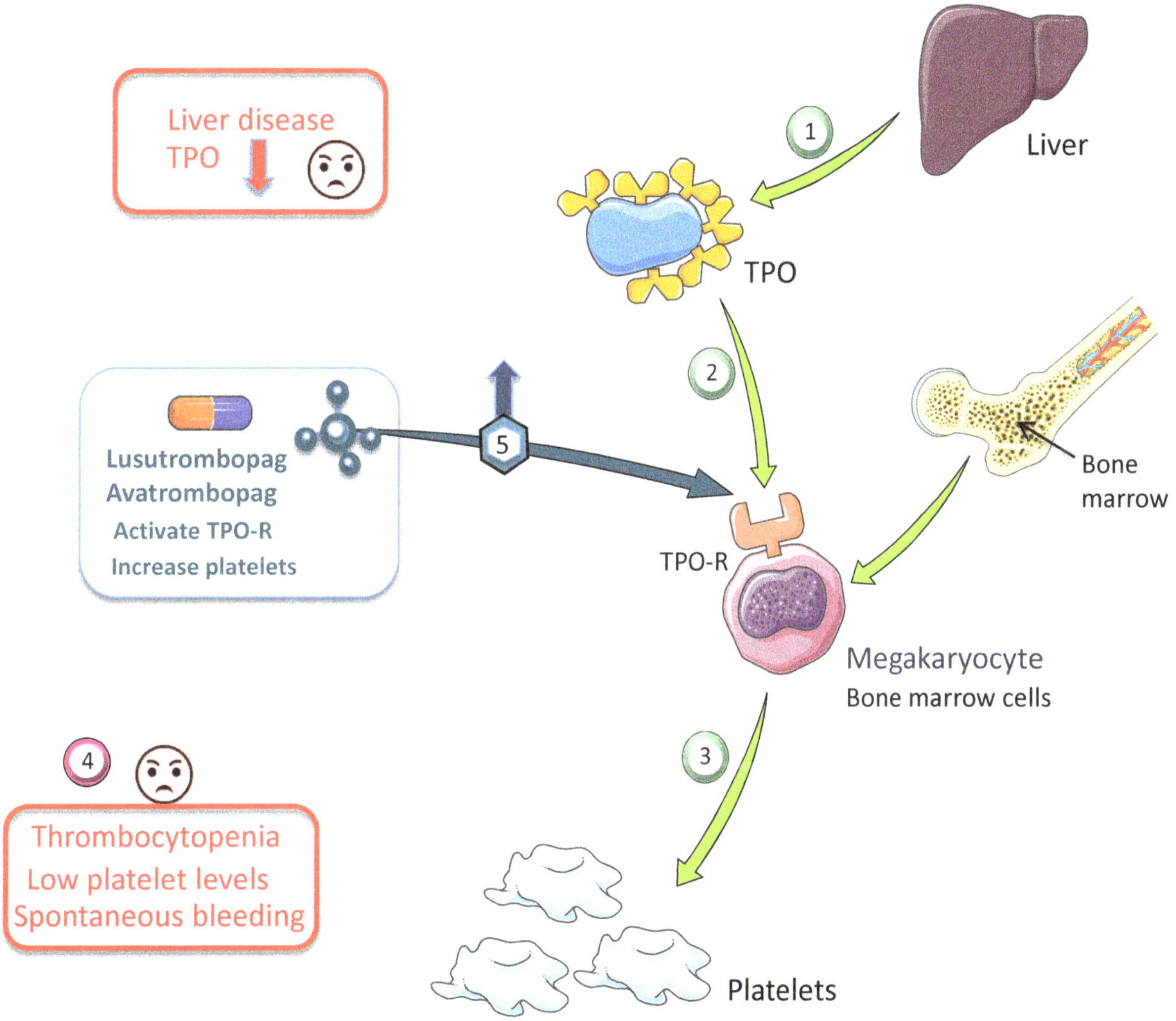

Liver disease
TPO
1
Liver
TPO
2
Lusutrombopag
Avatrombopag
Activate TPO-R
Increase platelets
5
Bone marrow
TPO-R
Megakaryocyte
Bone marrow cells
3
4
Thrombocytopenia
Low platelet levels
Spontaneous bleeding
Platelets

Blood cell disorders and medicines: Thrombocytopenia, Lusutrombopag, Avatrombopag,

The disease: Non-Hodgkin lymphoma

Non-Hodgkin **lymphoma** may arise in **lymph nodes** anywhere in the body. The most common type is refractory diffuse large B-cell lymphoma (DLBCL) an aggressive lymphoma that affects **B-lymphocytes**.

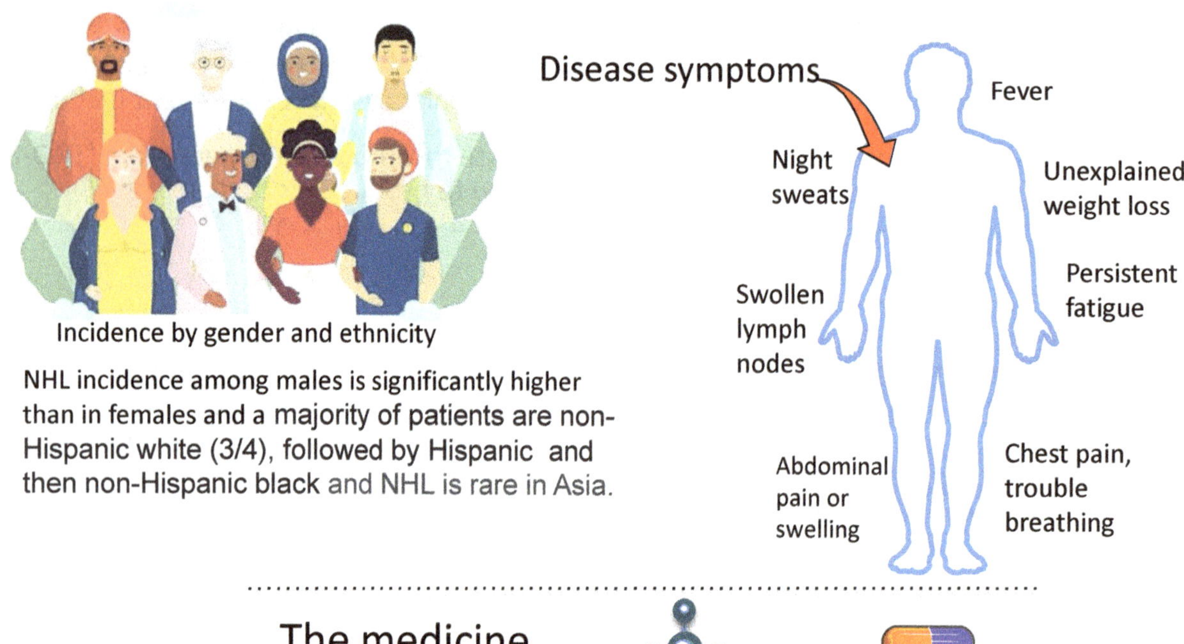

Incidence by gender and ethnicity

NHL incidence among males is significantly higher than in females and a majority of patients are non-Hispanic white (3/4), followed by Hispanic and then non-Hispanic black and NHL is rare in Asia.

The medicine

Polatuzumab, Polivy, FDA Approval 2018

Polatuzumab is an antibody linked to the chemotherapy drug auristatin E. Cleavage of the linker inside tumor cells by cathepsin activates auristatin E (~3.5 molecules/antibody).

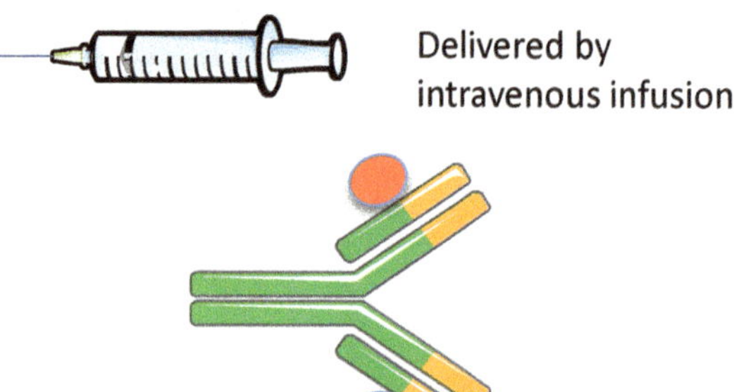

Delivered by intravenous infusion

Vincristine, Oncovin, FDA Approval 1963

Vincristine, isolated from Madagascar periwinkle, produces a cytotoxic effect on leukemic cells but not on normal lymphocytes. Inhibits leukocyte production and maturation.

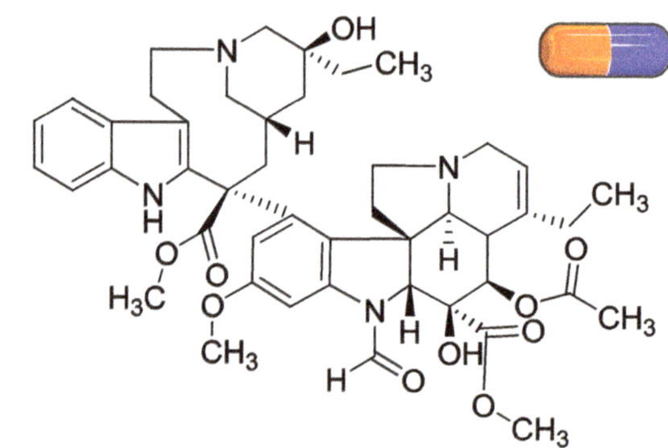

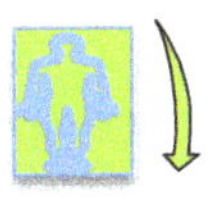

Microtubule blockage causes the cell to be unable to separate its chromosomes during the metaphase. The cell then undergoes apoptosis.

Auristatin E is derived from peptides occurring in a marine mollusk and **interferes** with the formation of **microtubules** by binding to the β-subunit of α-β tubulin dimers in the cytoplasm.

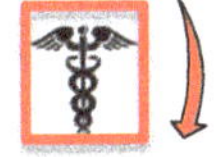

Non-Hodgkin's lymphoma begins in the lymphatic system. **Lymphocytes can grow** abnormally and form tumors throughout the body.

Polatuzumab binds to a B-cell specific antigen receptor (CD79b) critical for B-cell function followed by releasing the auristatin (chemotherapy drug) into those cells.

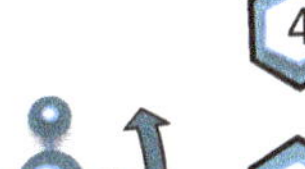

5 **Release of** auristatin by cleavage of linker by **cathepsin** (an enzyme involved in protein recycling in the lysosome).

Vincristine works by binding to the **tubulin protein**, stopping the tubulin dimers from polymerizing to form microtubules.

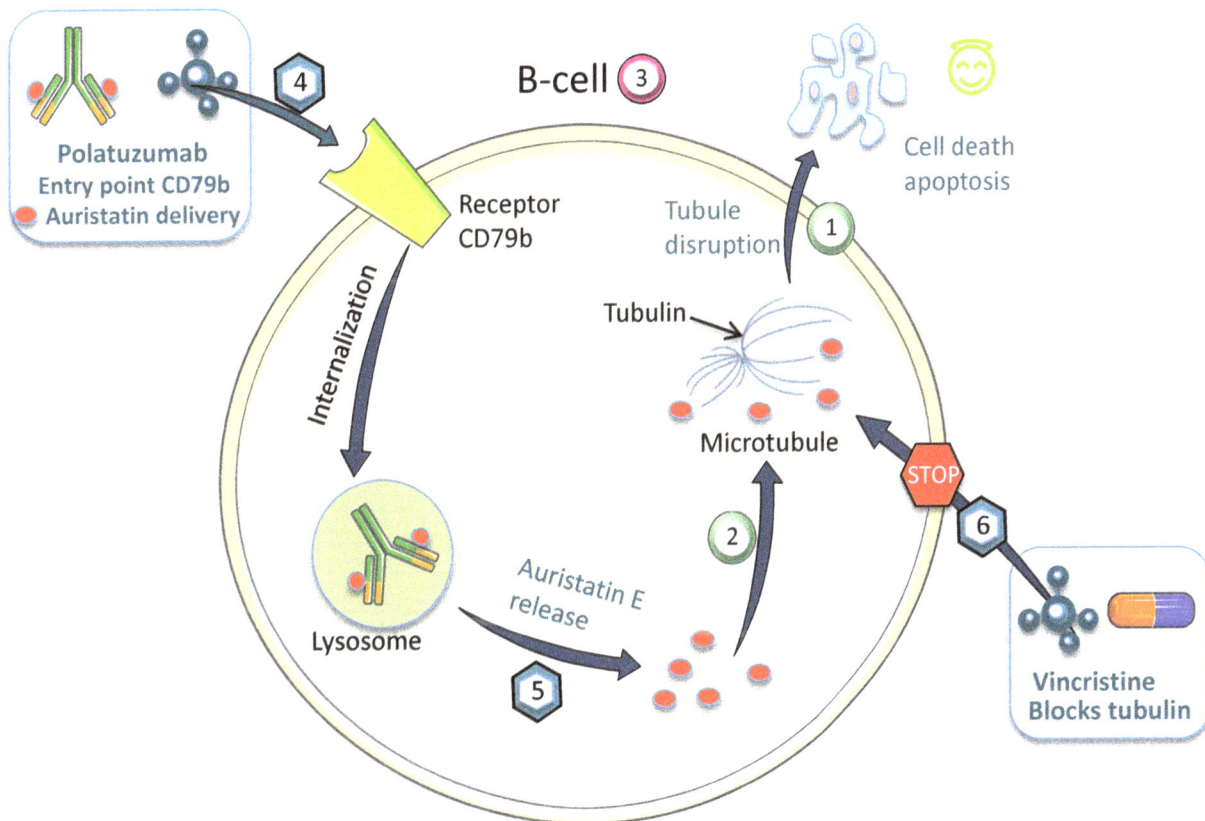

Polatuzumab
Entry point CD79b
Auristatin delivery
4
B-cell 3
Cell death
apoptosis
Receptor
CD79b
Tubule
disruption
1
Internalization
Tubulin
Microtubule
STOP
6
2
Lysosome
Auristatin E
release
5
Vincristine
Blocks tubulin

The disease: Multiple myeloma

Multiple myeloma is a cancer of plasma cells in which abnormal plasma cells multiply uncontrollably in the bone marrow.

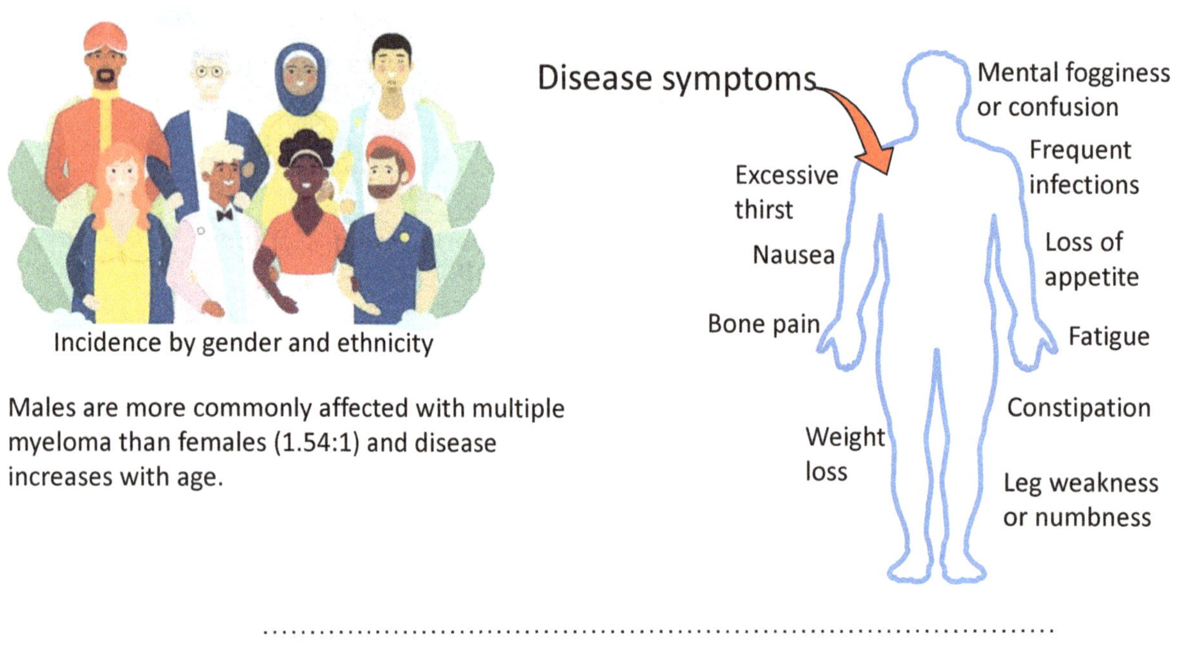

Incidence by gender and ethnicity

Males are more commonly affected with multiple myeloma than females (1.54:1) and disease increases with age.

The medicine

Selinexor; Xpovio, FDA Approval 2019

XPOVIO is used to treat multiple myeloma and is used **in combination with dexamethasone** (a corticosteroid) in patients with no other treatment options with refractory cancer.

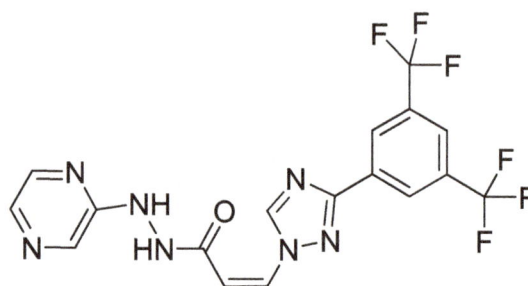

Action of Selinexor on cell and disease biology

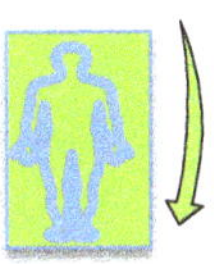

1 **Exportin 1 (XPO1)** is a nuclear protein, which is a chaperone and exports >250 proteins out the nucleus.

2 **XPO1 specifically exports and inactivates tumor suppressor proteins** (TSPs), which blocks tumor growth, such as tumor protein RB and p53.

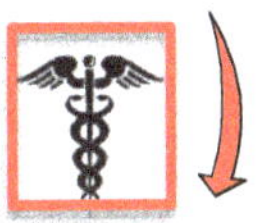

3 **Retinoblastoma protein (Rb)** is a TSP that prevents excessive cell growth by inhibiting cell cycle progression.

4 **Tumor protein p53** regulates cell division by keeping cells from growing in an uncontrolled way.

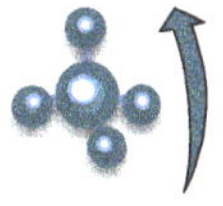

5 **Selinexor is an inhibitor of XPO1**, which results in the retention of multiple TSPs in the nucleus leading to tumor suppression and cell death.

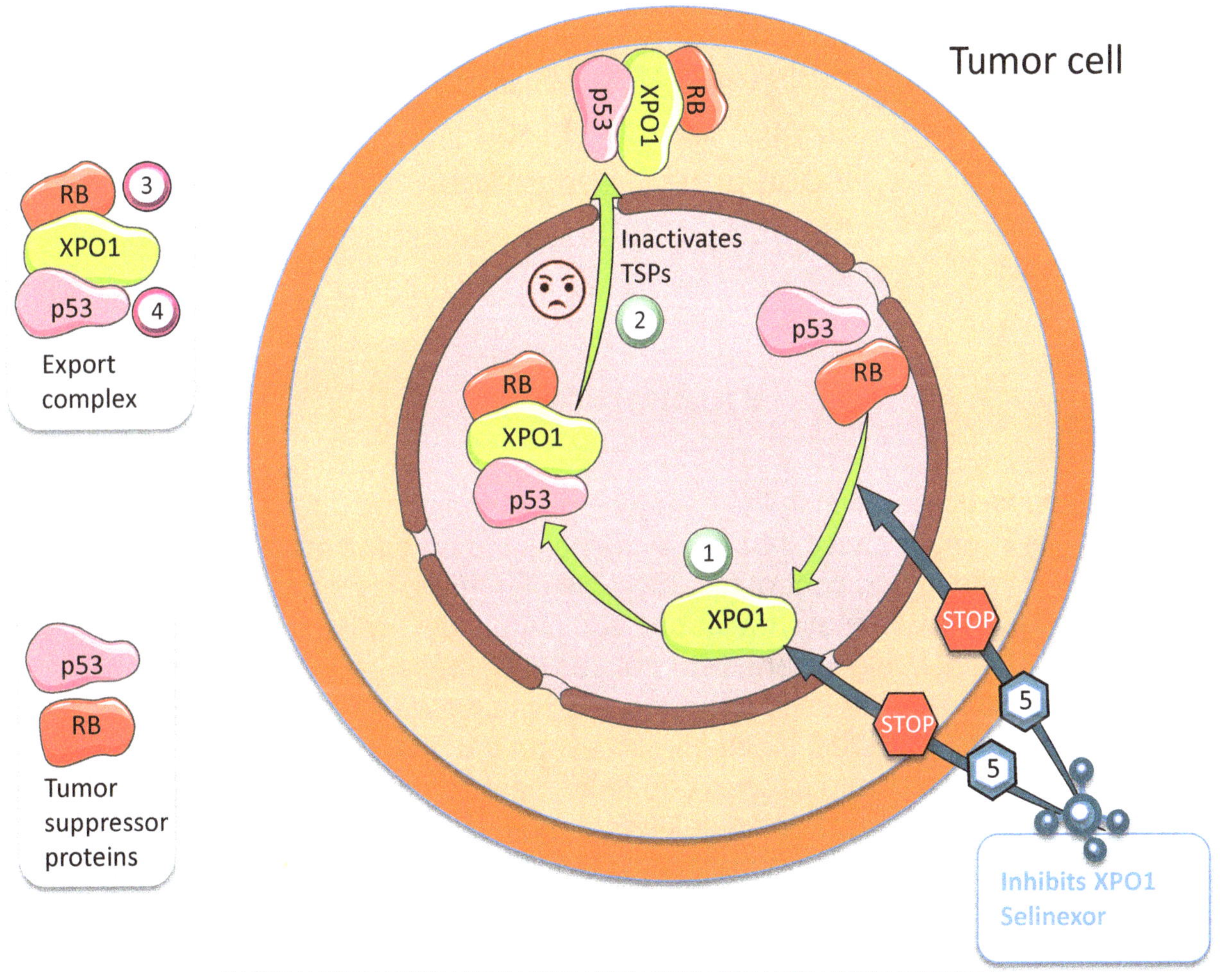

Tumor cell
RB
XPO1
p53
Export complex
p53
RB
Tumor suppressor proteins
Inactivates TSPs
STOP
STOP
Inhibits XPO1
Selinexor

Chapter 4 Homeostasis of the body's physiology

Physiological homeostasis is the maintenance of critical physiological parameters of the body's internal environment within a values set.

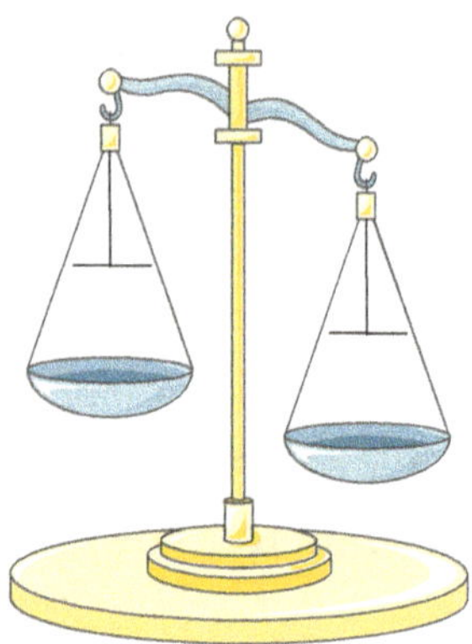

Body temperature regulation
Oxygen levels in blood
Blood pressure regulation
Regulation of blood glucose levels
Inflammation, aging, and cancer

Overview

Homeostasis is essential to the healthy functioning of the body and an imbalance in one of these intricate systems is the origin of many diseases. For example, in aging, the control mechanisms of homeostasis can operate at reduced efficiency. Genetic mutations and certain life styles can also result in diseases related to significant disturbances in homeostasis. This chapter will describe drugs that are used to treat prevalent diseases, namely, anemia, hypothyroidism, diabetes, blood pressure, and the disease cluster of inflammation, aging, and cancer. The drugs selected in this book represent both recently approved drugs resulting from medical innovations but are currently used in restricted patient groups and drugs, which have been the mainstay of healthcare for many years and are widely prescribed to the US population. Many of the drugs described in this chapter represent top selling brands for common diseases such as hypothyroidism, diabetes, blood pressure, and inflammation.

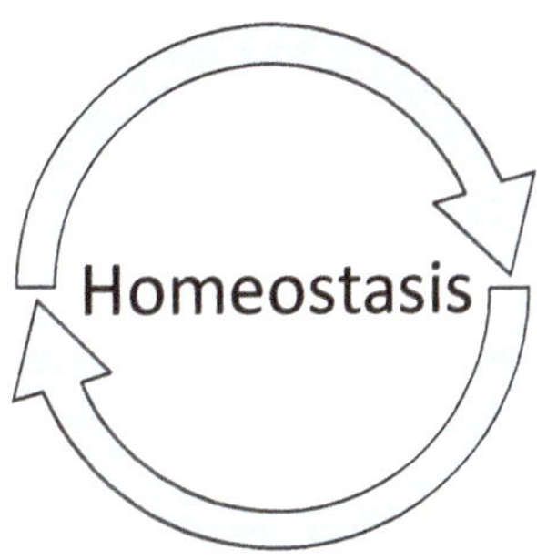

Figure: Selected drugs approved by the FDA.
✓ = Drugs approved recently (2007–2020) (Brand name)

Body metabolism
Hypothyroidism
- Synthroid

Blood oxygen levels
Anemia
- Epogen

Blood pressure
- Zestril
- Lopressor
- Norvasc
- Microzide

Blood glucose levels
Diabetes
- Lantus
- Jardiance
- Metformin
- Amaryl

Inflammation, aging, cancer
Inflammatory diseases
- Bayer 81
- Rayos

Rheumatoid arthritis
- Rinvoq ✓

Prostate cancer
- Erleada ✓

Bladder cancer
- Balversa ✓

Prostatic hyperplasia
- Flomax

Coronary artery disease
- Colcrys

Hormones are an important part of homeostasis acting as chemical messengers sent from cells throughout the body to regulate cells in other regions.

1 **Pineal gland** produces the hormone **melatonin**, regulates circadian rhythm and reproductive hormones.

2 **Pituitary gland and hypothalamus** are the **command and control centers**, directing hormones to other glands and throughout the body.

3 **Thyroid gland** regulates the **body's metabolism**, free calcium levels, and importantly energy levels, growth, development, and reproduction.

4 **Thymus gland** plays a central role with the production of progenitor cells, which mature into **T-cells** (thymus-derived cells).

5 **Adrenal glands** produce **epinephrine,** norepinephrine, regulate metabolism, immune system, blood pressure, **response to stress**.

6 **Pancreas** regulates **digestion and energy homeostasis** by releasing various digestive enzymes and pancreatic hormones such as **insulin and glucagon**.

7 **Ovary gland** secretes **estrogen and progesterone**, which act on skeletal muscle, liver, adipose tissue, decreases insulin secretion and sensitivity, and inflammation.

8 **Testis secretes testosterone** for production of new blood cells as well as maintenance of bone density and muscle mass.

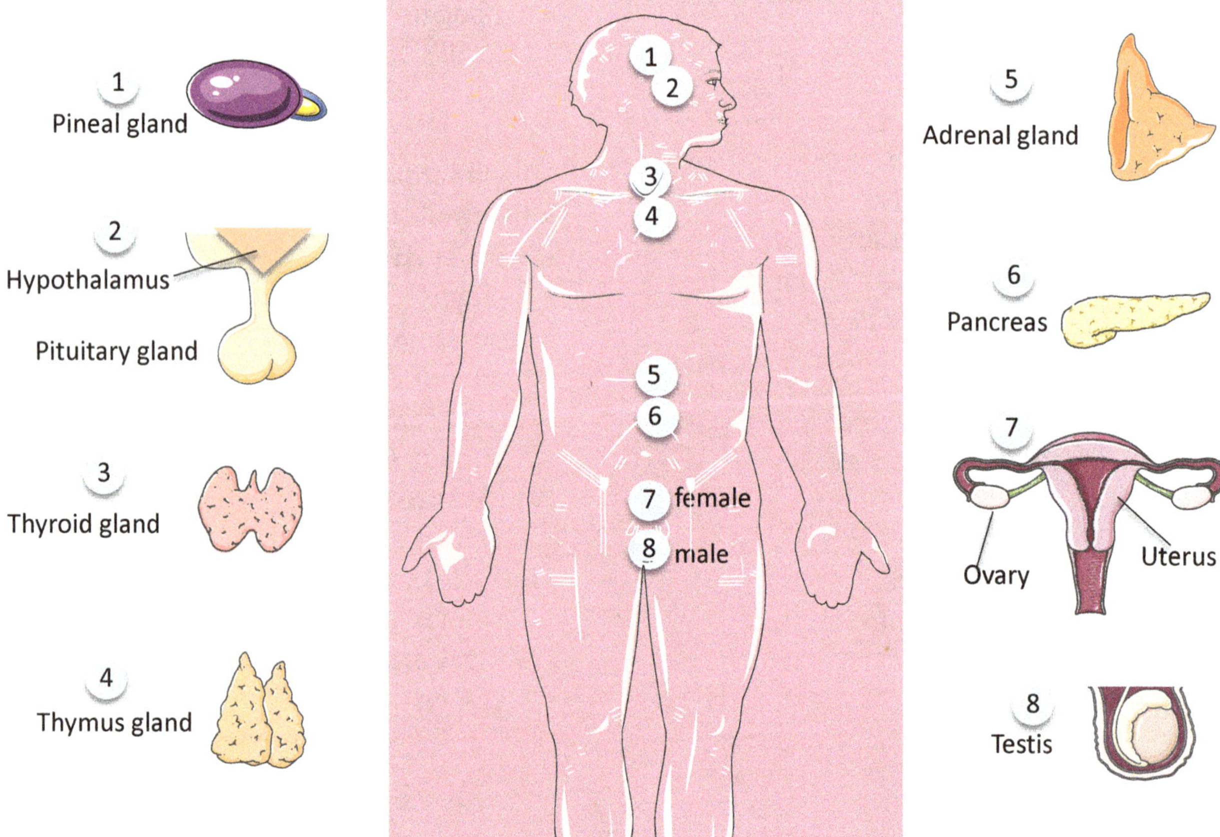

Introduction: The glands of the body and hormones

Homeostasis and body temperature

High temperatures will be detected by nerve cells with endings in your skin and brain and relayed to a **temperature-regulatory control center** in your brain.

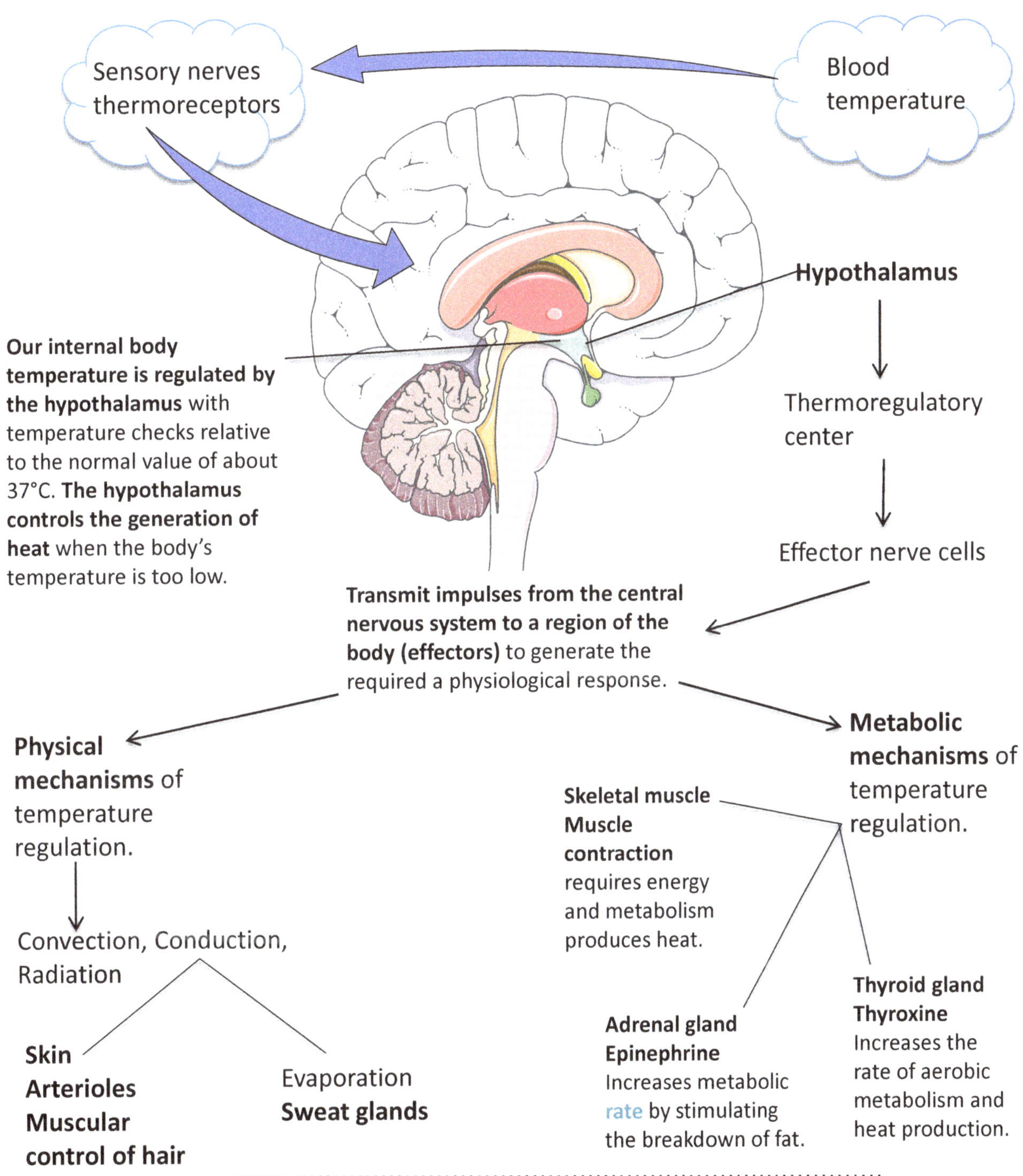
Sensory nerves thermoreceptors
Blood temperature
Hypothalamus
Thermoregulatory center
Effector nerve cells
Our internal body temperature is regulated by the hypothalamus with temperature checks relative to the normal value of about 37°C. **The hypothalamus controls the generation of heat** when the body's temperature is too low.
Transmit impulses from the central nervous system to a region of the body (effectors) to generate the required a physiological response.
Physical mechanisms of temperature regulation.
Metabolic mechanisms of temperature regulation.
Convection, Conduction, Radiation
Skin
Arterioles
Muscular control of hair
Evaporation
Sweat glands
Skeletal muscle
Muscle contraction requires energy and metabolism produces heat.
Adrenal gland
Epinephrine
Increases metabolic rate by stimulating the breakdown of fat.
Thyroid gland
Thyroxine
Increases the rate of aerobic metabolism and heat production.

Homeostasis: Body temperature

The disease: Hypothyroidism

Hypothyroidism is caused by **underactivity of the thyroid gland, inadequate** production of thyroid hormones (**T3 and T4**), and a slowing of vital body functions. The most **common** cause of hypothyroidism is an **autoimmune disorder** (Hashimoto's thyroiditis), as well as an iodine deficient diet, over-response to hyperthyroidism treatment, and surgery.

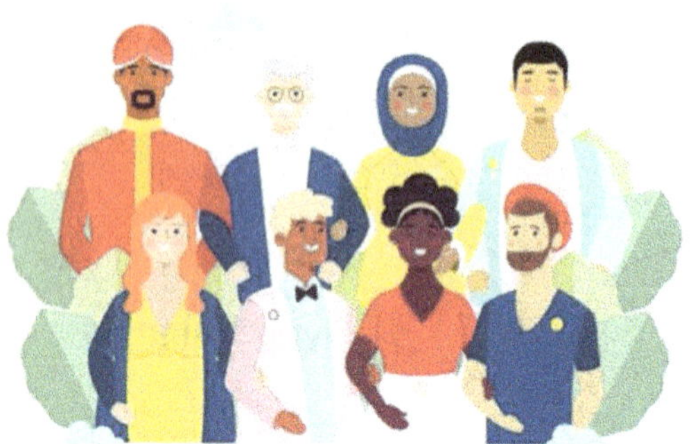

Incidence by gender and ethnicity

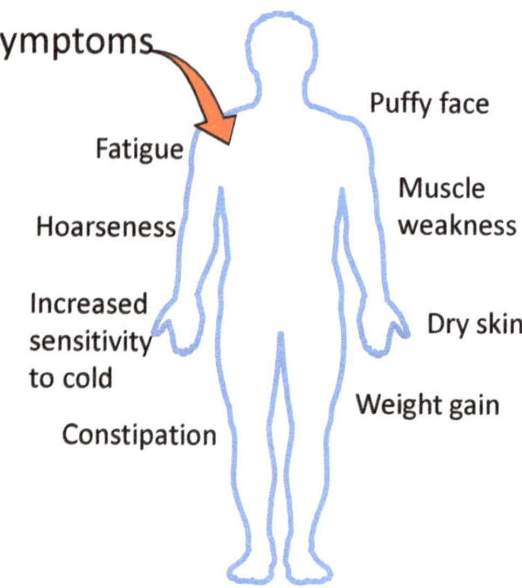

Thyroid disease is much more common in females than in males, ranging from 2 to 8 times higher prevalence. Hashimoto thyroiditis incidence is highest in whites and lowest in blacks and Asian/Pacific Islanders. The disease may occur in young women, but often develops at 30–50 years old.

The medicine

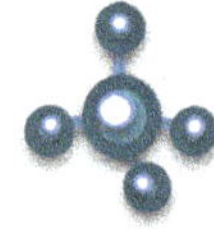

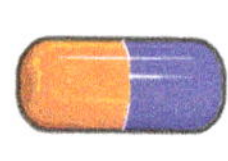

Second Most US Prescribed Drug, (2019), 103 million prescriptions

Levothyroxine; Synthroid, FDA Approval 2000

Synthroid (Levothyroxine) is a synthetic version of thyroxin (T4) and is used to **treat hypothyroidism** by replacing the thyroid gland hormone T4 and usually to be taken for life.

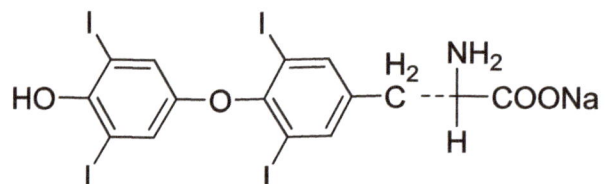

Temperature regulation, Hypothyroidism, Levothyroxine

1 **The hypothalamus** releases **thyrotropin-releasing hormone** to act on the anterior pituitary and secrete **thyroid-stimulating hormone** (TSH), which acts on the thyroid gland to release a mixture of **thyroxine**, T4 (80%), and **triiodothyronine**, T3 (20%), to **regulate basal metabolic rate**.

2 During circulation **T4 is converted to T3** by enzymatic **de-iodination** (via deiodinases [DI] in the liver and kidney).

3 **T3 and T4 act to increase the basal metabolic rate** of the body by regulating protein, fat, and carbohydrate metabolism, as well regulating development of the body's cells.

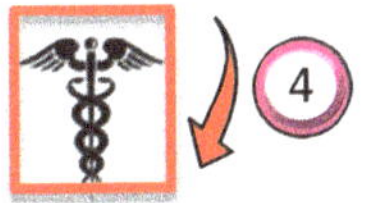

4 Hashimoto's thyroiditis is an **autoimmune disease** where antibodies attack and destroy the thyroid gland.

5 **Levothyroxine** is a synthetic version of T4.

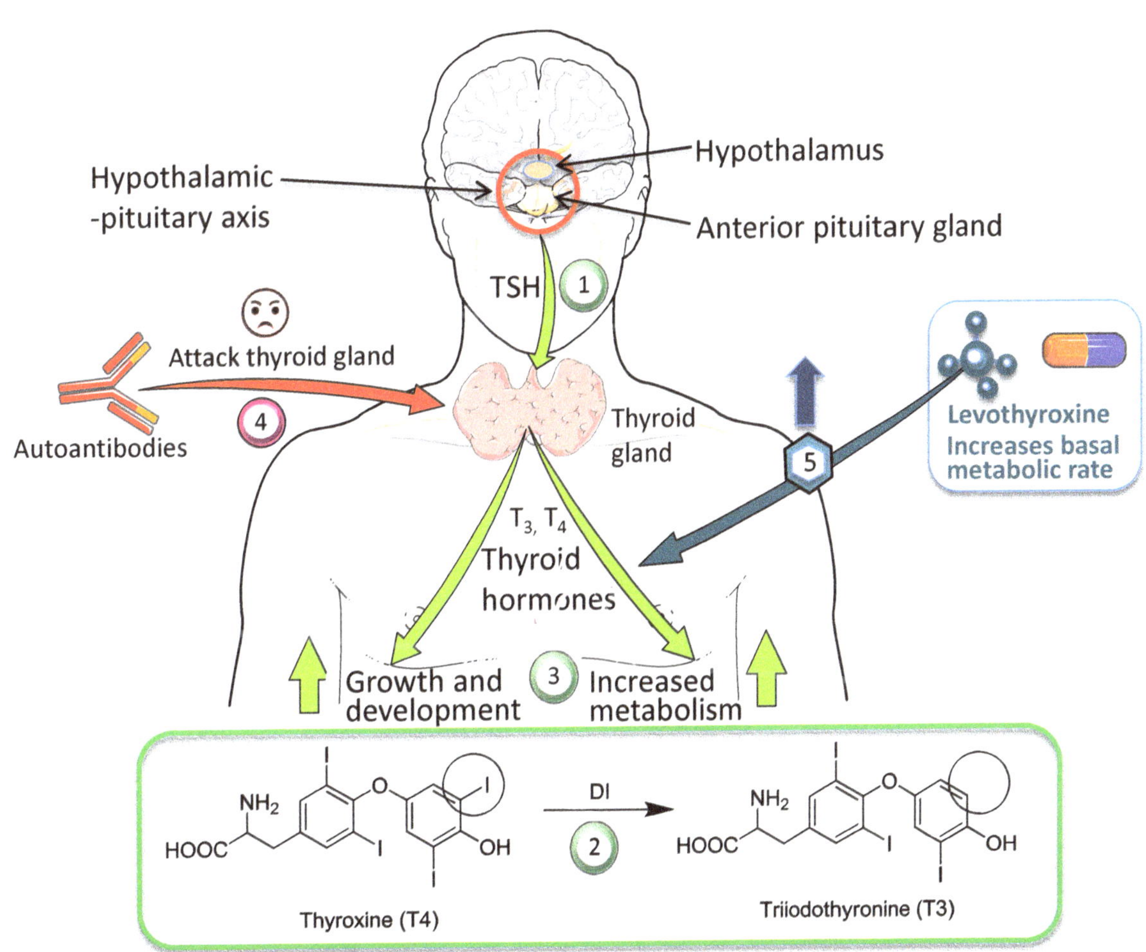

Temperature regulation, Hypothyroidism, Levothyroxine

Homeostasis—Oxygen levels in blood

Oxygen is tightly regulated within the body because below-normal level of oxygen in arteries can result in adverse effects on organ systems such as the brain, heart, and kidneys.

Below-normal level of oxygen in the blood

As an example, **toxin damage to the kidney or the bone marrow** interferes with the production of red blood cells with resulting anemia (low RBCs).

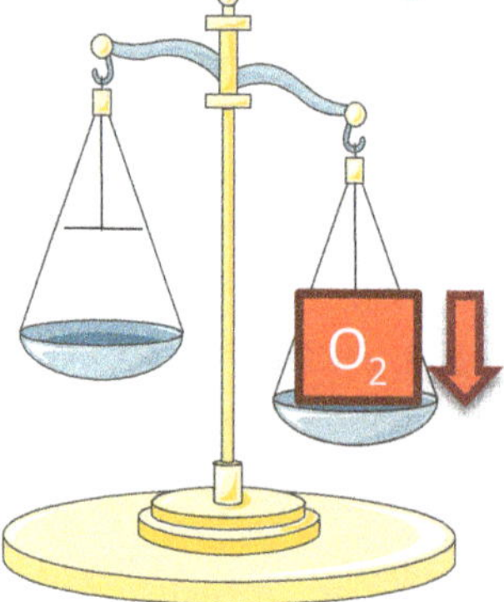

Reduced oxygen levels in circulation signals the kidney to produce and secrete erythropoietin (EPO) .

Increased oxygen levels

Stimulation of the bone marrow to increase red blood cells (RBCs) and hemoglobin will raise oxygen levels in the blood and other tissues.

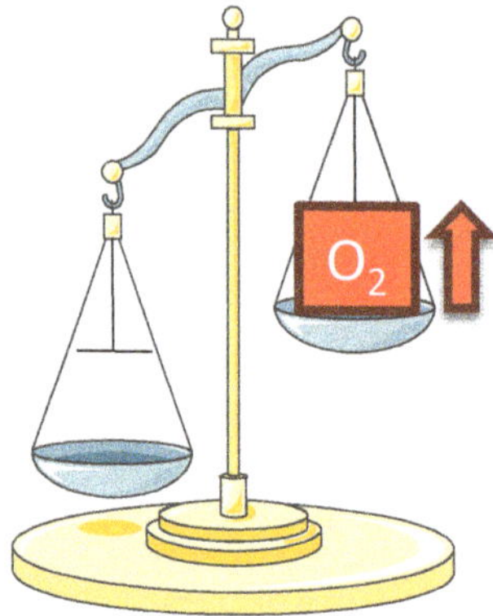

Raise oxygen levels in the blood and other tissues.

Restoring oxygen levels in blood

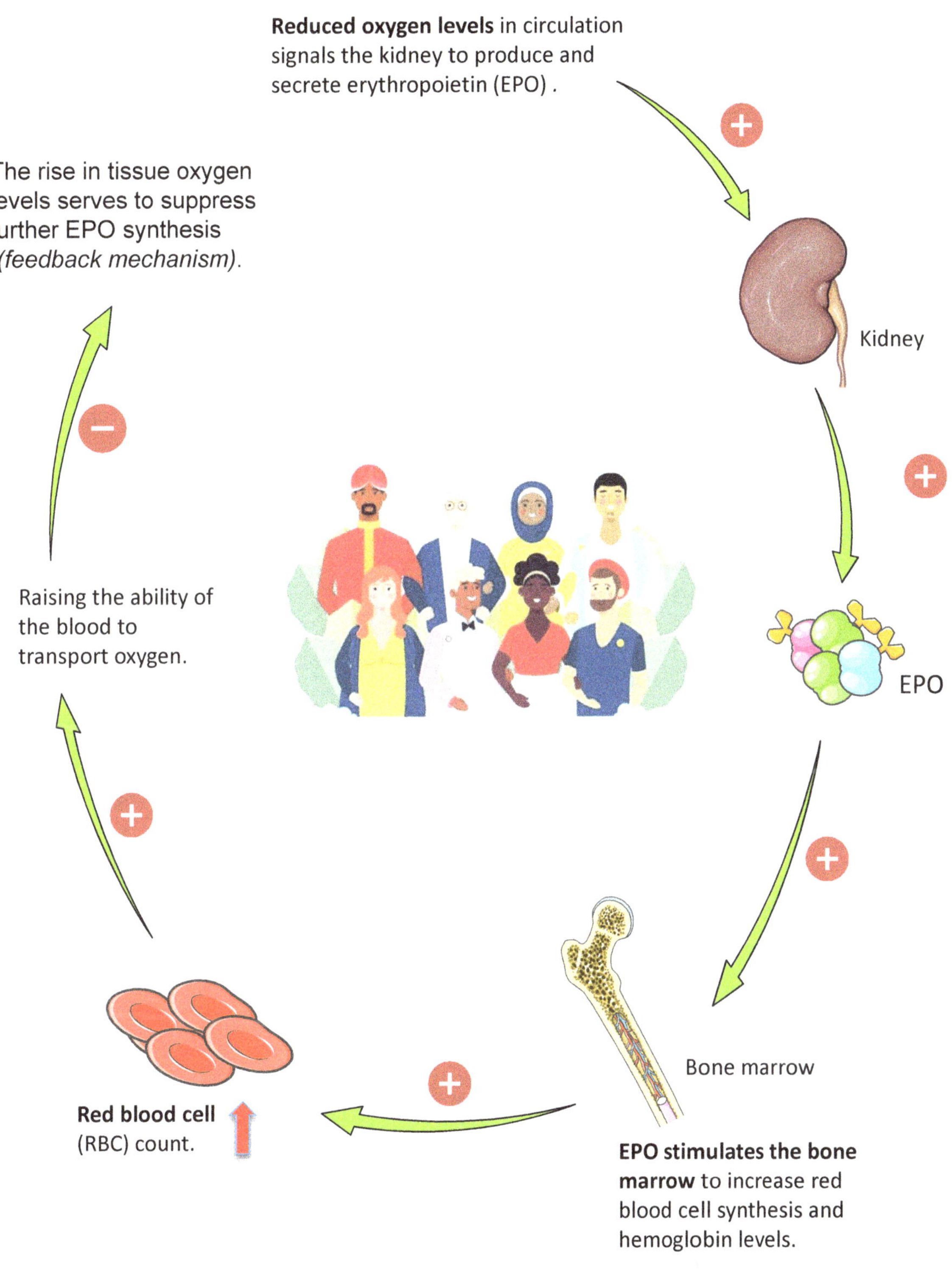

Reduced oxygen levels in circulation signals the kidney to produce and secrete erythropoietin (EPO) .
Kidney
EPO
Bone marrow
EPO stimulates the bone marrow to increase red blood cell synthesis and hemoglobin levels.
Red blood cell (RBC) count.
Raising the ability of the blood to transport oxygen.
The rise in tissue oxygen levels serves to suppress further EPO synthesis *(feedback mechanism)*.

The disease: Anemia

If the body does not produce enough Erythropoietin (EPO), severe anemia can occur (insufficient healthy red blood cells). Anemia results from chronic renal failure (dialysis) and immunosuppressive chemotherapy.

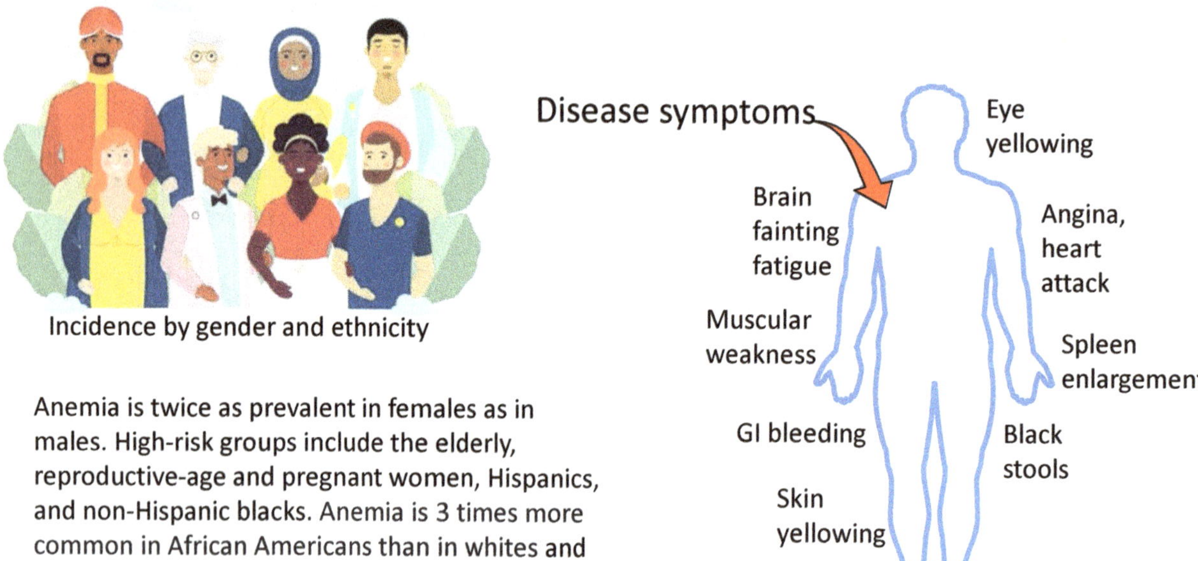

Incidence by gender and ethnicity

Anemia is twice as prevalent in females as in males. High-risk groups include the elderly, reproductive-age and pregnant women, Hispanics, and non-Hispanic blacks. Anemia is 3 times more common in African Americans than in whites and anemia was prevalent in Southeast Asia.

The medicine

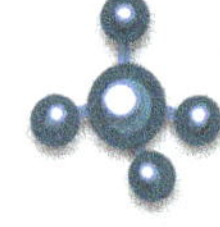

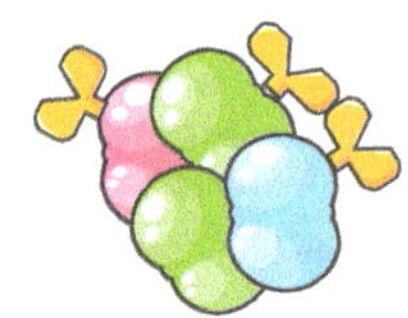

Epoetin alfa; Epogen, FDA Approval 1989

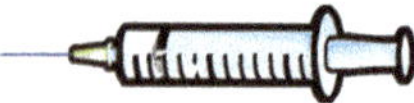

Administered as a subcutaneous injection

Epoetin alfa is used to **treat anemia** (low red blood cell count) in patients with long-term serious kidney disease (chronic kidney failure), or patients with some HIV and cancer chemotherapy treatments.

Erythropoietin (EPO) is a glycoprotein made by **recombinant manufacturing** in a hamster cell line (CHO). These cells allow the production of a biosynthetic hormone with glycan side chains highly similar to the natural human form.

Oxygen levels: Anemia, Epoetin alfa

Action of Epoetin alfa on cell and disease biology

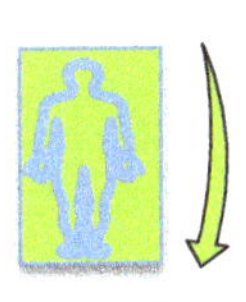
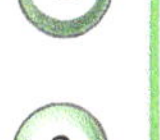

1 **Erythropoietin** (EPO) is **produced** primarily in the **kidney,** circulates in blood, and binds to cell-surface **receptors** in the **bone marrow**.

2 **EPO** controls **red blood cell (RBC) production** by regulating differentiation and proliferation of erythroid progenitor cells in bone marrow.

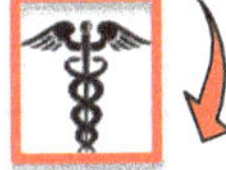
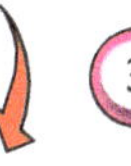

3 **Insufficient** production by renal **EPO-producing cells** causes renal **anemia** and anemia associated with chronic disorders.

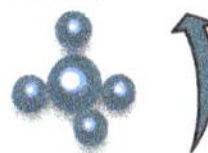

4 **Epoetin stimulates** the **bone marrow** to produce red blood cells.

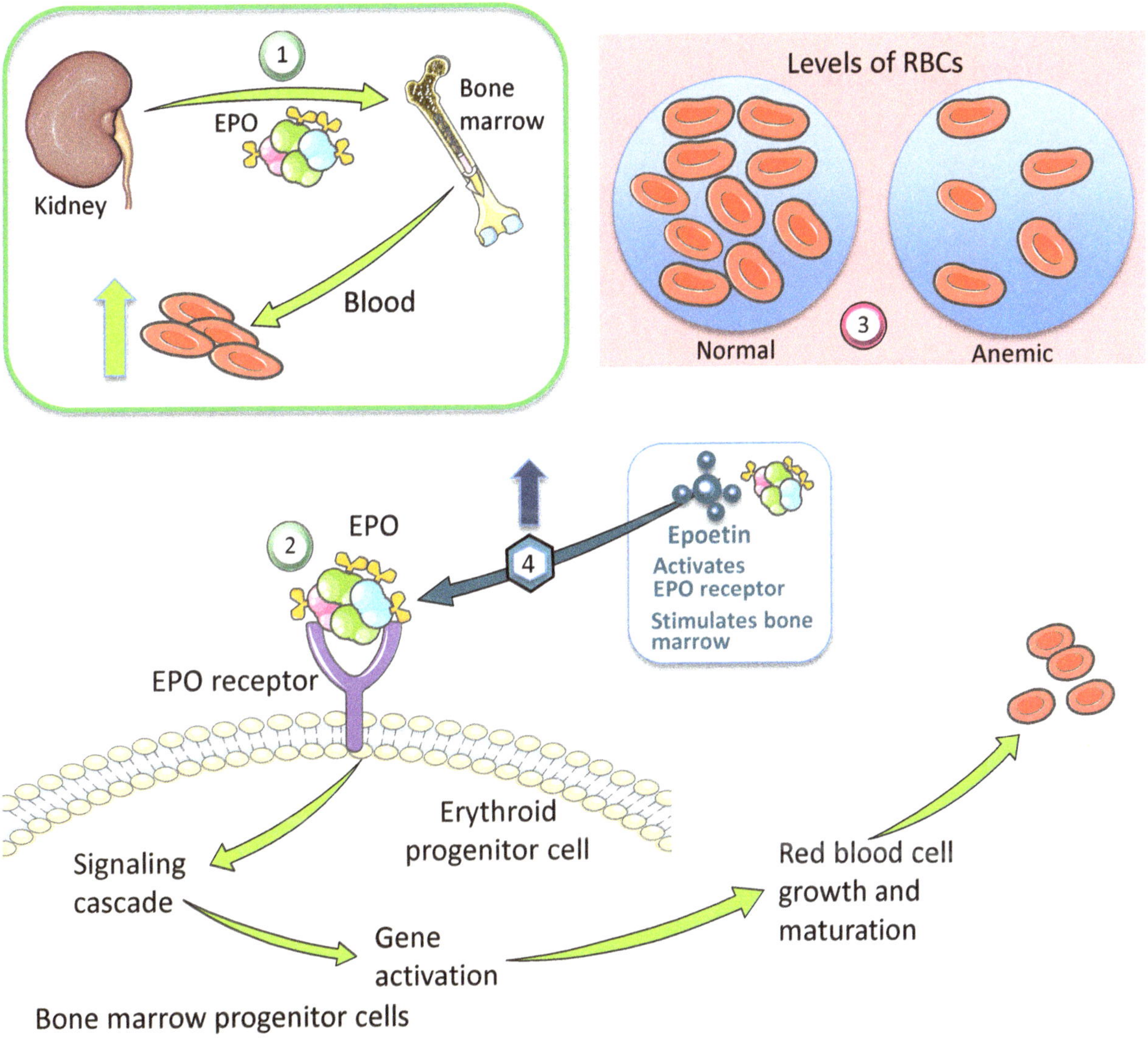

1
EPO
Kidney
Bone marrow
Blood

Levels of RBCs
Normal
3
Anemic

EPO
2
EPO receptor
4
Epoetin
Activates EPO receptor
Stimulates bone marrow
Erythroid progenitor cell
Signaling cascade
Gene activation
Red blood cell growth and maturation
Bone marrow progenitor cells

Oxygen levels: Anemia, Epoetin alfa

Homeostasis—Regulate the body's blood pressure

Blood pressure is a powerful example of homeostasis, which needs to be **tightly controlled** within a narrow range via a feedback loop to ensure adequate blood flow to organs throughout the body.

Amount of blood pumped

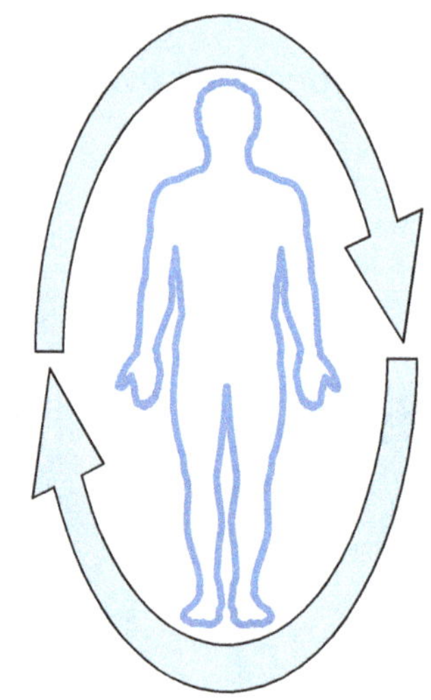

Arterial resistance

The pressure is determined by the **amount of blood pumped** and **resistance to the flow in the arteries**. A greater blood flow and narrower arteries will raise blood pressure.

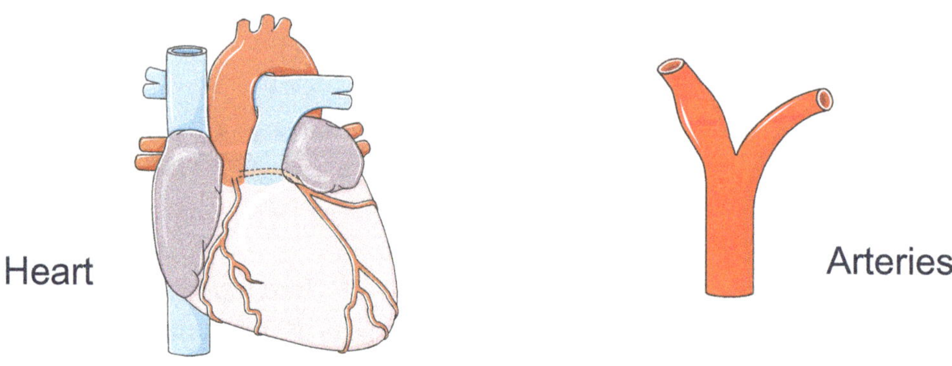

Homeostasis: Blood pressure control

Regulation of blood pressure

1 **The brain stem** (midbrain, pons, and medulla oblongata) controls the flow of messages between the brain and the rest of the body and helps **regulate breathing, heart rate, blood pressure**.

2 **Arterial blood pressure control is accomplished by negative feedback systems** incorporating pressure sensors (baroreceptors), which are mainly located in the neck (carotid sinus).

5 **Epinephrine binds to the alpha- and beta-receptors** to constrict the arteries and increase the heart contractile force and heart rate.

3 **If blood pressure decreases, the kidneys decrease their excretion of sodium and water,** so that blood volume increases and blood pressure returns to normal.

3 **The kidneys maintain the body's fluid balance** by regulating the **chemical balance of the blood** (sodium, potassium, and calcium). The kidneys regulate blood pressure by **removing waste products** and **excess water**.

4 **The renin–angiotensin–aldosterone system** (RAAS) regulates blood pressure and fluid and electrolyte balance.

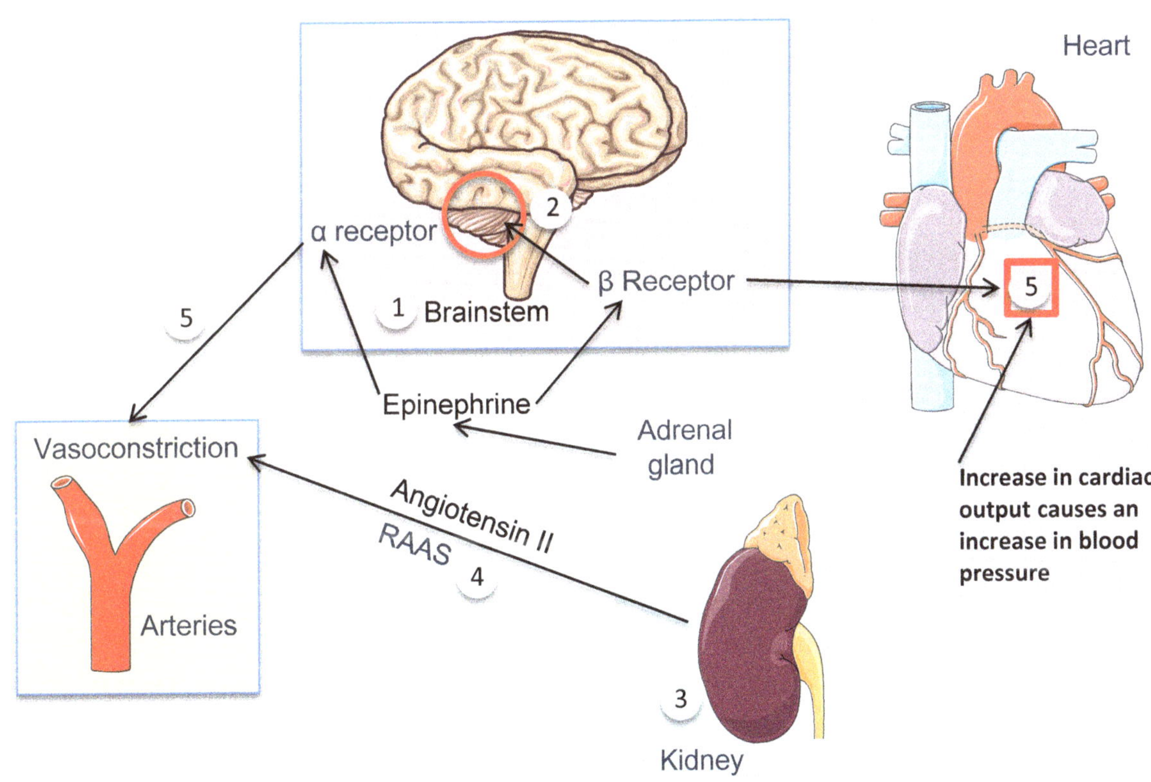

Homeostasis: Blood pressure control

The disease: Hypertension

Hypertension or high blood pressure is a long-term medical condition in which the **blood pressure** of the arteries is persistently **elevated.**

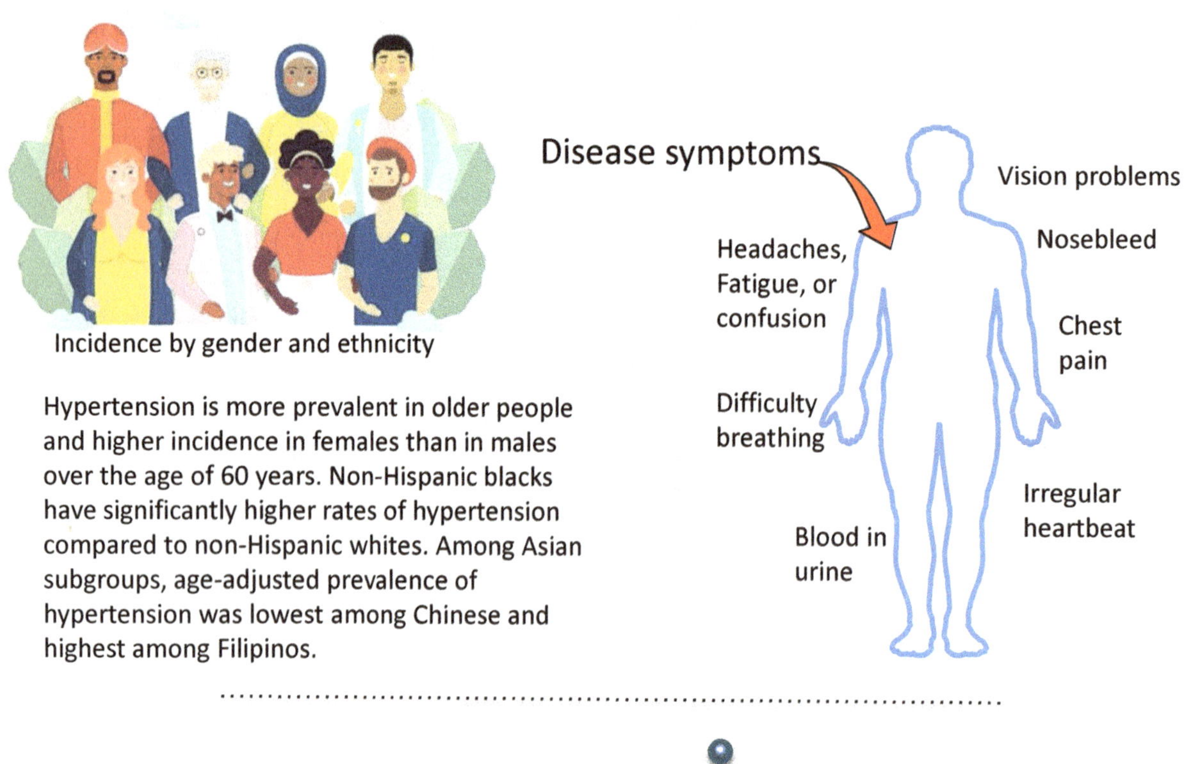

Incidence by gender and ethnicity

Hypertension is more prevalent in older people and higher incidence in females than in males over the age of 60 years. Non-Hispanic blacks have significantly higher rates of hypertension compared to non-Hispanic whites. Among Asian subgroups, age-adjusted prevalence of hypertension was lowest among Chinese and highest among Filipinos.

The medicine

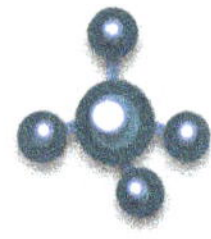

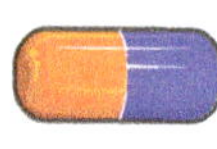

Third Most US Prescribed Drug, (2019), 91.9 million prescriptions

Lisinopril; Zestril, FDA Approval 1987

Lisinopril lowers blood pressure by **relaxing blood vessels** and **increasing blood flow** and oxygen supply to the heart.

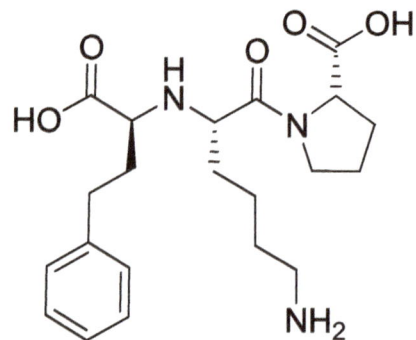

Blood pressure: Hypertension, Lisinopril

1 **Reduced renal blood pressure** or flow, **releases renin** from the kidneys to produce Angiotensin I (ATI) from angiotensinogen in the liver.

2 **Angiotensin-converting enzyme (ACE)** from the kidney catalyzes the conversion of ATI to the **vasoconstrictor** Angiotensin II (**AT II).**

3 **Angiotensin II** raises blood pressure by **narrowing of blood vessels** by smooth muscle cells (vasoconstriction).

4 **Angiotensin II** stimulates **aldosterone secretion** by the adrenal cortex to cause the renal tubules of the **kidney** to increase **reabsorption of sodium and water** coupled to potassium excretion.

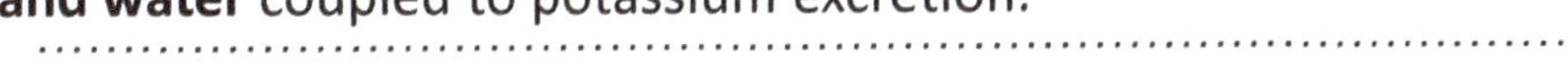

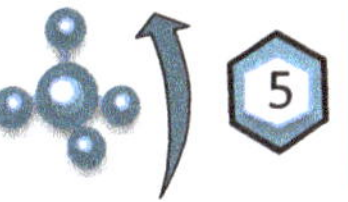

5 **Lisinopril inhibits ACE** and production of angiotensin II and results **in lower aldosterone secretion** due to a decrease in angiotensin II levels .

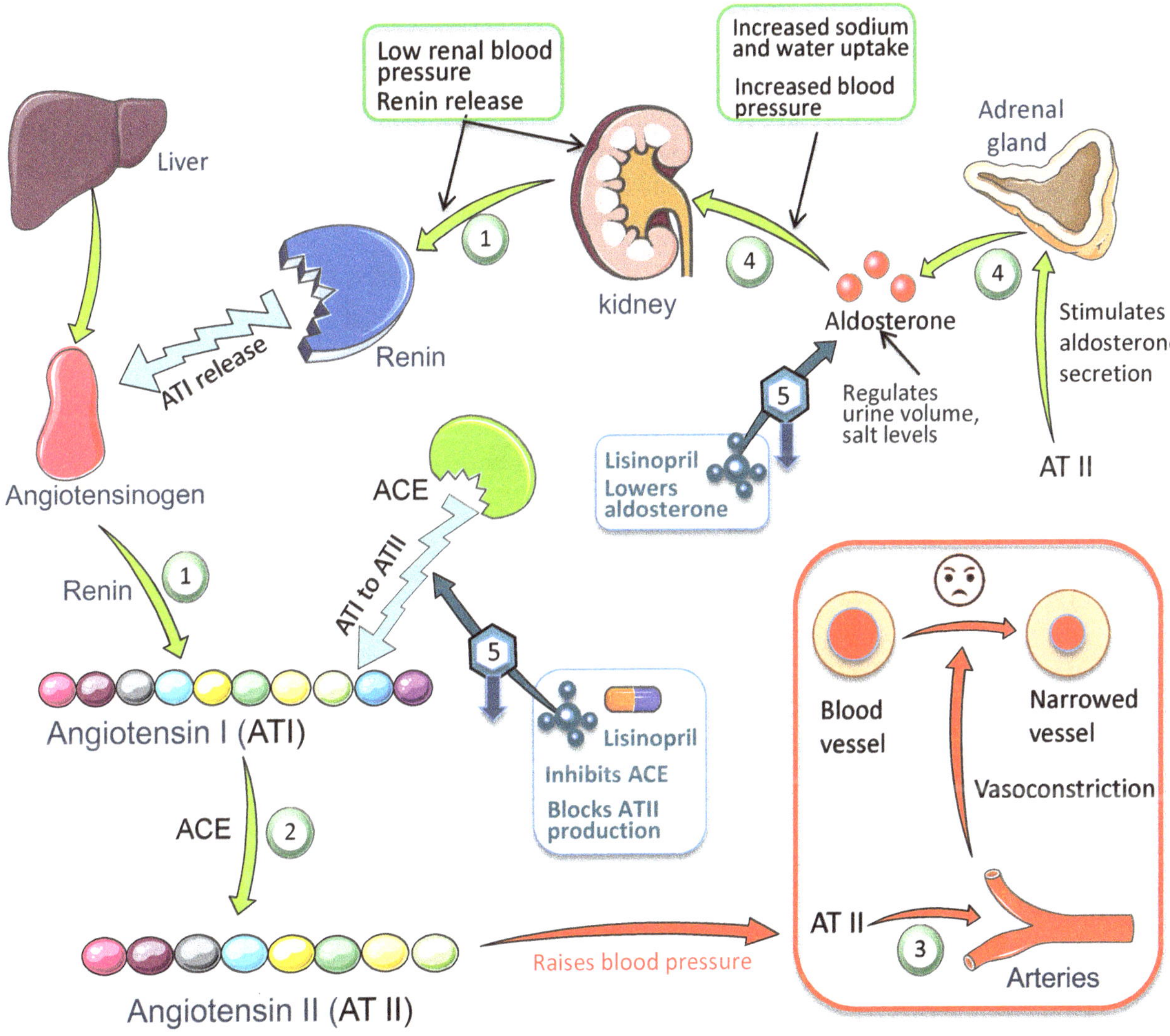

Low renal blood pressure
Renin release
Increased sodium and water uptake
Increased blood pressure
Liver
Adrenal gland
kidney
Renin
ATI release
Aldosterone
Stimulates aldosterone secretion
Regulates urine volume, salt levels
AT II
Lisinopril Lowers aldosterone
Angiotensinogen
ACE
ATI to ATII
Renin
Angiotensin I (ATI)
Lisinopril
Inhibits ACE
Blocks ATII production
Blood vessel
Narrowed vessel
Vasoconstriction
ACE
AT II
Arteries
Raises blood pressure
Angiotensin II (AT II)

The disease: High blood pressure

High blood pressure with **associated chest pain** due to **poor blood flow to the heart**, and other heart conditions, which involve an abnormally fast heart rate.

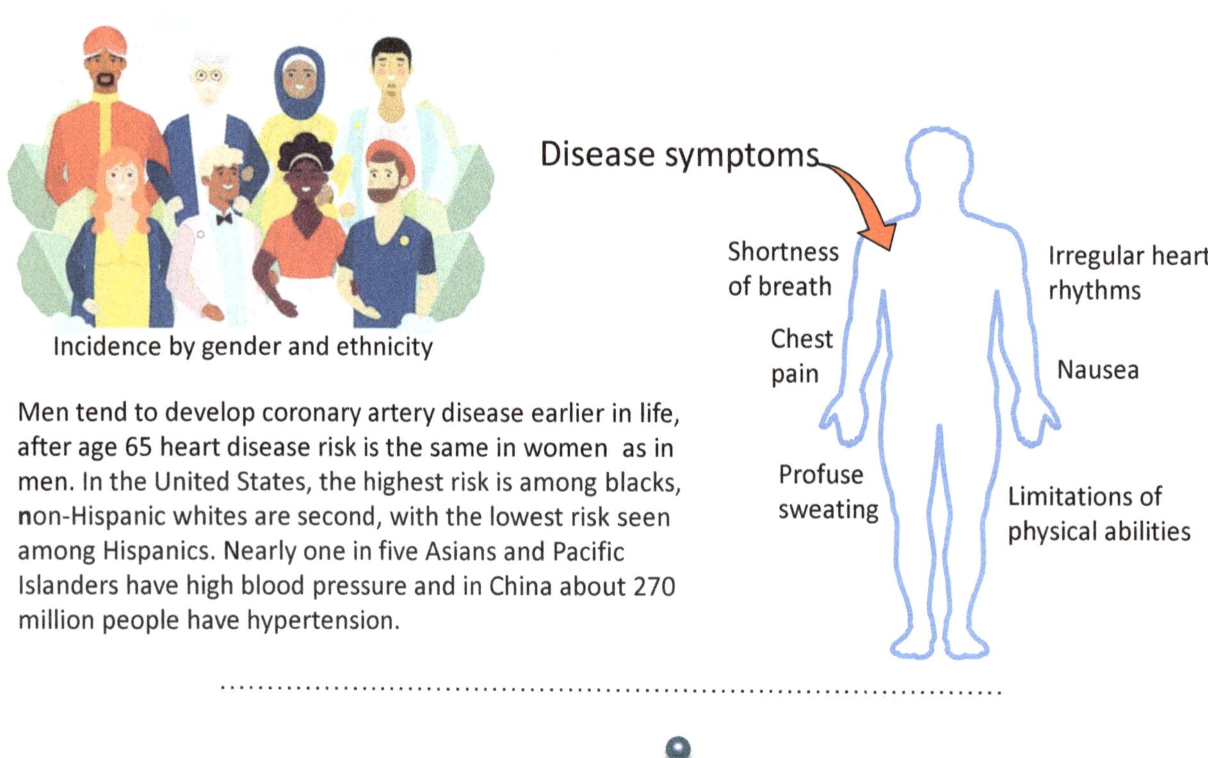

Incidence by gender and ethnicity

Men tend to develop coronary artery disease earlier in life, after age 65 heart disease risk is the same in women as in men. In the United States, the highest risk is among blacks, **n**on-Hispanic whites are second, with the lowest risk seen among Hispanics. Nearly one in five Asians and Pacific Islanders have high blood pressure and in China about 270 million people have hypertension.

The medicine

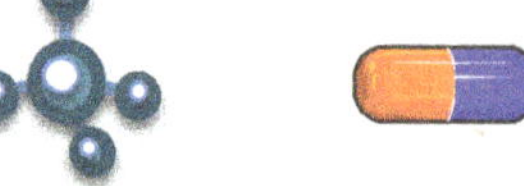

Fifth Most US Prescribed Drug, (2019) 74.6 million prescriptions

Metoprolol; Lopressor, FDA Approval 1982

Metoprolol is a beta-blocker that causes the heart to beat more slowly with less force which **lowers blood pressure** and also used to treat angina. Metoprolol provides relief of hypertension for patients with complications from myocardial infarction, ischemic heart disease, or congestive heart failure.

OH H N CH_3 CH_3 O H_3CO

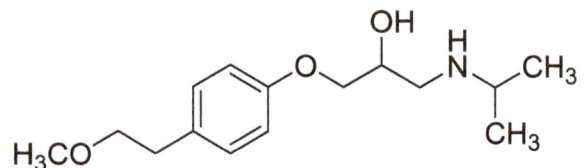

Blood pressure: Hypertension, Metoprolol

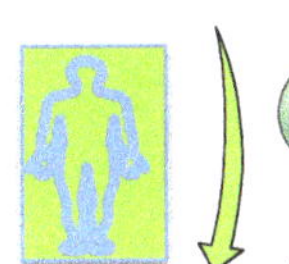

1 The **beta-1 adrenergic receptor** is the dominant receptor for heart function, **activated** by the hormone **epinephrine** (EPI, adrenal gland).

2 Beta-1 receptor activation **increases muscular firing of the heart**, heart rate, and contractility with increased stroke volume and cardiac output.

3 **G-proteins** activate ATP-derived signaling that causes **increased calcium entry** into the cells, **release of calcium** by the **sarcoplasmic reticulum** in heart muscle cells, resulting in **contraction of the myocyte**.

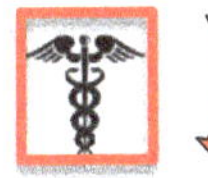

4 **Heart conditions** such as heart failure, thickening of the heart muscle can be caused by **high blood pressure** (heart working under increased pressure).

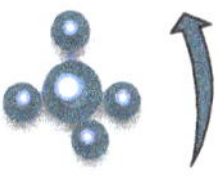

5 **Metoprolol blocks** binding of **epinephrine** to the beta-1 adrenergic receptor, relaxing blood vessel smooth muscles and lowering blood pressure.

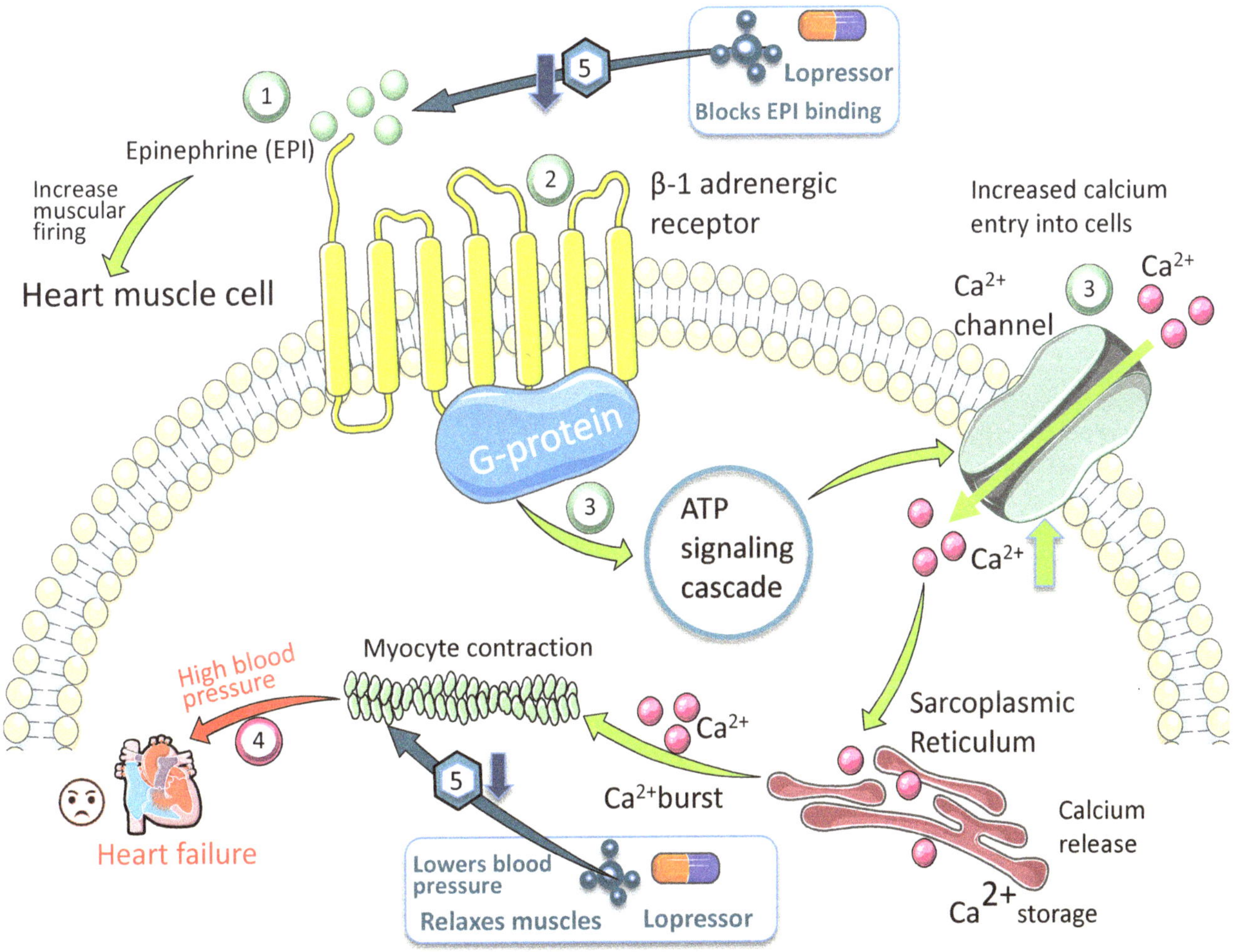

5 Lopressor
Blocks EPI binding
1 Epinephrine (EPI)
Increase muscular firing
Heart muscle cell
2 β-1 adrenergic receptor
G-protein
Increased calcium entry into cells
Ca^{2+} channel
3 Ca^{2+}
3 ATP signaling cascade
Ca^{2+}
Myocyte contraction
High blood pressure
4
Heart failure
Ca^{2+}
Ca^{2+}burst
Sarcoplasmic Reticulum
Calcium release
Ca^{2+} storage
5
Lowers blood pressure
Relaxes muscles
Lopressor

The disease: High blood pressure

Uncontrolled high blood pressure can **cause damage to arteries** and decreased flow of blood and oxygen to the heart with resulting **chest pain** (angina) and heart failure.

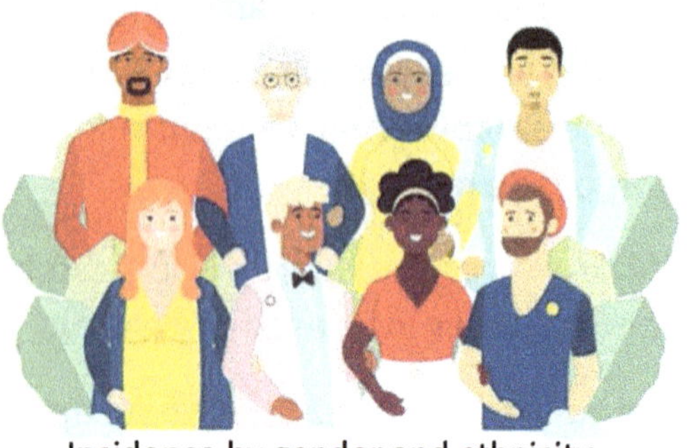

Incidence by gender and ethnicity

Men tend to develop coronary artery disease earlier in life, after age 65 heart disease risk is the same in women as in men. In the United States. the highest risk is among blacks, non-Hispanic whites are second, with the lowest risk seen among Hispanics. Nearly one in five Asians and Pacific Islanders have high blood pressure and in China, about 270 million people have hypertension.

Disease symptoms

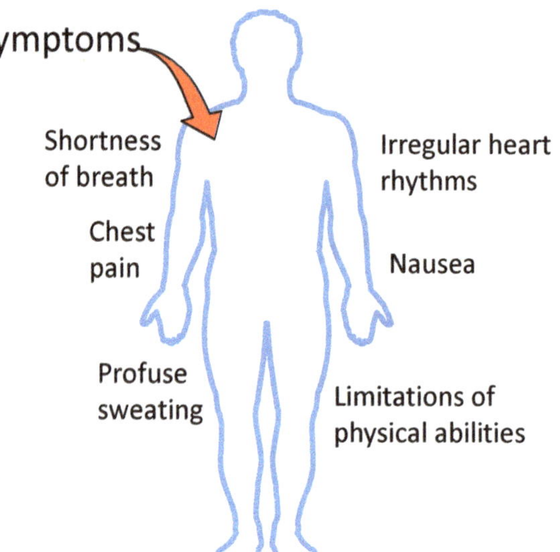

The medicine

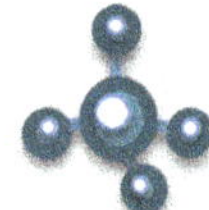

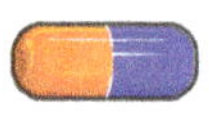

Sixth Most US Prescribed Drug (2019), 73.5 million prescriptions

Amlodipine; Norvasc, FDA Approval 1992

Amlodipine is used to treat high blood pressure (hypertension) and to treat chest pain (angina) and other conditions caused by coronary artery disease. **Amlodipine** is a **long acting calcium channel blocker** that **dilates** the main coronary and systemic arteries with **increased blood flow** and oxygen delivery to the myocardial tissue, and **decreased total peripheral resistance.**

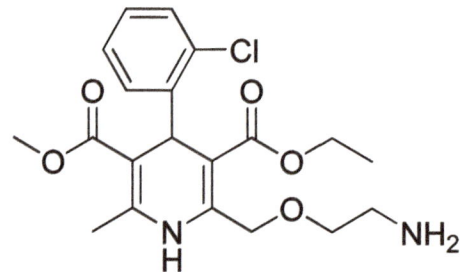

Cl O O O O O N H NH_2

Blood pressure: Hypertension, Amlodipine

Action of Amlodipine on cell and disease biology

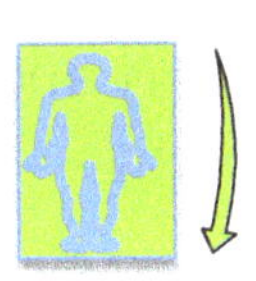

1 The L (long-lasting activation)-type high-voltage-activated **calcium channel** in **cardiac and smooth muscle cells and dihydropyridine (DHP) receptor**

2 functions as the **voltage sensor** for the Ca^{2+} channel.

Calcium channel blockers (CCBs) act as **potent vasodilators** because of their ability to bind to and block the L-type calcium channel.

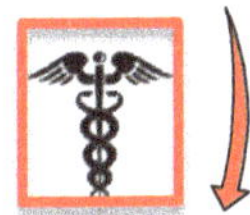

3 With high blood pressure the heart works harder to pump blood, **heart muscle thickens,** muscles may not get enough oxygen causing **angina** (chest pain), the heart can weaken over time leading to **heart failure.**

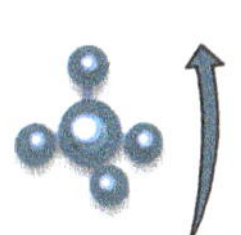

Amlodipine penetrates the plasma membrane to **inhibit the DHP receptor,** blocks the influx of extracellular calcium ions into smooth muscle cells, induces long-lasting channel closings which **results in relaxation of smooth muscle** cell muscles and **dilation of the blood vessel walls.**

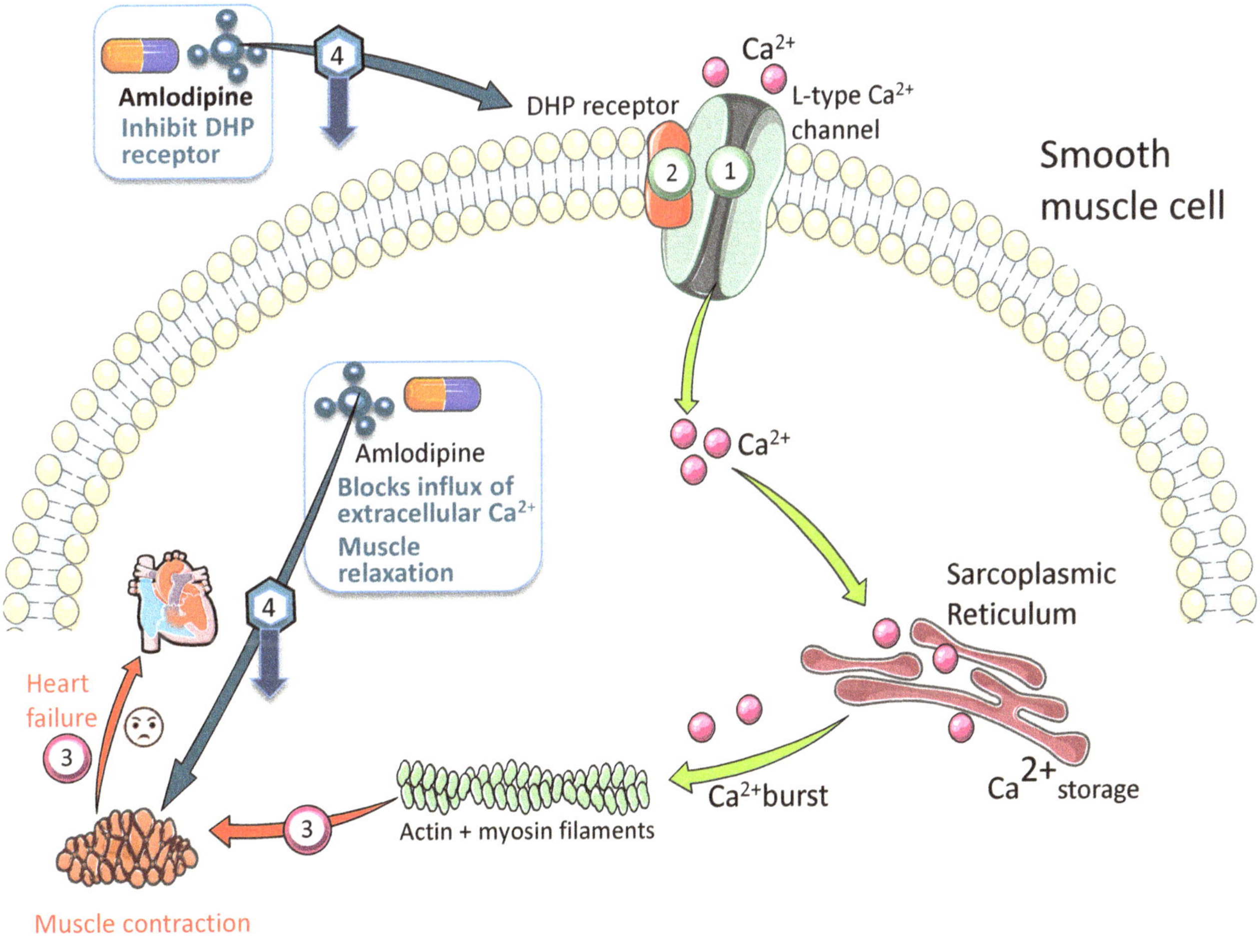

Amlodipine
Inhibit DHP receptor
4
DHP receptor
Ca^{2+}
L-type Ca^{2+} channel
2
1
Smooth muscle cell
Amlodipine
Blocks influx of extracellular Ca^{2+}
Muscle relaxation
Ca^{2+}
Sarcoplasmic Reticulum
4
Heart failure
3
Ca^{2+}burst
Ca^{2+} storage
3
Actin + myosin filaments
Muscle contraction

Blood pressure: Hypertension, Amlodipine

The disease: High blood pressure

Hypertension increases **risk of serious health problems** including heart failure, coronary and peripheral artery disease, stroke, kidney, and liver disease and hypertensive retinopathy.

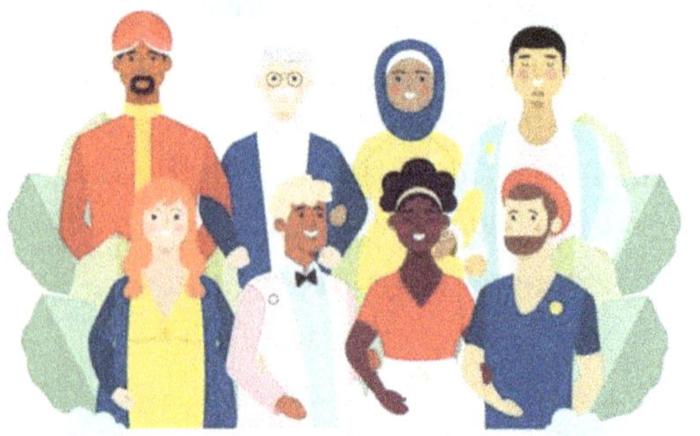

Incidence by gender and ethnicity

Men tend to develop coronary artery disease earlier in life, after age 65 heart disease risk is the same in women as in men. In the United States, the highest risk is among blacks, non-Hispanic whites are second, with the lowest risk seen among Hispanics. Nearly one in five Asians and Pacific Islanders have high blood pressure and in China, about 270 million people have hypertension.

Disease symptoms

Shortness of breath

Chest pain

Profuse sweating

Irregular heart rhythms

Nausea

Limitations of physical abilities

The medicine

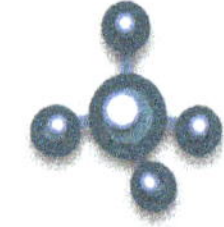

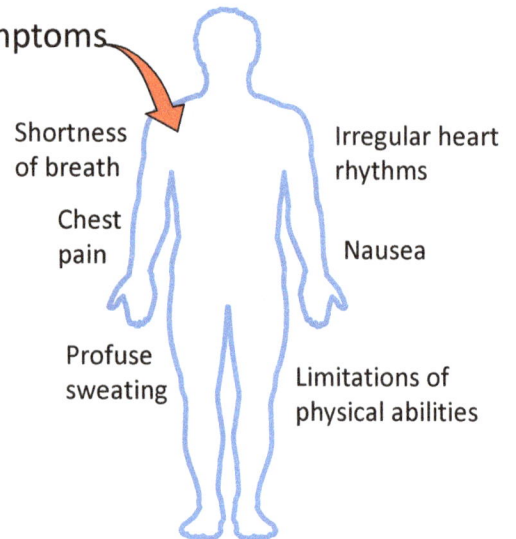

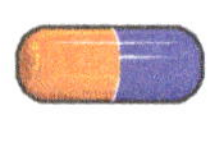

11th Most US Prescribed Drug (2019), 38.6 million prescriptions

Hydrochlorothiazide; Microzide, FDA Approval 1982

Hydrochlorothiazide (HCTZ) is used to treat hypertension, fluid retention in congestive heart failure, cirrhosis of the liver, or kidney disorders. **Hydrochlorothiazide lowers peripheral vascular resistance** and **inhibits vasoconstriction** by depletion of blood volume.

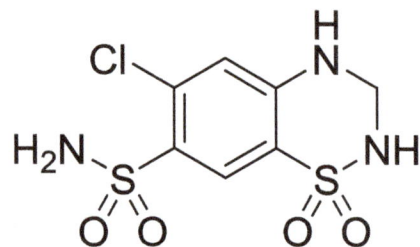

Blood pressure: Hypertension, Hydrochlorothiazide

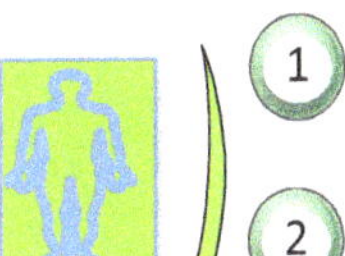

1. **Bulk reabsorption** of water as well as 60%–70% of total Na^{+} back into the plasma occurs from the **proximal tubule**.
2. The **NaCl cotransporter** (epithelial cell plasma membrane) **reabsorbs sodium and chloride ions** from tubular fluid into cells of the distal tubule.

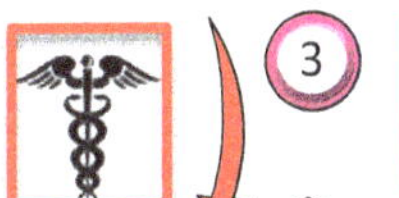

3. A **salt increase** causes **constriction of blood vessels**, expands blood volume by retaining fluids. High dietary sodium damages the endothelial layer.

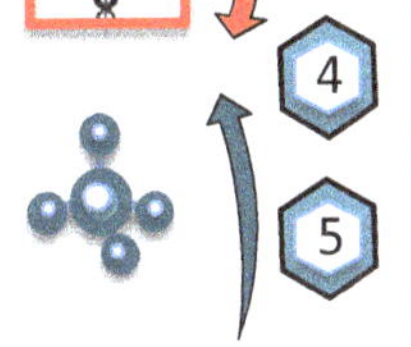

4. **Thiazides** increase urine output by **NaCl cotransporter inhibition** (chloride site competition), an increase in sodium excretion, reduced reabsorption.
5. **HCTZ** acts by **decreasing** the **kidneys' ability to retain water,** reducing blood volume and blood return to the heart.

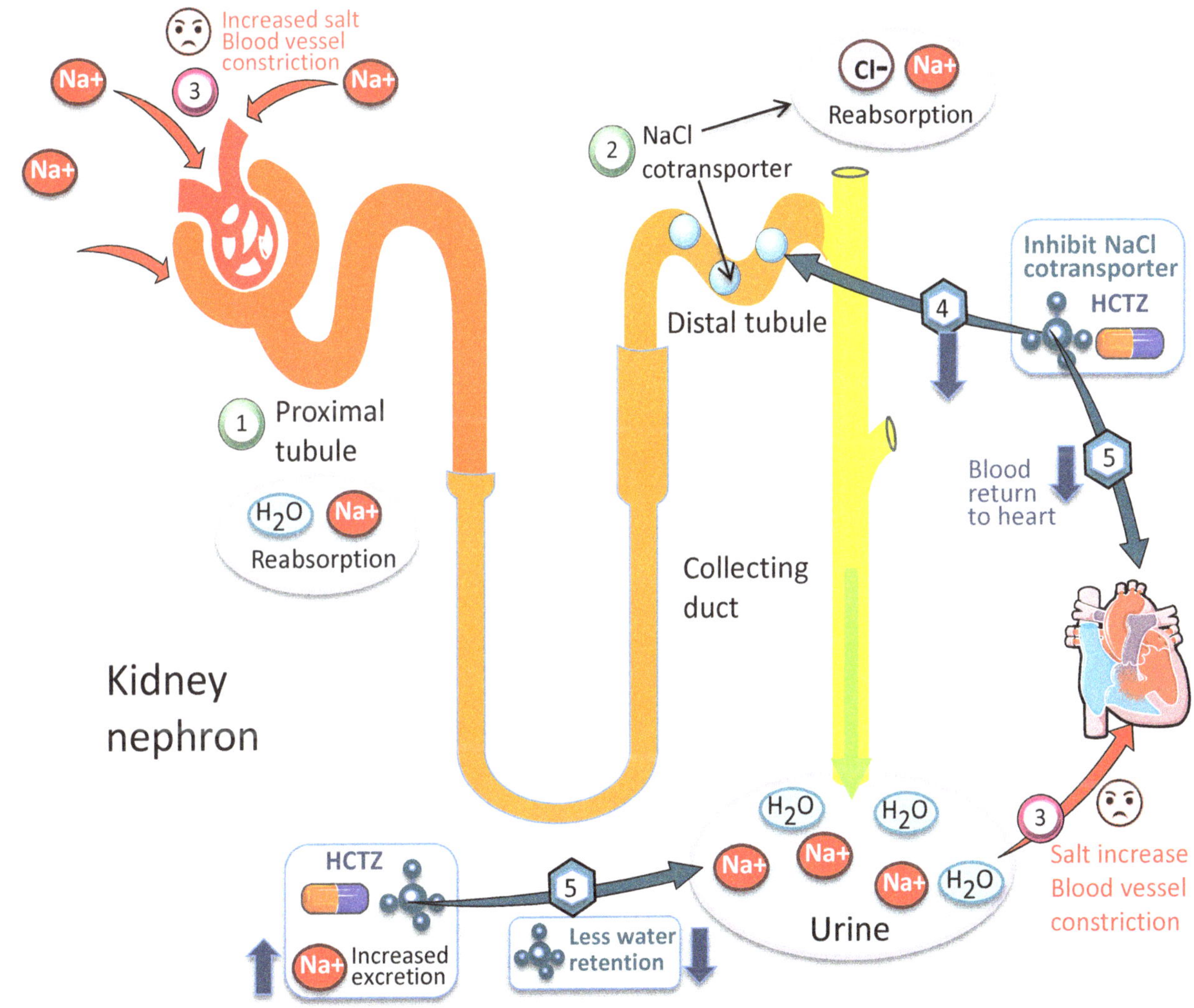

Increased salt
Blood vessel constriction
3
Na+
Na+
Na+
Cl-
Na+
Reabsorption
2 NaCl cotransporter
Distal tubule
Inhibit NaCl cotransporter
HCTZ
4
1 Proximal tubule
H_2O Na+
Reabsorption
Blood return to heart
5
Collecting duct
Kidney nephron
H_2O
H_2O
Na+
Na+
Na+
H_2O
Urine
3
Salt increase
Blood vessel constriction
HCTZ
Na+ Increased excretion
5
Less water retention

Blood pressure: Hypertension, Hydrochlorothiazide

Homeostasis—How we regulate the body's glucose levels

Hyperglycemia (high blood glucose levels)

Blood glucose concentration rises after a meal (the stimulus).

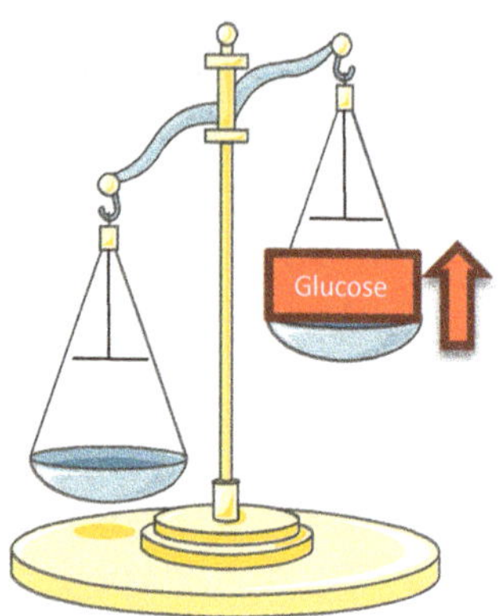

Hypoglycemia (low blood glucose levels)

Often related to diabetes treatment, drugs, or other rare conditions.

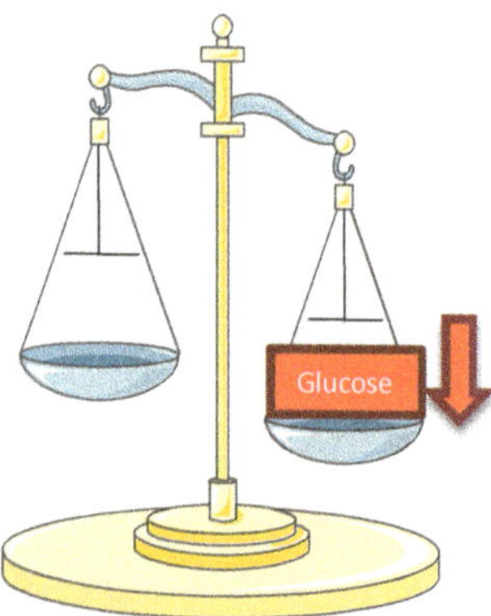

Homeostasis—How we regulate the body's glucose levels

Control of blood glucose levels by the pancreas and other body organs.

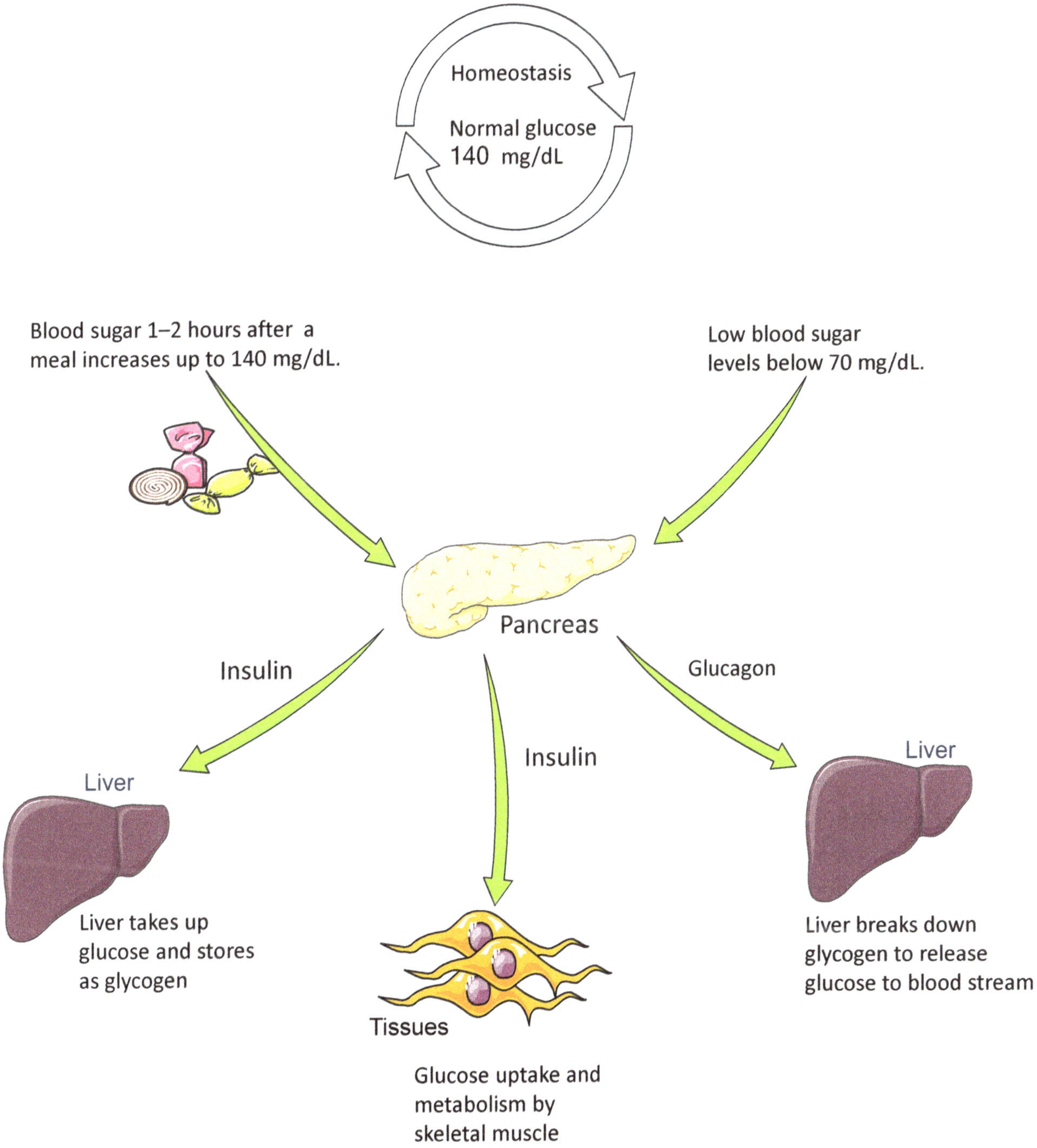

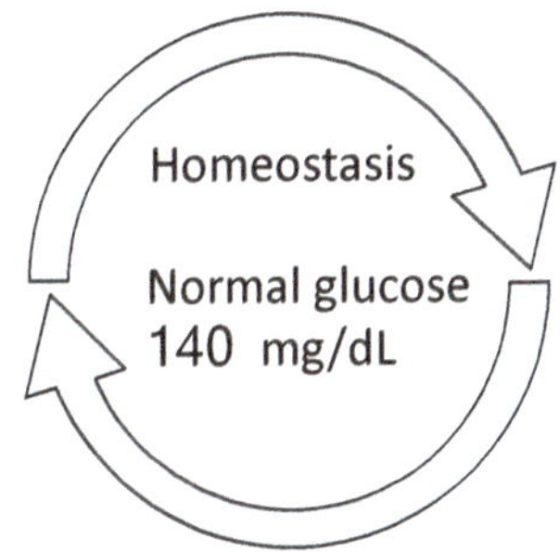

Homeostasis
Normal glucose
140 mg/dL
Blood sugar 1–2 hours after a meal increases up to 140 mg/dL.
Low blood sugar levels below 70 mg/dL.
Pancreas
Insulin
Insulin
Glucagon
Liver
Liver takes up glucose and stores as glycogen
Tissues
Glucose uptake and metabolism by skeletal muscle
Liver
Liver breaks down glycogen to release glucose to blood stream

Homeostasis: Glucose levels

The disease: Type 2 diabetes

Type 2 diabetes (T2D) is characterized by persistent **hyperglycemia** as a result of β-cell dysfunction coupled with **insulin resistance. Overweight or obesity** is considered a primary risk factor for diabetes.

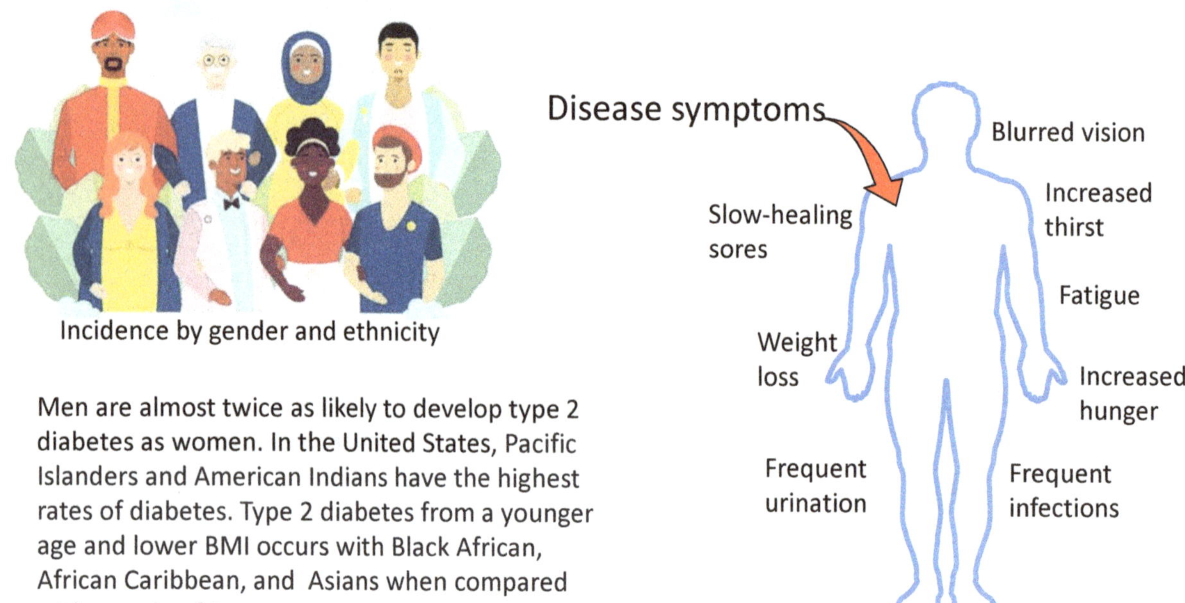

Incidence by gender and ethnicity

Men are almost twice as likely to develop type 2 diabetes as women. In the United States, Pacific Islanders and American Indians have the highest rates of diabetes. Type 2 diabetes from a younger age and lower BMI occurs with Black African, African Caribbean, and Asians when compared with people of European ancestry. .

The medicine

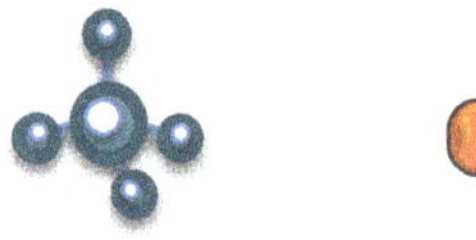

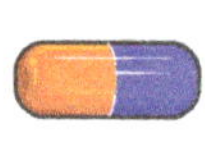

146th most US Prescribed Drug (2019),
4.5 million prescriptions

Empagliflozin; Jardiance, FDA Approval 2014

Empagliflozin is used to treat type 2 diabetes. It may be used together with other medications such as metformin or insulin. It is not recommended for type 1 diabetes. Empagliflozin **inhibits glucose reabsorption** from the kidney nephron into bloodstream.

HO O Cl O O HO OH OH

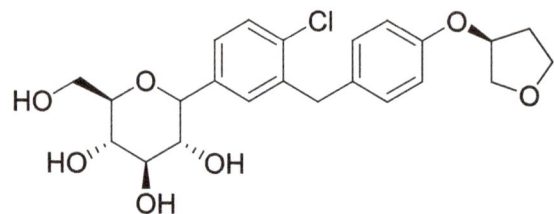

Glucose levels: Diabetes, Empagliflozin

Action of Empagliflozin on cell and disease biology

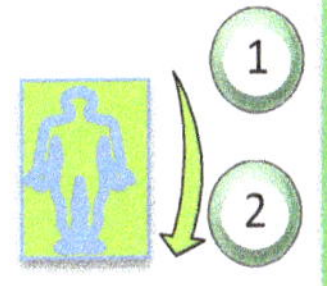

1 **SGLT2** is a sodium-dependent **glucose transport protein** in the proximal tubule of the kidneys, responsible for 90% of glucose reabsorption.

2 **Inhibition of SGLT2 decreases blood glucose levels** due to the increase in renal glucose excretion.

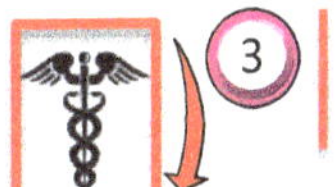

3 **Type 2 diabetics** have **higher levels of SGLT2** with greater reabsorption of glucose into the bloodstream and higher blood levels .

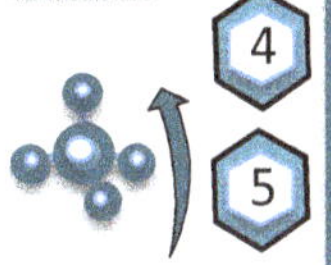

4 **Empagliflozin is** a potent **inhibitor of renal SGLT2 transporters** and blocks the reabsorption of glucose by the kidneys.

5 **Empagliflozin increases glucose excretion** in urine**,** lowers blood sugar levels in people with diabetes.

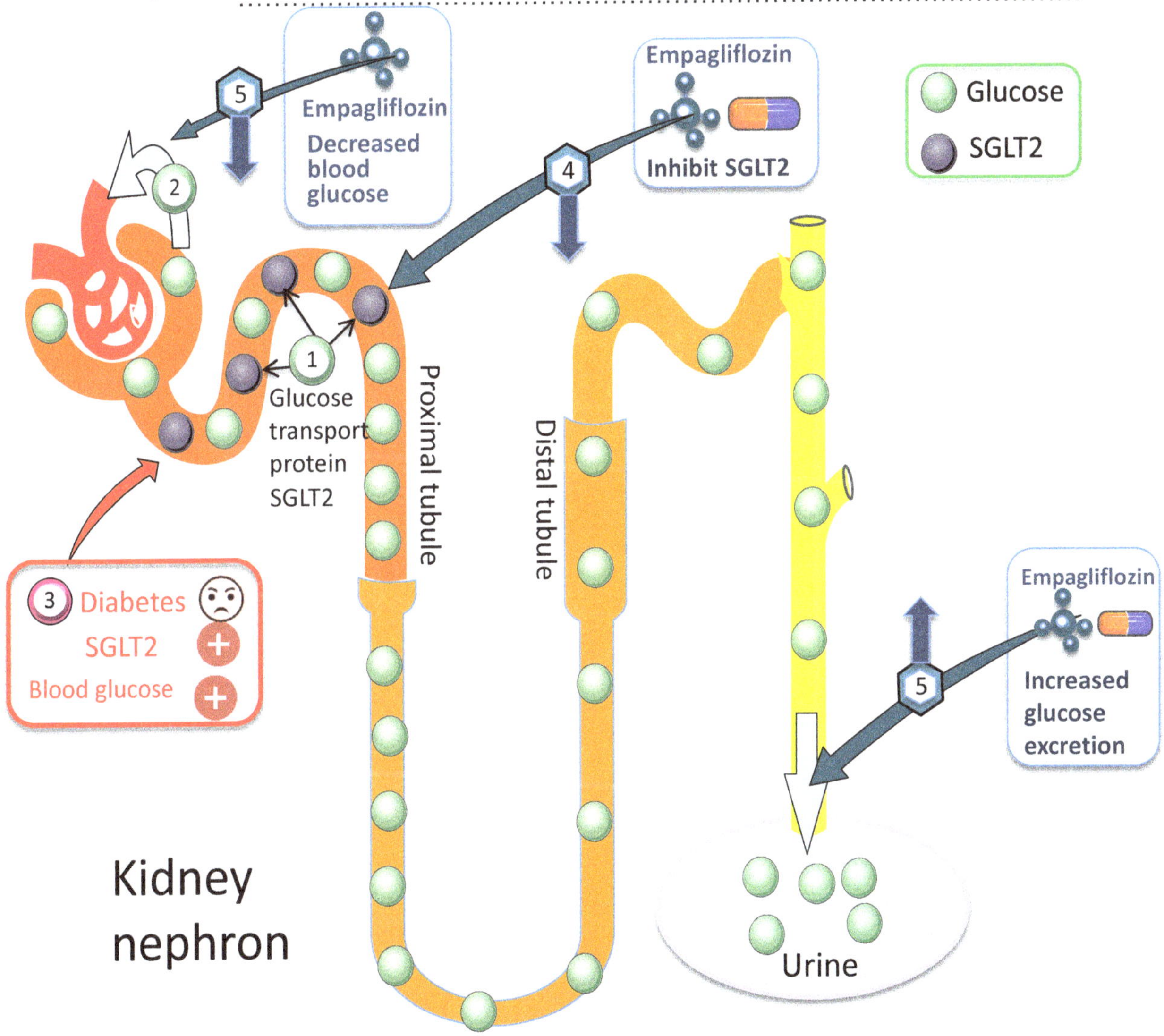

Glucose levels: Diabetes, Empagliflozin

The disease: Diabetes

In **Type 1 diabetes (T1D)** is a chronic condition in which the pancreas produces little or no insulin. **Type 2 diabetes (T2D)** is characterized by **high blood sugar**, diminished ability of cells to respond to the action of insulin (**insulin resistance**).

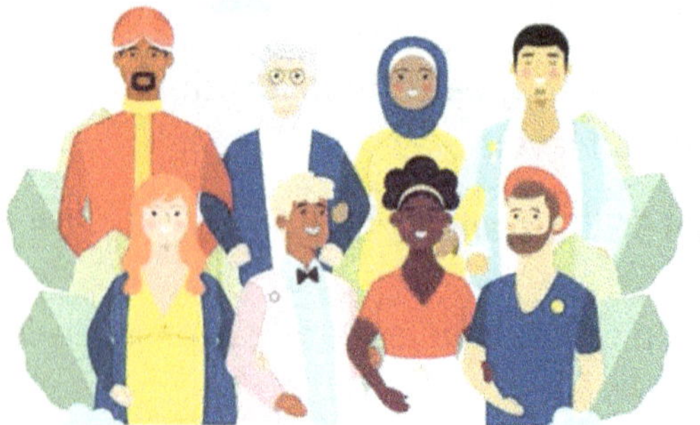

Incidence by gender and ethnicity

Caucasians seem to be more susceptible to type 1 than African-Americans and Hispanic-Americans. Chinese people have a lower risk of developing type 1, as do people in South America. Type 1 diabetes, unlike other autoimmune diseases, affects both males and females equally. Although women generally have lower mortality than men.

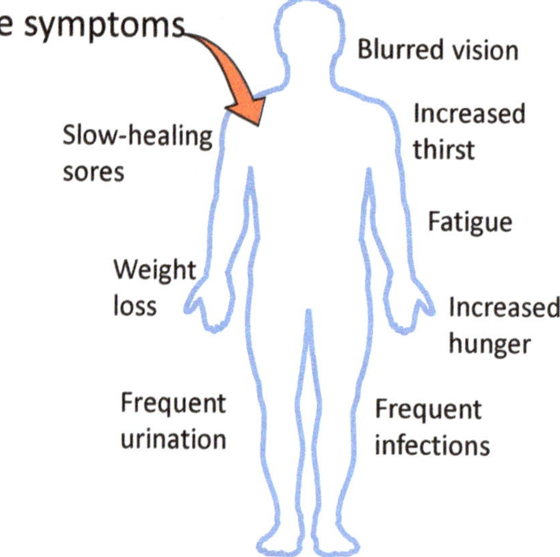

The medicine

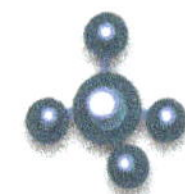

Fourth Most US Prescribed Drug (2019), 86 million prescriptions

Metformin; Glucophage, FDA Approval 1998

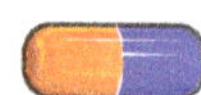

Metformin is an **oral blood glucose-lowering agent** to manage type 2 diabetes and can be used in combination with insulin.

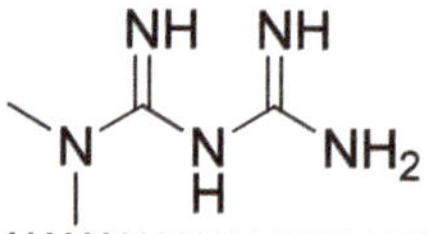

26th Most US Prescribed Drug, (2019), 25 million prescriptions

Insulin glargine; Lantus, FDA Approval 2000

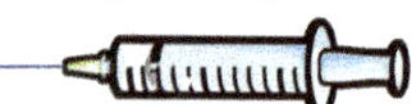

Administered as a subcutaneous injection

Lantus (insulin glargine) is a **long-acting insulin** with two extra arginine residues at the C-terminus. **Lantus promotes glucose utilization and storage** by increasing glucose transport and glycogen synthesis and injected once a day to control glucose levels.

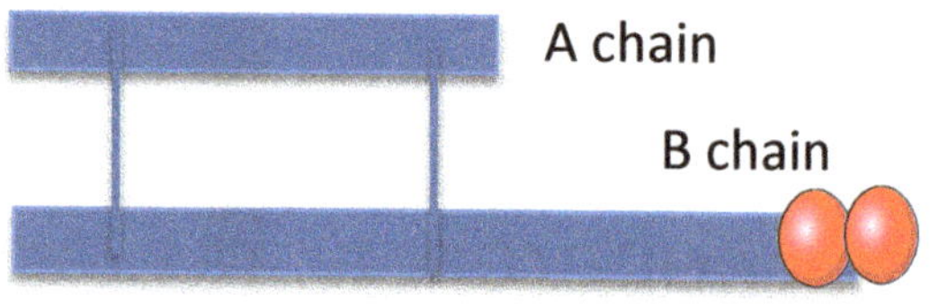

Glucose levels: Diabetes, Lantus, Metformin

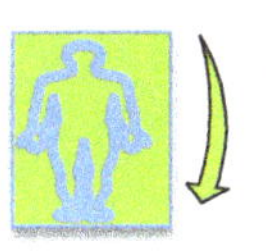

1 The **insulin signaling cascade** results in increased glucose transport activity by translocation and fusion of the **glucose transporter (GLUT4) storage vesicle**s to the plasma membrane.

2 **Insulin** exerts all of its known physiological effects by binding to **the insulin receptor** on the plasma membrane of target cells.

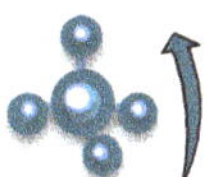

3 **Metformin** can **increase** insulin receptor **signaling activity**, enhance glycogen synthesis, and increase the activity of GLUT4 transporters.

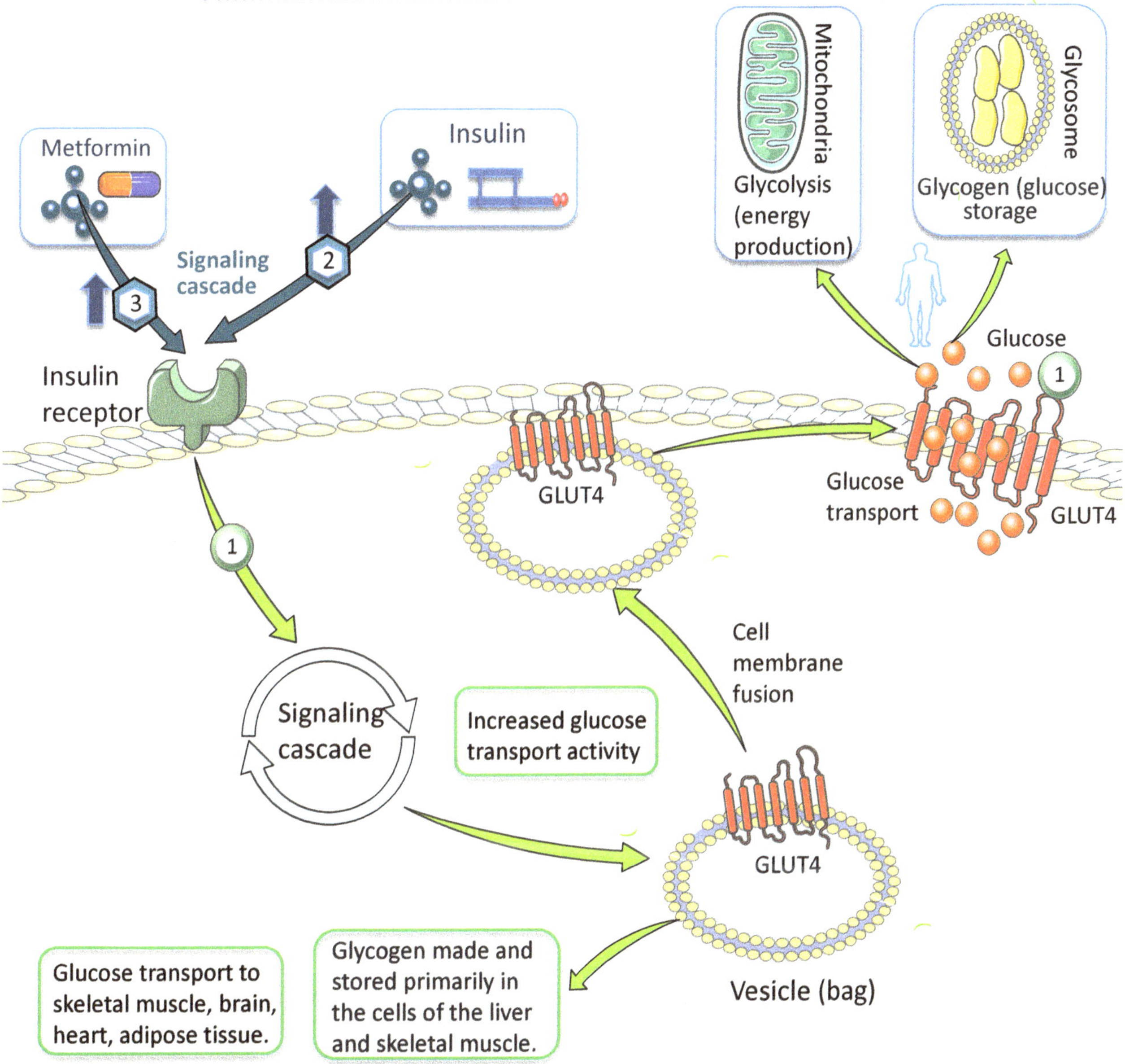

Glucose levels: Diabetes, Lantus, Metformin

The disease: Type 2 diabetes

Type 2 diabetes (T2D) is characterized by persistent **hyperglycemia** as a result of β-cell dysfunction coupled with **insulin resistance.**

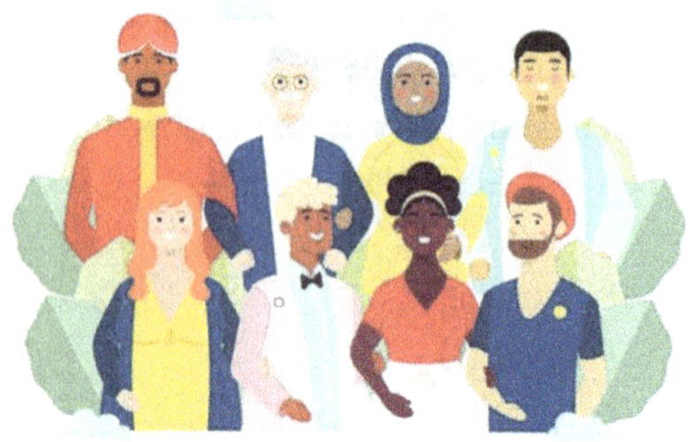

Incidence by gender and ethnicity

Men are almost twice as likely to develop type 2 diabetes as women. In the United States, Pacific Islanders and American Indians have the highest rates of diabetes. Type 2 diabetes from a younger age and lower BMI occurs with black African, African Caribbean, and Asians when compared with people of European ancestry. .

Disease symptoms

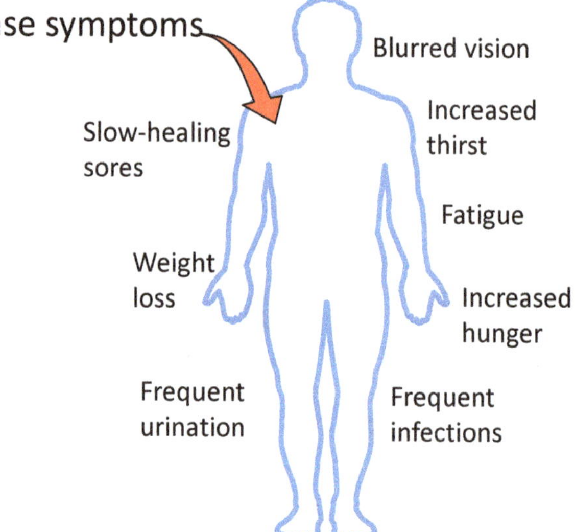

The medicine

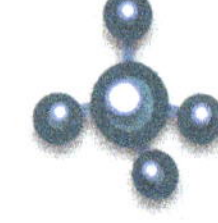

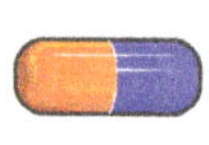

62nd Most US Prescribed Drug, (2019), 11.5 million prescriptions

Glimepiride; Amaryl, FDA Approval 1999

Glimepiride improves glycemic control with type 2 diabetes and reduces the risk of cardiovascular death. Glimepiride binds to **sulfonylurea receptors** (SUR-1) on functioning pancreatic beta-cells to acutely lower plasma glucose by stimulating the release of insulin.

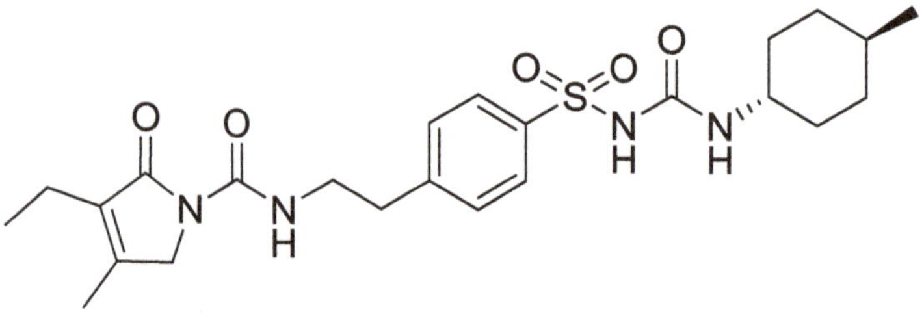

Glucose levels: Diabetes, Glimepiride

Action of Glimepiride on cell and disease biology

1. **Glucose transporter 2 (GLUT2),** glucose transporter in pancreatic beta cells.

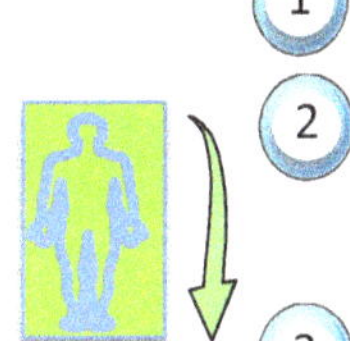

2. Pancreatic **β-cell ATP channel has** two subunits (channel and sulfonylurea receptor, SUR1), links ATP generation to insulin secretion, open **ATP channels blocks insulin secretion.**
3. **Closure of the ATP channel** causes membrane depolarization, **rise in cytosolic Ca^{2+}**, **insulin** secretory granules to the cell surface and **secretion**.

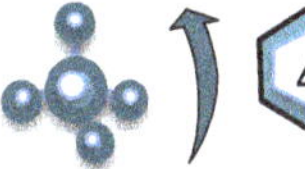

4. **Glimepiride** promotes insulin secretion by binding to the **regulatory sulfonylurea receptor-1 (SUR1) subunit, closes the ATP channels**.

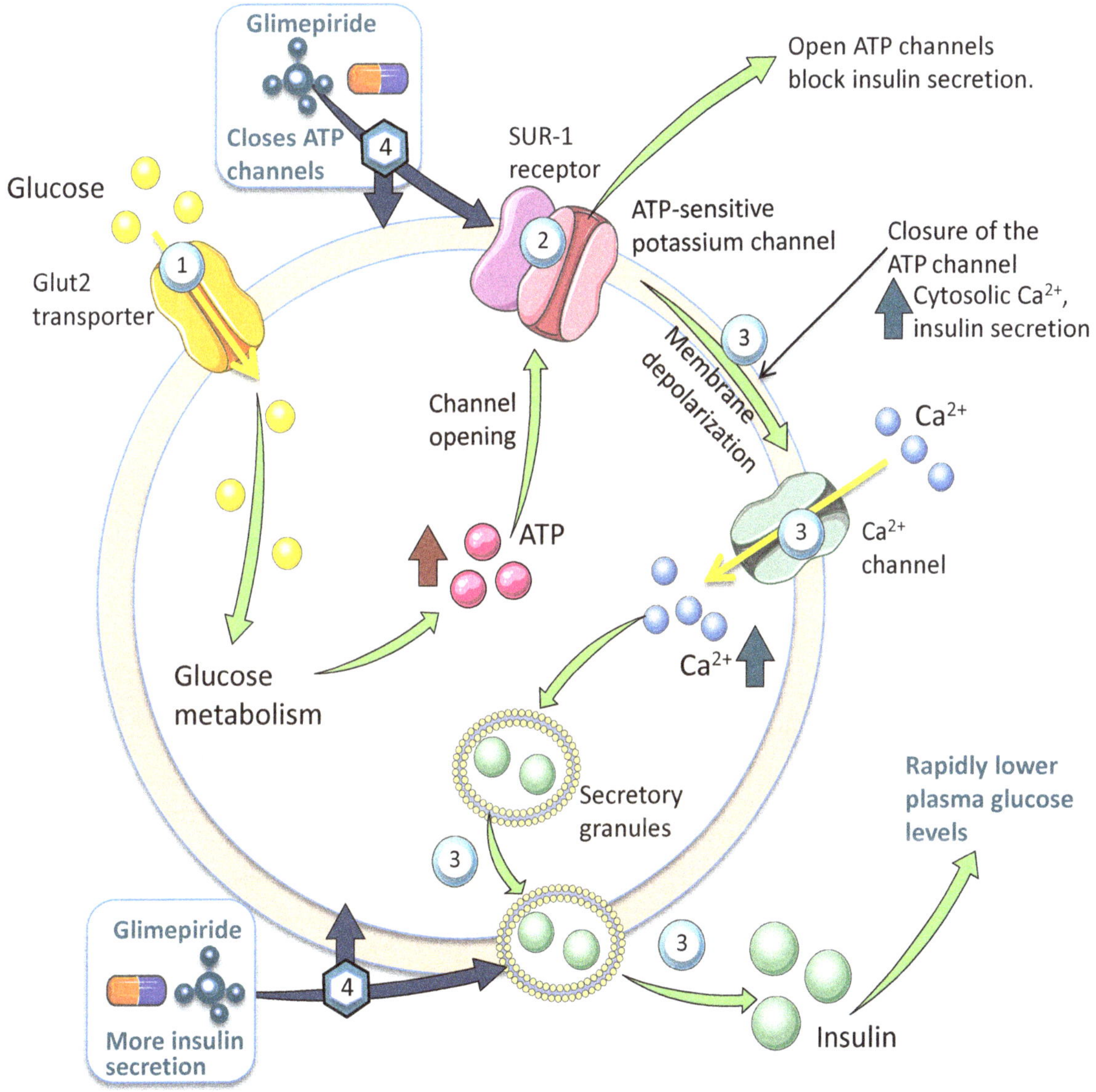

Glimepiride

Closes ATP channels

4

Open ATP channels block insulin secretion.

SUR-1 receptor

Glucose

ATP-sensitive potassium channel

2

1

Glut2 transporter

Closure of the ATP channel

Cytosolic Ca^{2+}, insulin secretion

3

Membrane depolarization

Channel opening

Ca^{2+}

ATP

3

Ca^{2+} channel

Glucose metabolism

Ca^{2+}

Secretory granules

Rapidly lower plasma glucose levels

3

3

Glimepiride

4

More insulin secretion

Insulin

Glucose levels: Diabetes, Glimepiride

Homeostasis—Inflammation, aging, and cancer

- While lifespan has increased, there has been an **increasing prevalence of diseases such as obesity, hypertension, and type 2 diabetes.**
- Such acquired diseases can occur when **homeostasis breaks down** and are associated with **chronic inflammation.**
- In addition, ageing with chronic and systemic low-grade inflammation is a major risk factor for **cancer** development.
- Inflammation can influence all cancer stages from cell transformation to metastasis.

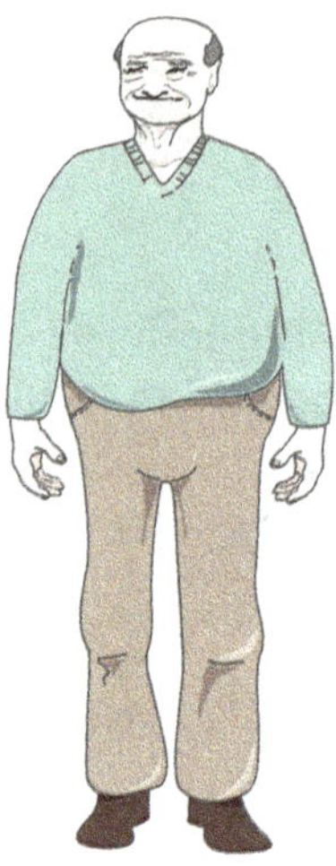

Aging is a gradual, continuous process of natural change with a decline in many bodily functions. **The response of cellular networks and protein pathways to environmental factors can slow aging. Networks that resist stress are critical** in the aging process and if disrupted contribute to chronic disease.

Aging can result from homeostatic imbalance due to a weakening of feedback loops, which results in an unstable internal environment. A deficiency in the homeostasis of a network will increase the risk of illness and resulting physical changes.

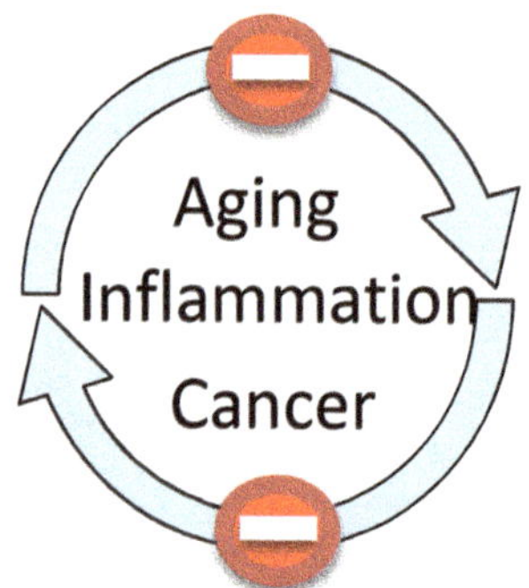

Deregulation of homeostatic processes can result in **abnormal tissue growth** which is not coordinated with normal surrounding tissue and results in **cancer.**

Homeostasis: Inflammation in aging and disease

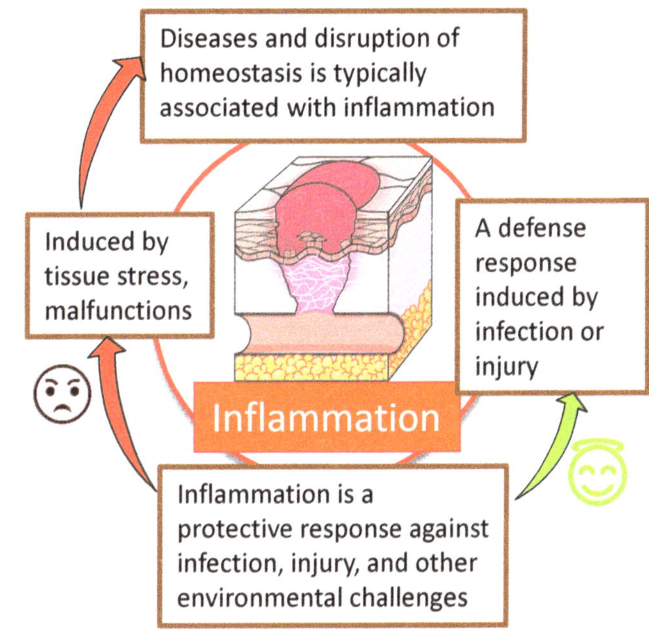

Two examples of age-associated cancers with FDA-approved drugs.

Bladder cancer occurs mainly in older people with the average age at the time of diagnosis of 73. People have a higher risk for bladder cancer from **exposure to tobacco or other cancer-causing agents** or drugs such as cyclophosphamide. Workplace **exposure of certain industrial chemicals** can also increase the risk for bladder cancer.

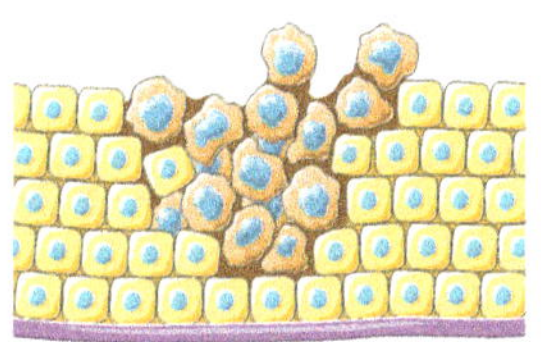

Prostrate cancer. The most common risk factor is age, which increases the chance of getting prostate cancer. A **high fat diet** and **high testosterone levels** may stimulate dormant prostate cancer cells into activity and may promote advanced prostate cancer. Another factor is **mutations acquired during a person's life** and are present only in certain cells of the prostrate.

The disease: Chronic inflammation

Chronic inflammation has a prolonged response with a progressive change in the type of cells present at the site of inflammation. It is characterized by the simultaneous **destruction and repair of the tissue** resulting from the **inflammatory process**.

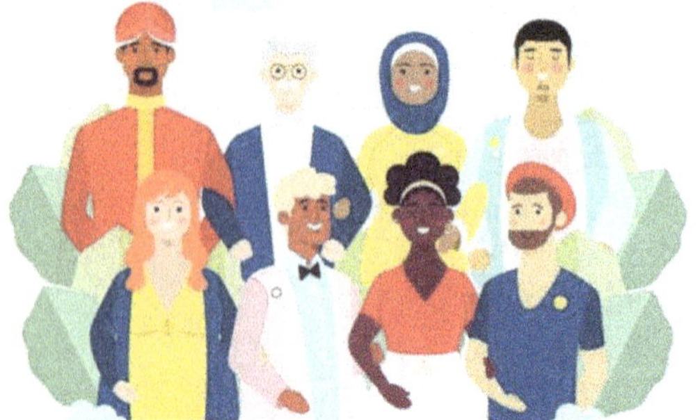

Incidence by gender and ethnicity

Inflammation pain is greater and more variable for women than for men and may present differently. Metabolic dysfunctions differ by race and gender, with higher incidence in African Americans and males. Elevated C-reactive protein (inflammation marker) is primarily due to obesity, smoking status, physical activity, and socioeconomic disadvantage.

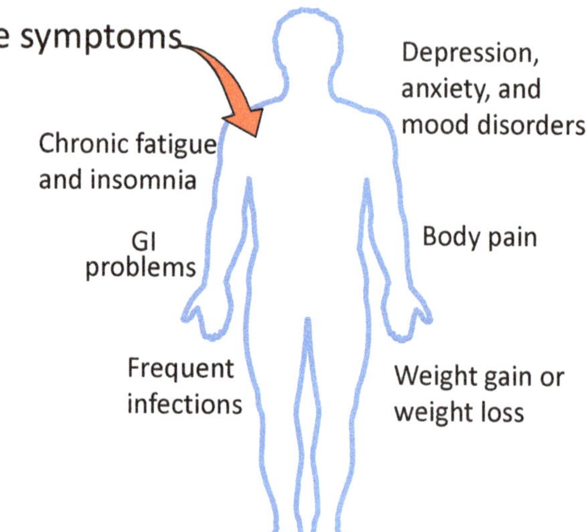

The medicine

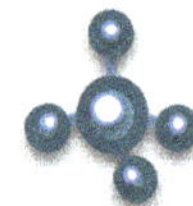

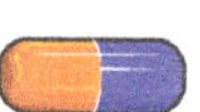

Aspirin: Bayer 81

Aspirin is a nonsteroidal **anti-inflammatory drug** (NSAID) for both acute and long-term inflammation in diseases such as rheumatoid arthritis. Prostaglandins form around an injury to increase blood flow which results in inflammation. **Aspirin blocks prostaglandin formation**, reducing inflammation. **Aspirin** may **prevent cancers** such as colorectal through its anti-inflammation activity.

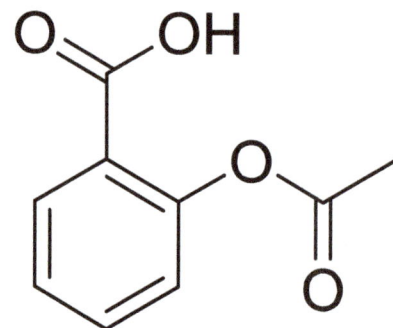

Chronic inflammation, Aspirin

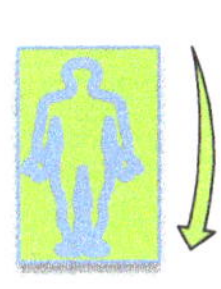

1. The biosynthesis of **15-epi-lipoxin A_4 (LXA4)** from metabolites of arachidonic acid is **initiated by aspirin acetylation of COX-2**.
2. COX-2–containing **endothelial cells act** as the donor cell to synthesize and release the **intermediate HETE**.
3. **Leukocytes** act as the accessory cell to take up the intermediate HETE and process with a **lipoxygenase** enzyme to make and release LXA4.

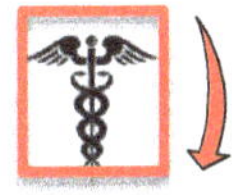

4. **Cyclooxygenase(COX)-2 catalyzes** formation of arachidonic acid derived prostaglandins that promote pain, fever, and **inflammation**.

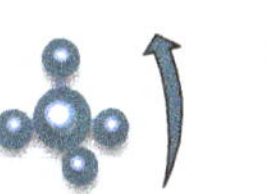

5. Low-dose **aspirin** inhibits COX-2 production of prostaglandins, **stimulates LXA4 production** with protective, anti-inflammatory actions and inhibits generation of pro-inflammatory cytokines.

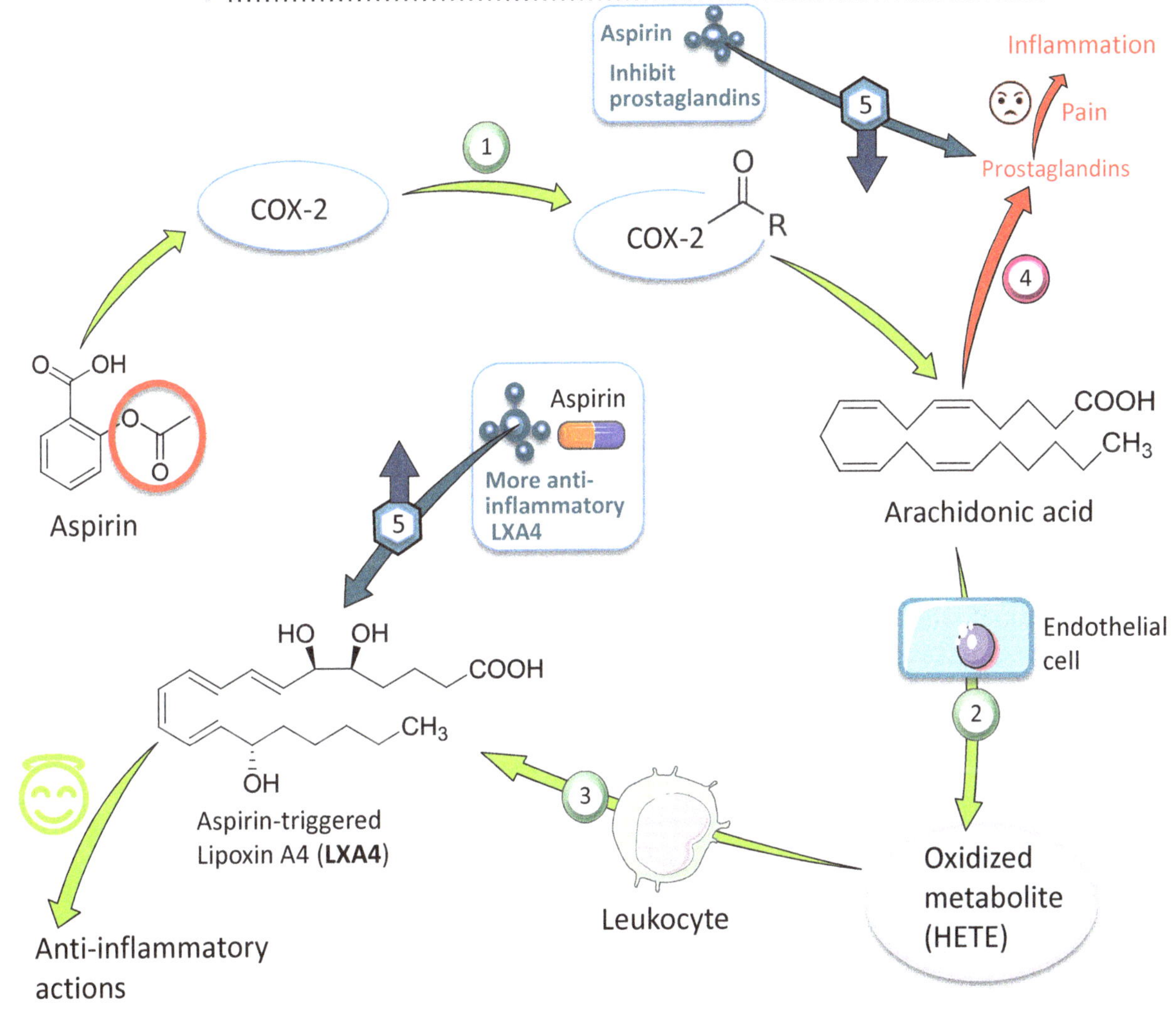

Aspirin
Inhibit prostaglandins
5
Inflammation
Pain
Prostaglandins
1
COX-2
COX-2
O
R
4
O
OH
O
O
Aspirin
Aspirin
More anti-inflammatory LXA4
5
COOH
CH_3
Arachidonic acid
Endothelial cell
2
HO
OH
COOH
CH_3
OH
Aspirin-triggered Lipoxin A4 (**LXA4**)
3
Leukocyte
Oxidized metabolite (HETE)
Anti-inflammatory actions

The disease: Chronic Inflammation

Inflammatory diseases that are caused by overproduction or inappropriate production of certain **cytokines.**

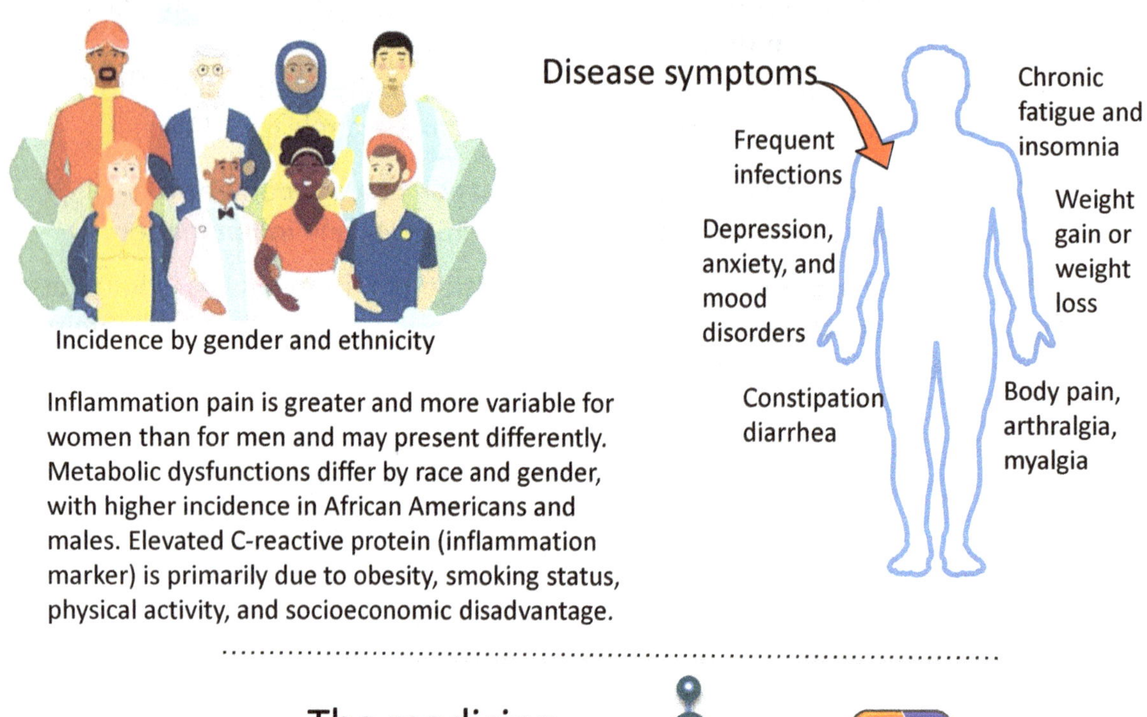

Incidence by gender and ethnicity

Inflammation pain is greater and more variable for women than for men and may present differently. Metabolic dysfunctions differ by race and gender, with higher incidence in African Americans and males. Elevated C-reactive protein (inflammation marker) is primarily due to obesity, smoking status, physical activity, and socioeconomic disadvantage.

The medicine

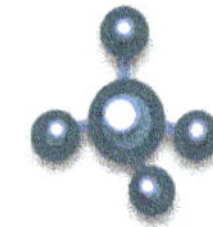

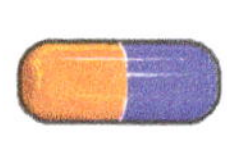

27th Most US Prescribed Drug, (2019), 23 million prescriptions

Prednisone; Rayos, FDA Approval 2012

Prednisone is a **delayed-release corticosteroid** used to treat a broad range of diseases including rheumatic, dermatologic, allergic states, ophthalmic, respiratory, hematologic, gastrointestinal, multiple sclerosis, arthritis, and skin diseases.

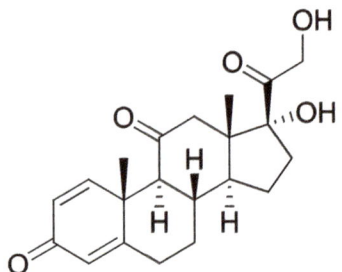

Liver

Reduction

Prednisone is a prodrug

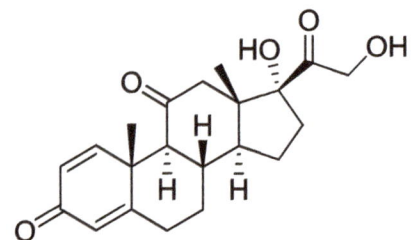

Prednisolone, active steroid

Chronic inflammation, Prednisone

Action of Prednisone on cell and disease biology

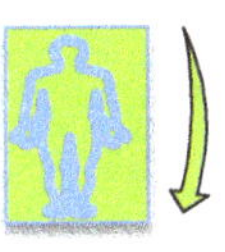

1. **Glucocorticoids actions** are mediated by an intracellular **glucocorticoid receptor (GR),** a nuclear-activating factor widely expressed in tissues.

2. **GR cycles** between the **cytoplasm and nucleus** to regulate the nuclear glucocorticoid-responsive genes and modulates proinflammatory genes.

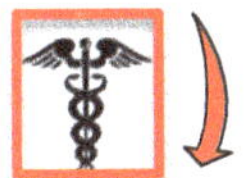

3. **Chronic neutrophil-driven inflammation** of tissue is linked to autoimmune diseases and cancer with more aggressive disease and a poorer prognosis.

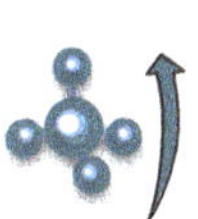

4. **Prednisone represses** expression of **pro-inflammatory cytokines** by immune cells, suppresses migration of neutrophils to inflammation site. **Prednisone reverses** increases in **capillary permeability**, which occurs in acute allergic reactions.

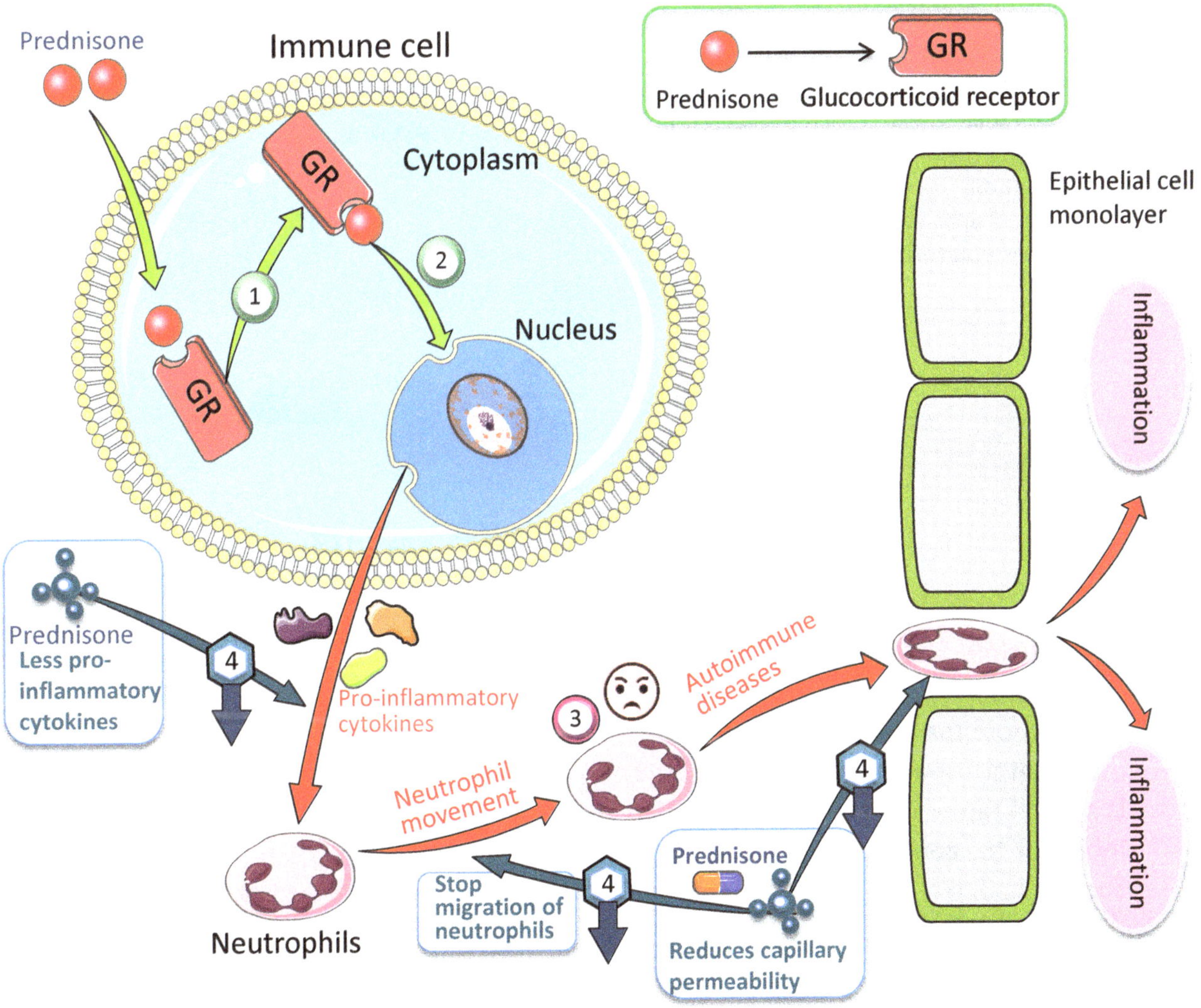

Prednisone
Immune cell
Prednisone → GR Glucocorticoid receptor
GR
Cytoplasm
1
2
GR
Nucleus
Epithelial cell monolayer
Inflammation
Prednisone Less pro-inflammatory cytokines
4
Pro-inflammatory cytokines
3
Autoimmune diseases
Neutrophil movement
4
Neutrophils
Stop migration of neutrophils
4
Prednisone
Reduces capillary permeability
Inflammation

Chronic inflammation, Prednisone

The disease: Rheumatoid arthritis

Rheumatoid arthritis (RA) is a progressive **autoimmune and inflammatory disease** which commonly affects the lining of joints of the hands, feet, and wrists.

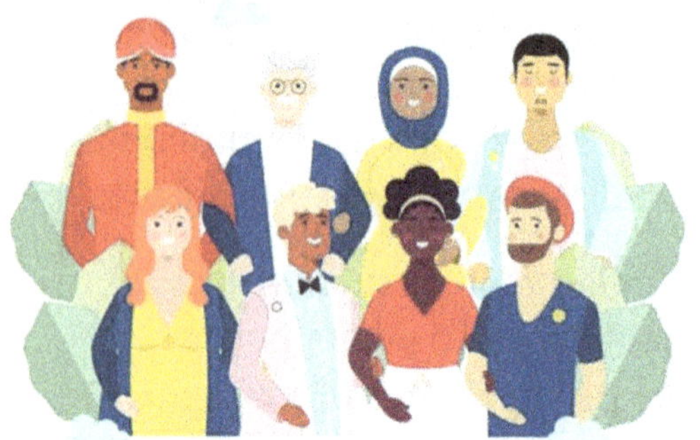

Incidence by gender and ethnicity

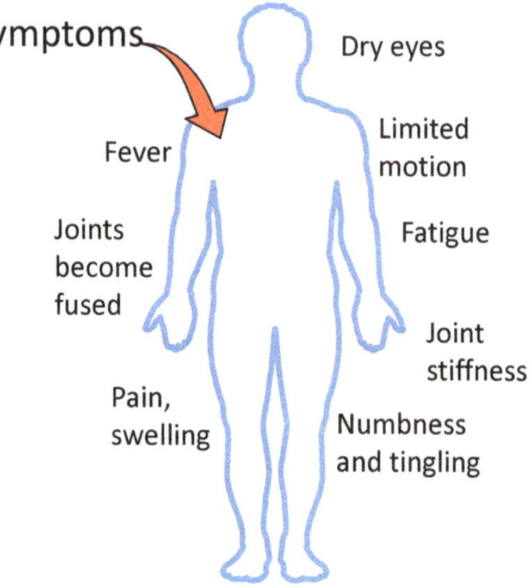

The prevalence of RA is higher in females than males (four to five times higher below the age of 50 and 2-fold higher above 60–70 years. Caucasians have the highest rate but knee osteoarthritis is more common in African Americans in the United States. Pain and functional limitations are greater for African Americans than Caucasians. Asians have a lower risk than Caucasians for osteoarthritis of most joints, except for knee joints.

The medicine

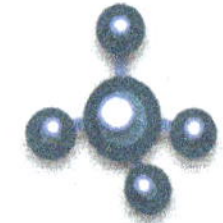

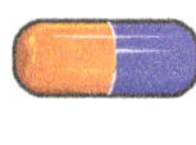

Upadacitinib; Rinvoq, FDA Approval 2019

Upadacitinib is used to **slow down disease progression** in moderately to severely active RA in whom the common treatment with the drug methotrexate (MTX) was not successful. **It** is an **oral Janus kinase (JAK)1-selective inhibitor** to **reduce** production of **cytokines** such as IL-6, IFN, IL-2 and IL-15.

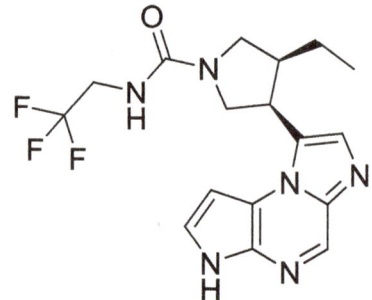

Inflammation, Rheumatoid arthritis, Upadacitinib

Action of Upadacitinib on cell and disease biology

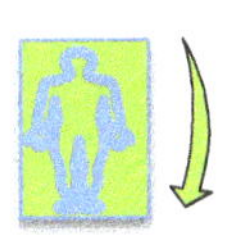

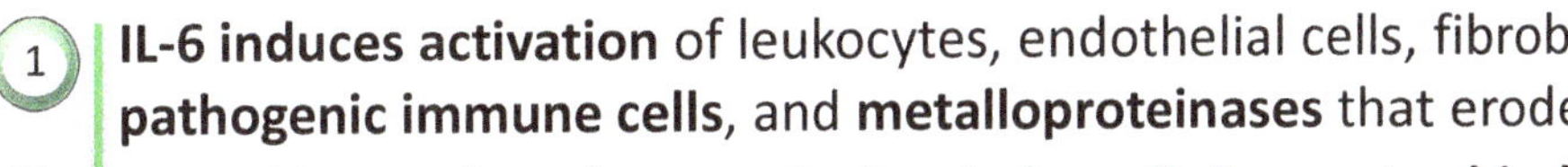

1 **IL-6 induces activation** of leukocytes, endothelial cells, fibroblasts, **pathogenic immune cells**, and **metalloproteinases** that erode the joint.

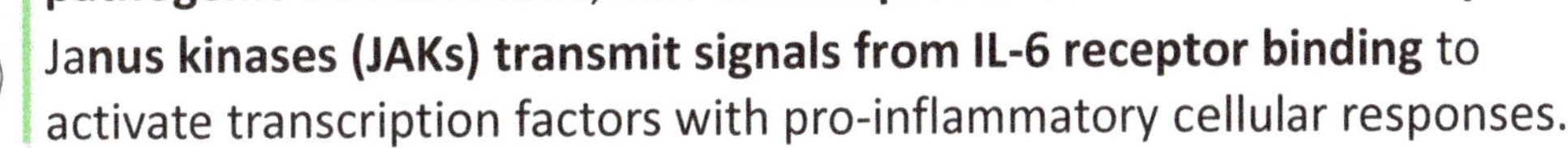

2 **Janus kinases (JAKs) transmit signals from IL-6 receptor binding** to activate transcription factors with pro-inflammatory cellular responses.

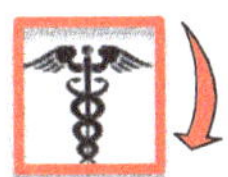

3 **Interleukin 6 (IL-6) is abundant in the synovial fluid of rheumatoid arthritis (RA) patients,** correlates with the disease severity and joint destruction.

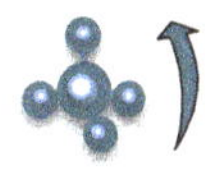

4 **Upadacitinib** selectively **targets JAK1** and inhibits downstream gene activation to decrease activity of immune cells and reduce inflammation.

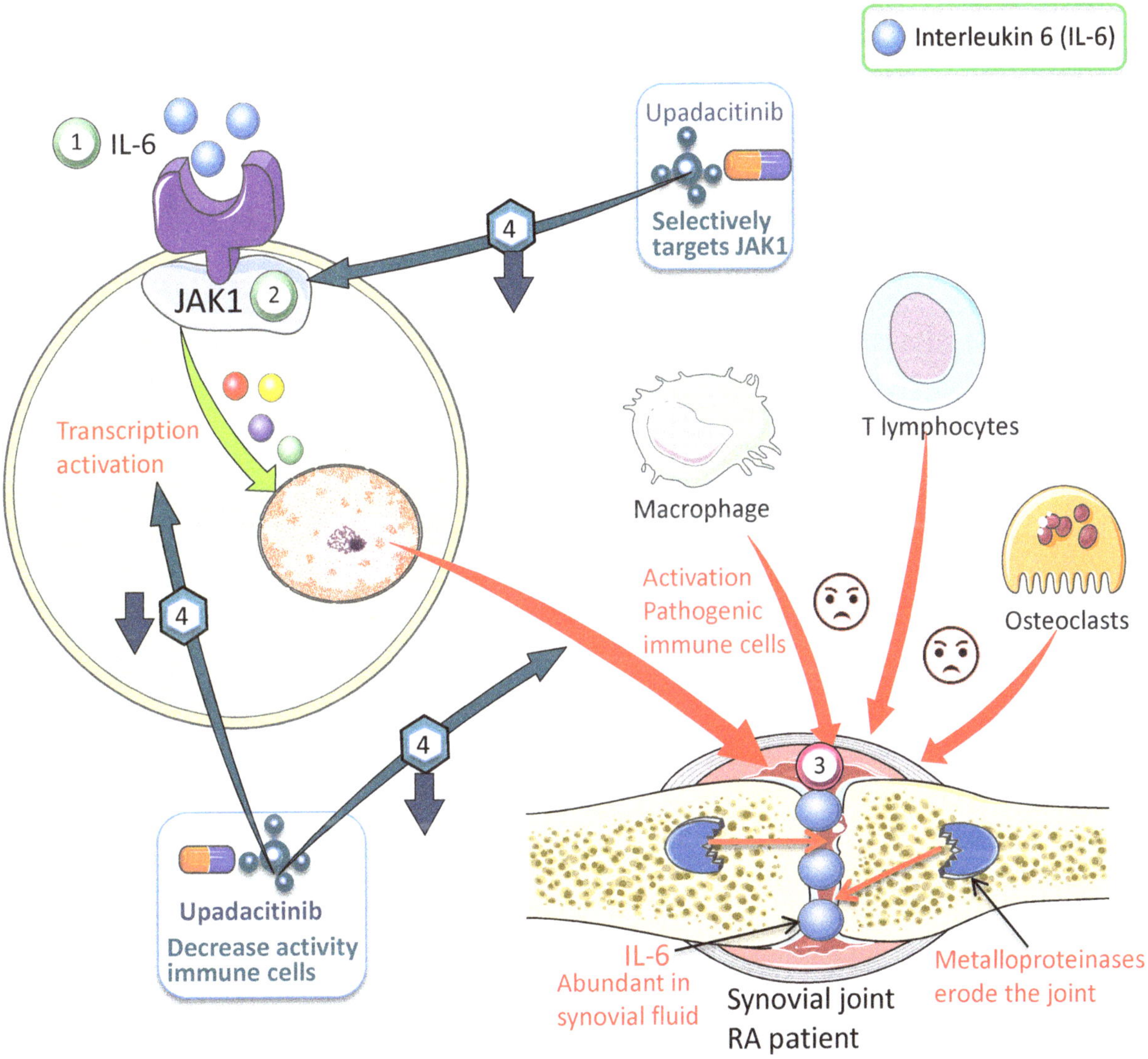

Interleukin 6 (IL-6)
1 IL-6
JAK1 2
Upadacitinib
Selectively targets JAK1
4
Transcription activation
4
4
Upadacitinib
Decrease activity immune cells
Macrophage
T lymphocytes
Osteoclasts
Activation Pathogenic immune cells
3
IL-6
Abundant in synovial fluid
Synovial joint
RA patient
Metalloproteinases erode the joint

Inflammation, Rheumatoid arthritis, Upadacitinib

The disease: Prostate cancer

Non-metastatic, castration-resistant prostate cancer that continues to grow despite treatment with hormone therapy and with increasing levels of prostate specific antigen (PSA).

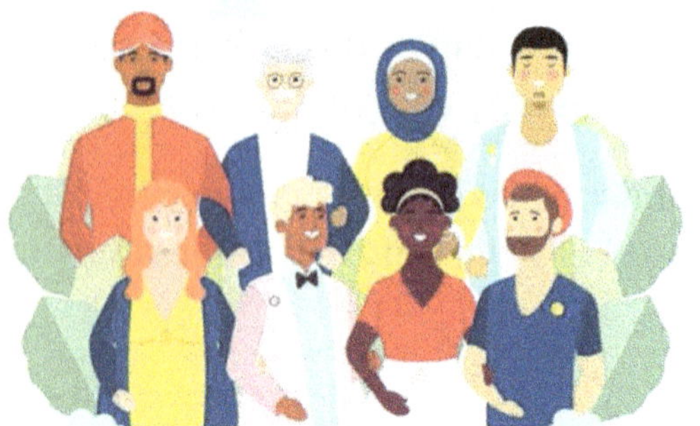

Incidence by gender and ethnicity

Prostate cancer is more likely to develop in older men (60–65 or older) and develop more often in men of African ancestry and at a younger age. Prostate cancer occurs less often in Asian American and Hispanic/Latino men, incidence and mortality in native Asian populations have gradually increased, but are one-third lower than in corresponding Asian American groups.

Disease symptoms

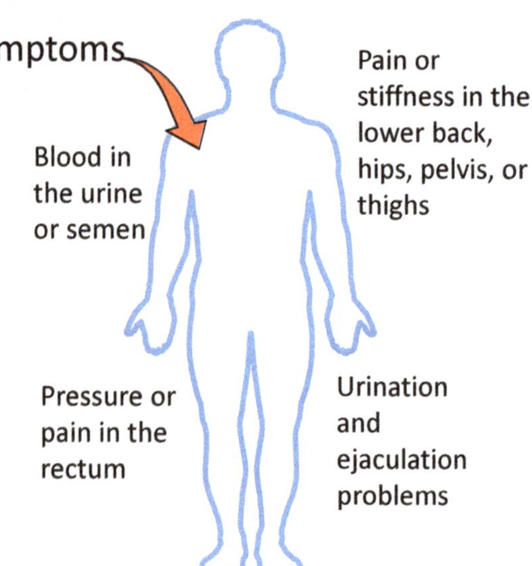

The medicine

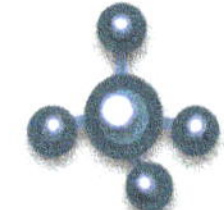

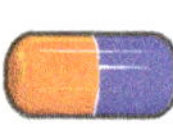

Apalutamide; Erleada, FDA Approval 2019

Apalutamide is a potent and competitive second-generation **anti-androgen agent** that **inhibits the androgen receptor** (AR). Used for treatment of patients who cancers become resistant to androgen deprivation and castration. **Apalutamide** was approved to **delay occurrence of metastatic disease.**

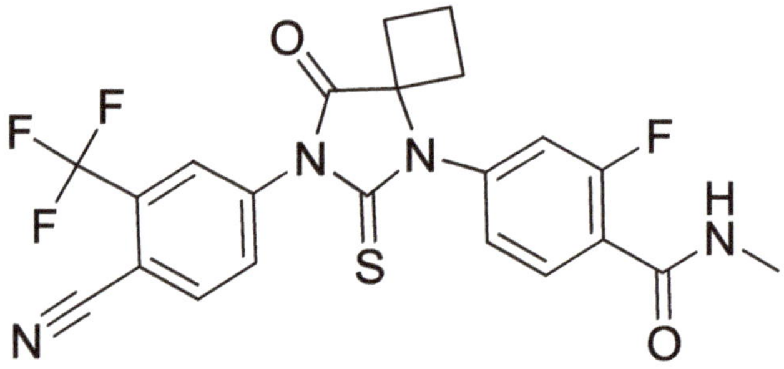

Aging, Prostate cancer, Apalutamide

Action of Apalutamide on cell and disease biology

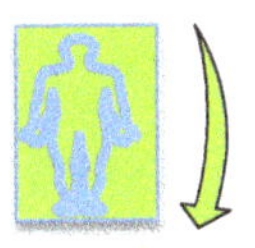

1 **Androgen**-responsive genes **regulate prostate** epithelial cell proliferation, differentiation, and gland enlargement.

2 **Androgen receptor** (AR) regulates gene expression, binding testosterone in the cytoplasm then translocating into the nucleus.

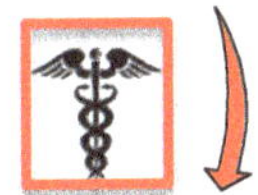

3 **Prostate cancer development is dependent on androgens** and growth factors and can develop **resistance** to castration by **AR overexpression** and receptor reactivation.

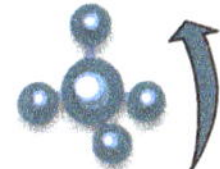

4 **Apalutamide** binds to the AR ligand-binding domain, **prevents AR activation,** DNA binding, and **androgen-regulated gene expression**.

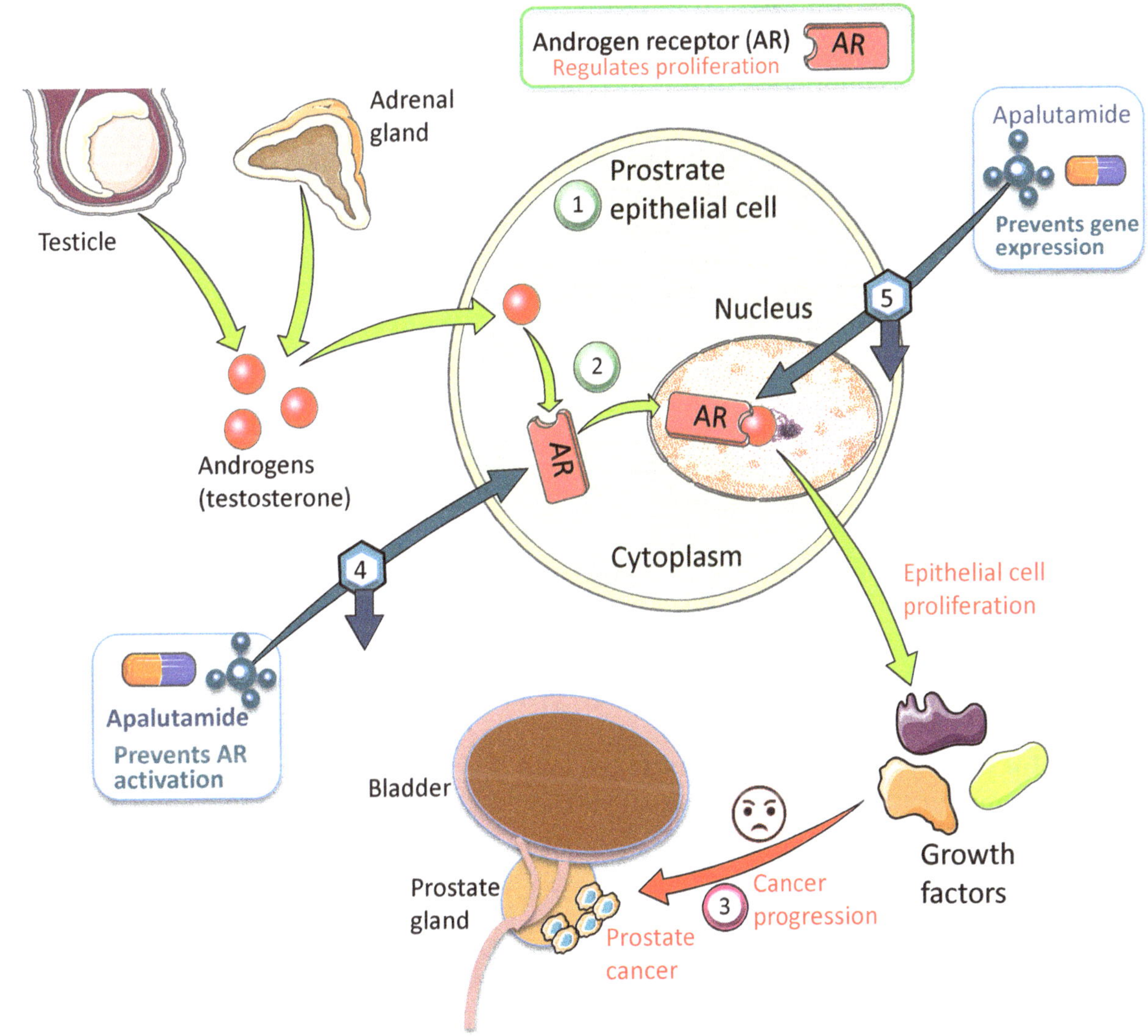

Androgen receptor (AR) AR
Regulates proliferation

Testicle
Adrenal gland
Androgens (testosterone)
Prostrate epithelial cell (1)
Nucleus
(2) AR
Cytoplasm
Apalutamide
Prevents gene expression (5)
Apalutamide
Prevents AR activation (4)
Epithelial cell proliferation
Growth factors
(3) Cancer progression
Bladder
Prostate gland
Prostate cancer

Aging, Prostate cancer, Apalutamide

The disease: Bladder cancer

Bladder cancer, which is locally advanced or metastatic and has a **genetic alteration FGFR3 or FGFR2,** which is resistant to platinum-based chemotherapy. Age and chemical exposure increase the risk of bladder cancer.

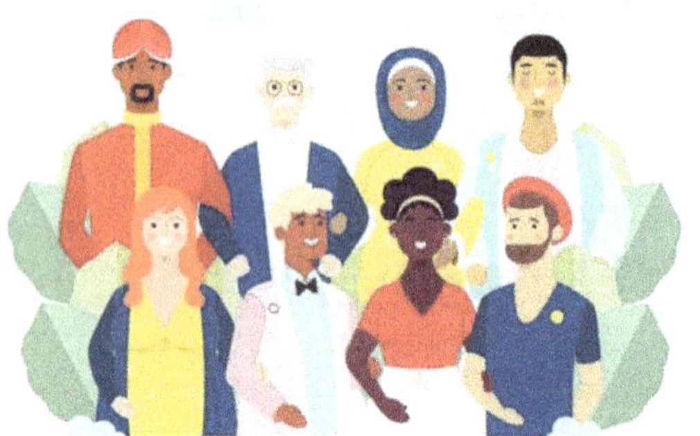

Incidence by gender and ethnicity

Disease symptoms

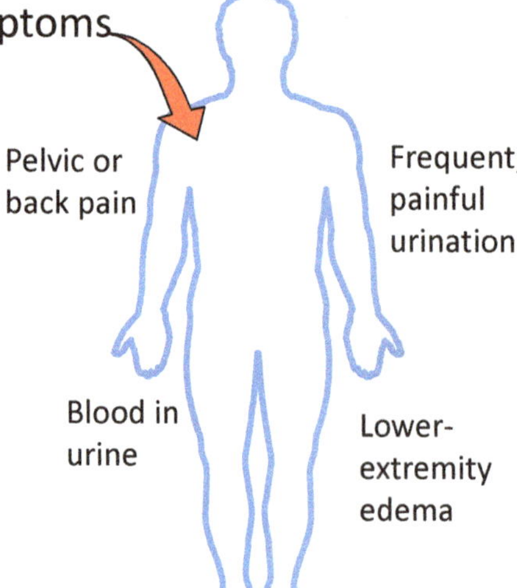

Bladder cancer incidence is three to four times greater in men than in women. White people are more than twice as likely to be diagnosed with bladder cancer as black people, followed by Hispanic whites, and Asian and Pacific Islanders. Black people are twice as likely to die from the disease, but non-Hispanic whites have the highest incidence rate.

The medicine

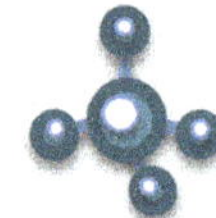

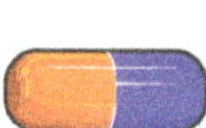

Erdafitinib; Balversa, FDA Approval 2019

Erdafitinib is a small molecule inhibitor of fibroblast growth factor receptor (FGFR) variants. FGFR **genes are mutated** in 20%–60% of common bladder cancers, especially FGFR3 (15%) and influence tumor cell differentiation, proliferation, angiogenesis, and cell survival.

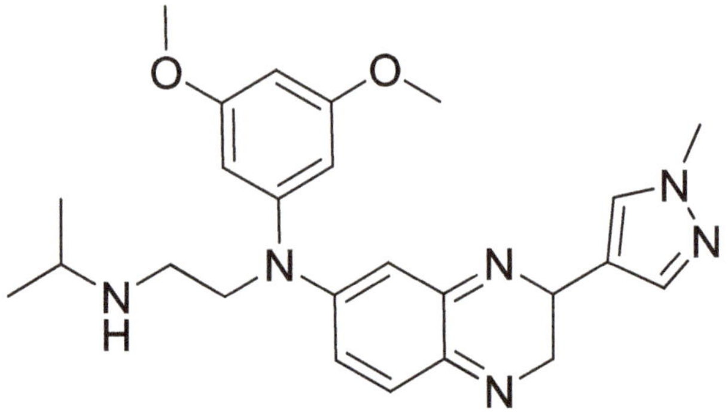

Homeostasis: Bladder cancer , Erdafitinib

Action of Erdafitinib on cell and disease biology

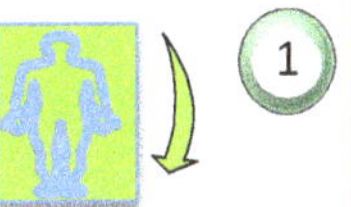

1 The **FGF/FGFR signaling pathway** made up of fibroblast growth factors (FGF) and receptors 2, 3 (FGFR) **regulates tissue homeostasis** and functions, including proliferation, differentiation, apoptosis, and migration.

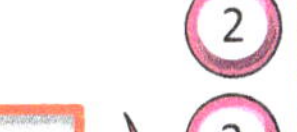

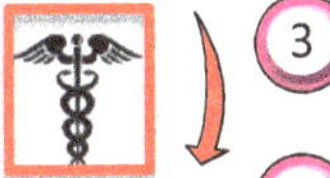

2 **Bladder cancer** often begins in the **urothelial cells** lining the bladder interior.

3 **Myofibroblasts** are abundant in solid tumors with a critical role in tumor growth, secretion of cytokines, which can result in resistance to treatment.

4 **FGFR mutations** contribute to higher rates of cancer cell proliferation in the urothelial lining and more invasive disease.

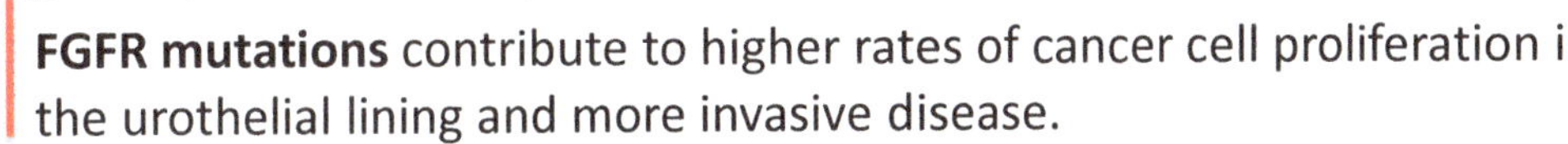

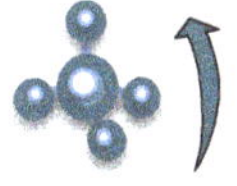

5 **Erdafitinib binds** to all **FGFR** members and **inhibits** the enzymatic activity of FGFR including **signaling pathways**.
The **anti-tumor activity of Erdafitinib** leads to the death of cancerous cells.

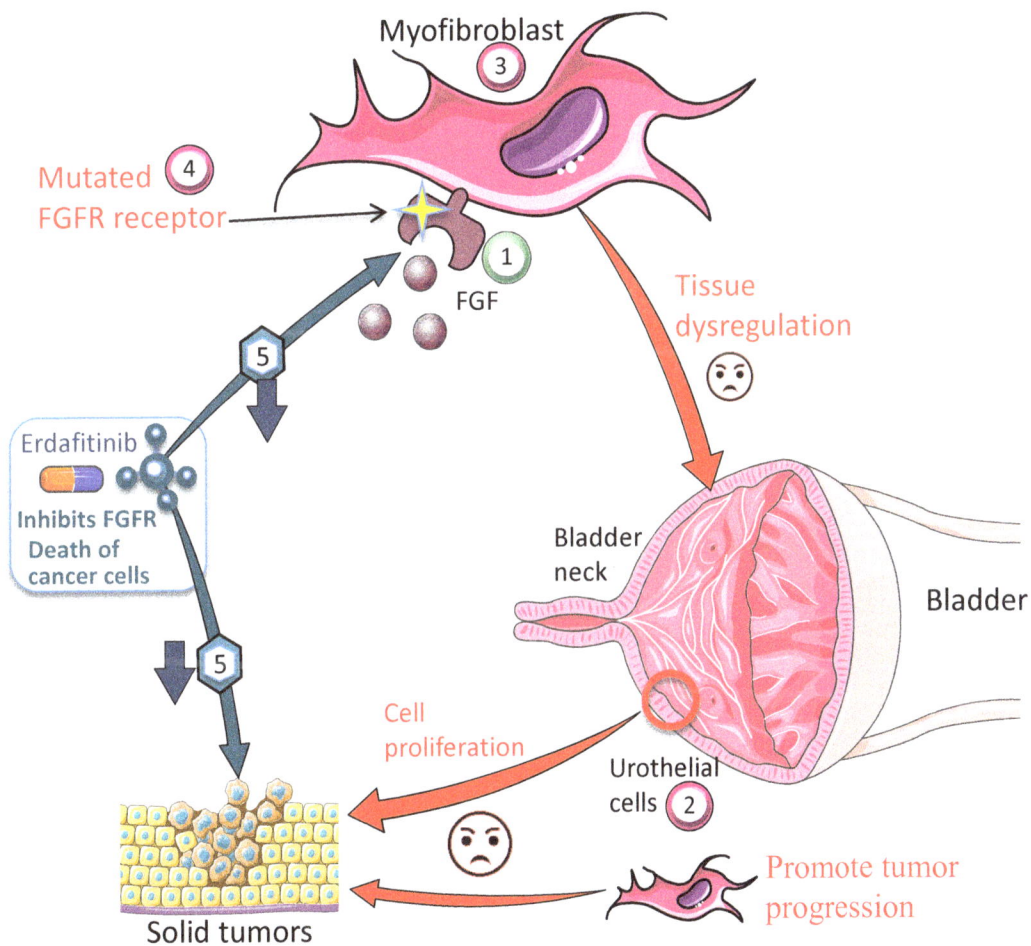

Homeostasis: Bladder cancer, Erdafitinib

The disease: Benign prostatic hyperplasia

Benign prostatic hyperplasia (BPH) is an **enlargement of the prostate gland** and is present in 50% of men >50 years. An enlarged prostate gland can cause uncomfortable urinary symptoms, such as blocking the flow of urine out of the bladder.

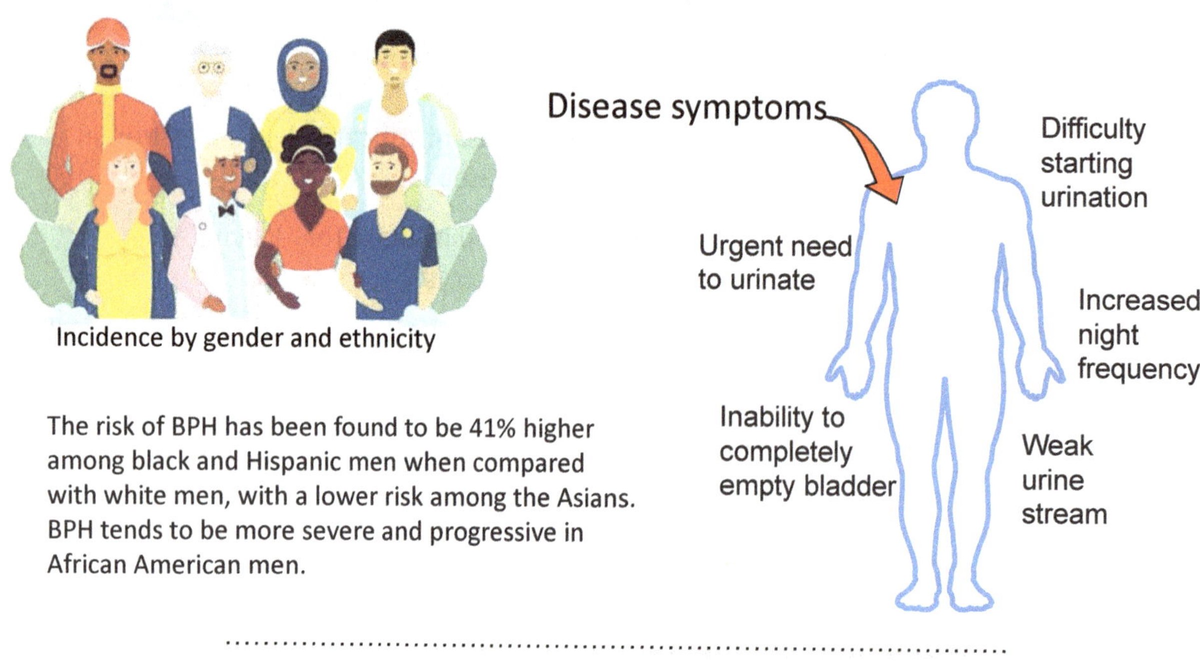

Incidence by gender and ethnicity

The risk of BPH has been found to be 41% higher among black and Hispanic men when compared with white men, with a lower risk among the Asians. BPH tends to be more severe and progressive in African American men.

The medicine

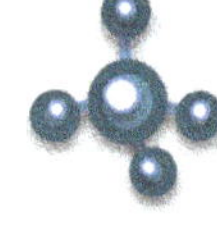

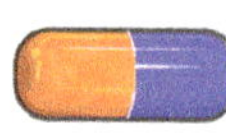

28th Most US Prescribed Drug (2019)
22 million prescriptions

Tamsulosin; Flomax, FDA Approval 1997

Tamsulosin is an alpha-blocker that **relaxes the muscles in the prostate** and bladder neck, making it easier to urinate. Tamsulosin is used to improve urination in men with benign prostatic hyperplasia (enlarged prostate).

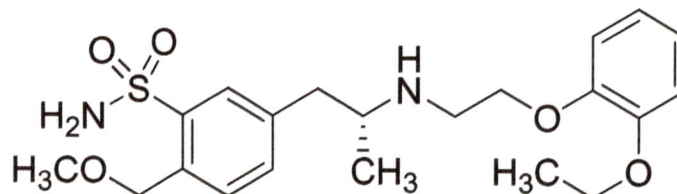

Action of Tamsulosin on cell and disease biology

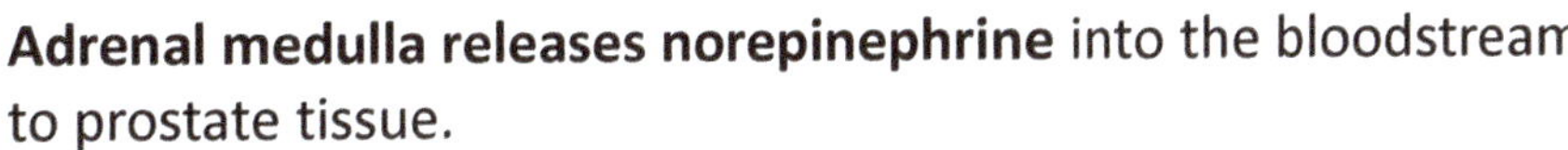

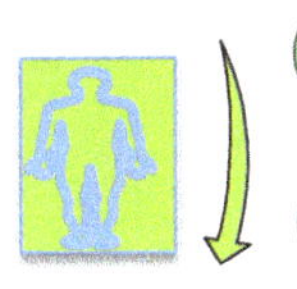

1. **Adrenal medulla releases norepinephrine** into the bloodstream to prostate tissue.
2. **Norepinephrine** binding to alpha-1A receptor will cause **constriction** of the **smooth muscle cells** resulting in decreased or inhibited urine flow.

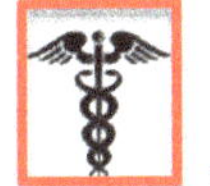

3. Increased prostate smooth **muscle contraction** can contribute to **bladder outlet obstruction** in patients with benign enlarged prostate gland.

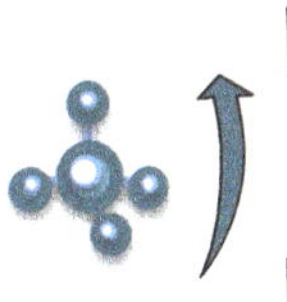

4. **Tamsulosin** is a selective **inhibitor** of **alpha-1A -adrenergic receptors** in the **smooth muscle cells** of the prostate gland and **inhibits norepinephrine** from binding to these receptors.
5. Tamsulosin **relaxes smooth muscles** in the **bladder neck** and lessens the prostate enlargement.

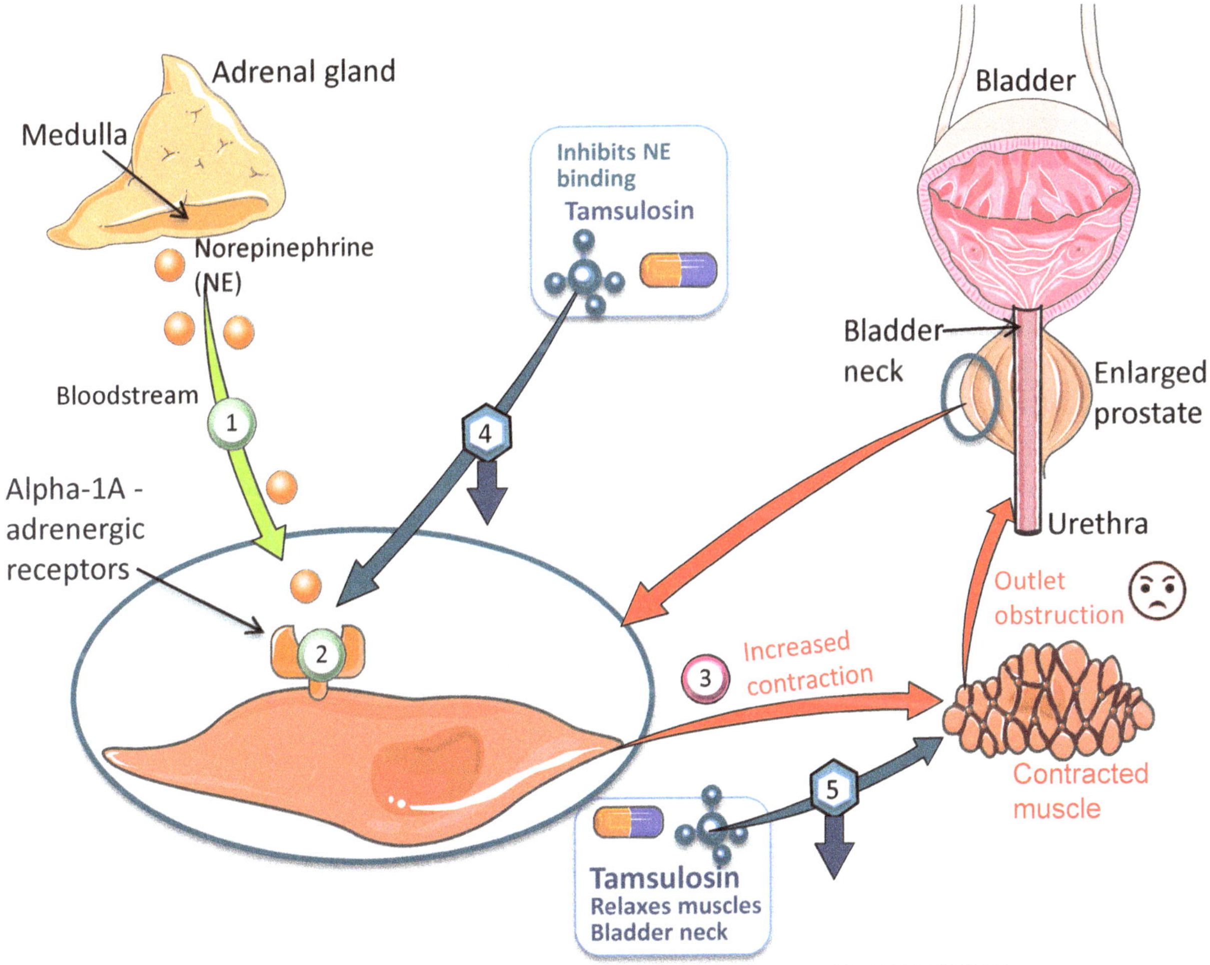

Adrenal gland
Medulla
Norepinephrine (NE)
Bloodstream
1
Alpha-1A - adrenergic receptors
2
Inhibits NE binding
Tamsulosin
4
Bladder
Bladder neck
Enlarged prostate
Urethra
Outlet obstruction
3
Increased contraction
Contracted muscle
5
Tamsulosin
Relaxes muscles
Bladder neck

Homeostasis: Benign prostatic hyperplasia, Tamsulosin

The disease: Coronary artery disease

Chronic coronary artery disease occurs with a **reduction of blood flow** to the heart muscle due to **build-up of cholesterol-containing plaques** (atherosclerosis) in the coronary arteries with symptoms such as angina and shortness of breath with physical activity.

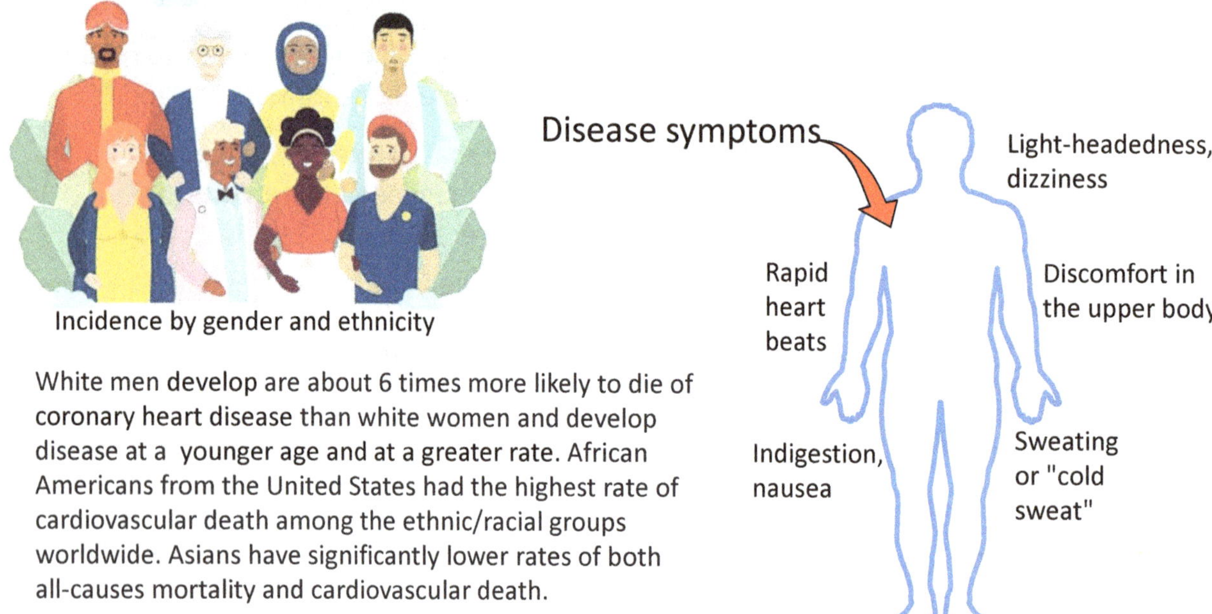

Incidence by gender and ethnicity

White men develop are about 6 times more likely to die of coronary heart disease than white women and develop disease at a younger age and at a greater rate. African Americans from the United States had the highest rate of cardiovascular death among the ethnic/racial groups worldwide. Asians have significantly lower rates of both all-causes mortality and cardiovascular death.

The medicine

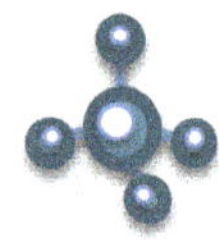

Colchicine; Colcrys, FDA Approval 2009

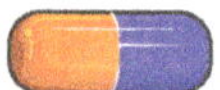

Colchicine is an anti-inflammatory agent and was approved by the FDA for the treatment of acute gout flares. Colchicine is capable of **reducing myocardial injury** in the infarcted area induced by elevated levels of **Interleukin 1 beta** (IL-1β) and neutralizes inflammatory activity by blocking its interaction with IL-1 receptors.

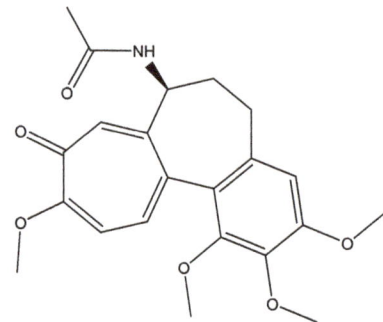

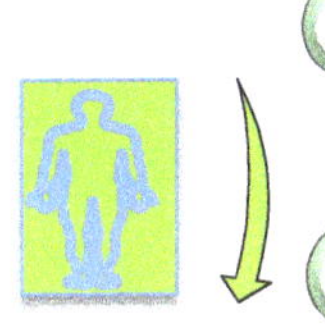

1 **Crystalized cholesterol** is highly immunogenic and activates the macrophage NLRP3 inflammasome, which is a multimeric protein complex that **triggers** the release of **proinflammatory cytokine IL-1β.**

2 In the **inflammasome complex**, the adaptor **bridges** between recognition receptors for the **foreign body and enzyme caspase**, which produces IL-1β.

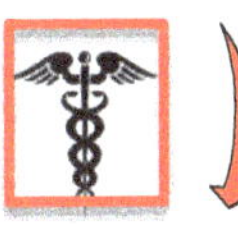

3 **Atherosclerosis** is a chronic inflammatory disease of the arterial wall with formation of **foam cells** (lipid-laden macrophages). **The inflammatory cascade** drives **plaque progression** and instability.

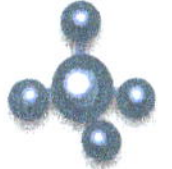

Colchicine inhibits tubulin polymerization, assembly, and activation of the macrophage NLRP3 inflammasome.

Homeostasis: Coronary artery disease, Colchicine

Chapter 5 Brain disorders and selected medicines

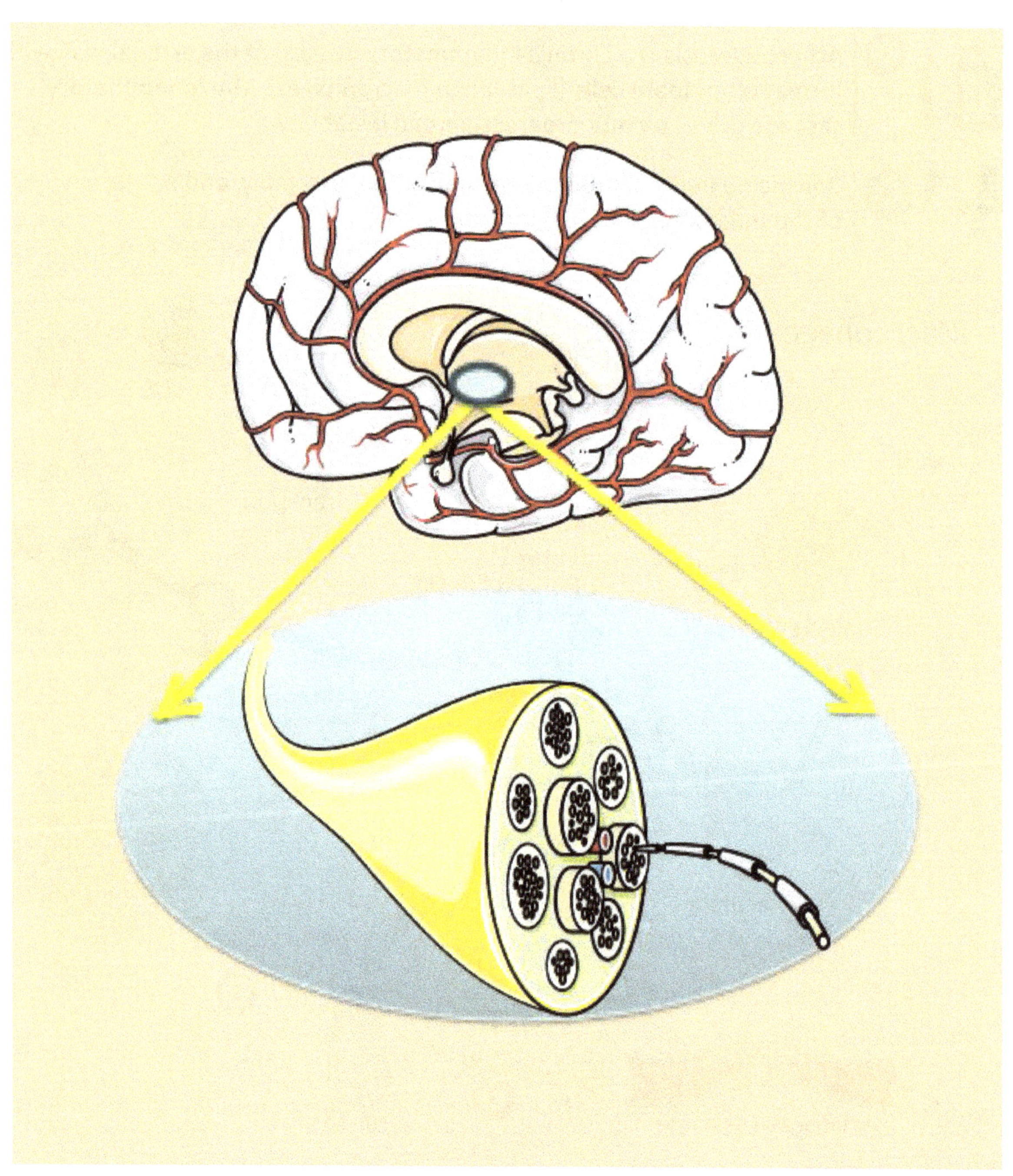

Diseases/disorders of the brain
Blood–brain barrier and infectious diseases
Neurotransmitter functions
Amine neurotransmitters
Amino acid neurotransmitters
Peptide and other neurotransmitters

Overview

Researchers are examining the biology behind disturbances of the brain and connections between distinct psychiatric conditions, such as "anxiety" or "psychosis." The concept of a clear demarcation between such conditions has largely been disproved. We now have the understanding that disorders shade into each other, there are no hard dividing lines and patients can exhibit a mixture of symptoms from different disorders. For example, a clear diagnosis of depression can be accompanied by another disorder such as anxiety.

In this context, the discovery of the biological basis of disorders will allow greater insights into commonalities and differences in brain disturbances. The chapter will describe both commonly prescribed drugs such as vicodin as well drugs recently approved by the FDA to treat a variety of disorders. New discoveries in biology has enabled the development of new therapies. An example is the calcitonin gene-related peptide, which is a potent vasodilator and has enabled the development of drugs for the treatment of migraine.

One group of drugs has been developed to treat diseases that result from disturbances of the blood–brain barrier as well as neurodegenerative diseases. Discussion of the treatment of psychiatric and neurological disorders will be organized on the basis of the associated neurotransmitters. Recent FDA approvals include drugs that target both the major excitatory and inhibitory neurotransmitters as well as dopamine, which can play either role depending on the location of a specific receptor in the nervous system.

Diseases/Disorders of the Brain

The brain is a principal source of disease and largest cause of disability-adjusted life years. Alzheimer disease, stroke, and Parkinson disease will be major future health challenges.

Disorder/Injuries

- Infections
- Traumatic brain injury
- Brain cancer
- Stroke and vascular Diseases

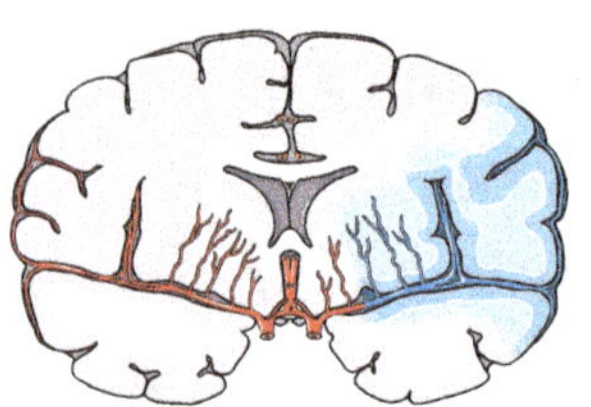

Neuropsychiatric

- Neurodegenerative conditions
- Epilepsy and other seizure disorders
- Mental disorders
- Dementias

Selected drugs approved by the FDA for brain diseases.
√ = Drugs approved recently (2017–2021)

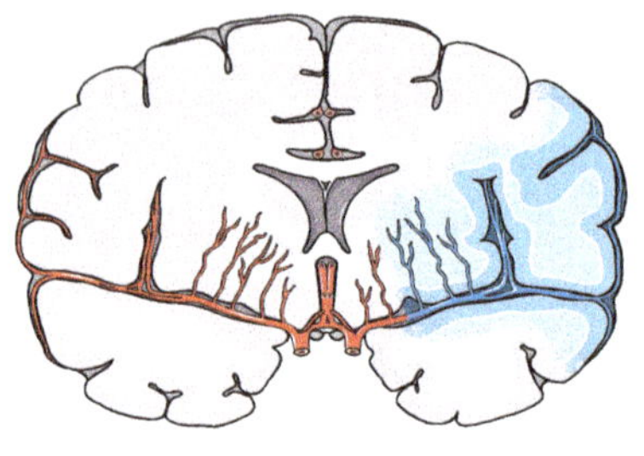

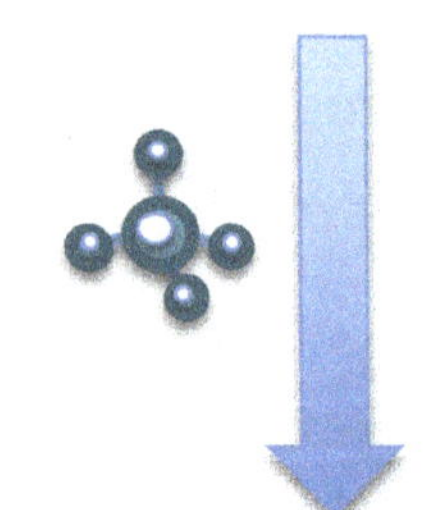

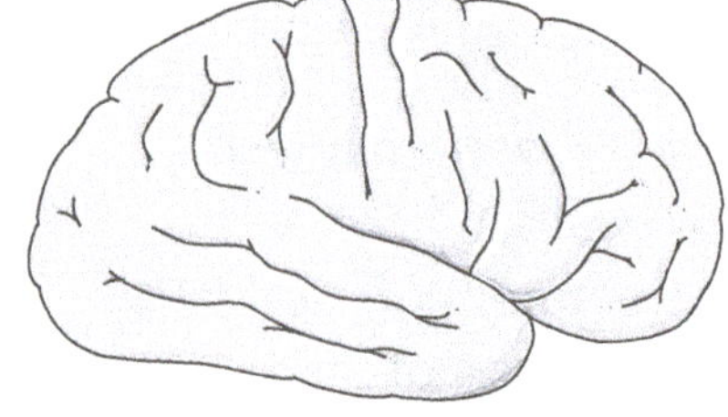

Disruption of the blood–brain barrier (BBB)

- Bacterial meningitis (Rocephin)
- Multiple sclerosis (Ocrevus √, Siponimod √)
- Amyotrophic lateral sclerosis (Radicava √)

Neurodegenerative diseases

- Parkinson disease (Xadago √, Nourianz √)
- Alzheimer disease (Aricept)
- Huntington disease (Austedo √)

Psychiatric disorders

- Anxiety disorders (Xanax)
- Postpartum depression (Zulresso √)
- Schizophrenia (Caplyta √)

Neurological disorders

- Migraine (Reyvow √, Emgality √, Ubrelvy √)
- Pain (Vicodin)
- Insomnia (Lunesta, Dayvigo √)
- Narcolepsy (Sunosi √, Wakix √)
- Epilepsy (Lamictal)

Types of of brain diseases/disorders and selected drugs

Blood–brain barrier (BBB)

The main function of the BBB is to **protect the brain and** maintain **homeostasis** of the most vital organ of the human body and keep it isolated from harmful toxins in the blood.

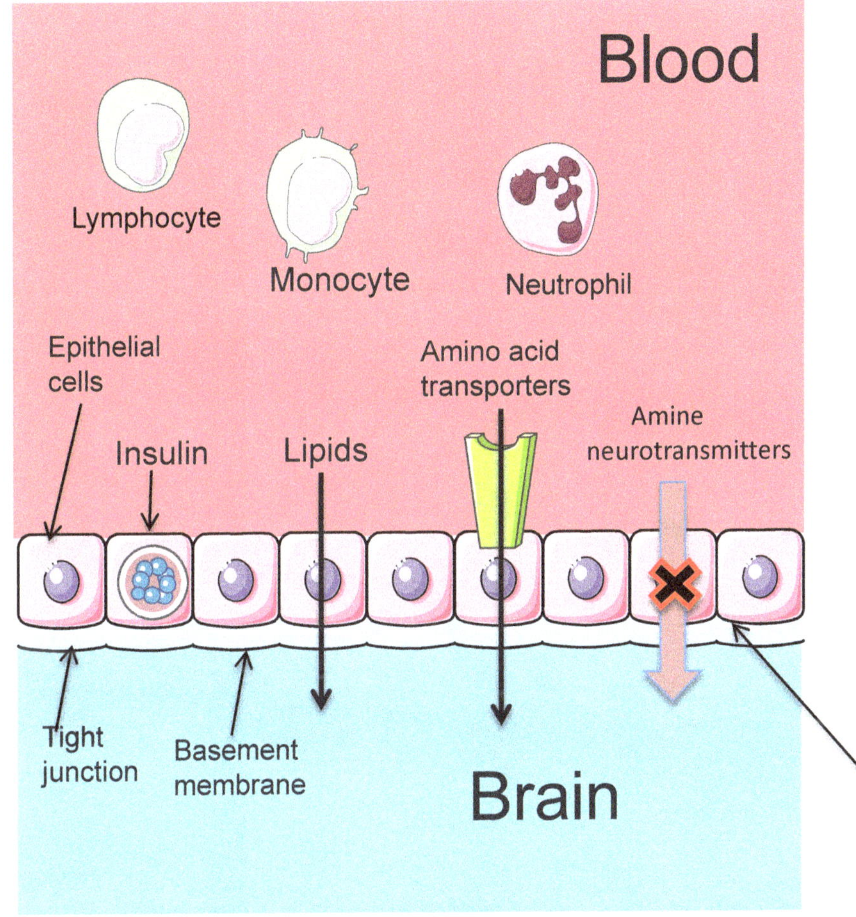

The **BBB becomes more permeable during inflammation**, which allows some antibiotics and phagocytes to move across the barrier but also some bacteria and viruses.

The BBB is formed by **tight junctions between epithelial cells** that surround brain tissue

Neurotransmitters such as dopamine or norepinephrine can not cross the blood–brain barrier. **Tryptophan,** an essential amino acid and a precursor for monoamine neurotransmitters, **must be transported across the BBB**.

98% of all small molecule drugs do not cross the BBB.

- The ideal compound to treat CNS infections is of a small molecular size and moderately lipophilic.
- A low level of plasma protein binding increases drug availability.
- Active efflux of the drug at the blood–brain or –CSF barrier needs to be minimized.

The disease: Bacterial meningitis

Bacterial meningitis affects the meninges, the membranes that surround the brain and the central nervous system (CNS). **Bacterial meningitis** is a condition that results in the **inflammation** of the protective blood–CSF/blood–brain barrier (**BBB**), which then **becomes leaky** by opening of intercellular tight junctions of the vessel walls. Symptoms include a fever, headache, and nausea.

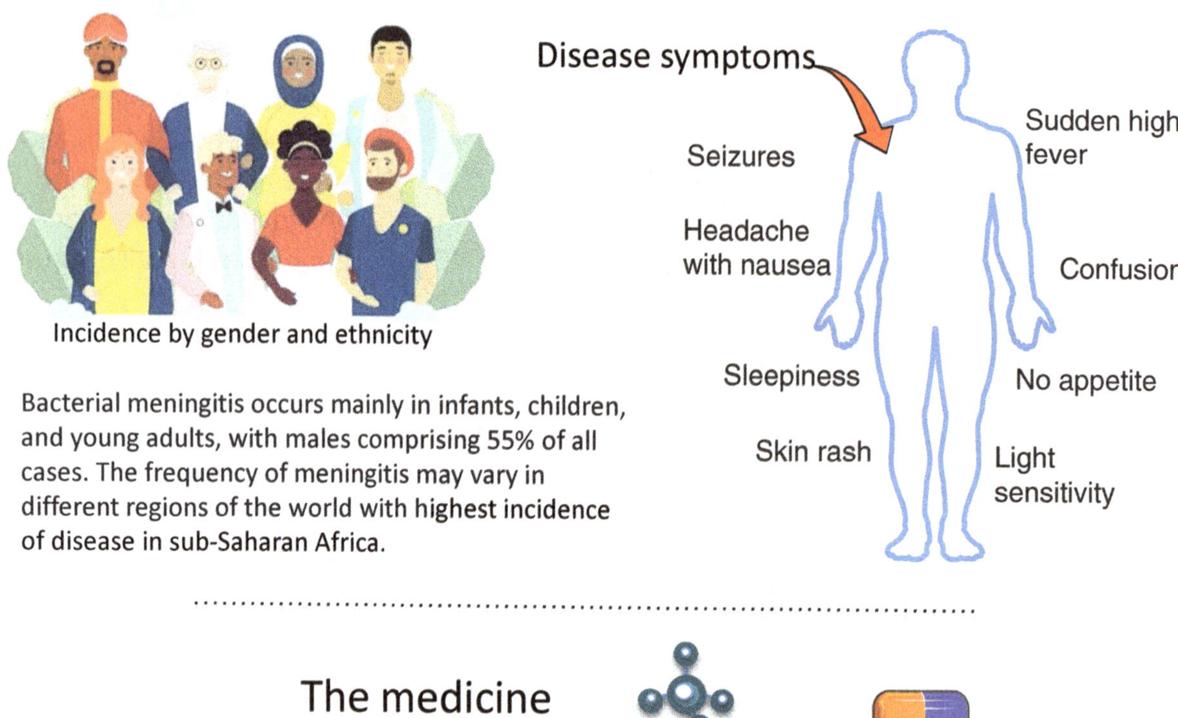

Incidence by gender and ethnicity

Bacterial meningitis occurs mainly in infants, children, and young adults, with males comprising 55% of all cases. The frequency of meningitis may vary in different regions of the world with highest incidence of disease in sub-Saharan Africa.

The medicine

Ceftriaxone; Rocephin, FDA Approval 2005

Ceftriaxone is a third-generation cephalosporin, which are **broad spectrum antibiotics** that have a beta-lactam ring. Rocephin is used to treat a variety of bacterial infections, especially meningitis. Two gram-positive bacteria are the most common causes of bacterial meningitis; Streptococcus pneumoniae (in adults), Streptococcus agalactiae (in neonates), and Neisseria meningitidis, a gram-negative bacterium.

Ceftriaxone has a long half life with higher serum concentrations and **penetration** through the inflamed **blood–brain barrier**.

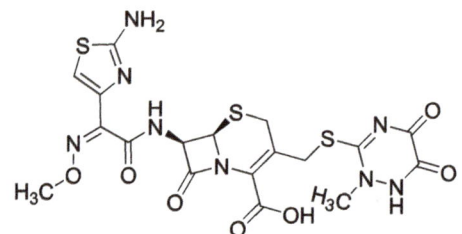

Brain diseases: Infection, bacterial meningitis, Ceftriaxone

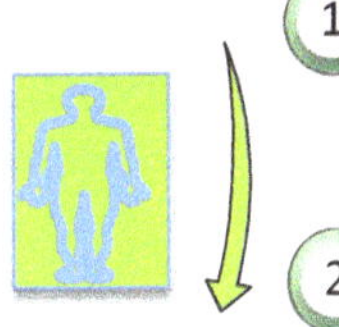

1 **Penicillin-binding proteins** (**PBPs**) are bacterial components, characterized by the ability to bind penicillin. PBPs are **transpeptidases** that are involved in bacterial cell wall synthesis.

2 When **penicillins** and cephalosporins **bind** to the **transpeptidas**e enzyme, the formation of **peptide cross-links is blocked** with rupture of the bacterium.

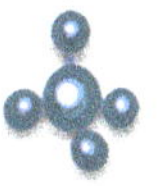

3 **Ceftriaxone interferes** with **bacterial cell wall synthesis** by binding to penicillin-binding proteins, eventually leading to cell lysis and death.

Bacterial cell wall

Peptide bridge

1 Penicillin-binding protein

3 Ceftriaxone
Blocks penicillin-binding proteins

2 Transpeptidase enzyme

Transpeptidase enzyme inhibited

Bacterial cell wall synthesis

Peptide bridge

Block peptide cross-links

Bacterium rupture

Bacterial cell wall

The disease: Multiple sclerosis

In multiple sclerosis (MS) the patients suffer symptoms such as **vision loss, pain, and impaired coordination.** The body's **immune cells attack and damage the myelin sheath** surrounding nerves (brain and spinal cord), blocks communication between the brain and body. In all forms of MS, patients experience inflammation in the nervous system and permanent loss of nerve cells in the brain, spinal cord, or optic nerves.

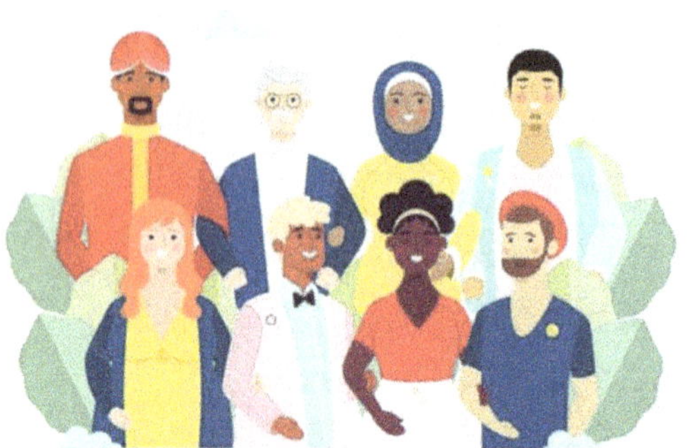

Incidence by gender and ethnicity

MS is more common in women than men (3.5–1.0) and increasing over time. Women have more inflammatory lesions, but men have a faster development of disability and worse relapse recovery. MS occurs in most ethnic groups, but is most common amongst people of European descent and is rare in Africa and Asia. MS is uncommon in the Asia Pacific region (China, Korea, Taiwan, South East Asia) as well as India.

Disease symptoms

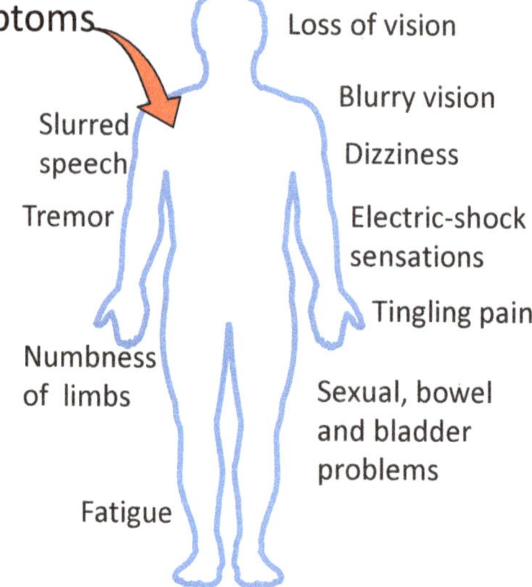

The medicine

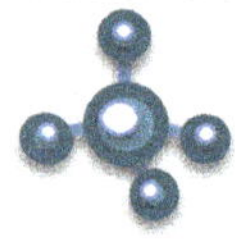

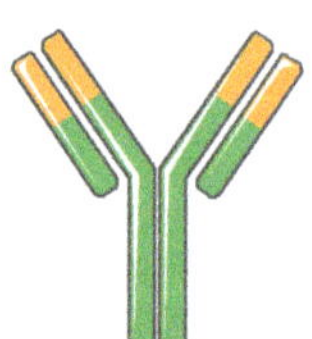

Ocrelizumab; Ocrevus, FDA Approval 2017

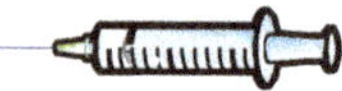

Administered as an intravenous infusion

Ocrelizumab is approved to treat **relapsing** (RMS) or **primary progressive** (PPMS, **a highly disabling form** of **MS**). Ocrevus achieves profound **suppression of inflammation** in RMS patients and a reduction in the progression of disability in PPMS.

Ocrelizumab is a humanized monoclonal **antibody (Ab) that targets the large extracellular loop of CD20**, which is a distinct epitope on CD20 that differentiates Ocrelizumab from the other CD20-depleting agents such as rituximab.

Action of Ocrelizumab on cell and disease biology

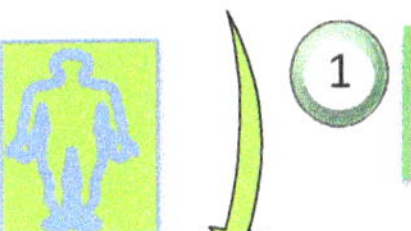

1 **CD20 functions** on resting **B cells** as a **gatekeeper** but B cells, which do not have CD20 as a surface marker, still can fight infections.

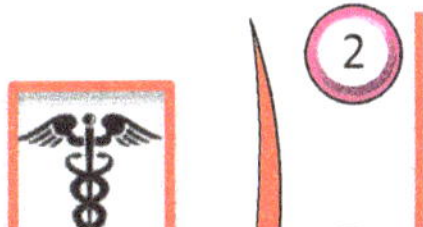

2 **Activated T-cells and B-cells** can cross the compromised blood–brain barrier (BBB) to cause **inflammation** and destroy myelin. The BBB can be disrupted by stress, inflammation, drugs, air pollution, or smoking.

3 **B cells recognize myelin fragments**, which are then presented as an antigen to proliferating T cells, signaling the launch of an immune attack.

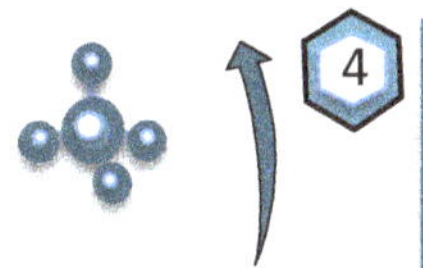

4 A single dose of **Ocrelizumab depletes CD20 containing B cells**. When B-cells are killed a highly activated subset of T-cells (CD20+) stop proliferating.

Other B cells, which do not have CD20 as a surface marker, still have the **capacity to fight infections**.

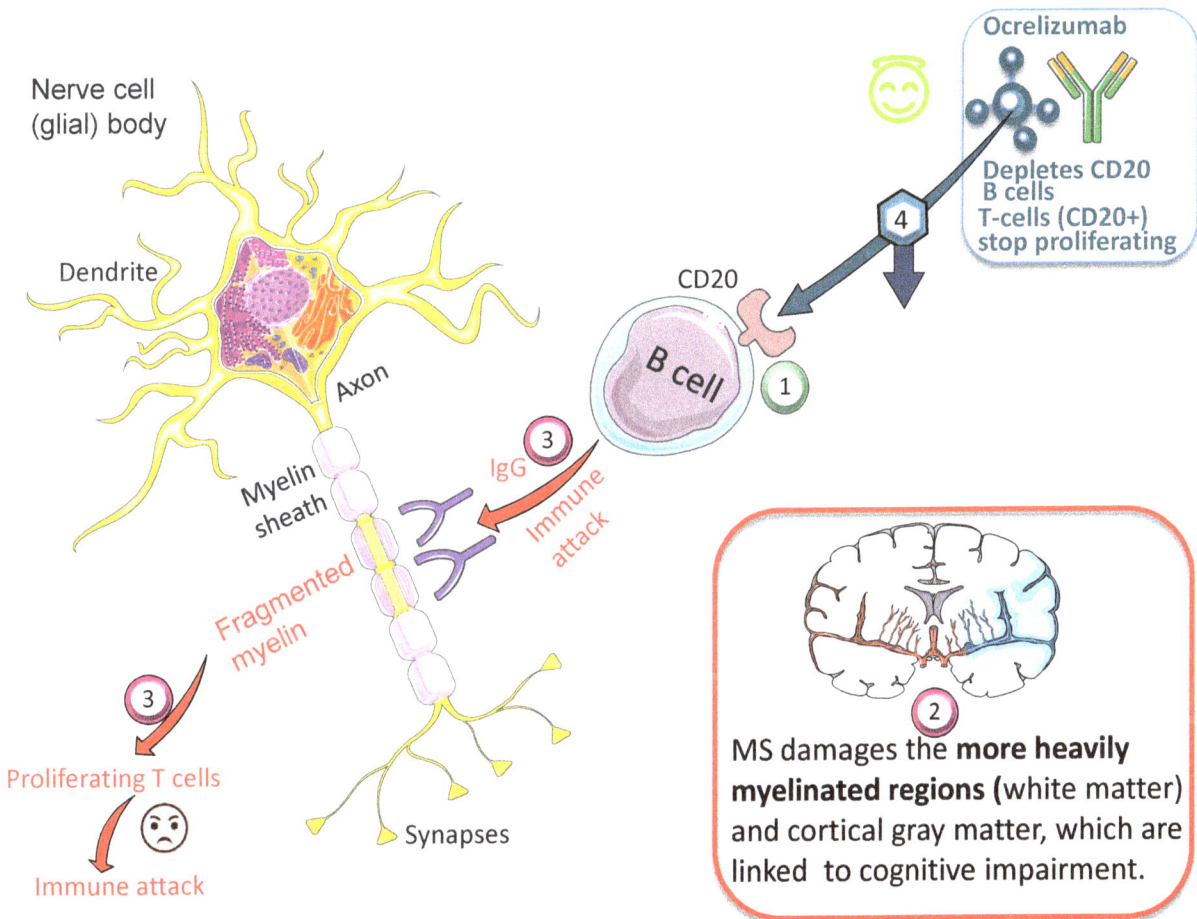

Brain diseases: Inflammation, multiple sclerosis, Ocrelizumab

The disease: Multiple sclerosis

In **multiple sclerosis**, the normally impenetrable blood–brain barrier (BBB) is breached and **activated lymphocytes enter the CNS** with an "inflammatory cascade." The resulting damage to myelin results in scarring of de-myelinated areas.

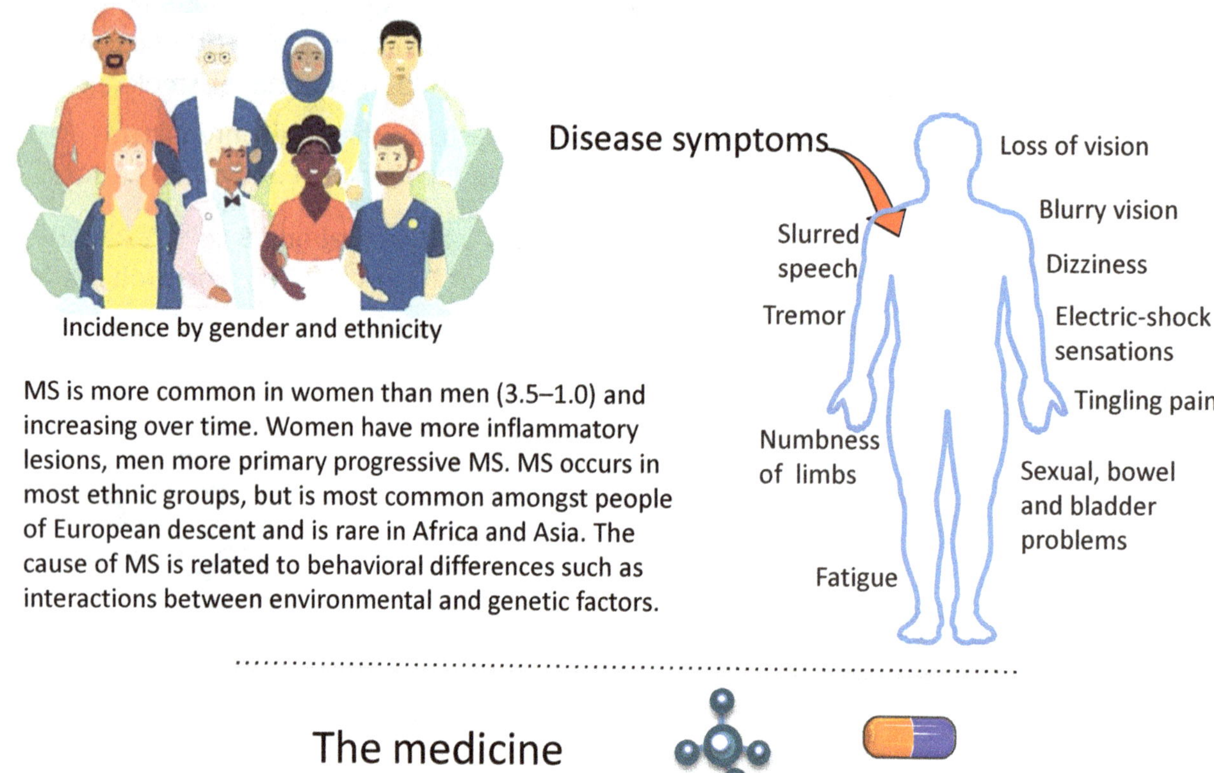

Incidence by gender and ethnicity

MS is more common in women than men (3.5–1.0) and increasing over time. Women have more inflammatory lesions, men more primary progressive MS. MS occurs in most ethnic groups, but is most common amongst people of European descent and is rare in Africa and Asia. The cause of MS is related to behavioral differences such as interactions between environmental and genetic factors.

The medicine

Mayzent; Siponimod, FDA Approval 2019

In **multiple sclerosis,** the normally impenetrable BBB is breached and **activated lymphocytes enter the CNS** with an "inflammatory cascade." The resulting damage to myelin results in scarring of de-myelinated areas.

Mayzent is a modulator of sphingosine 1-phosphate (S1P) receptors on surface of lymphocytes. Mayzent modulates glia reactivity and **reduces** neuronal **injury**.

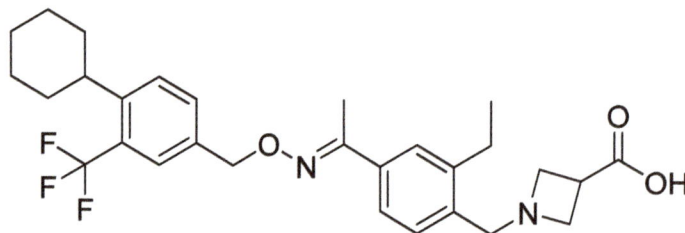

F F F O N N O OH

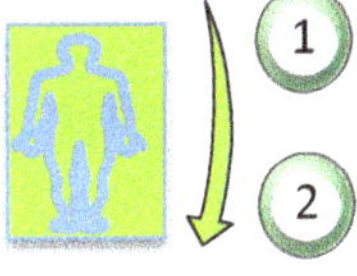

1 **Sphingosine-1-phosphate** (S1P) is a **signaling lipid**, which regulates proliferation, survival, migration of astrocytes, microglia, oligodendrocytes.

2 Endothelial cells and astrocytes are the principal BBB cellular constituents and express **S1P receptors** located **at the plasma membrane**, thus inducing biological responses

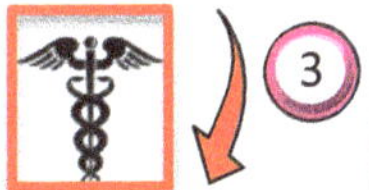

3 Sphingosine-1-phosphate (**S1P**) promotes **infiltration of peripheral immune cells** in the CNS during neuroinflammation and T- cell trafficking.

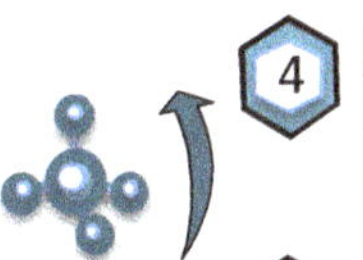

4 **Mayzent internalizes the S1P1 receptor,** inhibits efflux of lymphocytes from lymph nodes, which results in lymphocytes being sequestered and **inhibits migration** to the location of inflammation.

5 Mayzent **stabilizes the blood–brain barrier** and reduces peripheral immune cell recruitment.

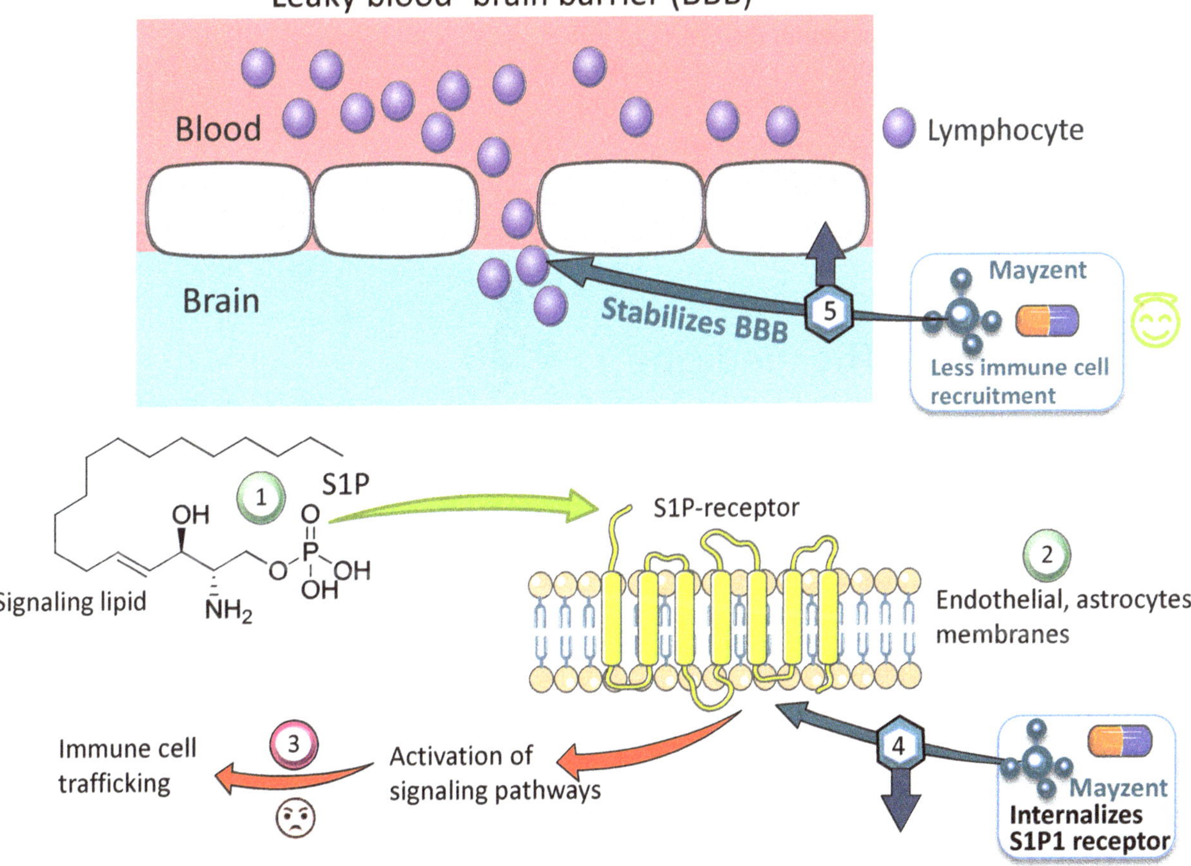

Brain diseases: Inflammation, multiple sclerosis, Mayzent

The disease: Amyotrophic lateral sclerosis

Amyotrophic lateral sclerosis (ALS) or Lou Gehrig's disease involves **degeneration of motor neurons** in the spinal cord, brainstem, and cerebral cortex, leading to progressive paralysis of voluntary muscles with death from respiratory failure. Most cases have no genetic association (**sporadic ALS),** but 10% of cases have mutations in over 20 genes, such as superoxide dismutase which converts reactive oxygen to harmless water.

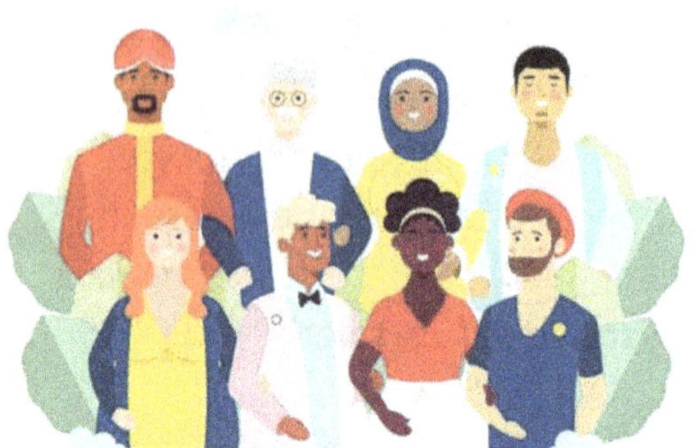

Incidence by gender and ethnicity

The prevalence of ALS are greater in men than in women and men predominate in the younger age groups of patients with ALS. As people age, the difference between men and women disappears. ALS rates are higher among Caucasians in Western countries compared with those of African, Asian, and Hispanic descent.

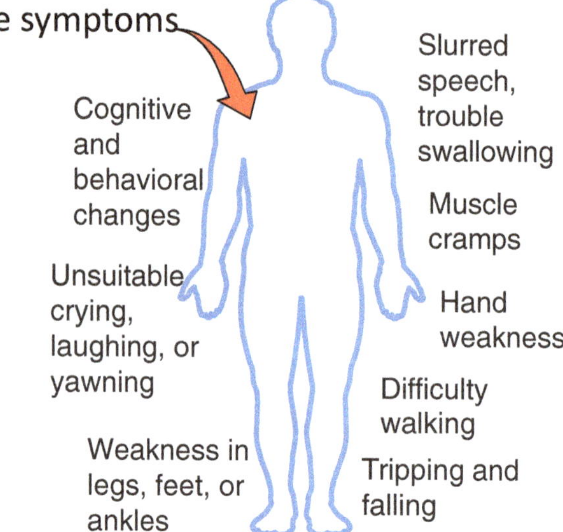

The medicine

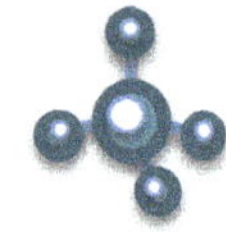

Edaravone; Radicava, FDA Approval 2017

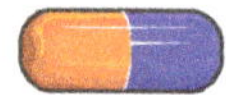

Edaravone reduces the effects of **oxidative stress**, which may be related to the death of motor neurons (nerve cells) in people with amyotrophic lateral sclerosis (ALS). Keeping **motor neurons healthy** may help to preserve muscle function.

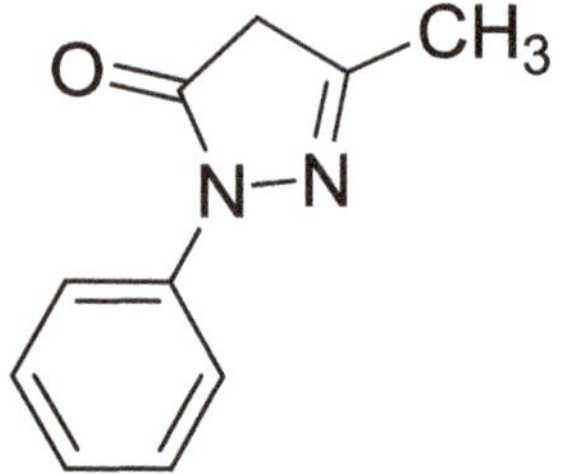

Action of Edaravone on cell and disease biology

In **amyotrophic lateral sclerosis** (ALS), alterations in the blood-central nervous system (CNS) barrier aggravate motor neuron damage.

1 **In ALS, oxidative damage of the motor neuron** is triggered by increased **production of reactive oxygen species** (ROS), such as **superoxide** (O_2^-), with increases in metal ions (copper, iron).

2 **Free radicals** that accumulate over time increase the production of **mutated DNA** that can be related to the disease process.

3 **Mitochondria exist in high numbers due to metabolic demand in the motor neurons** and are vulnerable to cumulative oxidative stress.

4 **Lipids are major targets of oxidative stress**, lipid peroxidation increases **membrane leakiness,** intracellular Ca^{2+} contents with disrupted signaling.

5 **Edaravone** is a neuroprotective agent, acts as a free radical scavenger to reduce oxidative stress (ROS), and damage to neurons and cell membranes to inhibit the progression of ALS .

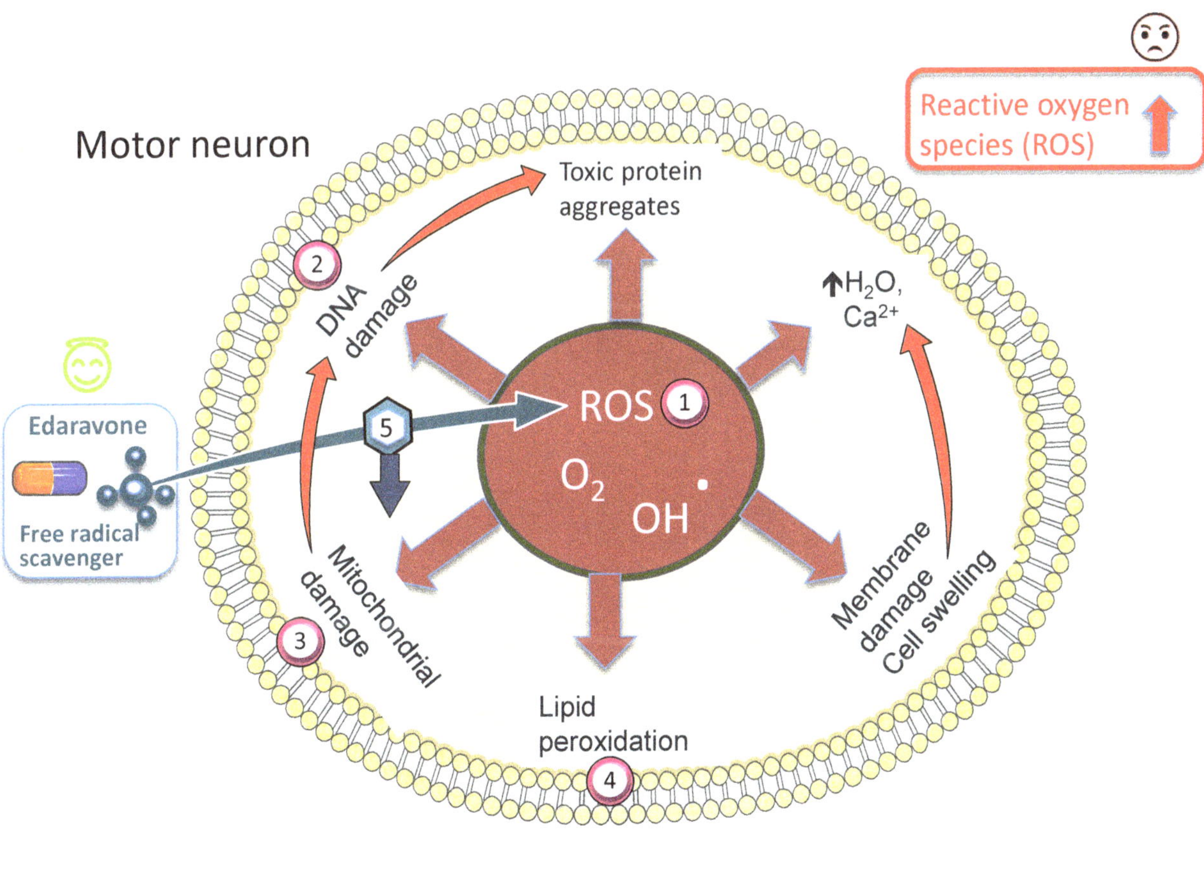

Neurotransmitters

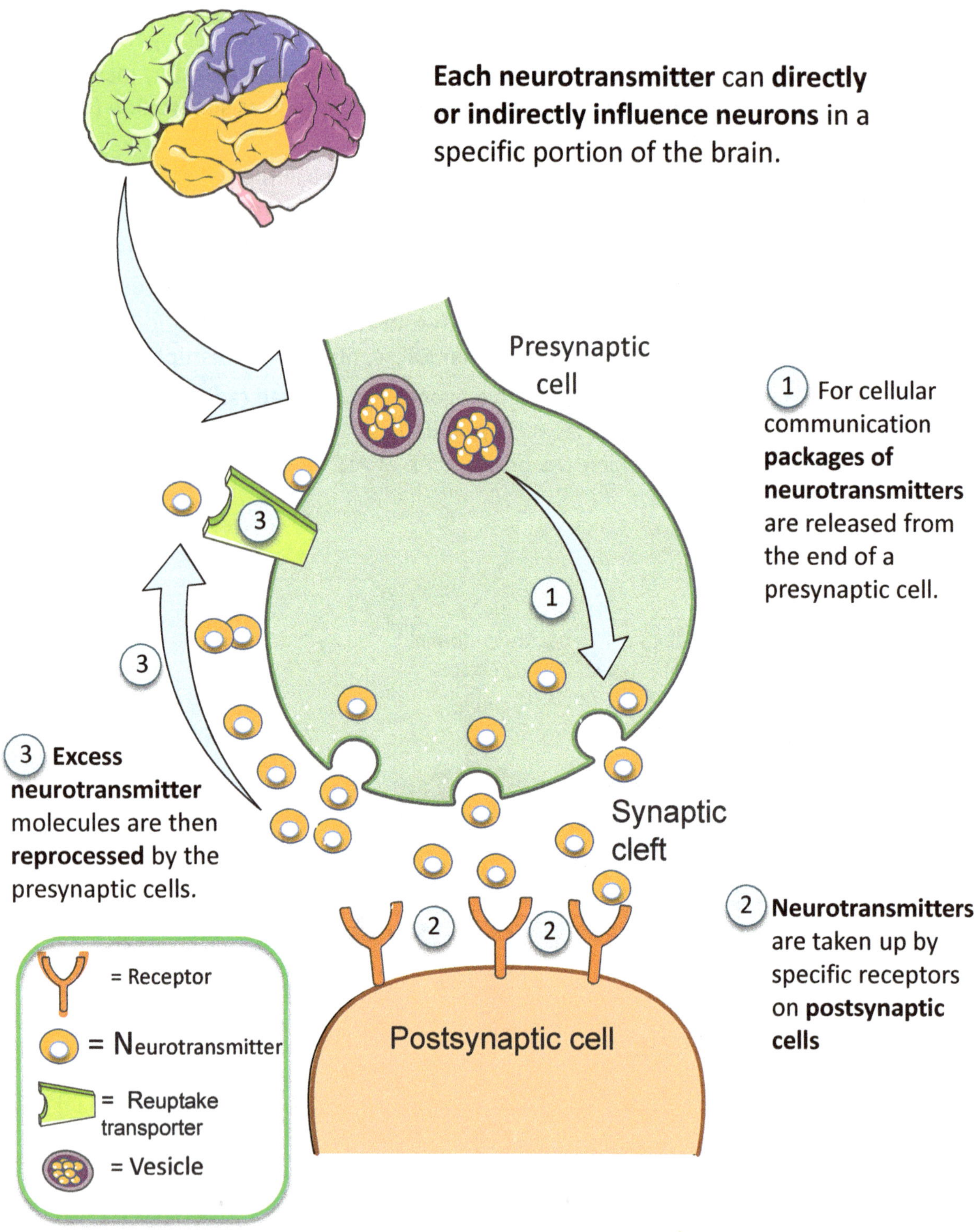

Each neurotransmitter can **directly or indirectly influence neurons** in a specific portion of the brain.
Presynaptic cell
1 For cellular communication **packages of neurotransmitters** are released from the end of a presynaptic cell.
3
1
3
3 **Excess neurotransmitter** molecules are then **reprocessed** by the presynaptic cells.
Synaptic cleft
2
2
2 **Neurotransmitters** are taken up by specific receptors on **postsynaptic cells**
Postsynaptic cell
= Receptor
= Neurotransmitter
= Reuptake transporter
= Vesicle

Excitatory and inhibitory neurotransmitters

Major **excitatory neurotransmitters**
- Acetylcholine
- Glutamate
- Norepinephrine
- Epinephrine
- Histamine

Dopamine functions as both an inhibitory and excitatory neurotransmitter depending upon the type and location of the receptor.

Important **inhibitory neurotransmitters**
- Gamma-aminobutyric acid (GABA)
- Serotonin
- Glycine

Serotonin is involved in cognition, memory, regulation of mood, appetite and digestion, the sleep-wake cycle, and social behavior. **Low levels** of serotonin are **associated with depression.**

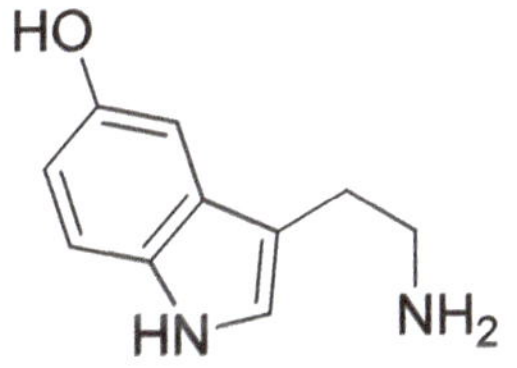
HO
HN
NH_2

Dopamine creates **positive feelings** associated with reward or reinforcement and may be associated with schizophrenia, depression, and the sleep-wake cycle. Dopamine **regulates our reward circuitry** and dopamine production is stimulated by drugs like cocaine, opiates, and alcohol.

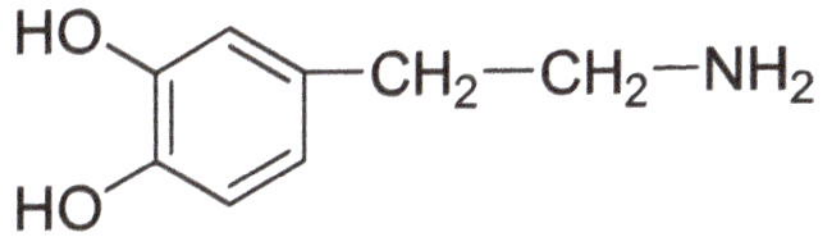
HO
HO
$-CH_2-CH_2-NH_2$

Gamma-aminobutyric acid (GABA) plays a **prominent role in the brain control of stress and hence mood.** Major depressive disorders are accompanied by reduced brain concentrations of GABA.

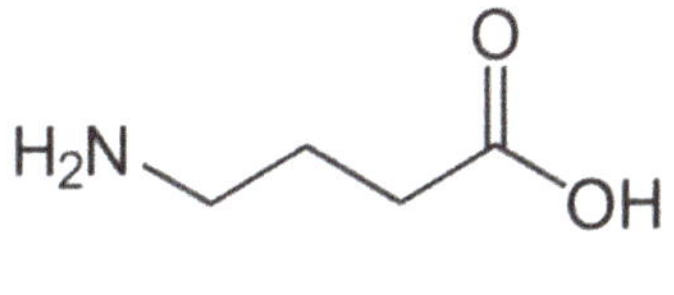
H_2N
O
OH

Norepinephrine has effects on attention, arousal, and emotional memory. Norepinephrine pathways can modulate synthesis of GABA. Some **depressions occur when there is too little norepinephrine** in certain brain circuits. Alternatively, mania results when there is too much in the brain.

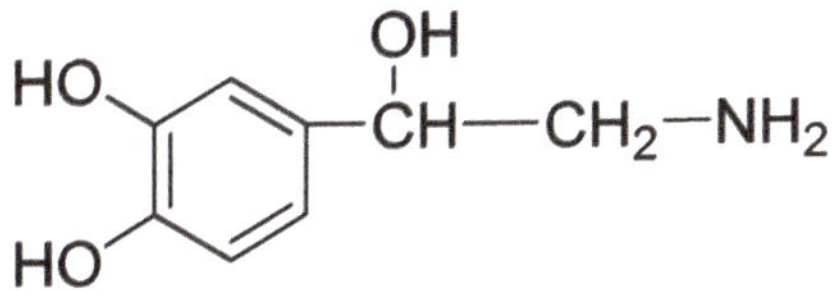
OH
HO
HO
$-CH-CH_2-NH_2$

Brain diseases: Neurotransmitter functions

Amine Neurotransmitters

- Dopamine 1
  (3,4-dihydroxyphenethylamine)
- Norepinephrine (noradrenaline) 2
- Epinephrine (adrenaline) 3
- Serotonin 4
  (5-hydroxytryptamine, or 5-HT)
- Histamine 5

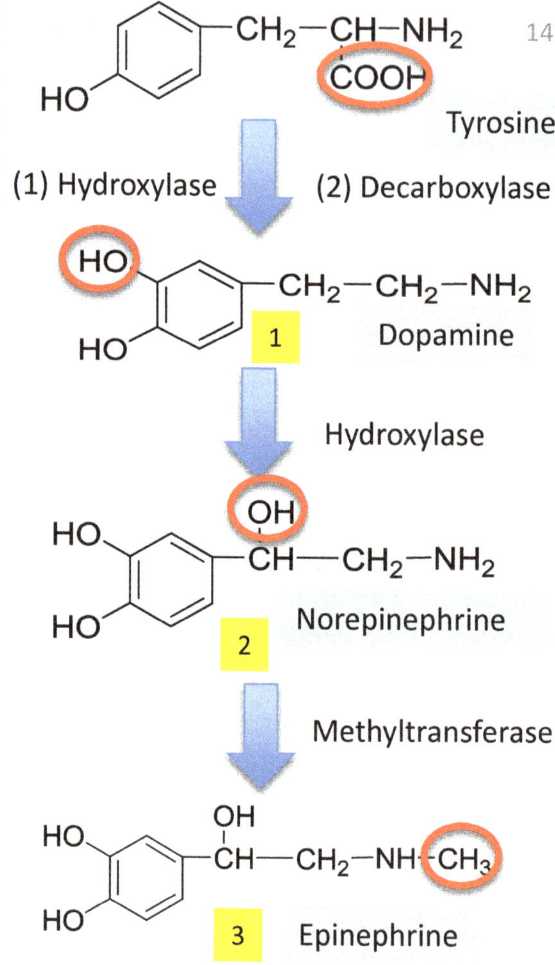

Drug effects on levels of neurotransmitters as a result of disease therapies (see later for detailed descriptions).

Neurotransmitter	↑↓ **Drug**	Disease
Dopamine		
	↑ **Caplyta**	Schizophrenia
	↑ **Sunosi**	Narcolepsy
	↑ **Xadago**	Parkinson's disease
	↓ **Austedo**	Tardive dyskinesias
Norepinephrine	↑ **Sunosi**	Narcolepsy
Serotonin	↑ **Reyvow**	Migraine
Histamine	↓ **Wakix**	Narcolepsy

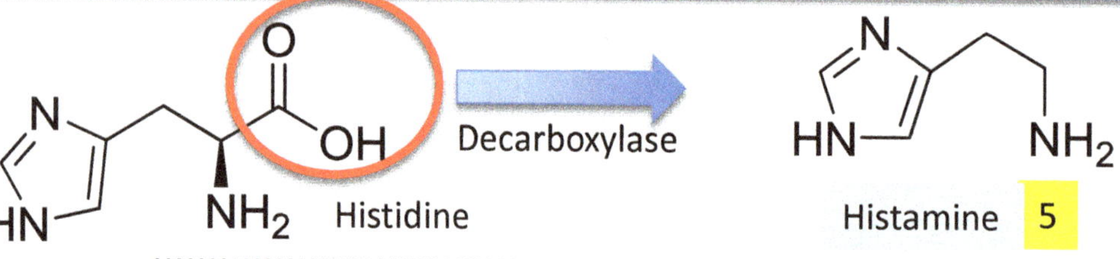

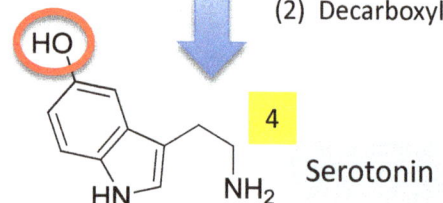

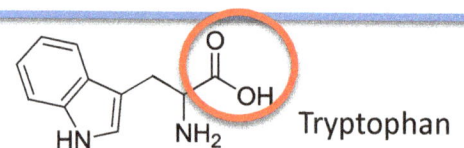

Brain diseases: Pathways for production

Divergence in neurotransmitter systems

The **release of neurotransmitters** is controlled by specialized receptors on a target cell.

Neurons synthesize these neurotransmitters and **package them in vesicles** located at the ends of axons.

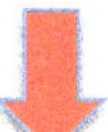

Neuronal activation causes the **release of neurotransmitters** from the axonal terminals onto **dendrites** (branch-like projections in adjacent neurons).

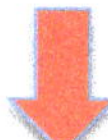

Every neurotransmitter can activate **multiple receptor subtypes.**

For example**, dopamine** and **serotonin** may directly **inhibit GABA-A** receptors that are adjacent to dopamine release sites in the striatum (forebrain).

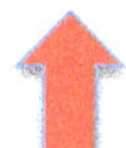

Divergence is the ability of one transmitter to activate **more than one subtype** of a receptor and resulting synaptic response.

Serotonin can be co-localized with other neurotransmitters which allows reciprocal interactions.

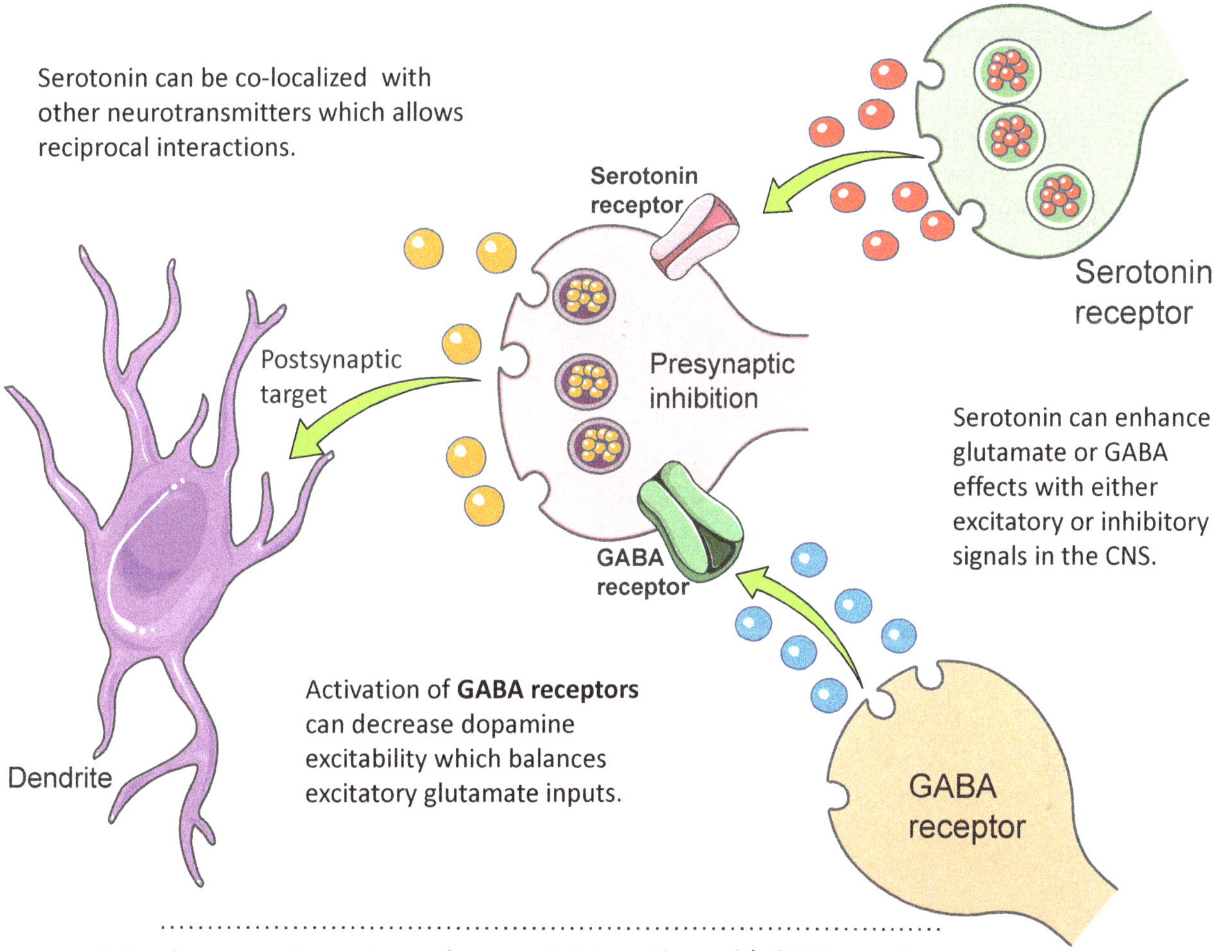

Serotonin receptor

Serotonin receptor

Postsynaptic target

Presynaptic inhibition

Serotonin can enhance glutamate or GABA effects with either excitatory or inhibitory signals in the CNS.

GABA receptor

Activation of **GABA receptors** can decrease dopamine excitability which balances excitatory glutamate inputs.

Dendrite

GABA receptor

The disease: Schizophrenia

Schizophrenia is a **complex brain disorder** that impacts 1% of the population. The symptoms include an individual hearing voices and becoming suspicious or withdrawn.

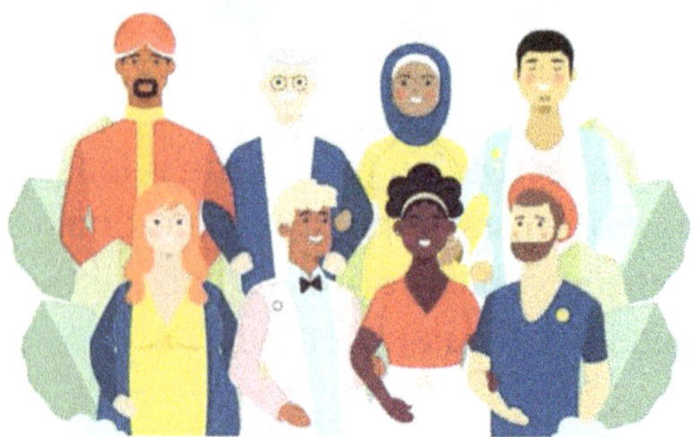

Incidence by gender and ethnicity

The incidence of schizophrenia was two to three times higher among males than females and the average age of onset tends to be in late teens to early 20s for men, and the late 20s to early 30s for women (uncommon to be diagnosed in a person younger than 12 or older than 40). Latino Americans where more than three times more likely to be diagnosed with Schizophrenia than Euro-Americans and self-reported psychotic symptoms is lowest in Asian Americans.

Disease symptoms

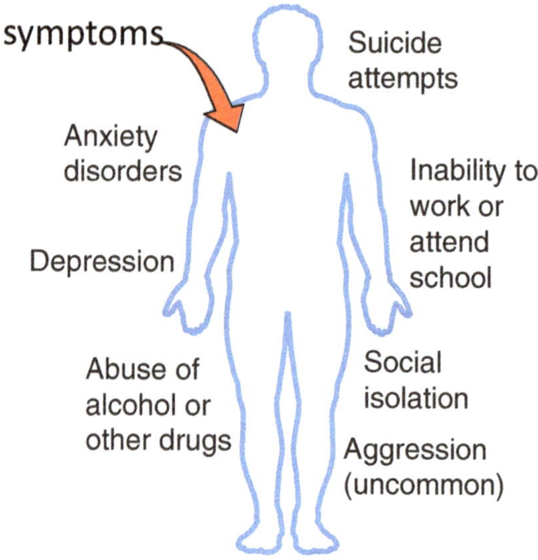

The medicine

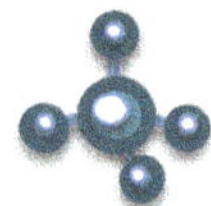

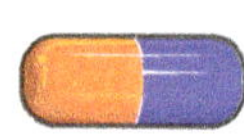

Lumateperone; Caplyta, FDA Approval 2019

Caplyta is a second-generation **antipsychotic** for the treatment of schizophrenia potentially through **blocking** activity at **serotonin and dopamine receptors.**

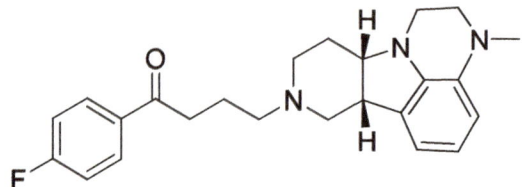

Amine neurotransmitters: Schizophrenia, Lumateperone

Action of Lumateperone on cell and disease biology

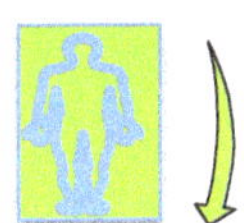

Dopamine D2 receptors are present in the midbrain/**basal forebrain** with **D2 pathways in** the **midbrain, prefrontal cortex, and limbic system**.

Serotonin pathways project from the **brain stem** (pons) and **midbrain** (raphe nuclei) **to the cortex and limbic system (**thalamus and hypothalamus).

Serotonin receptors (S) are in the **prefrontal cortex** and limbic system; **hypothalamus** (anxiety, stress response); **hippocampus** (learning and memory deficits, seizures, depression); **brain stem (Raphe nuclei).**

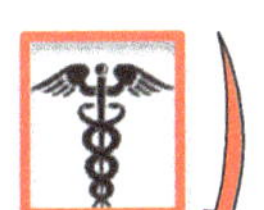

In psychosis, **dopamine signals are typically abnormal**. Stress in schizophrenia patients causes an increased release of dopamine in the prefrontal cortex.

Serotonin 2A receptor has been implicated in **mental disorders**, in processes such as learning, memory, and in neurogenesis.

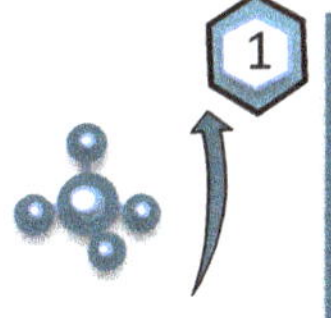

Lumateperone is selective for **dopamine (D2) receptors, modulates glutamate, serotonin and dopamine**, all related to schizophrenia pathophysiology.

Lumateperone's action may be due to a combination of **blocking activity** in **the central nervous system of both serotonin 2A receptors** and **postsynaptic** localized **dopamine D2 receptors.**

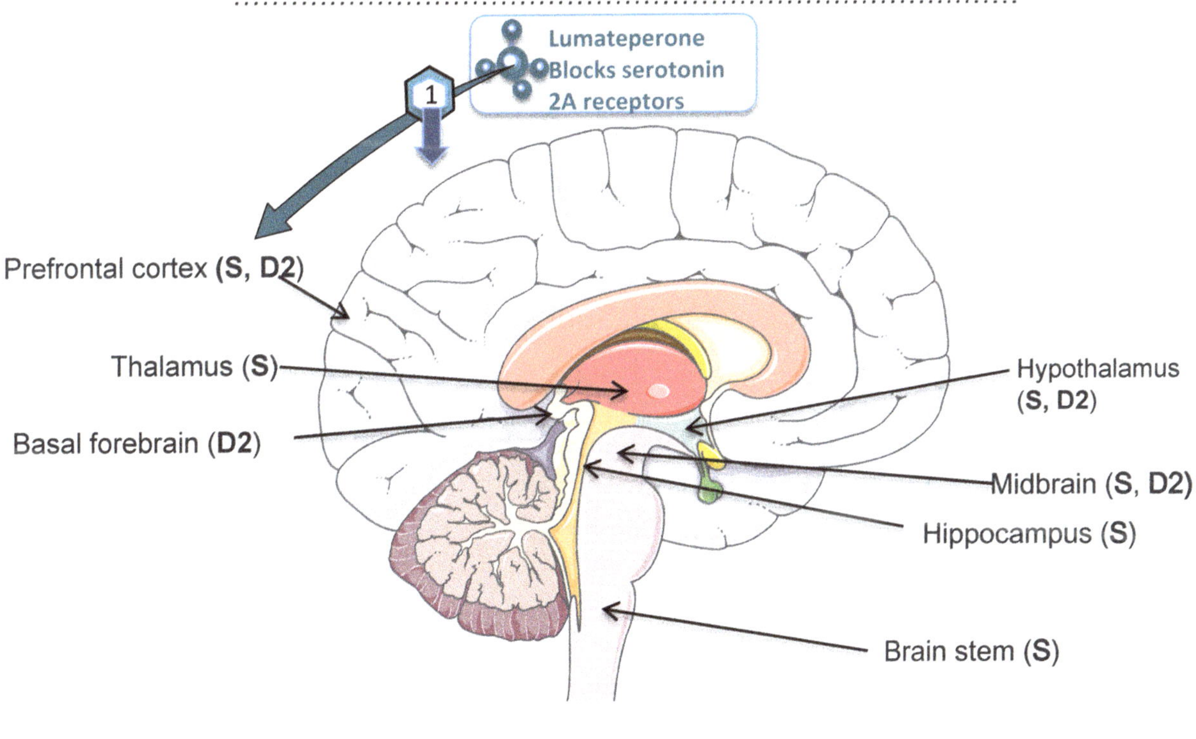

The disease: Narcolepsy

Narcolepsy is a rare excessive sleep disorder that affects the brain's ability to regulate the normal sleep-wake cycle, leading to **excessive daytime sleepiness**. Some patients also experience **sudden episodes of cataplexy**. Narcolepsy may be due to "**sleep state instability**" with both fragmented wakefulness during the daytime or at night.

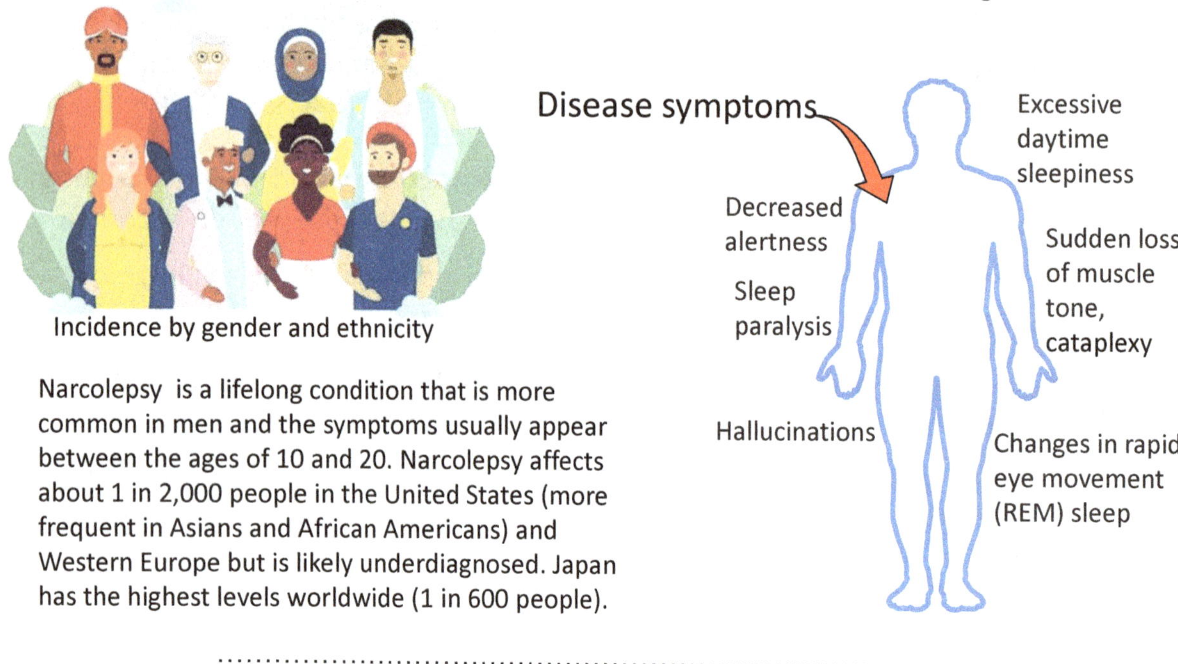

Incidence by gender and ethnicity

Narcolepsy is a lifelong condition that is more common in men and the symptoms usually appear between the ages of 10 and 20. Narcolepsy affects about 1 in 2,000 people in the United States (more frequent in Asians and African Americans) and Western Europe but is likely underdiagnosed. Japan has the highest levels worldwide (1 in 600 people).

The medicine

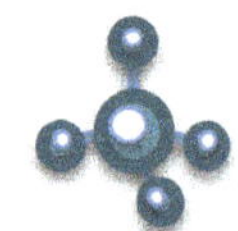

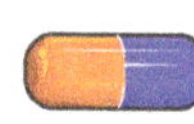

Solriamfetol; Sunosi, FDA Approval 2019

Solriamfetol improves wakefulness in patients with excessive daytime sleepiness associated with **narcolepsy** or obstructive sleep apnea by **blocking** the action of the norepinephrine and the dopamine **transporter receptor**.

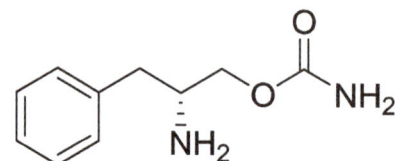

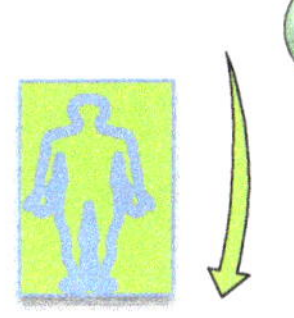

1 **Monoamine transporters** are responsible for **reuptake of extracellular norepinephrine (NE) and dopamine (DA)** to regulate concentrations in the synaptic cleft.

During normal **wakefulness**, hypothalamic neuropeptides **(orexins)** send long-lasting signals to other neurons that produce **norepinephrine, serotonin, and dopamine,** which **sustain alertness** and wakefulness.

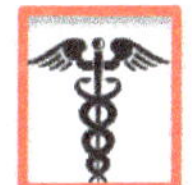

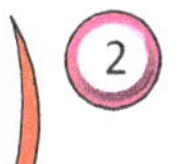

2 **Dopamine and norepinephrine are stimulatory neurotransmitters** and their dysregulation play a role in wakefulness and sleep.

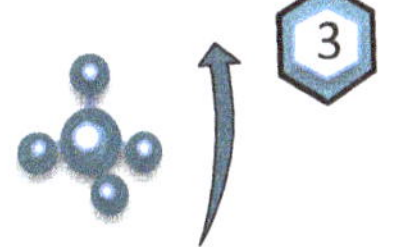

3 **Solriamfetol blocks** the action of the norepinephrine and the dopamine **transporter receptor,** inhibits dopamine and norepinephrine reuptake.

Inhibiting reuptake results in increased concentrations of dopamine and norepinephrine in the synaptic clefts and an **increase in dopamine-type neurotransmission**.

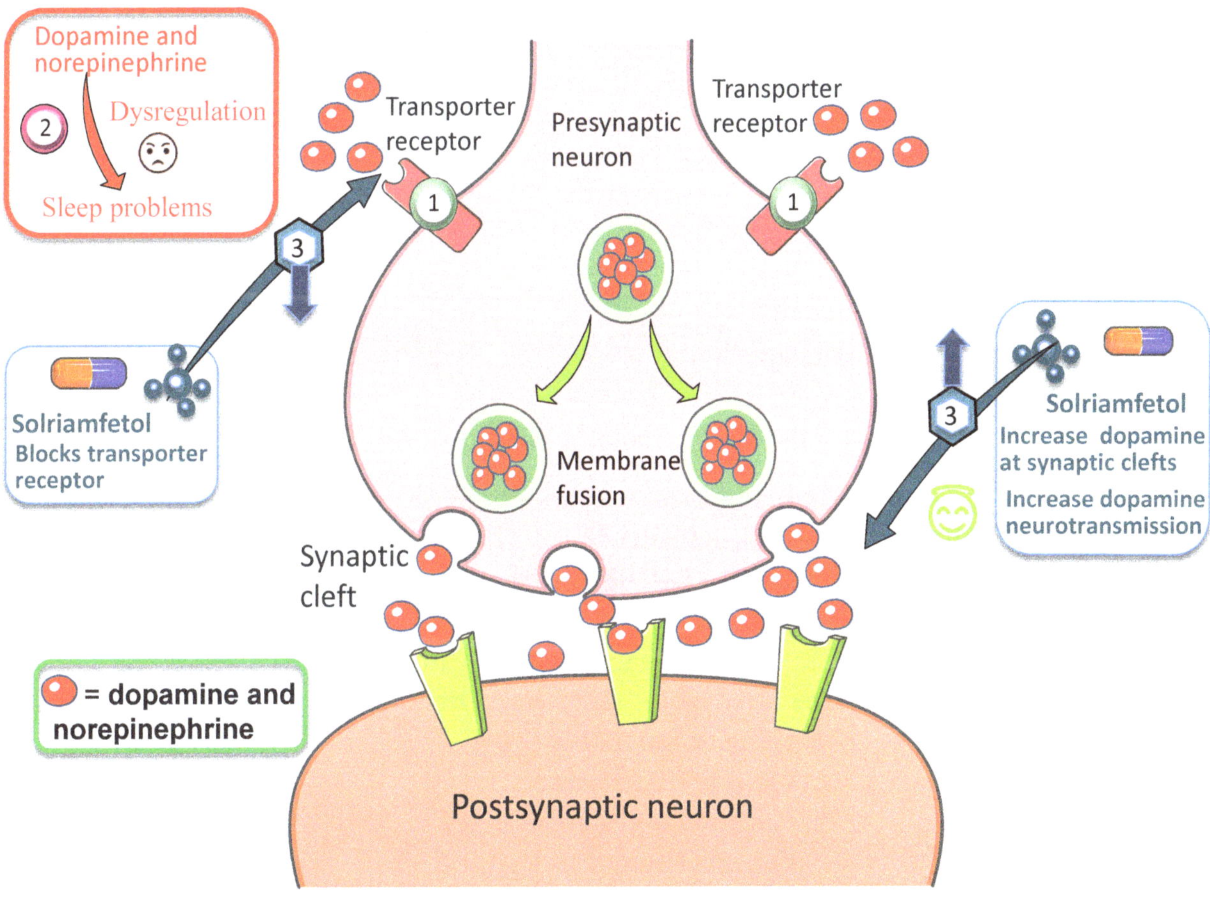

The disease: Parkinson's disease

Parkinson's disease (PD) is a progressive nervous system disorder that affects movement. Tremors are common as well as stiff muscles, slow movement, and problems with balance. The **nerve cells** in the brain **do not produce enough of the neurotransmitter dopamine**, which aids control and coordination of body movements. Classical motor features of PD such as rigidity and tremor develops when about 50%–80% of **dopaminergic neurons** in regions of the **midbrain** and base of the **forebrain are lost.**

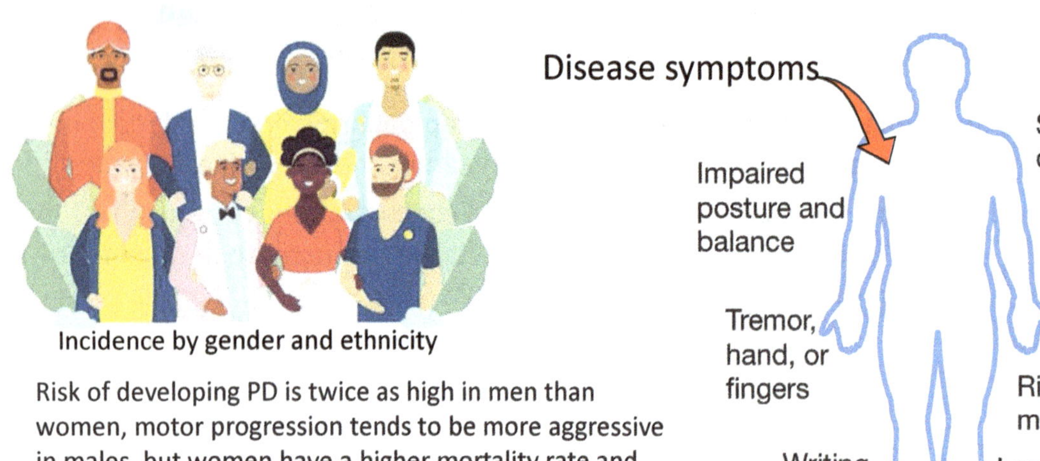

Incidence by gender and ethnicity

Risk of developing PD is twice as high in men than women, motor progression tends to be more aggressive in males, but women have a higher mortality rate and faster progression of the disease. In the United States, PD is twice as common in whites and Hispanics as for blacks and Asians. In Asia, there is a lower prevalence in Japan, Singapore and China

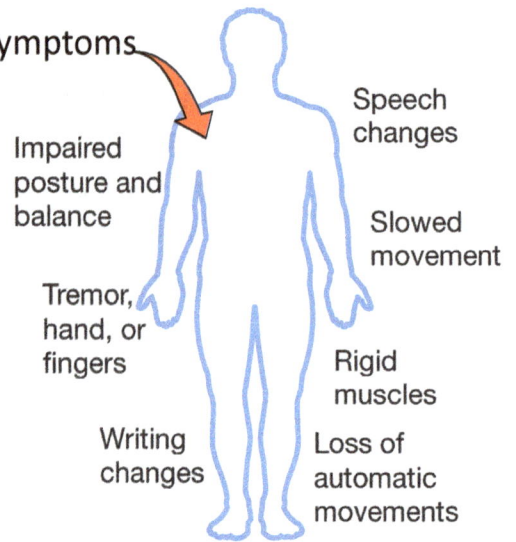

The medicine

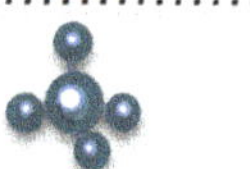

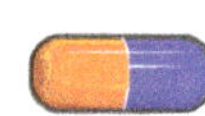

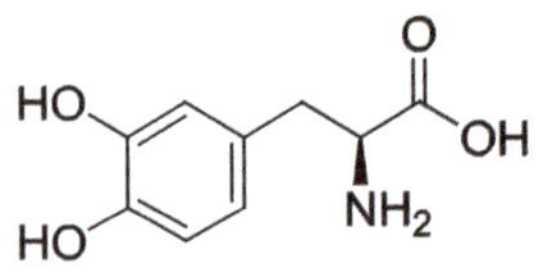

Levodopa (dopamine precursor is used **to replace the missing dopamine**)

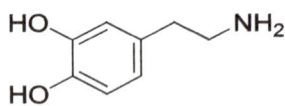

HO
HO
NH_2

Dopamine

Safinamide, Xadago; FDA Approval 2017

Safinamide inhibits monoamine oxidase-B (MAO-B), which **blocks** the **catabolism of dopamine** with an increase of dopamine levels and activity in the brain (regions shown). **The addition of Safinamide to a stable dose of levodopa** significantly **improves PD symptoms** and reduces periods with tremors.

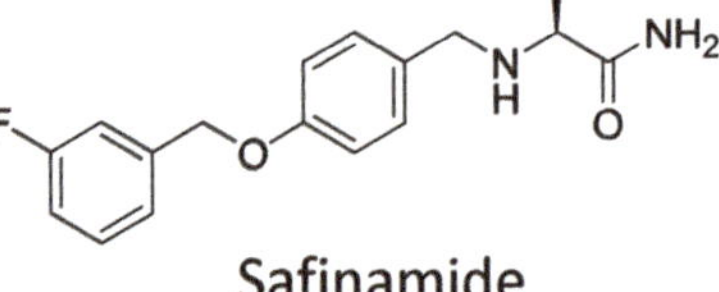

Safinamide

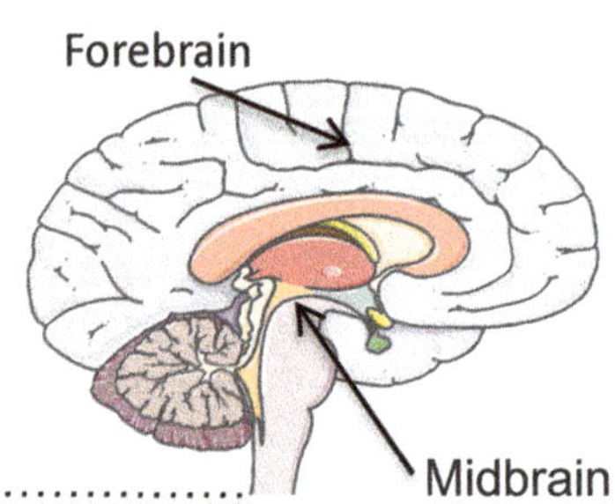

Amine neurotransmitters: Parkinson's disease, Safinamide

Action of Safinamide on cell and disease biology

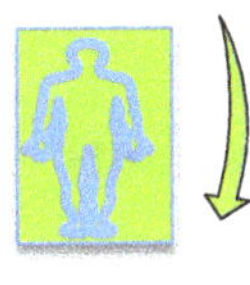
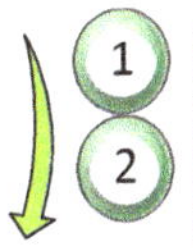

1 Monoamine oxidase B (**MAOB**) **degrades** dopamine in the brain

2 **Dopamine** may **inhibit GABA-A** receptors that are adjacent in the forebrain. Gamma-aminobutyric acid (**GABA**) plays a prominent role in the brain control of stress and influences the **activity of dopamine neurons.**

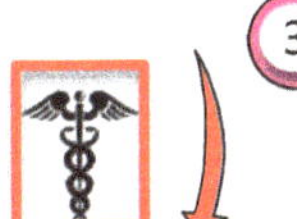
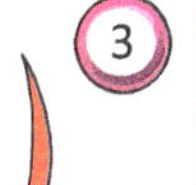

3 In **mid-to-late PD,** there is a profound **depolarization of the Glu postsynaptic membrane** due to persistent sodium channel and calcium channel opening, which can contribute to axonal degeneration.

4 **Stress triggers abnormal release of glutamate** (Glu) which plays a prominent role in the brain control.

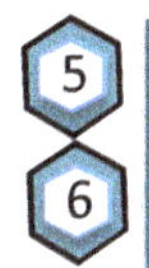

5 **Safinamide** reversibly **inhibits MAOB** and increases dopamine levels

6 **Safinamide** blocks Na^+, Ca^{2+} channels, which **inhibits Glu and GABA release** from overactive Glu and GABA terminals, **reduces neuronal hyperexcitability,** and may slow the progression of PD.

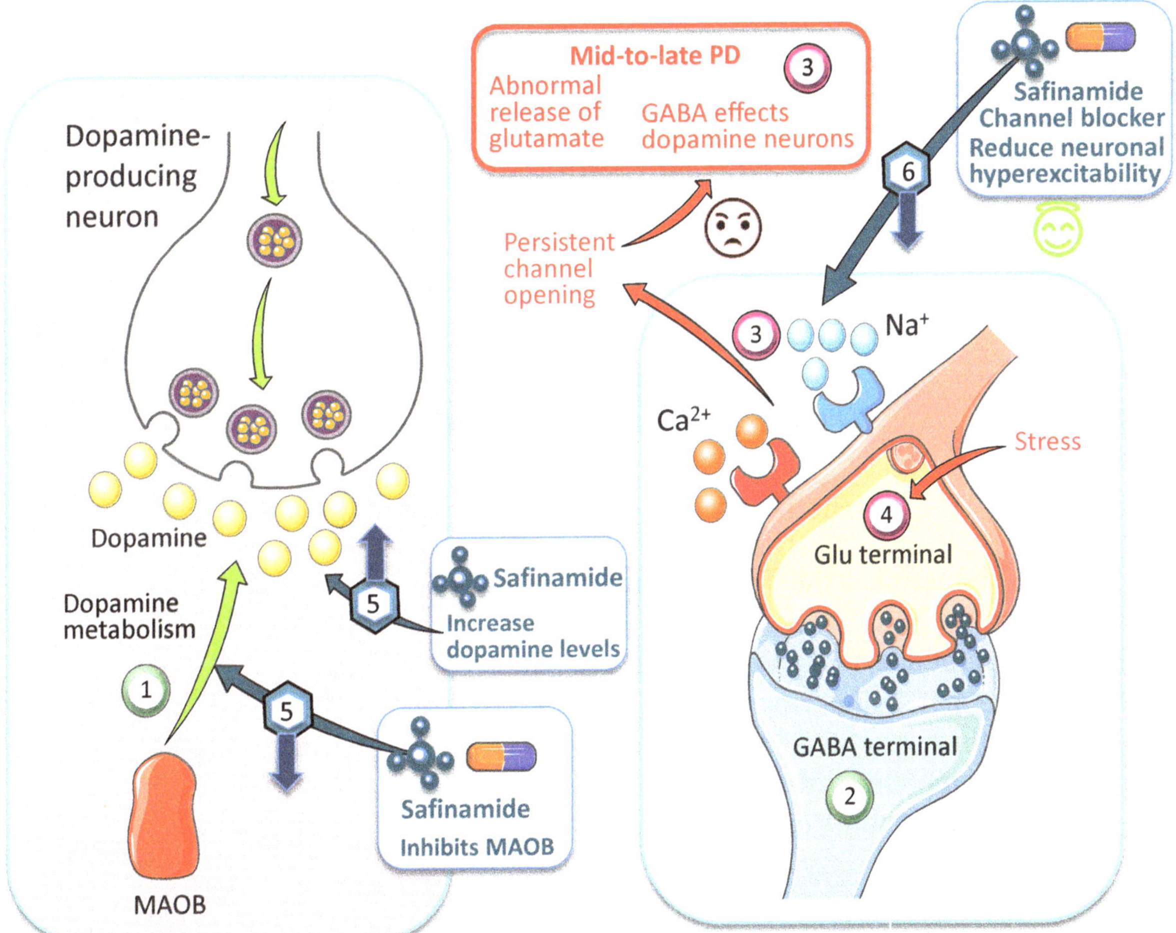

The disease: Huntington's disease

Huntington's disease (HD) is caused by **glutamine repeats in the Huntington gene.** **Patients** exhibit **tardive dyskinesias** characterized by **involuntary repetitive movements** and **disabling facial and trunk movements** and chorea (involuntary, irregular, unpredictable muscle movements). In the early stages of HD with hyperkinetic movements, there is an **increase in dopamine neurotransmission.** Symptoms can be alleviated by depleting dopamine levels.

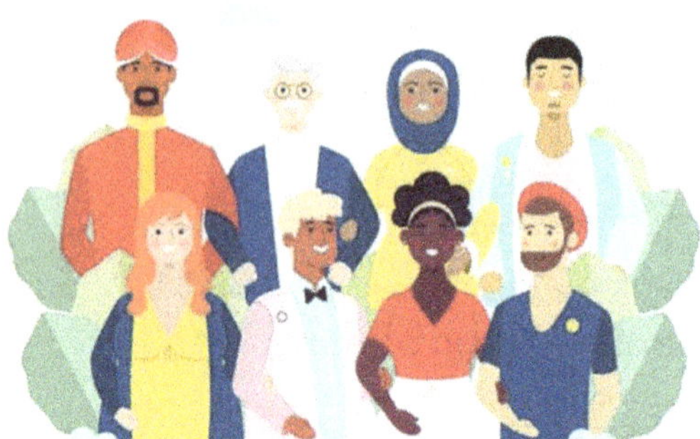

Incidence by gender and ethnicity

HD has a higher prevalence in women than in men. Huntington's disease primarily affects people of European ancestry and is less common in other populations, such as Japanese, Chinese, and African. Egypt has the highest prevalence of Huntington's disease.

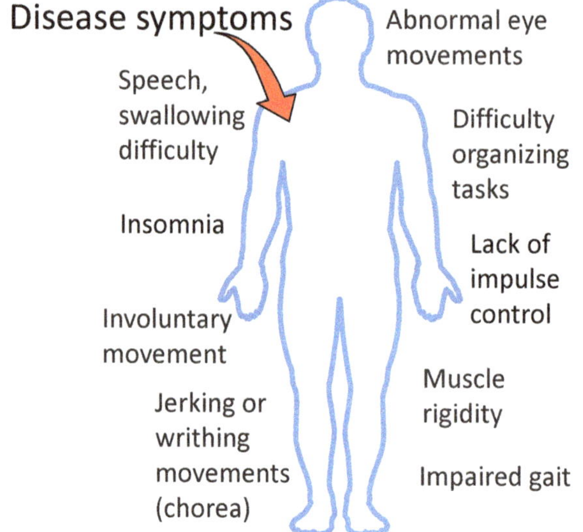

The medicine

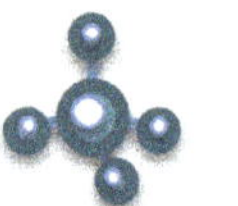

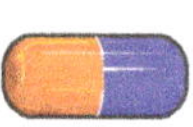

Deutetrabenazine; Austedo, FDA Approval 2018

Deutetrabenazine is the **first deuterated drug** approved by FDA. The presence of **deuterium decreases metabolism** and increases the half-live of the active metabolite, which allows lower dosing and fewer adverse reactions. **Deutetrabenazine is used to treat movement disorders**, including tardive dyskinesia and chorea caused by Huntington's disease.

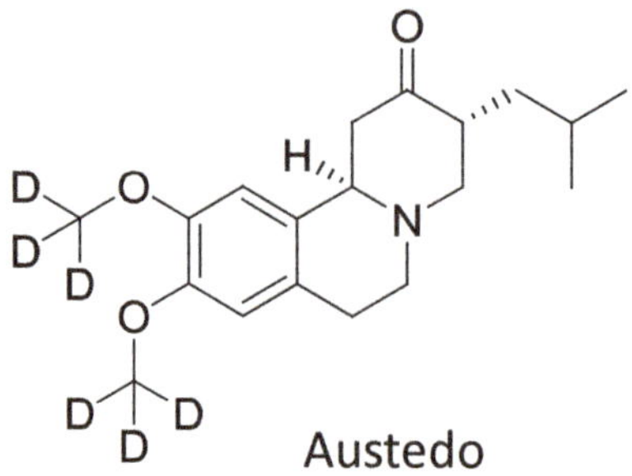

Austedo

Amine neurotransmitters: Huntington's disease, Deutetrabenazine

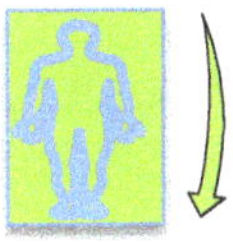

Action of Deutetrabenazine on cell and disease biology

Neuronal connections of dopamine pathways are used to transport dopamine to different areas of the brain.

1 **Vesicular monoamine transporter 2 (VMAT2) transports dopamine** from the cellular cytosol into vesicles (small sacs) **where dopamine is released** from the vesicles **into the synaptic cleft.**

2 **VMAT2 inhibition blocks release of dopamine** into the vesicles and **reduces levels** of **dopamine** in the synaptic cleft.

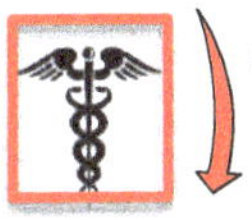

3 **Dysfunction** of dopamine pathways and dopamine levels in **neurological disorders. Unusually high levels** of dopamine cause chorea (involuntary jerking or writhing movements) in Huntington's patients.

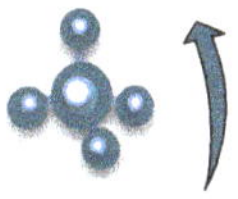

4 **Deutetrabenazine is a selective inhibitor of synaptic vesicular monoamine transporter 2** (VMAT2), which results in a depletion of neuroactive monoamines especially dopamine in nerve terminals.

Deutetrabenazine
Inhibits VMAT2
Blocks dopamine release
4
Dopamine
1
Monoamine transporter 2
VMAT2
Dopamine transport
2
Vesicle
Deutetrabenazine
Depletion of dopamine in nerve terminals
4
3
Huntington's disease
Excess dopamine causes jerking and writhing.
Dopamine
Synaptic cleft
Dopamine receptors

Amine neurotransmitters: Huntington's disease, Deutetrabenazine

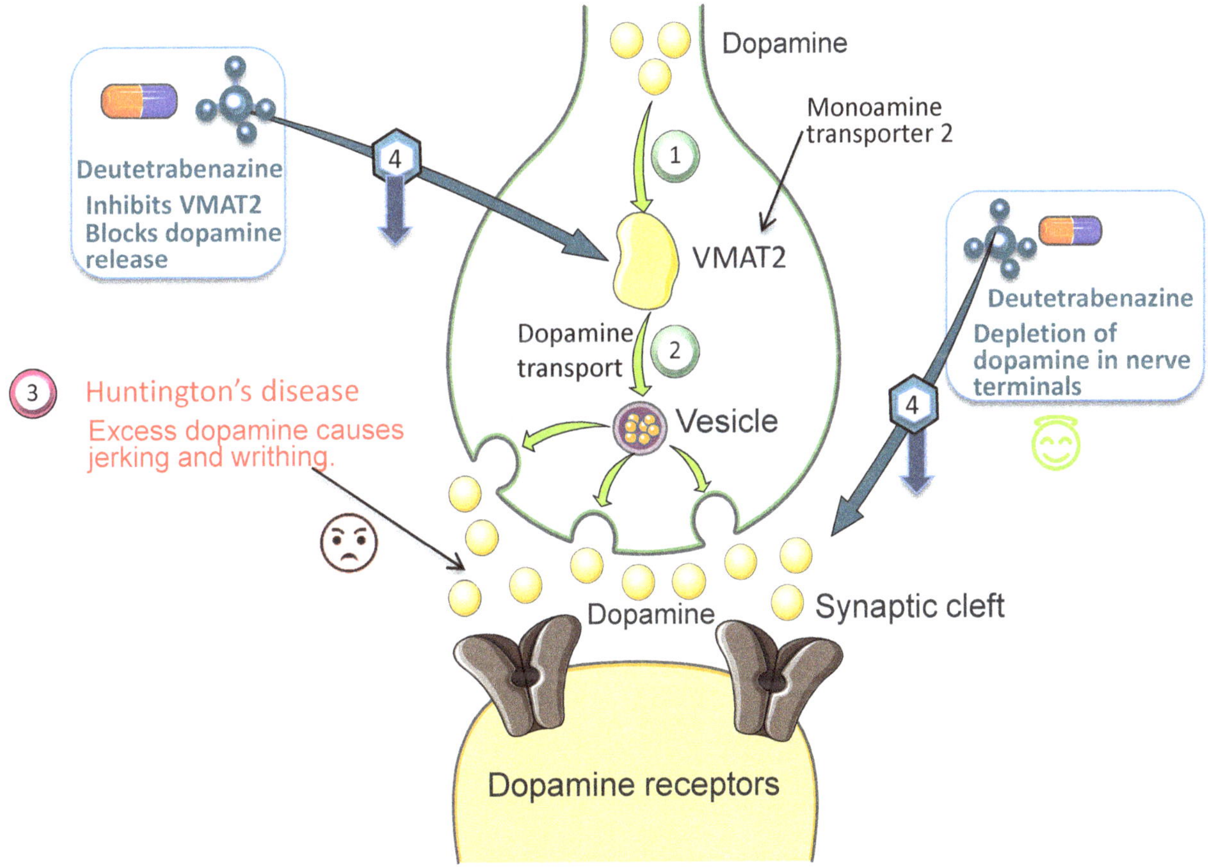

The disease: Migraine pain

Migraine pain is often described as an **intense throbbing or pulsing pain** in one area of the head. Additional symptoms include nausea and sensitivity to light/sound and can be triggered by stress, hormonal changes, and diet. Approximately, one-third of individuals also experience aura.

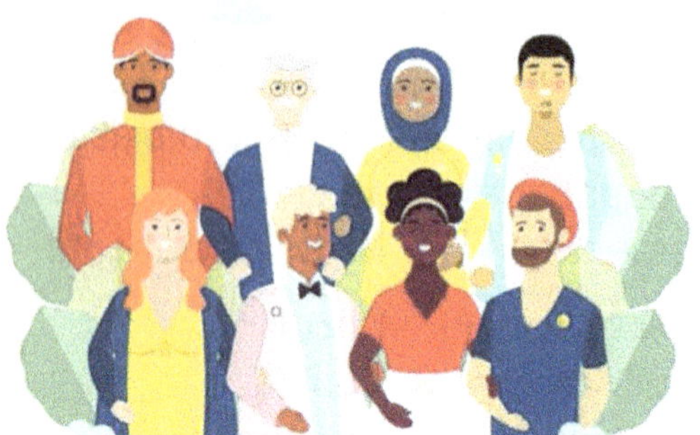

Incidence by gender and ethnicity

Migraine is most common between the ages of 18 and 44 and can afflict men, women, and children, but women have two to three times greater incidence, highest in their 30s and linked to estrogen. Whites have a higher prevalence than African Americans and Asian Americans and highest in North America, then South and Central America, Europe, Asia, and Africa.

Disease symptoms

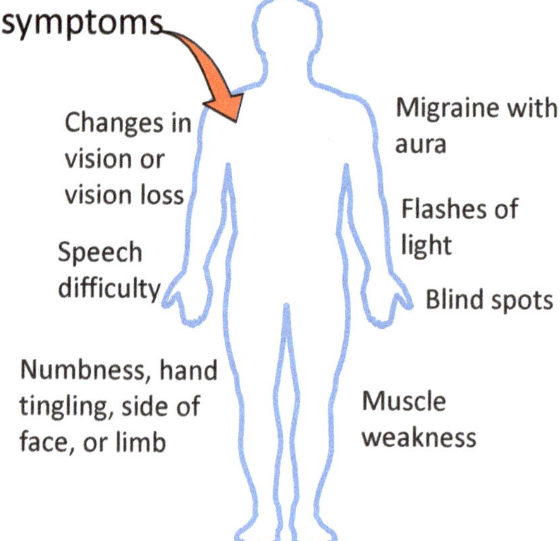

The medicine

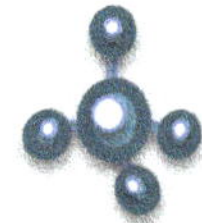

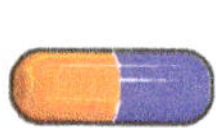

Lasmiditan; Reyvow, FDA Approval 2019

Lasmiditan is for the **acute** (active but short-term) **treatment of migraine** with or without aura (a sensory phenomenon with visual disturbance) in adults.

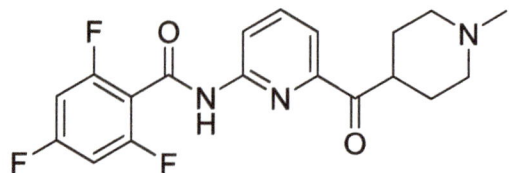

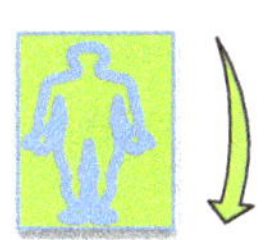

Serotonin receptors, located on the trigeminal system, can be divided into 7 families to mediate both excitatory and inhibitory neurotransmissions and participate in **blocking migraine pain transmission**.

The **trigeminal nerve,** the largest of the cranial nerves with three major branches, is responsible for facial motor functions. **The nerves supply the cerebral blood vessels** and is a **major trigger point for migraines.**

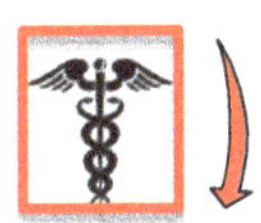

Calcitonin gene-related peptide (CGRP) is abundant in **trigeminal neurons** to **transmit responses to harmful stimuli** in the nervous system. Serotonin constricts smooth muscle cells in cerebral blood vessels, which can cause migraine.

Lasmiditan stimulates serotonin-1F receptors on trigeminal fibers with antimigraine actions and without constriction of human coronary arteries.

Lasmiditan has a direct action on the central descending pain inhibiting pathways and **modulates CGRP release**.

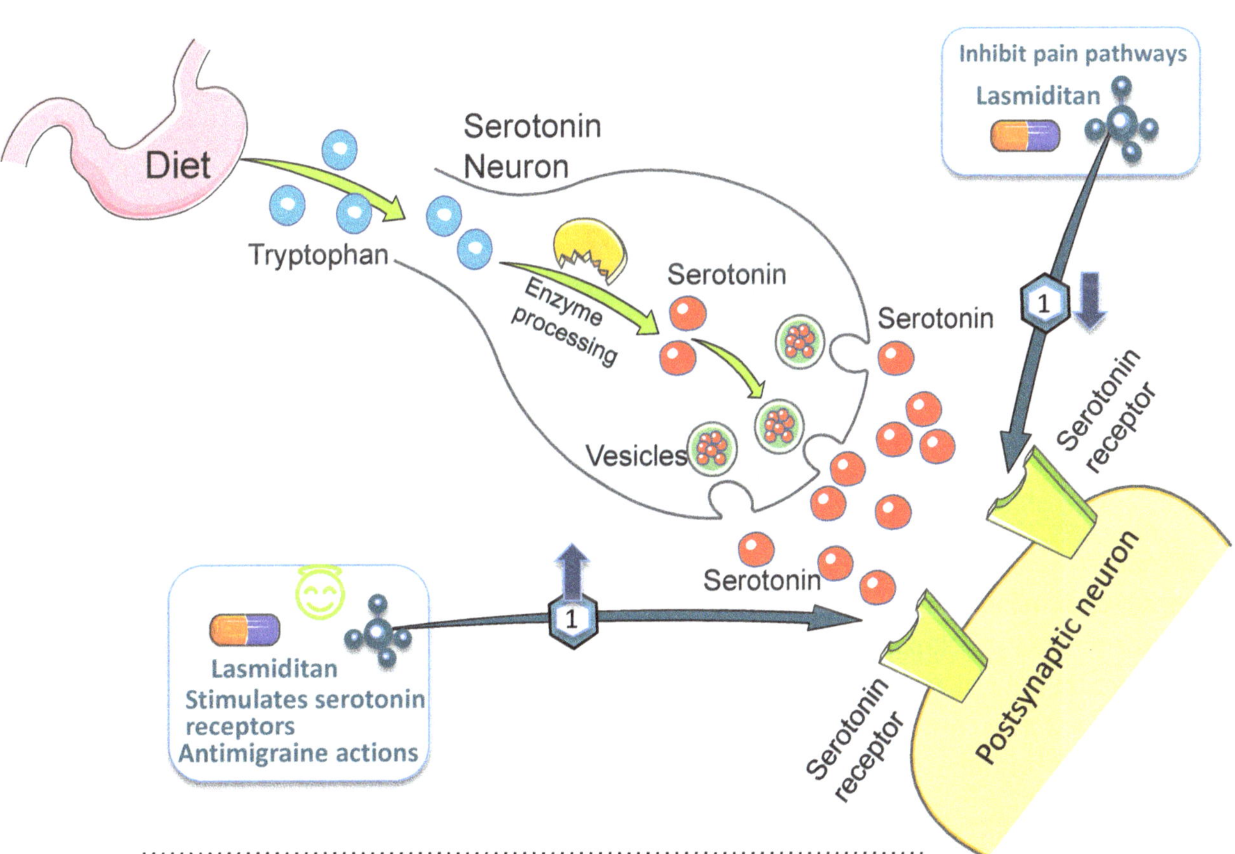

Amine neurotransmitters: Migraine pain, Lasmiditan

The disease: Narcolepsy

Narcolepsy is a chronic sleep disorder that affects the brain's ability to regulate the normal sleep-wake cycle, leading to **excessive daytime sleepiness**. Some patients also experience episodes of cataplexy, which is a sudden, brief loss of voluntary muscle tone.

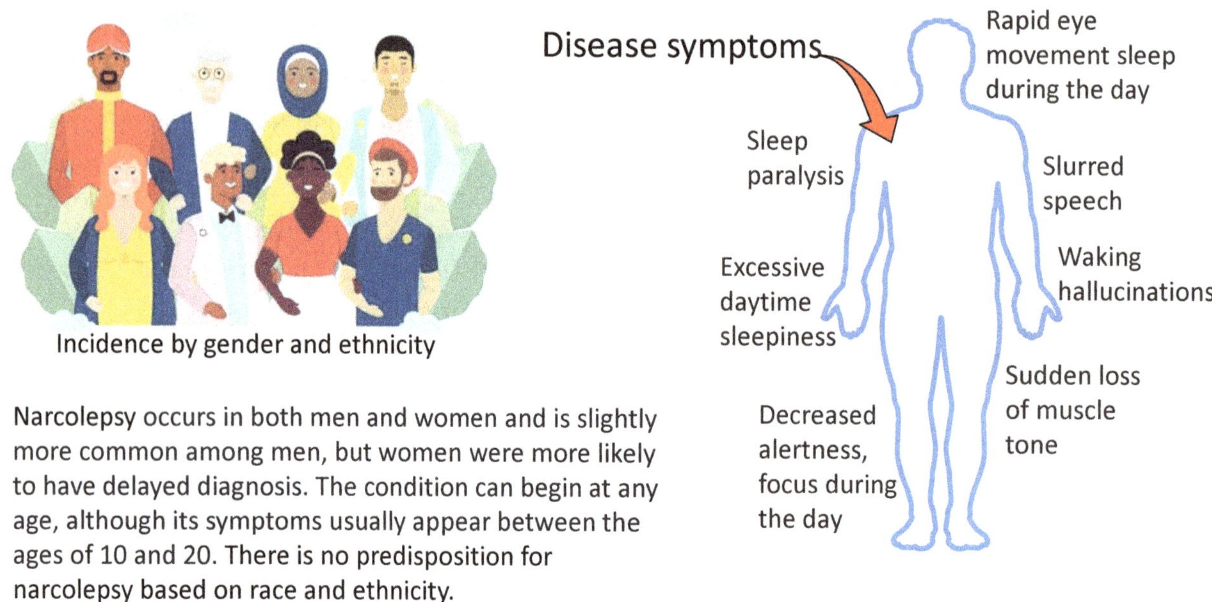

Incidence by gender and ethnicity

Narcolepsy occurs in both men and women and is slightly more common among men, but women were more likely to have delayed diagnosis. The condition can begin at any age, although its symptoms usually appear between the ages of 10 and 20. There is no predisposition for narcolepsy based on race and ethnicity.

The medicine

Pitolisant; Wakix, FDA Approval 2020

Pitolisant is a **histamine-3 (H_3) receptor blocker (antagonist)** for the treatment of narcolepsy. Pitolisant, the first treatment for EDS, is not categorized as a controlled substance with the potential to be habit-forming.

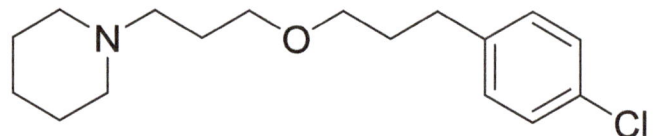

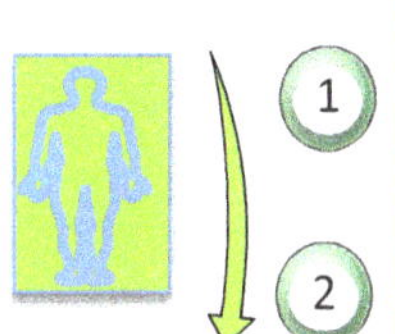

Neurons project through ascending bundles to forebrain structures, and a descending bundle to the spinal cord.

Histamine-regulating neurons in the the hypothalamus are involved with the control of arousal, learning, memory, sleep, and energy balance.

Histamine is a wake-promoting neurotransmitter that **activates the histamine H1 receptor** as well as glutamate and GABA-A receptors.

Histamine H3 receptor (H3R) is an **inhibitory receptor** located on presynaptic nerve terminals, which modulates the release of histamine by **blocking** the activity of **histidine decarboxylase.** .

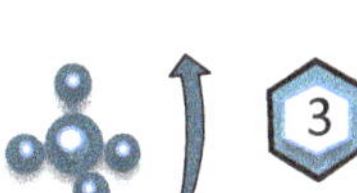

Pitolisant is a **H3 receptor inhibitor** and enhances histamine release in the brain, leading to increased wakefulness and alertness.

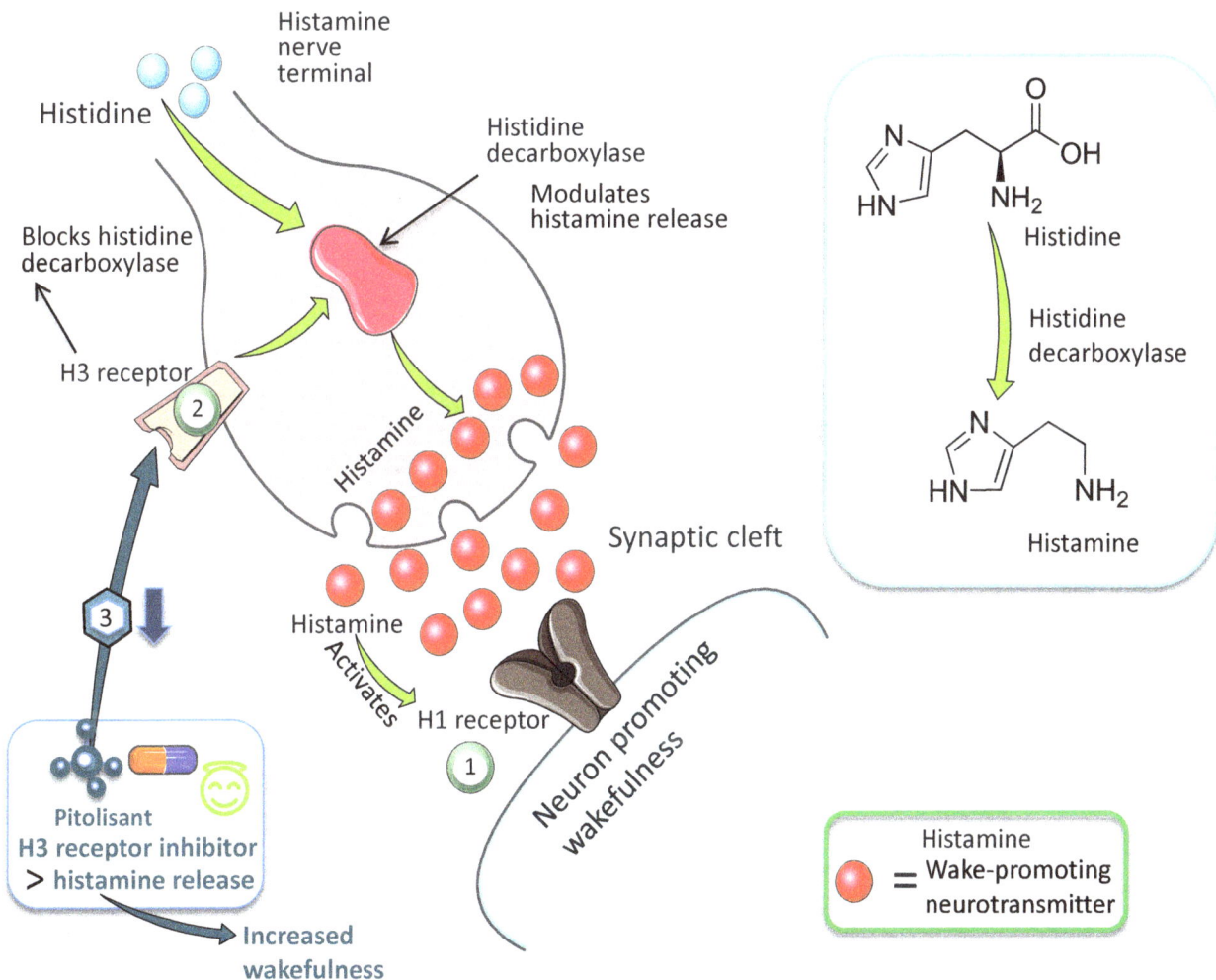

Histamine nerve terminal
Histidine
Histidine decarboxylase
Modulates histamine release
Blocks histidine decarboxylase
H3 receptor
2
Histamine
Synaptic cleft
3
Histamine
Activates
H1 receptor
1
Neuron promoting wakefulness
Pitolisant
H3 receptor inhibitor
> histamine release
Increased wakefulness

O
OH
N
HN
NH_2
Histidine
Histidine decarboxylase
N
HN
NH_2
Histamine

Histamine = Wake-promoting neurotransmitter

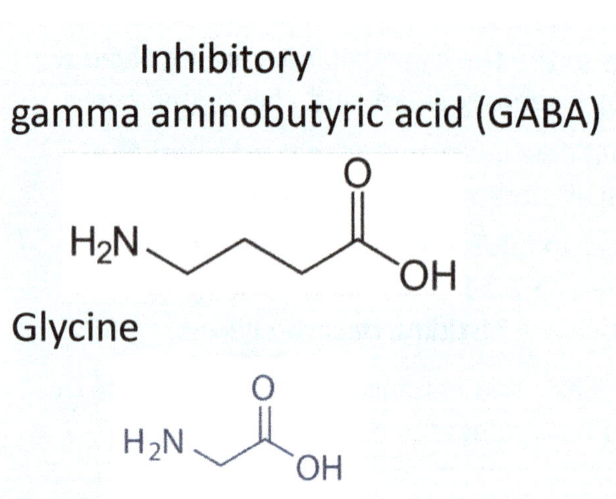

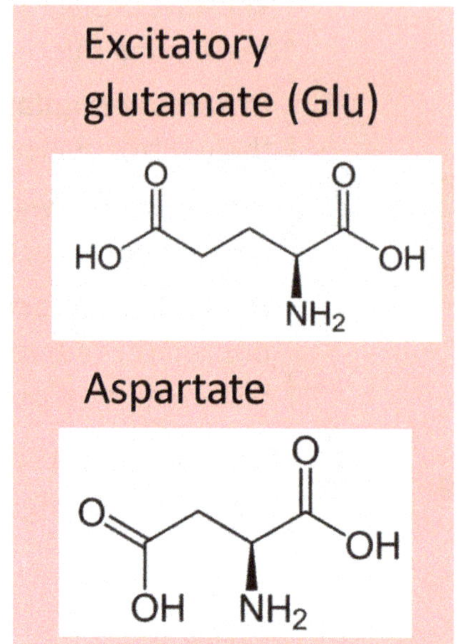

Drug-induced changes in levels of neurotransmitters in disease therapies.

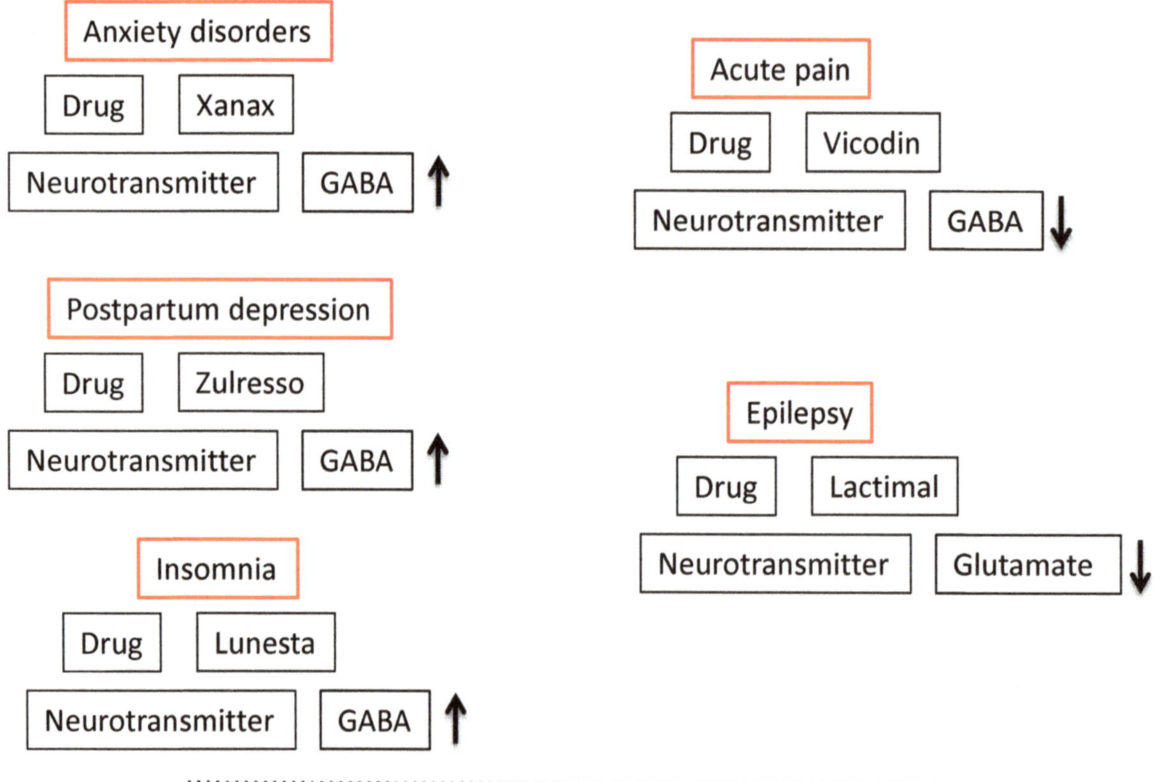

Glutamate Neurotransmitters

Glutamate is a **major mediator of excitatory signals** in over 90% of the synaptic connections in the human brain. The **levels of glutamate are strictly regulated** with the high levels of blood glutamate being excluded by the blood–brain barrier.

Glutamate is involved in **cognitive functions** such as learning and memory

Glutamate plays an important role in **nervous system reorganization**

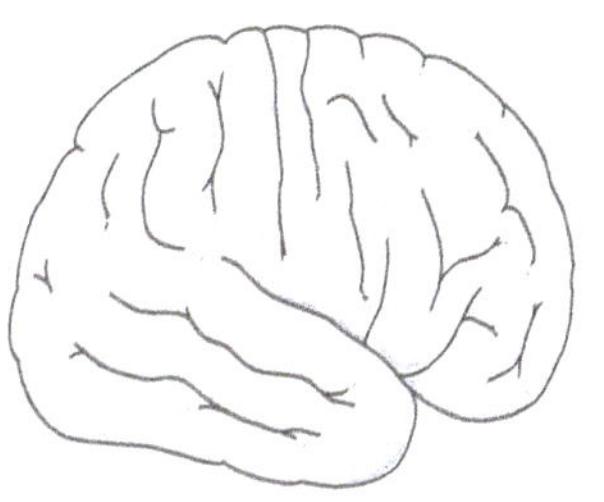

Glutamine transporters rapidly remove glutamate from the extracellular space for recycling

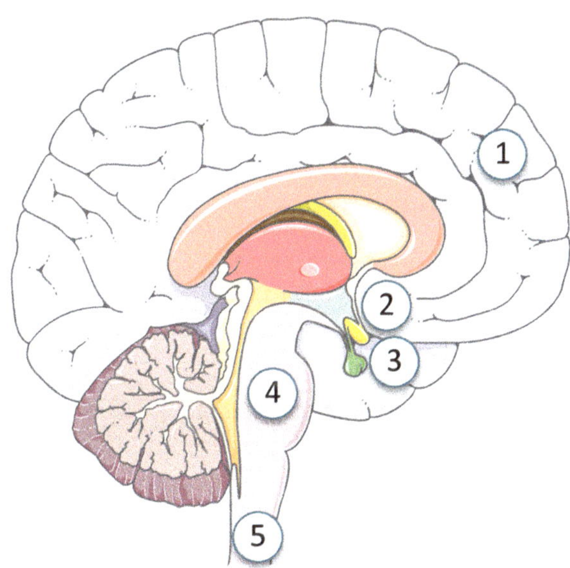

Glutamatergic neurons (G) are most densely concentrated in the **cerebral cortex**, hippocampus, basal ganglia including amygdala, brain stem, and spinal cord.

1. Cerebral cortex (G)
2. Hippocampus (G)
3. Amygdala (G)
4. Brain stem (G)
5. Spinal cord (G)

In **brain injury** or disease, the **transporters can reverse the process** with **excess glutamate accumulation** outside the cells. The result is neuronal damage and **cell death** caused by calcium ions entering the cells.

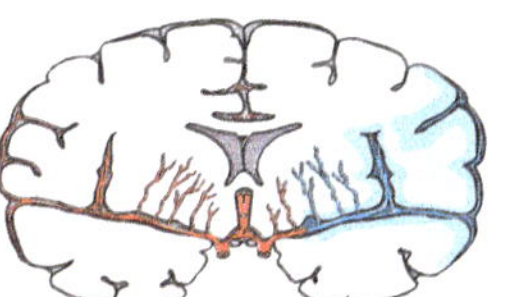

Excessive activation of glutamate receptors result in the death of nerve cells ("**excitotoxicity**").

Such **excitotoxicity** occurs during the **ischemic cascade** that is associated with stroke, forms of intellectual disability, as well as amyotrophic lateral sclerosis and Alzheimer's disease.

The disease: Epilepsy

Epilepsy is a chronic disorder characterized by recurrent seizures, which can range from minor symptoms to **severe and prolonged convulsions**.

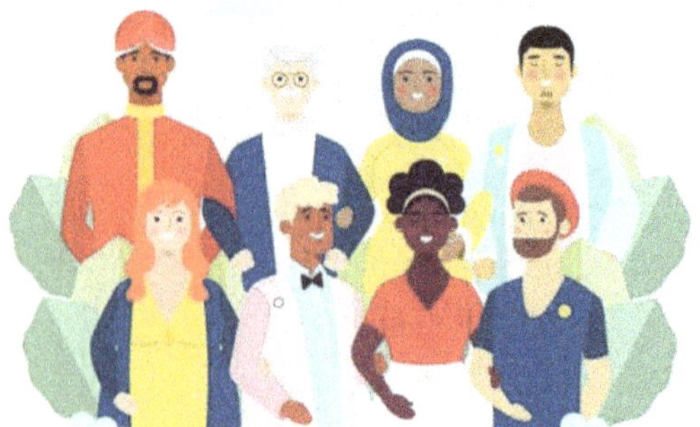

Incidence by gender and ethnicity

Disease symptoms

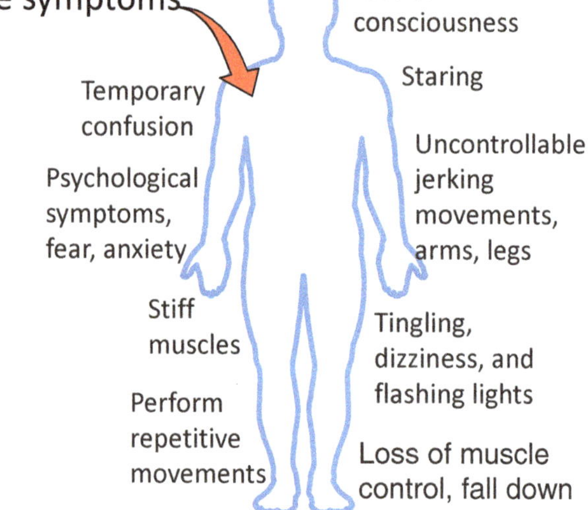

Males have a higher incidence of epilepsy than females and epilepsy is more common in people of Hispanic background than in non-Hispanics. Active epilepsy (seizures are not completely controlled) is more common in whites than in blacks but blacks are more likely than whites to develop epilepsy during their lifetime. The prevalence of epilepsy is particularly high in Latin America and in several African countries.

The medicine

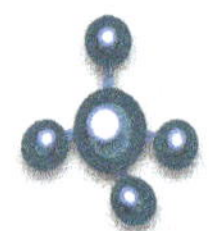

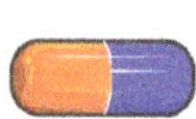

71st Most US Prescribed Drug,
10.7 million prescriptions

Lamotrigine; Lamictal, FDA Approval 1994

Lamotrigine is used to **treat epileptic seizures**, as an anticonvulsant and **manic depression** in adults with bipolar disorder. **Lamotrigine** is **more specific** than other anticonvulsants and does not have pronounced effects on **other neurotransmitter receptors**.

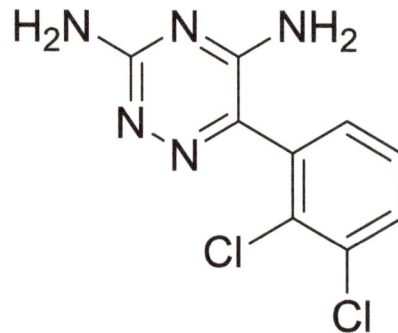

H_2N N NH_2 N N Cl Cl

Action of Lamotrigine on cell and disease biology

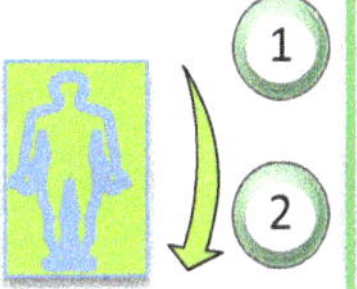

1 **Glutamine is freely permeable** into the glial and neuronal plasma membranes, whereas glutamate in unable to diffuse across membranes.

2 **Glutamate needs a transporter** for the synaptic space and is removed from the synapse by a **high-affinity uptake systems** in neurons and glia when neuronal activity is high.

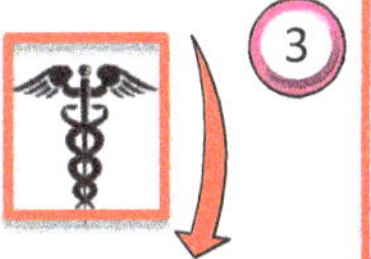

3 In **brain injury or seizures** glutamate transporters generate **excess glutamate accumulation** outside cells causing neuronal damage and **cell death.** **Chronic seizures** can alter neuronal and glial expression of glutamate receptors and uptake transporters. Such changes to the brain can cause neurons to fire in a hyper-synchronous manner, which is known as a seizure.

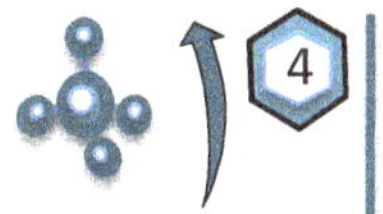

4 **Lamotrigine inhibits** the glutamate **transporters** to **blocks** the **release of glutamate,** which stabilizes neuronal membranes and reduces degeneration of nerve cells.

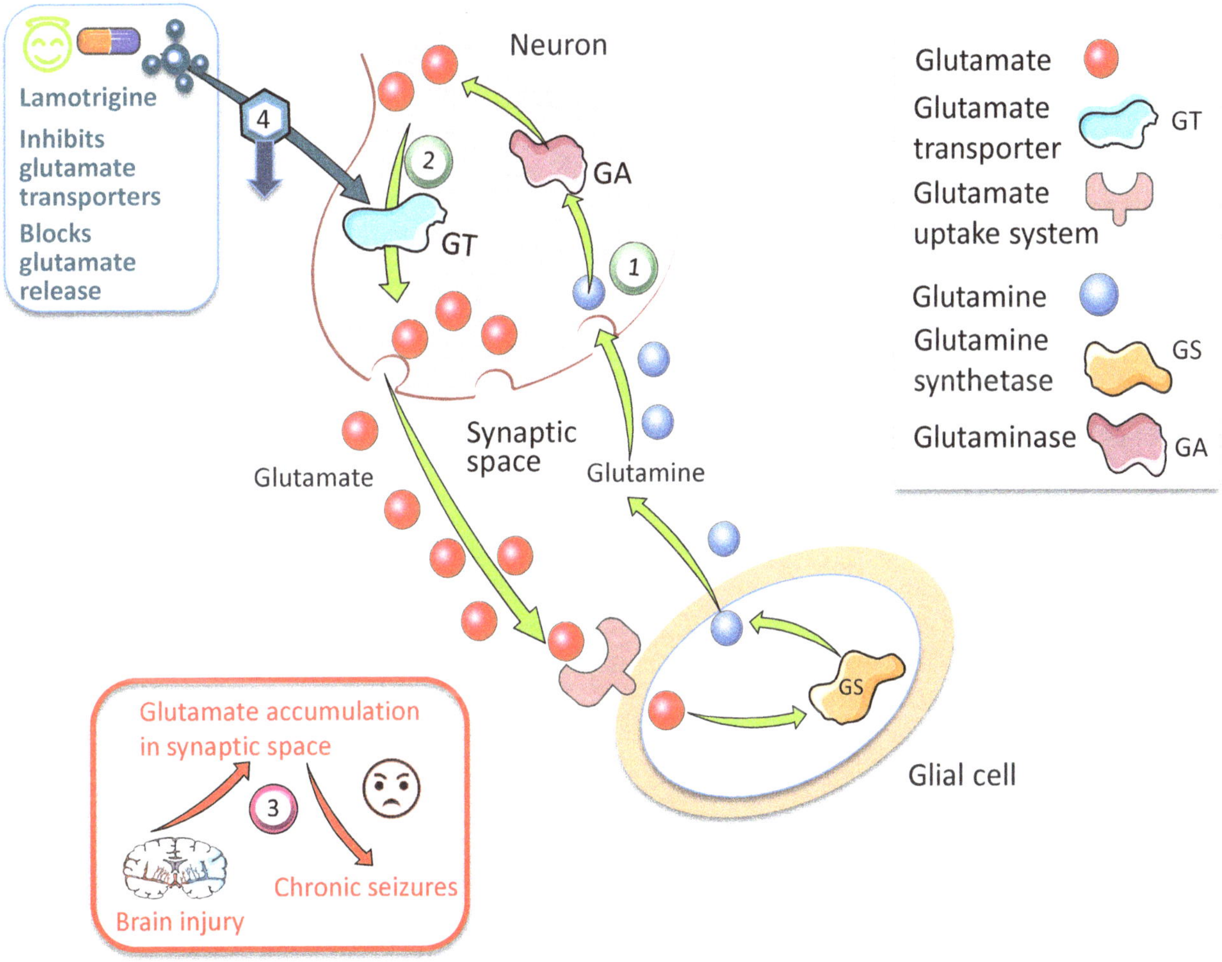

Lamotrigine
Inhibits glutamate transporters
Blocks glutamate release
4
Neuron
2
GT
GA
1
Glutamate
Synaptic space
Glutamine
GS
Glial cell
Glutamate accumulation in synaptic space
3
Brain injury
Chronic seizures

Glutamate
Glutamate transporter GT
Glutamate uptake system
Glutamine
Glutamine synthetase GS
Glutaminase GA

The disease: Anxiety disorders

Anxiety disorders with feelings of extreme worry, specifically panic disorders, strong feelings of fear or discomfort, and generalized anxiety disorder. Such conditions can **lead to depression** (feelings of sadness that do not go away).

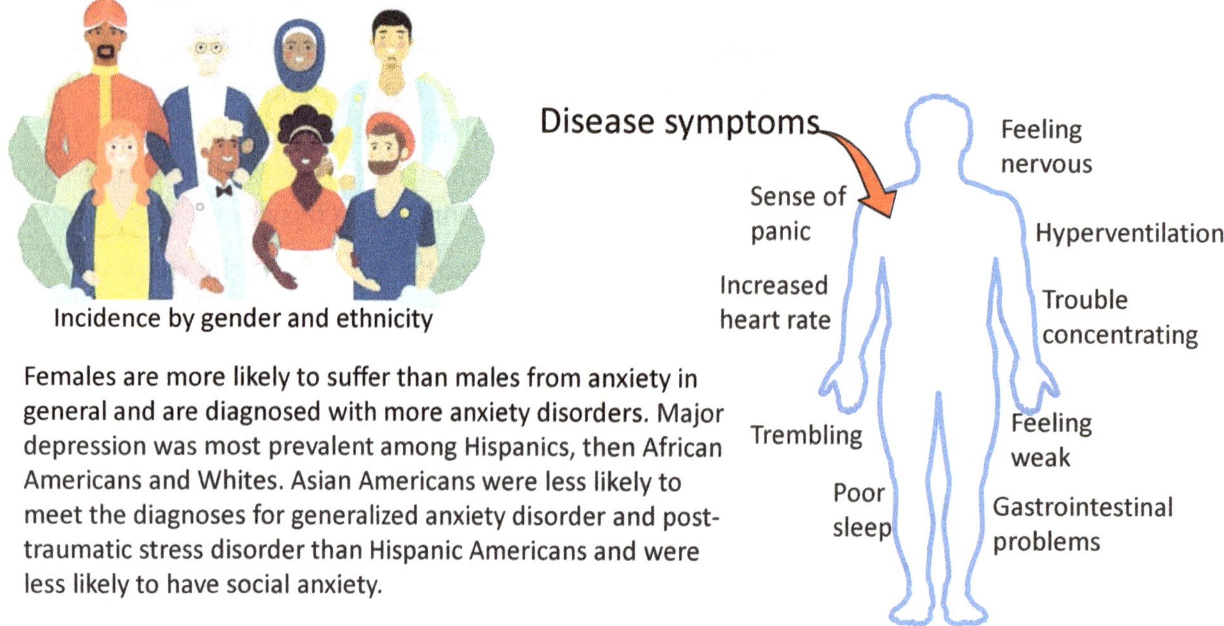

Incidence by gender and ethnicity

Females are more likely to suffer than males from anxiety in general and are diagnosed with more anxiety disorders. Major depression was most prevalent among Hispanics, then African Americans and Whites. Asian Americans were less likely to meet the diagnoses for generalized anxiety disorder and post-traumatic stress disorder than Hispanic Americans and were less likely to have social anxiety.

The medicine

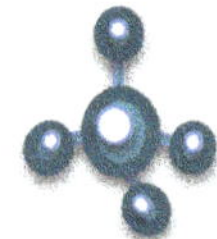

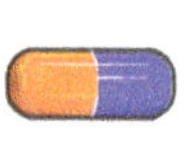

14th Most US Prescribed Drug in 2019, 21.5 million prescriptions

Alprazolam; Xanax, FDA Approval 1982

Alprazolam is approved for the treatment of **generalized anxiety disorders** and symptoms of anxiety, including anxiety associated with depression. Also prescribed for **panic disorders**, situational anxiety and **alcohol withdrawal**.

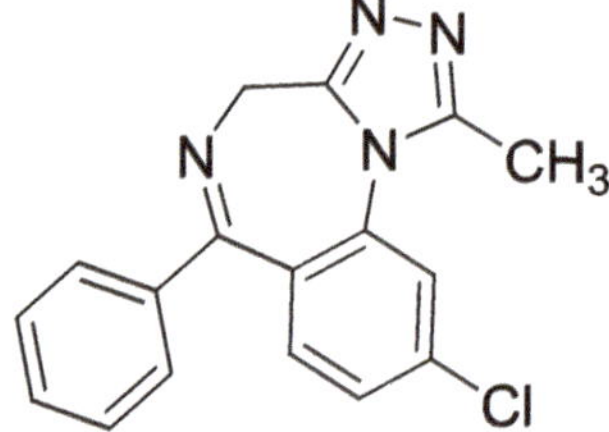

Benzodiazepines (also called "benzos") **specifically act on GABA-A receptors**.

Amine neurotransmitters: Anxiety disorders, Alprazolam

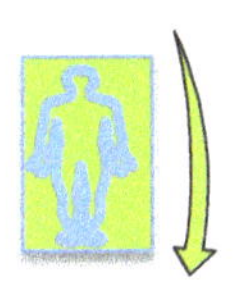

γ-aminobutyric acid (GABA) is the **major inhibitory neurotransmitter** in the CNS and activates the receptor on both pre- and postsynaptic membranes.

The **GABA-A receptor** is located in the hippocampus, thalamus, basal ganglia, hypothalamus, and brainstem regions of the CNS.

The **GABA-A receptor** is made up of **five subunit proteins,** which transverse the postsynaptic membrane and are arranged to form a **central pore**.

1 Drugs binding to the **benzodiazepine site** result in an **increased affinity of GABA** for the receptor and rapid inhibitory synaptic transmission.

2 GABA binding leads to an increase in the frequency of chloride-channel opening events with a resulting **decrease in neuronal excitability.**

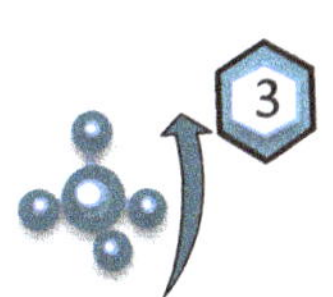

3 **Alprazolam binds** to the specific benzodiazepine binding site on the GABA-A receptor complex and causes a structural modification of the receptor to **enhance the affinity of GABA for the receptor.**

Alprazolam can be addictive by limiting the restraint of dopamine-producing neurons from releasing excessive amounts of dopamine.

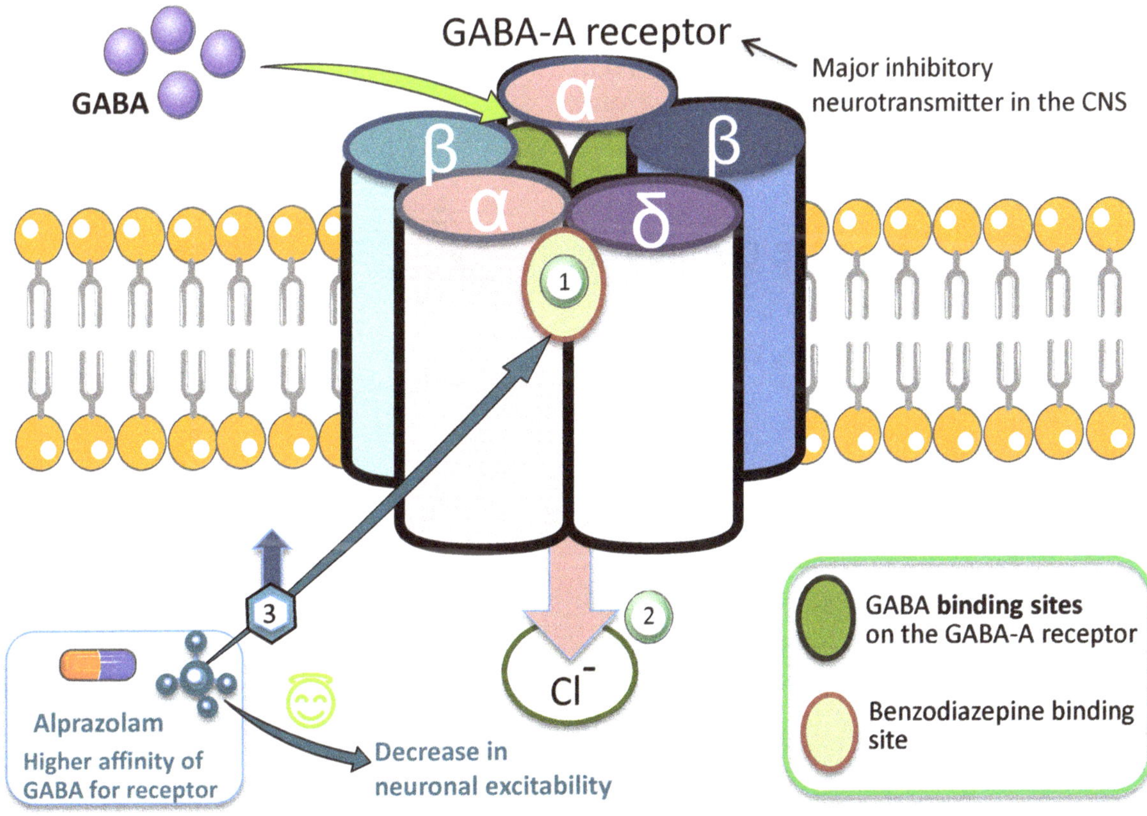

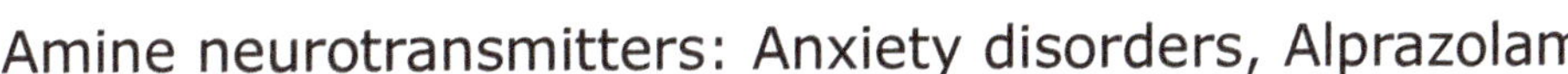

Amine neurotransmitters: Anxiety disorders, Alprazolam

The disease: Insomnia

Insomnia is defined as transient or **chronic inadequate sleep**

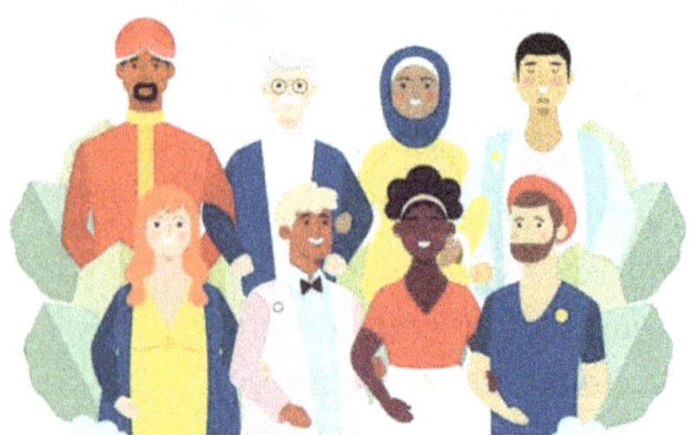

Incidence by gender and ethnicity

Women are 1.4 times as likely as men to report insomnia symptoms, with 40% of women between the ages of 40 and 55 years with sleep difficulty. Women report worse sleep quality than men and experience insomnia differently. Older women are at a higher risk of insomnia. African Americans have a higher prevalence and severity of sleep-disordered breathing, but that whites report more insomnia symptoms, whereas Asians report the least amount of sleep problems.

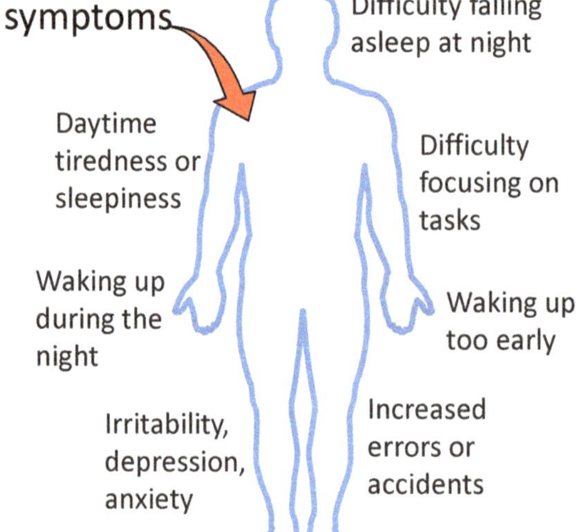

The medicine

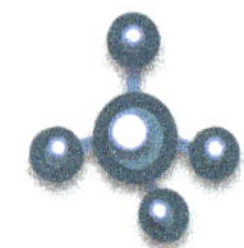

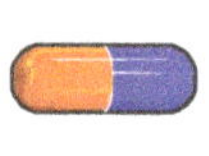

223rd Most US Prescribed Drug in 2019, 2.1 million prescriptions

Eszopiclone; Lunesta, FDA Approval 2004

Eszopiclone is a hypnotic, which is a nonbenzodiazepine (**very similar** to **benzodiazepine** pharmacodynamics), which is used for the **long-term treatment of insomnia** and is absorbed rapidly with an oral availability of 80%.

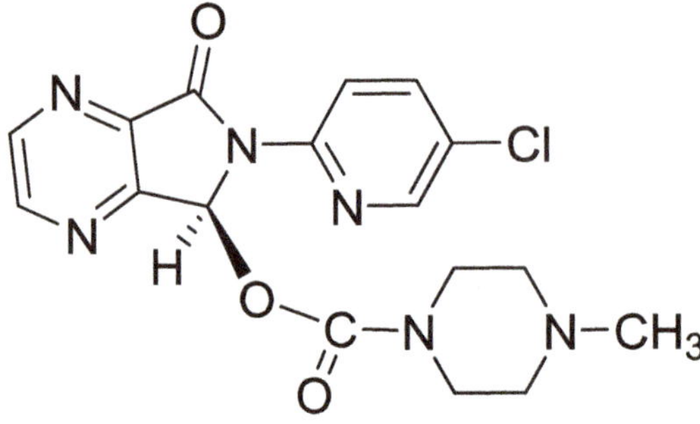

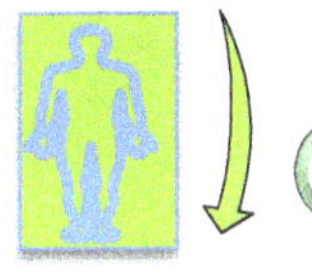

Benzodiazepine drugs result in an **increased affinity of GABA for the receptor**, activation of the chloride channel, and **rapid inhibitory synaptic transmission**.

1 Drugs binding to the **benzodiazepine site** locks the receptor into a **high GABA affinity** conformation.

2 GABA binding leads to an increase in the frequency of chloride-channel opening events with a resulting **decrease in neuronal excitability.**

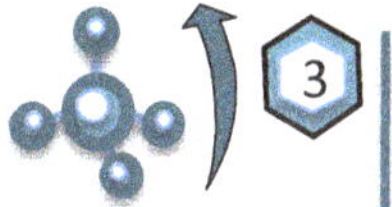

3 **Eszopiclone binds to a site on the GABA-A receptor** located adjacent or structurally coupled to benzodiazepine receptors and boost the levels of GABA.

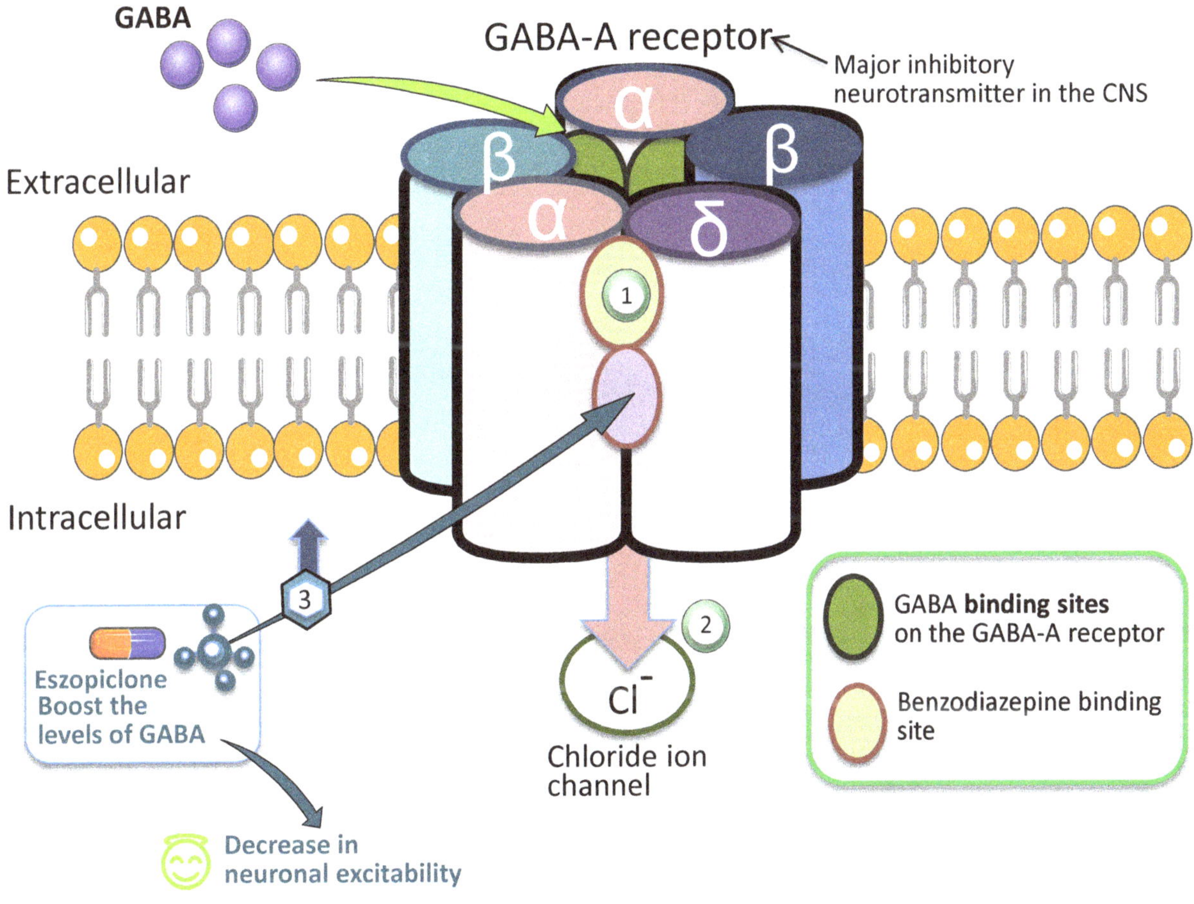

The disease: Postpartum depression

Postpartum depression is a mood disorder that can affect women after childbirth. **After childbirth, estrogen and progesterone quickly drop** with chemical changes in the brain that may trigger **mood swings** as well as sleep deprivation.

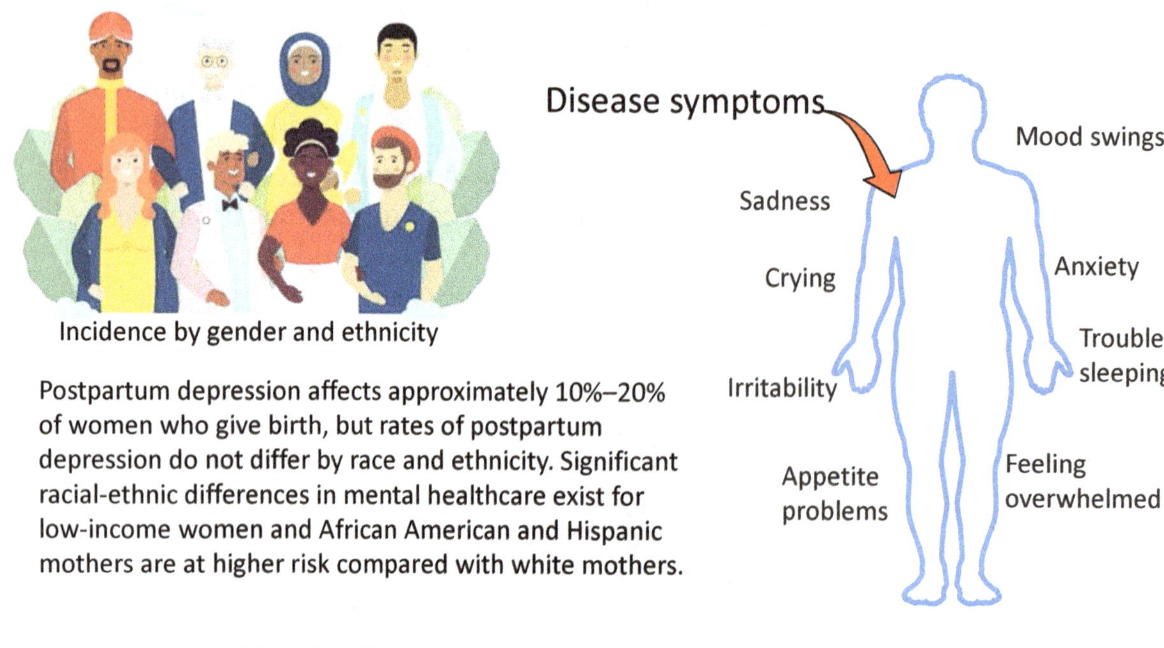

Incidence by gender and ethnicity

Postpartum depression affects approximately 10%–20% of women who give birth, but rates of postpartum depression do not differ by race and ethnicity. Significant racial-ethnic differences in mental healthcare exist for low-income women and African American and Hispanic mothers are at higher risk compared with white mothers.

The medicine

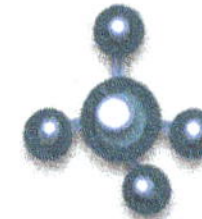

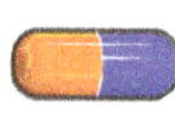

Brexanolone; Zulresso, FDA Approval 2019

Brexanolone is a neuroactive steroid, which acts as a transcriptional factor and is a formulation of **allopregnanolone,** which is a metabolite of progesterone. **Allopregnanolone** acts on the GABA receptor. The therapeutic use of Zulresso for depression may also **include effects on the hypothalamic pituitary adrenal (HPA) axis.**

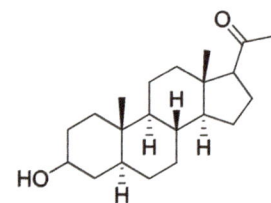

HO H H H H O

Allopregnanolone

Action of Brexanolone on cell and disease biology

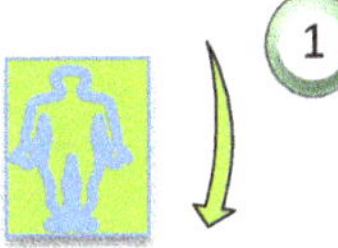

1 **Neurosteroids** binds to the "neurosteroid binding site" on the **GABA-A receptors and interacts** with neuronal membrane receptors to **promote network inhibition** in the brain.

Glial cells surround and support neurons and **synthesize neurosteroids** from cholesterol, as well as testosterone, estradiol, and Vitamin D.

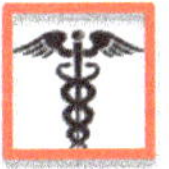

Reduced levels of allopregnanolone in the **cerebrospinal fluid** were associated with major **depression and anxiety disorders**.

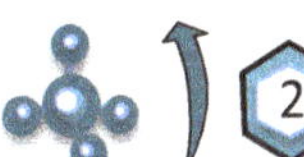

2 **Brexanolone** binds to the "neurosteroid binding site" on the **GABA-A receptor** with modulation of disrupted GABAergic activity in the CNS.

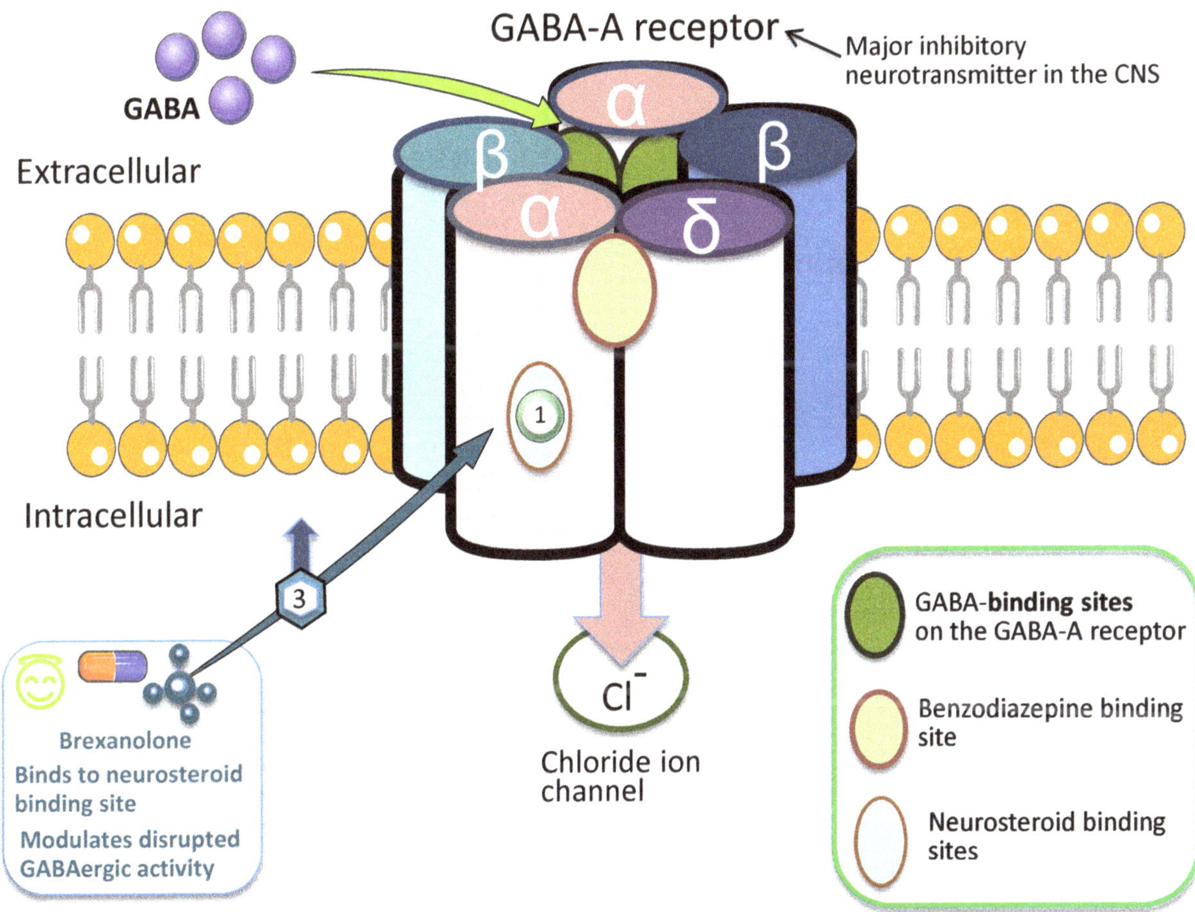

Peptide and other neurotransmitters

The hypothalamus maintains **homeostasis** via body temperature, hunger, attachment behaviors, thirst, fatigue, sleep, and circadian rhythms.

The **hypothalamus** produces releasing and inhibiting hormones to control production of other hormones throughout the body and is the link between the endocrine and nervous systems.

- Thyrotropin-releasing hormone
- Gonadotropin-releasing hormone
- Growth hormone-releasing hormone
- Corticotropin-releasing hormone
- Somatostatin
- Dopamine
- Vasopressin
- Oxytocin
- Dynorphins
- Orexins

Peptide neurotransmitters

- Opioids
- Orexin (hypocretin)
- Endorphins
- Somatostatin
- Oxytocin
- Vasopressin

Other neurotransmitters

- Acetylcholine
- Adenosine
- Nitric oxide

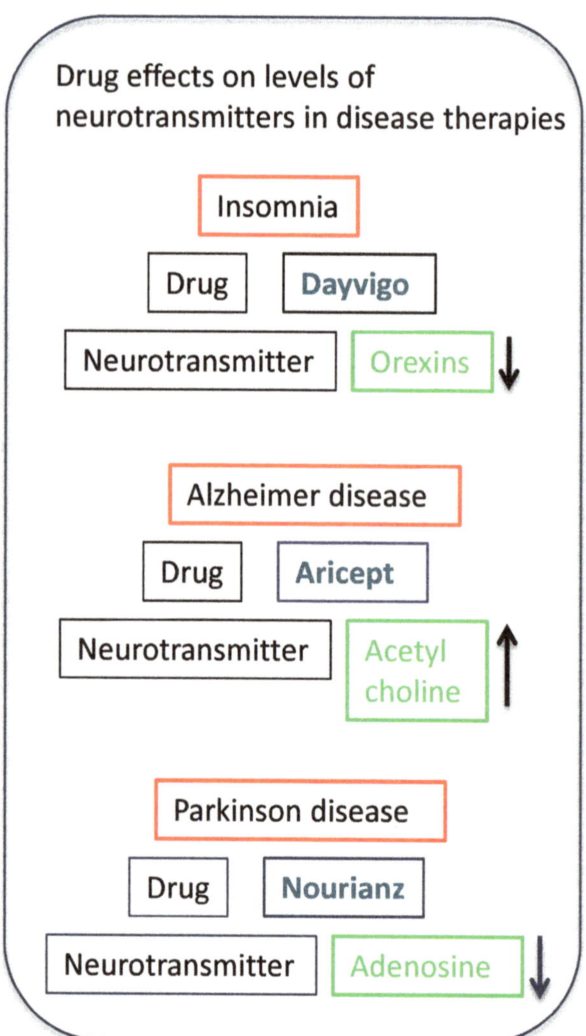

Opioid Neurotransmitters

The opioid system, activated by **enkephalins, dynorphins, and orexins** control pain and reward systems, which can result in addictive behaviors.

Locations of **mu opioid receptor** (MOR) in brain. Receptor activity in the brain is shown by the colored areas. Labeled locations are only approximate.

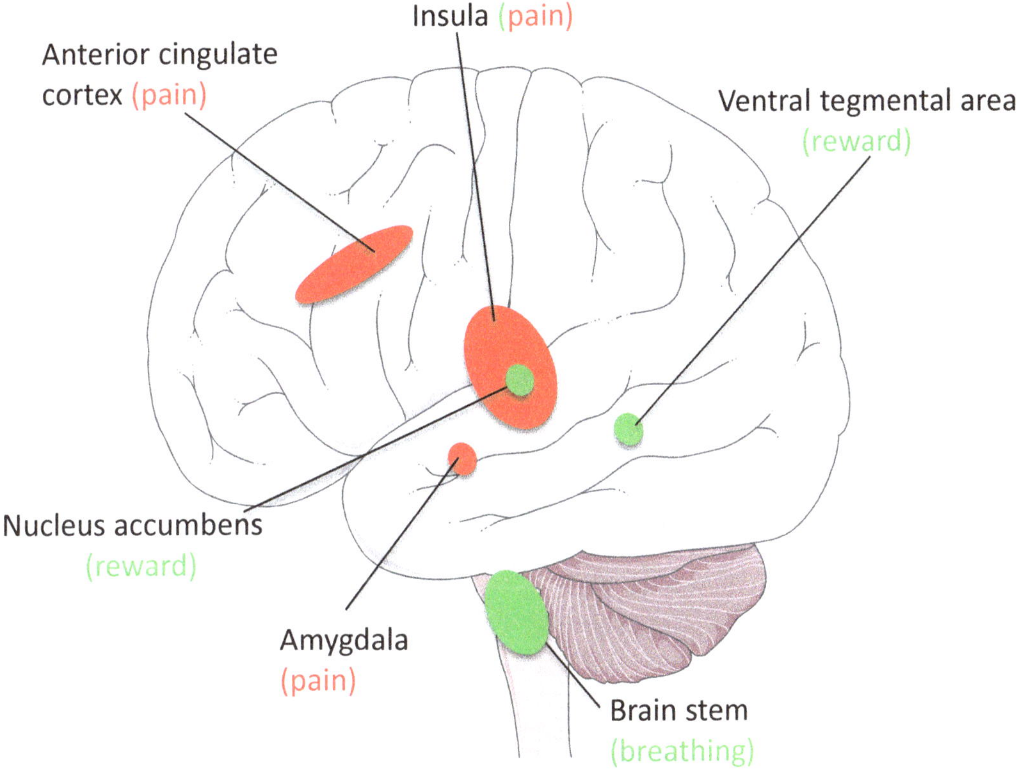

Opioids exert their pharmacological actions through three receptors, mu (MOR), kappa (KOR), and delta (DOR).

These receptors can be activated exogenously by plant based opiates, such as morphine, which acts as a painkiller through activating the μ-opioid receptor (MOR) in the central nervous system.

....

The disease: Migraine

Migraine is a neurological disorder that manifests as a debilitating headache associated with altered sensory perception. Episodic cluster headache in adults is the abrupt onset of severe pain on one side of the head. Pain is felt in the eye sockets (orbital), or immediately above (supraorbital), and/or back of the head and neck.

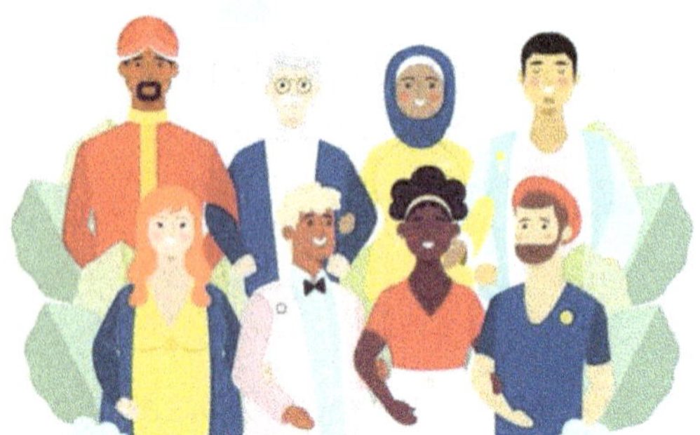

Incidence by gender and ethnicity

Women have two to three times the rate of migraines than men with a peak at age of 35 that can be linked to hormonal triggers. The rate then gradually tapers off until it declines steeply at menopause. The prevalence of migraine is lower among African Americans and Asian Americans than among whites. The adjusted prevalence of migraine is highest in North America, followed by South and Central America, Europe, Asia, and Africa.

Disease symptoms

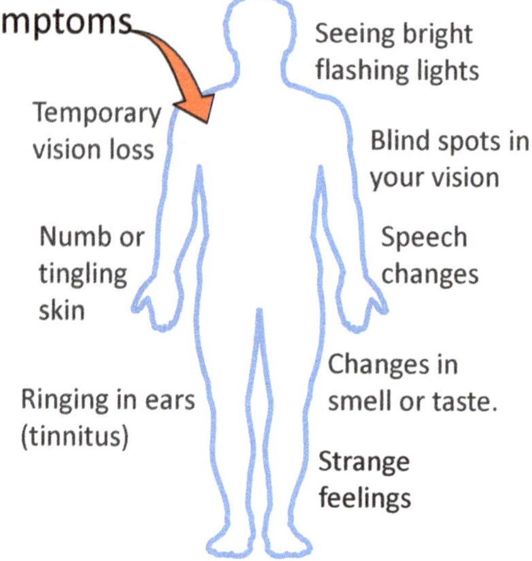

The medicine

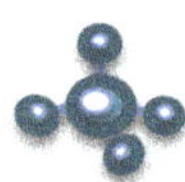
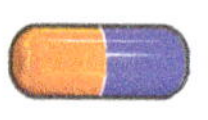

Ubrogepant ; Ubrelvy, FDA Approval 2019

Administered as a subcutaneous injection

Ubrogepant is an oral calcitonin gene-related peptide receptor antagonist for acute, short-term treatment migraine with or without aura (visual disturbance) in adults. **Ubrogepant does not constrict blood vessels** and thus can be prescribed for patients at risk of heart attacks or stroke.

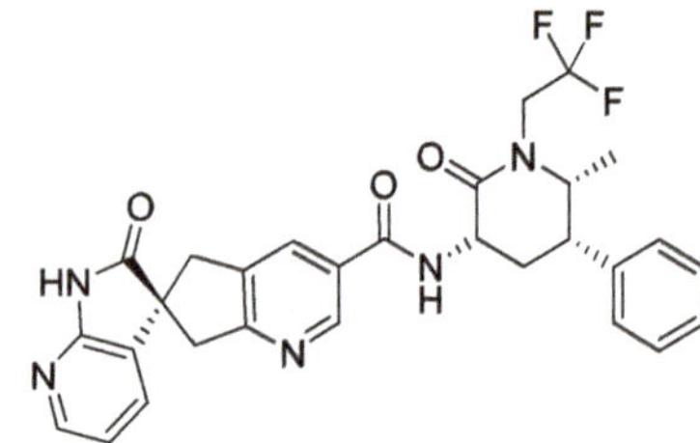

Galcanezumab; Emgality, FDA Approval 2018

Galcanezumab is for the preventive treatment of migraine in adults by injection. Is a humanized IgG4 monoclonal **antibody** (Mab) which is specific for **calcitonin-gene related peptide** (CGRP).

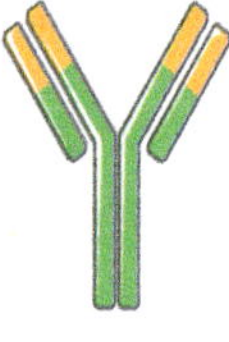

Action of Ubrogepant, Galcanezmab on cell and disease biology

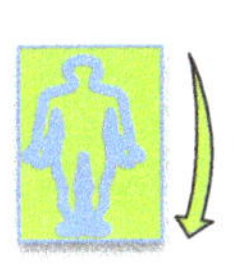
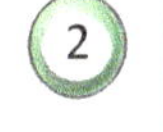

1 Calcitonin gene-related peptide (**CGRP**), produced in peripheral and central neurons, is a **potent vasodilator** causing widening of blood vessels near the surface of skin, leading to increased blood flow with flushing.

2 **CGRP receptor is a** seven-transmembrane receptor located in the cell membrane and CGRP **binding initiates a signaling** cascade.

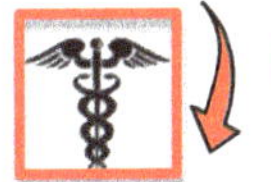

3 **Levels of CGRP in the blood rise** during migraine attacks and **CGRP infusion** results in **headache** in migraine patients.

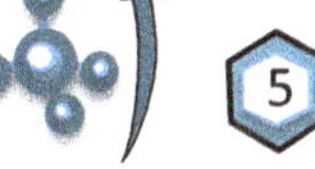

4 **CGRP antagonists inhibit neurogenic cranial vasodilatation** and inflammation by blocking the effects of CGRP

5 **Ubrogepant** is an **oral CGRP receptor antagonist,** which blocks CGRP binding to its receptors.

6 **Galcanezumab binds to endogenous CGRP** to block binding to CGRP receptors and reduce migraine activity.

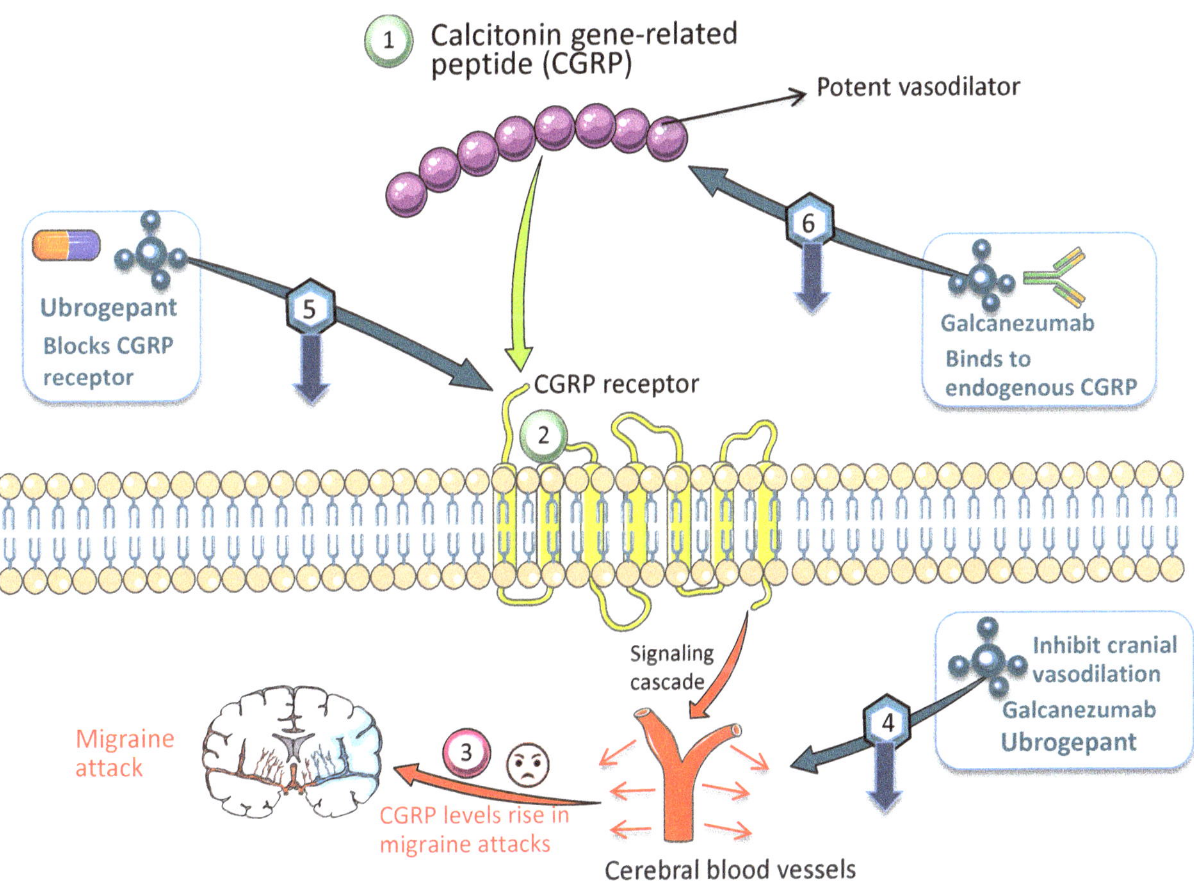

Peptide neurotransmitters: Migraine, Ubrogepant, Galcanezumab

The disease: Insomnia

Insomnia, which is trouble falling or staying asleep, is a prevalent sleep disorder that affects people ranging from childhood to old age and is the most common sleep disorder. **Insomnia** is likely driven not by the inability of the brain to "switch on" sleep-related circuits, but rather an **inability to "switch-off" wake-promoting circuits.**

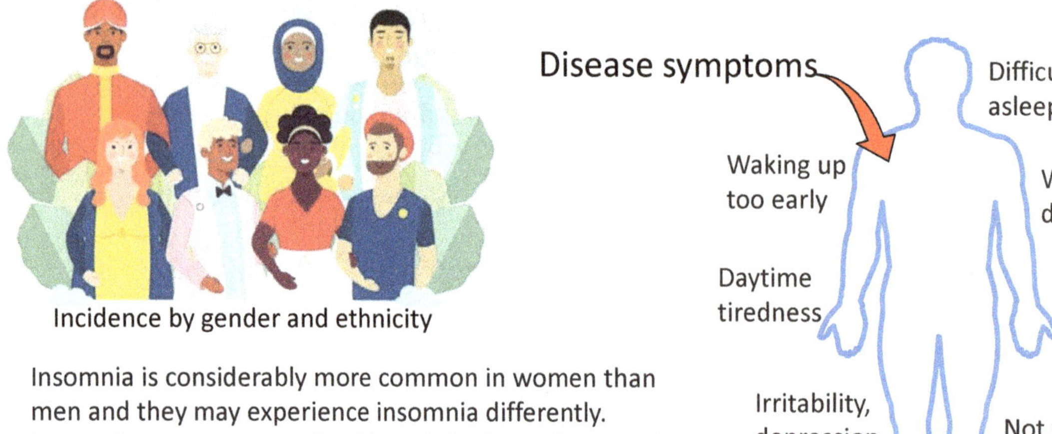

Incidence by gender and ethnicity

Insomnia is considerably more common in women than men and they may experience insomnia differently. Insomnia more common in older adults (over the age of 60–65 years old). Stress, menopause, and medical and mental health conditions are common causes of insomnia. Asians report less sleep problems, while insomnia is more prevalent in minority ethnic groups.

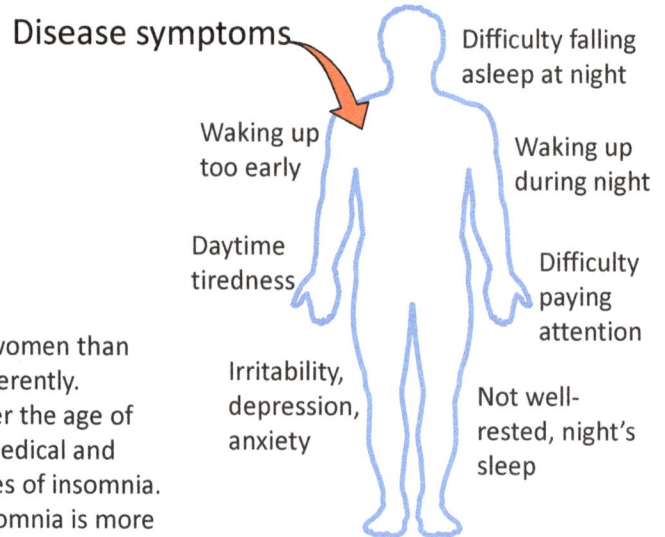

The medicine

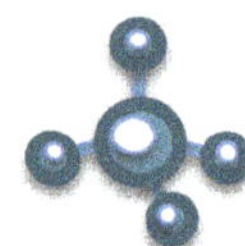

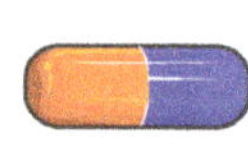

Lemborexant; Dayvigo, FDA Approval 2019

Lemborexant is a novel dual **orexin receptor blocker (antagonist)** and used in the **treatment of insomnia** characterized by difficulties with sleep onset and/or sleep maintenance. **Lemborexant counteracts inappropriate wakefulness** and stimulates sleep-promoting effects.

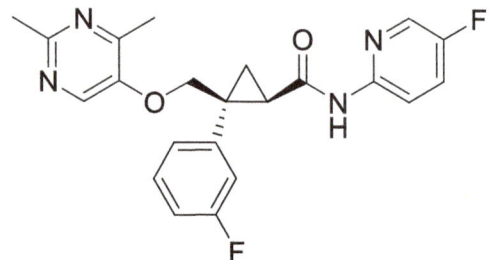

The **sleep-wake cycle** is a complex system of reciprocally regulating neural systems for stable transitions between states of wakefulness and sleep.

1 **Orexin neurons** in the hypothalamus, with axons throughout the brain, **function in wakefulness**, feeding, reward, and pain reception.

2 **Orexin A and B neuropeptides** regulate **transitions between arousal and sleep.** OX2R signaling primarily dictates arousal. OX1R and OX2R signaling is involved in shifting between sleep stages.
Orexin receptor 1 (OX1R) is specific for orexin A.
Orexin receptor 2 (OX2R) binds both orexin A and B.

3 **OX1R, OX2R signaling** acts to **increase intracellular calcium and** N-methyl-D-aspartate **(NDMA) receptors** on the cell surface with long-lasting **increases in neuronal excitability.**

4 **Lemborexant is a dual orexin receptor blocker** acting at both OX1R and OX2R.

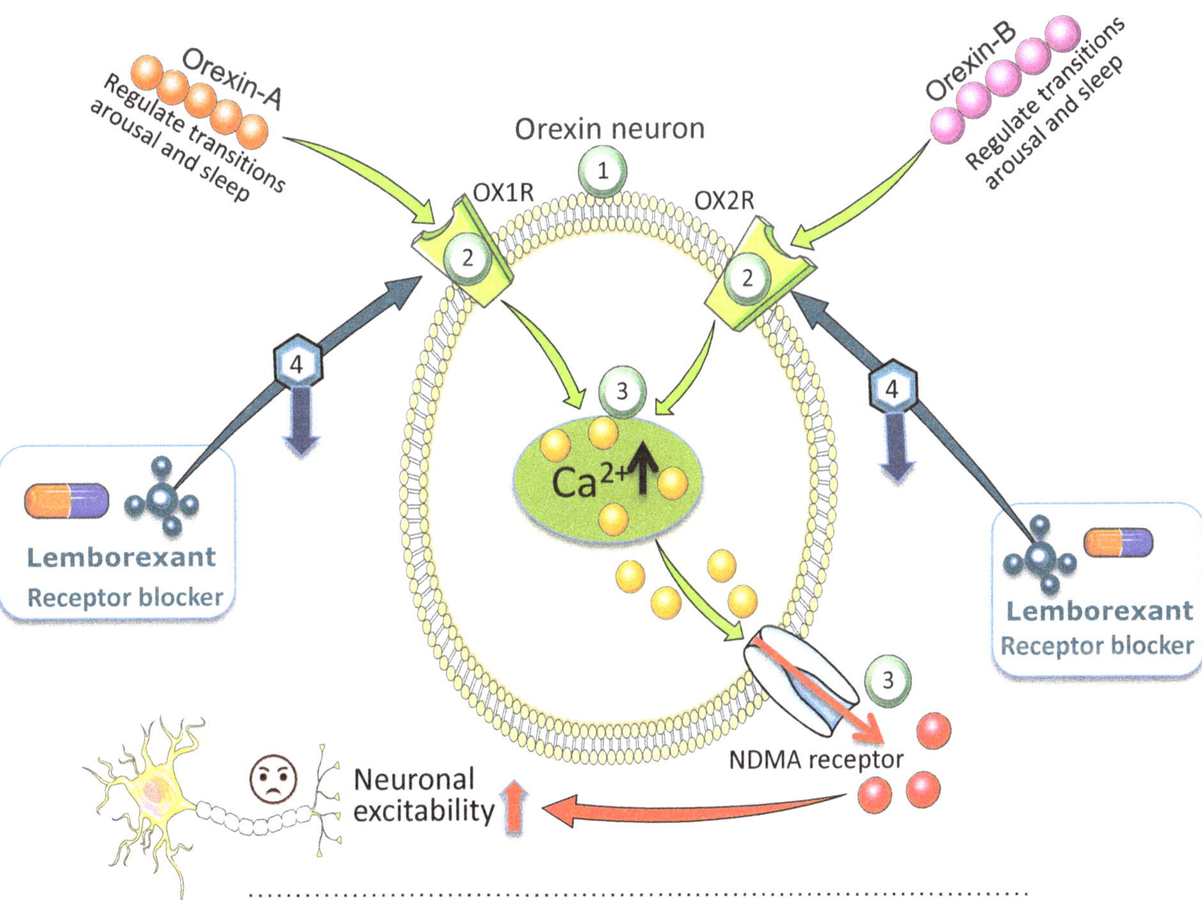

The disease: Parkinson's disease

Parkinson's disease (PD) is a **neurodegenerative disorder** with **reduced dopamine** levels in the mid-brain and when neurons that control body movement become impaired and/or die. Sleep-wake disturbances are common non-motor manifestations in PD due to an inability to "switch-off" wake-promoting circuits

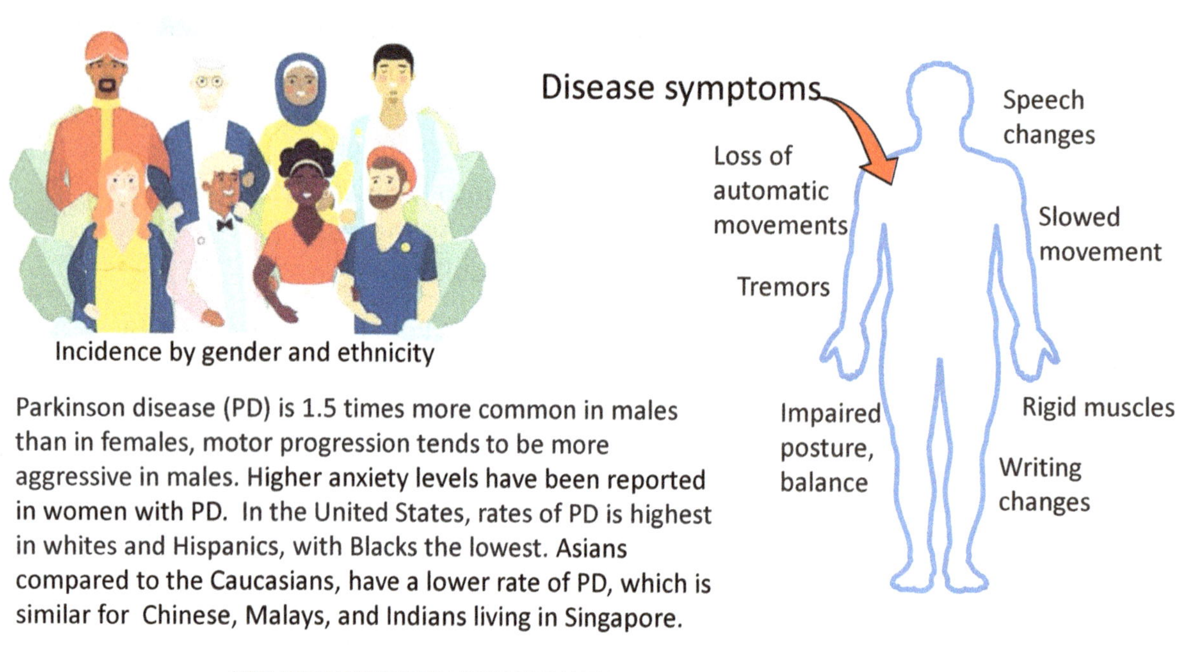

Incidence by gender and ethnicity

Parkinson disease (PD) is 1.5 times more common in males than in females, motor progression tends to be more aggressive in males. Higher anxiety levels have been reported in women with PD. In the United States, rates of PD is highest in whites and Hispanics, with Blacks the lowest. Asians compared to the Caucasians, have a lower rate of PD, which is similar for Chinese, Malays, and Indians living in Singapore.

The medicine

Istradefylline; Nourianz, FDA Approval 2019

Istradefylline is an **adjunctive treatment** to levodopa (L-DOPA) in both moderate and advanced stages of Parkinson's disease (PD) experiencing "off" episodes with movement symptoms, a common complication of chronic treatment with L-DOPA. Patients treated with **Istradefylline** can be used to **reduce l-dopa dosage** and side effects, such as dyskinesia. It is an **Adenosine A2A receptor inhibitor.**

O, CH_3, H_3C, N, N, OCH_3, O, N, N, OCH_3, H_3C

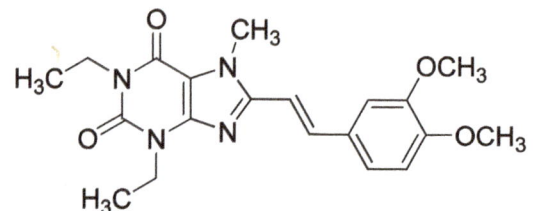

Other neurotransmitters : Parkinson's disease, Istradefylline

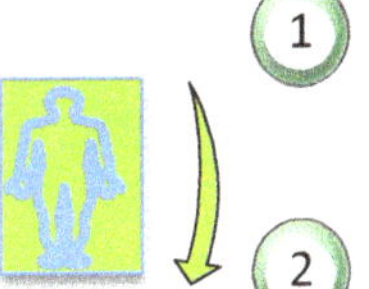

1 **Brain adenosine** is an **inhibitory neurotransmitter,** prolonged increased in neural activity in the brain triggers the release of adenosine. **Adenosine A2A receptors** are concentrated in the **dopamine rich areas of the brain.**

2 Adenosine receptor stimulation and interactions between **adenosine and dopamine receptors** regulate the **release of dopamine.**

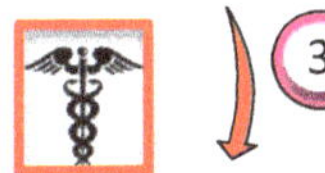

3 Parkinson's disease symptoms from **low levels of dopamine** in the striatum.

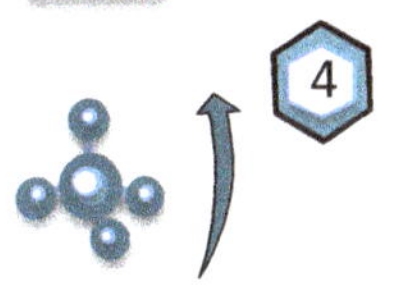

4 **Istradefylline inhibits** the adenosine **A2A receptor,** which results in improved symptoms and motor control.

Istradefylline increases the **release of GABA**, stabilizes a weakened blood–brain barrier as well as neuronal activity .

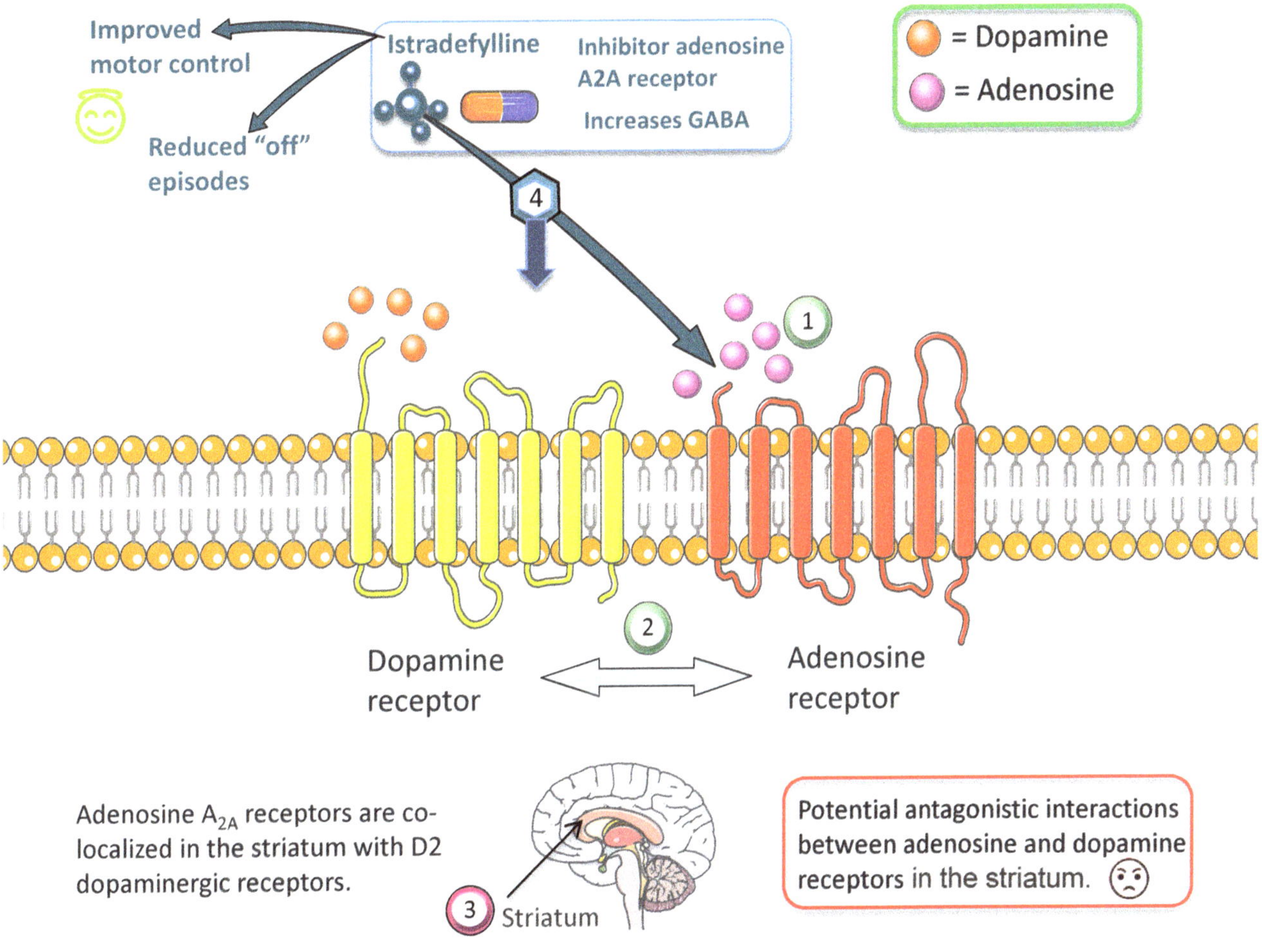

Improved motor control

Reduced "off" episodes

Istradefylline

Inhibitor adenosine A2A receptor

Increases GABA

= Dopamine

= Adenosine

4

1

2

Dopamine receptor

Adenosine receptor

Adenosine A_{2A} receptors are co-localized in the striatum with D2 dopaminergic receptors.

3 Striatum

Potential antagonistic interactions between adenosine and dopamine receptors in the striatum.

The disease: Acute pain

Acute pain, which derives from trauma such as broken bones, burns, birth or surgery.

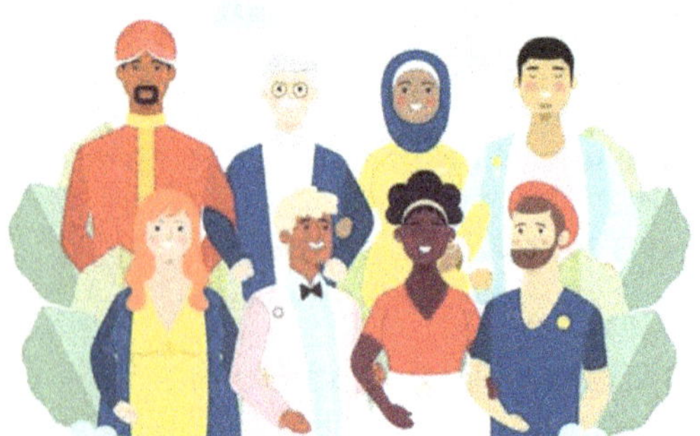

Incidence by gender and ethnicity

Men have higher pain thresholds and tolerance than women. The female body with a greater nerve density has a more intense natural response to painful stimuli. African American subjects reported higher levels of clinical pain and pain tolerance than Caucasians. Asian subjects such as Indian and Chinese have lower pain tolerances than Caucasians.

Disease symptoms

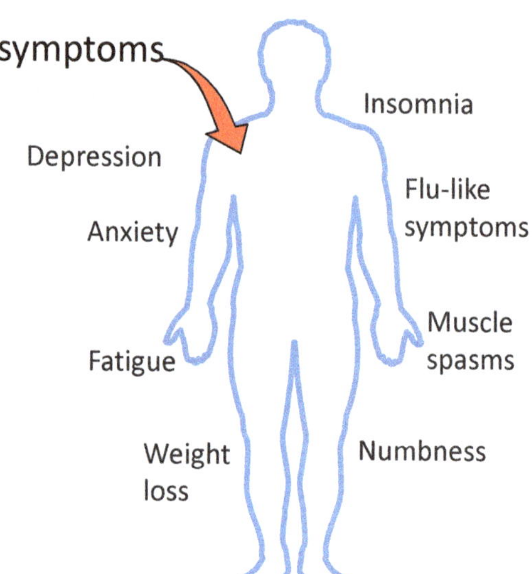

The medicine

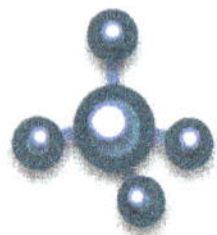

Hydrocodone; Vicodin, FDA Approval 1982

12th Most US Prescribed Drug in 2020, 40 million prescriptions

Codeine is typically used for the management of **pain severe** enough to require an opioid analgesic. Codeine is used for mild to moderate pain, whereas **Vicodin** is **more potent** and used for severe pain.

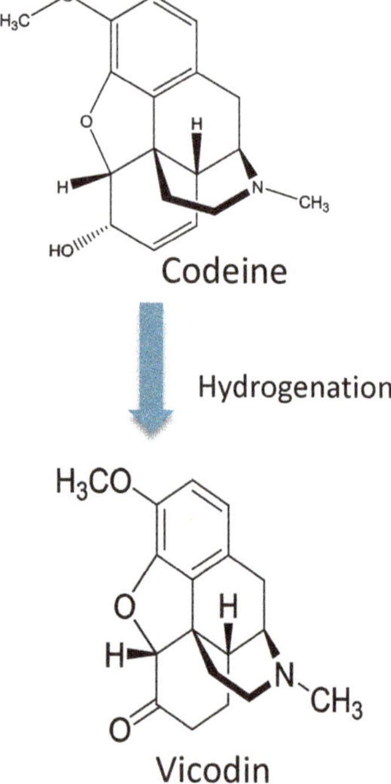

Other neurotransmitters: Acute pain, Hydrocodone

Action of Hydrocodone on cell and disease biology

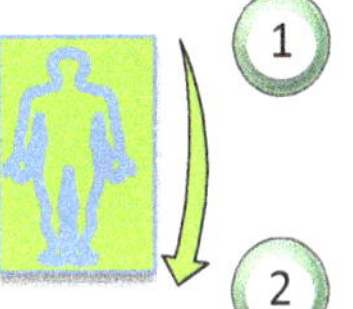

1 **Opioids bind** to the **Mu-opioid receptor** to **block pain messages** sent from the body through the spinal cord to the brain, reducing nerve cell excitability and pain transmission.

2 **Gamma-amino butyric acid** (GABA) is the primary **inhibitory neurotransmitter** and opioids inhibit GABA-mediated release and synaptic transmission in brain regions, reducing presynaptic neurotransmitter release.

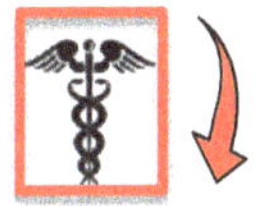

Acute pain is initiated by a harmful stimulus which directly or indirectly acts on **sensory nerve fibers** to generate an action potential and the pain signal is transmitted to the dorsal horn of the spinal cord.

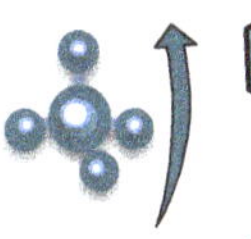

3 The pain-inhibitory neuron is indirectly activated by opioids and **hydrocodone is an opioid agonist,** which **activates the mu-opioid receptor** in the central nervous system.

4 A decrease in the neuron's action potential results in lack of excitation of nearby neurons and resulting pain states.

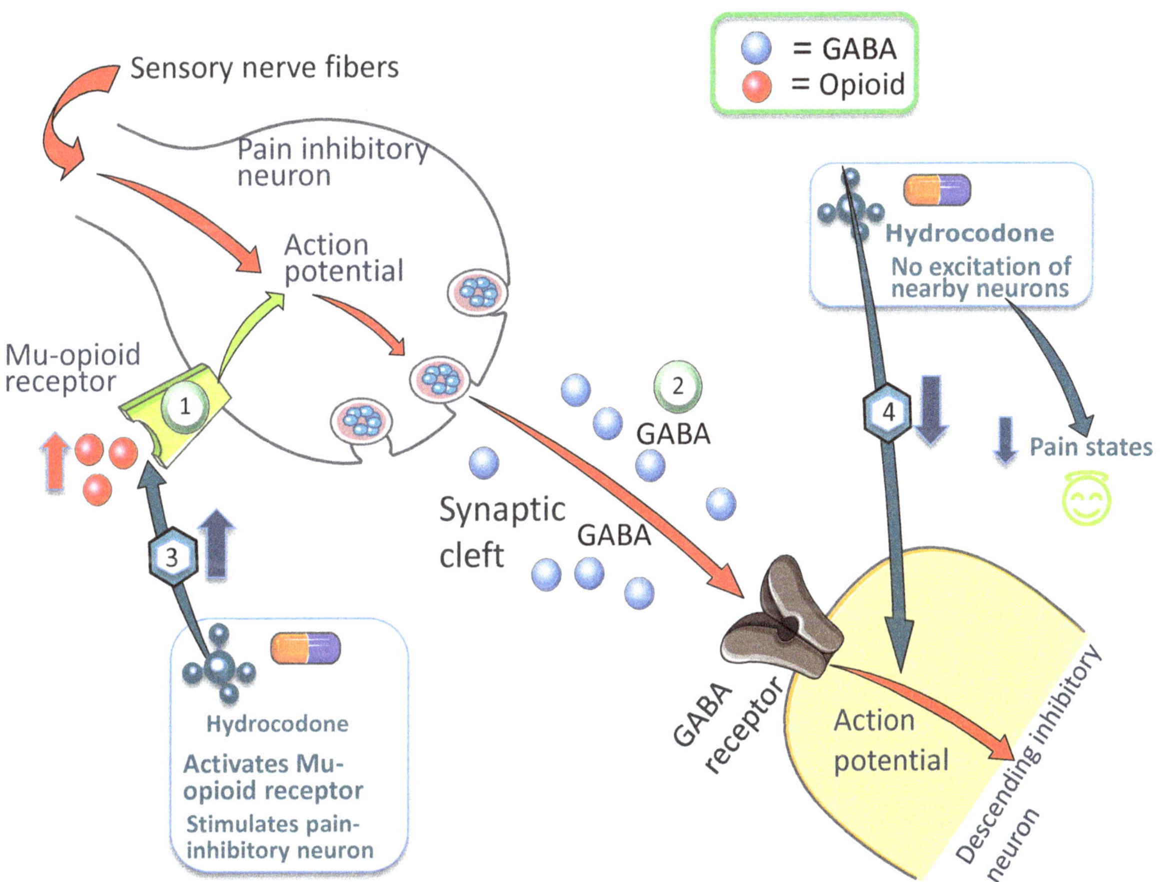

Other neurotransmitters: Acute pain, Hydrocodone

The disease: Alzheimer's disease

Alzheimer's disease (AD) is a progressive neurologic disorder that causes the brain to atrophy with **degeneration of brain cells** and dementia, with a continuous decline in thinking, behavioral and social skills that affects a person's ability to function independently. Alzheimer's disease is the most common cause of dementia.

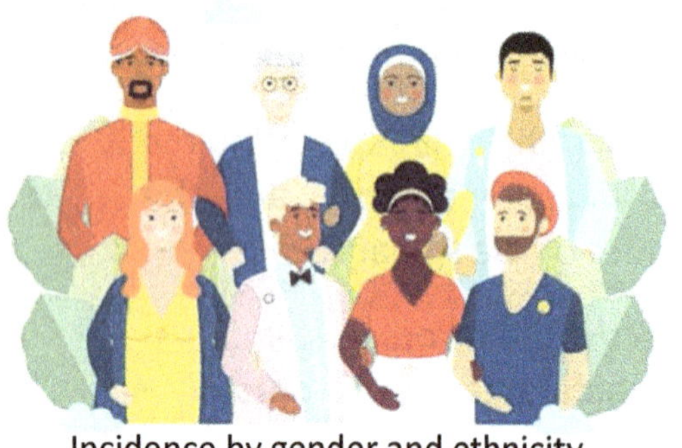

Incidence by gender and ethnicity

Disease increases with age in individuals who are 65 years or older. In the US more disease occurs in women and is higher in African-American and Hispanic communities, lower in non-Hispanic whites and lowest for American Indians and Asians. Disease is higher in Europe than Asia or India but increasing in Japan with an aging population.

Disease symptoms

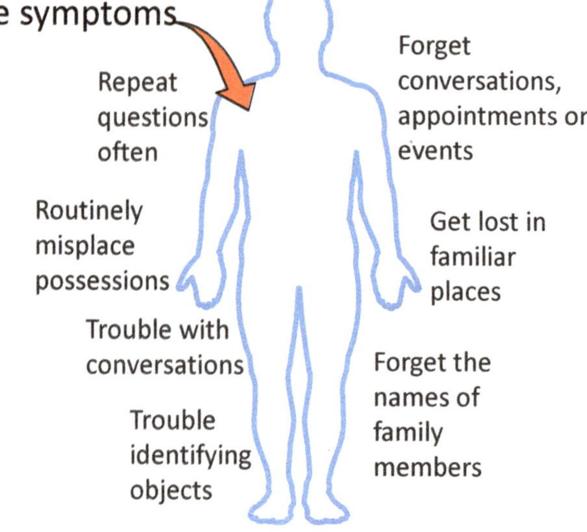

The medicine

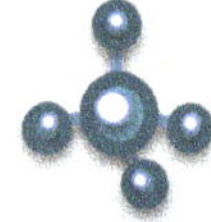

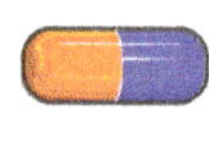

120th Most US Prescribed Drug (2019), 5.5 million prescriptions

Donepezil ; Aricept, FDA Approval 1996

Donepezil is an **inhibitor** of **acetylcholine esterase** that prevents **the breakdown of the neurotransmitter acetylcholine** (ACh). The resulting increase in levels of ACh in the brain is important for processes of memory and reasoning. Although **Donepezil improves cognition** and dementia **in Alzheimer patients** it **does not cure** the disease.

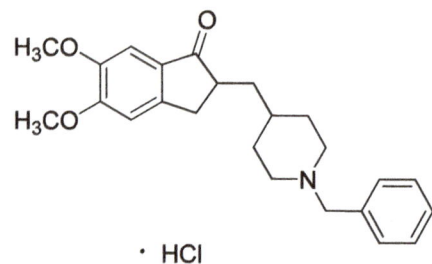

H_3CO H_3CO O N · HCl

Other neurotransmitters: Alzheimer disease, Donepezil

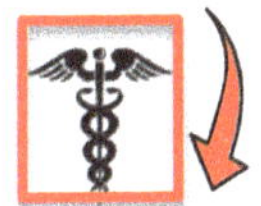

1 **Acetyl choline** (Ach) **functions** in projections from the basal **forebrain** to the **cerebral cortex and hippocampus** to support cognitive functions. The **brainstem** Ach containing neurons can send **excitatory inputs**.

2 ACh is synthesized in neurons from acetyl coenzyme A by the enzyme **choline acyltransferase (ChaT) .**

3 Acetylcholinesterase (AChE) is **anchored to membranes** at **cholinergic synapses in the central and peripheral nervous systems**.

In **Alzheimer's disease** there is **underactivity of cholinergic projections** to the hippocampus and cortex with loss of **long-term memory**.

4 **Donepezil inhibits** acetylcholinesterase (AChE) and **hydrolysis of acetylcholine**, increasing acetylcholine at synapses, **enhancing transmission.**

Surrogate markers of treatment are **reduced decline** in regional cerebral blood flow and slowing of hippocampal atrophy.

2 Enzymatic hydrolysis of acetyl choline

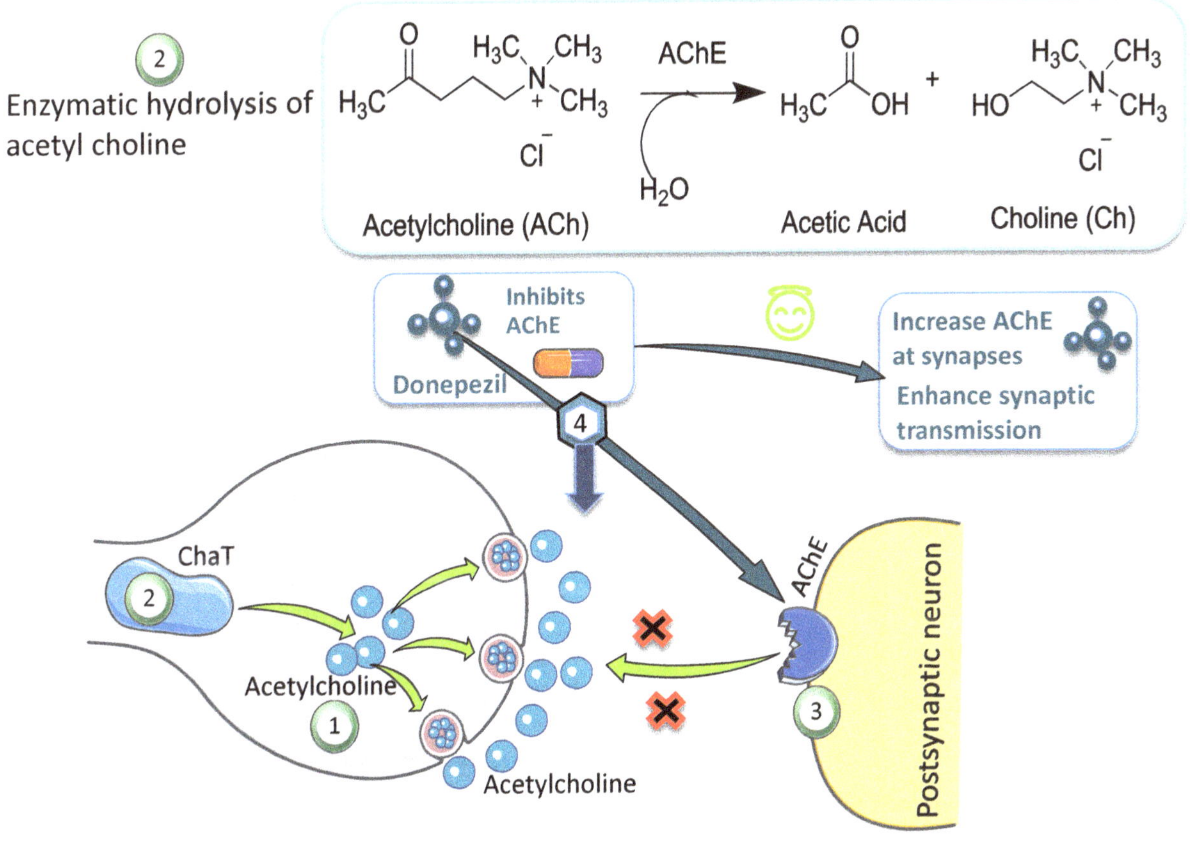

Chapter 6

Rare diseases
Small-molecule drugs
Antibody drugs
Peptide drugs
RNA drugs
Cell and gene therapy

Innovative medicines and breakthrough therapies
Recently approved by the FDA (2018 →)

Rare diseases
- Lennox–Gastaut and Dravet syndrome (Cannabidiol)
- Fabry disease (Galafold)
- Blastic plasmacytoid dendritic cell neoplasm (Tagraxofusp)
- Transthyretin-mediated amyloid cardiomyopathy (Tafamidis)
- Hutchinson–Gilford (progeroid) syndrome (Lonafarnib)
- Pro-opiomelanocortin (POMC) deficiency (Setmelanotide)
- X-linked hypophosphatemia (Burosumab)
- Primary hemophagocytic lymphohistiocytosis (Emapalumab)
- Types I and II hereditary angioedema (Lanadelumab)
- Acute hepatic porphyria (Givosiran)
- Duchenne muscular dystrophy (Golodirsen)
- Hereditary transthyretin amyloidosis (Patisiran)
- Primary hyperoxaluria type 1 (Lumasiran)
- Phenylketonuria (Pegvaliase)
- Adenosine deaminase deficiency (Elapegademase)
- Spinal muscular atrophy (Zolgensma)

Small-molecule drugs
- Cannabidiol
- Galafold
- Talzenna
- Vyndamax
- Piqray
- Zokinvy
- Elzonris

Antibody drugs
- Burosumab
- Emapalumab
- Lanadelumab
- Romosozumab
- Naxitamab
- Emicizumab

RNA drugs
- Givosiran
- Golodirsen
- Patisiran
- Lumasiran

Peptide drugs
- Semaglutide
- Setmelanotide

Cell and gene therapy
Yescarta
Zolgensma

Breakthrough therapies
The development of drugs which may address serious or life-threatening diseases and which lack effective treatments can be facilitated by an accelerated review by the FDA. Treatment of resistant disease such as advanced metastatic or relapsed/refractory disease can be facilitated by the availability of preliminary evidence of a clinically significant endpoint with can expedite the drug review process.

Rare diseases
The development of new technologies such as the analysis of single cell genomes and transcriptomes has started to guide precision medicine and the identification of rare diseases. Currently in America alone, there are 7000 such diseases that effect up to 30 million patients with only 5% of these patients having access to approved drugs. The FDA has created development incentives for drugs that treat rare or "orphan" diseases that affect 200,000 or fewer Americans. By 2019, the FDA has approved drugs and biologics for some 750 rare disease indications.

Small-molecule drugs
The rapid and multi-disciplinary advances of pharmaceutical sciences together with powerful new chemical synthetic approaches have resulted in significant innovations in the development of small molecule drugs. The developments encompass the exploration of chemical space around a ligand and target with new imaging approaches, use of artificial intelligence and machine learning, as well as high-throughput screening of multifaceted and novel small-molecule libraries.

Antibody and peptide drugs
Recent therapeutic antibody drugs exhibit reduced side effects and high target specificity, such as delivery of cytotoxic molecules into cancer cells. Immunogenicity of the drug has been minimized by developments such as human versions of the antibodies and the use of less immunogenic antibody fragments (lack of Fc domain). Other developments include antibody–drug conjugates (ADCs) and bispecific antibodies which links two antigen-binding domains. Peptide drugs developments include multifunctional and cell penetrating peptides, peptide drug conjugates, and oral delivery using permeation enhancers and reduced degradation by gut and other enzymes.

DNA, RNA, and cell therapy drugs
RNA-based therapeutics have been enabled by manufacturing improvements and novel delivery methods which include antisense oligonucleotides, aptamers, and small interfering RNAs.
DNA-based drugs now use a nonintegrating viral vectors such as adeno-associated virus (AAV) for the delivery of large DNA cargos which can code for a therapeutic protein. The modified AAV contains a linear single-stranded DNA with key AAV viral genes removed and the therapeutic gene is inserted, which enables delivery to the target cell and then expression.
Cell therapies use a DNA vector to transfect a patient cells *ex vivo,* which are then expanded and delivered in a single dose to the patient.
CAR-T cell therapy uses enriched T cells isolated from a patient's peripheral blood, which are treated with a lentiviral or retroviral vector that contains a chimeric antigen receptor (CAR). Subsequently, the modified T cells are expanded, cryopreserved, and later infused into the patient to kill the targeted disease cells.

The disease: Lennox–Gastaut syndrome and Dravet syndrome

Treatment of seizures associated with two rare, severe, and strongly drug-resistant epileptic syndromes that occur in childhood: Lennox–Gastaut syndrome (LGS) and Dravet syndrome (DS). **DS** appears during the first year of life with frequent fever-related seizures. **LGS** begins with multiple types of seizures including tonic seizures, which cause the muscles to contract uncontrollably.

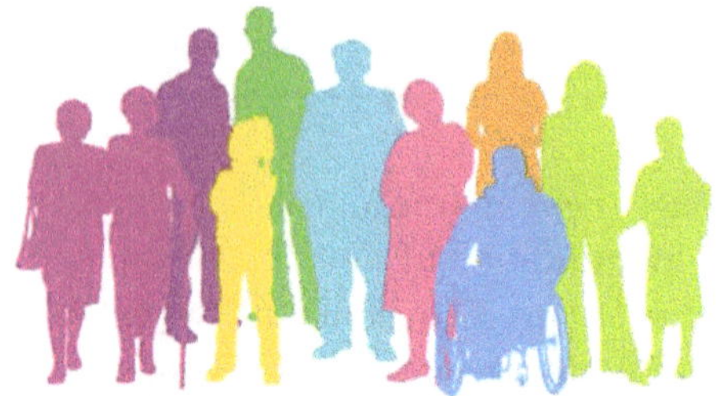

Incidence by gender and ethnicity

LGS and DS (LGS) begin in childhood and continue into adulthood with significant impact. Unprovoked seizures are more common in men, but some forms of epilepsy are more common in women. Hispanics have more epilepsy but whites have more uncontrolled episodes.

Disease symptoms

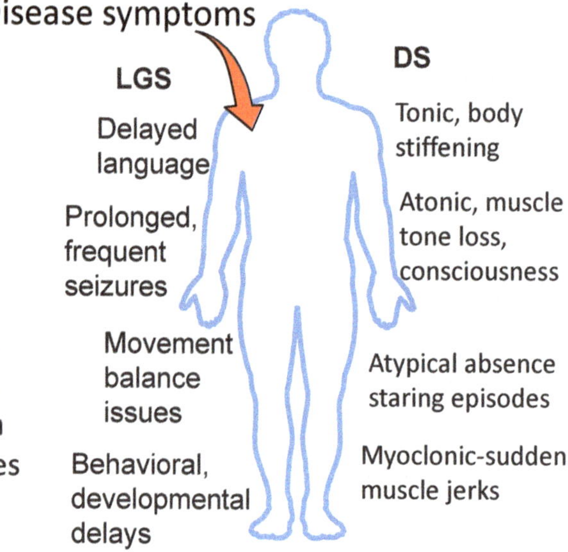

The medicine

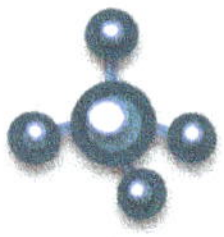

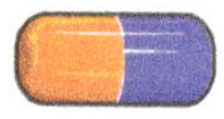

Epidioloex: Cannabidiol , FDA Approval 2020

Cannabidiol (CBD) is a highly-purified cannabinoid that is a nonpsychoactive component of the Cannabis sativa plant. CBD is related to endocannabinoids produced within the body (endogenous ligands of cannabinoid receptors, CB1 and CB2).

Small molecule drugs: Seizures, Epidioloex

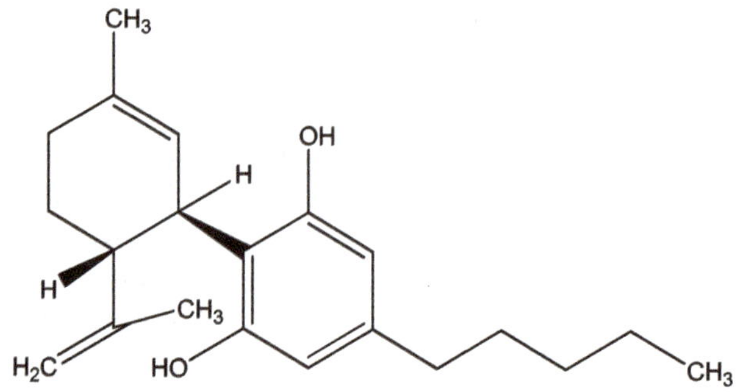

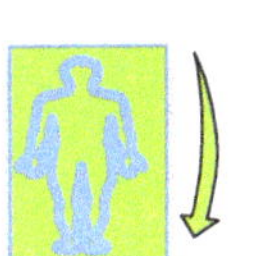

1 **Serotonin** can be **co-localized with other neurotransmitters** with reciprocal interactions.

2 Gamma-aminobutyric acid **(GABA)** and GABAA receptors form the major inhibitory neurotransmitter system and **depresses excitatory synapses.**

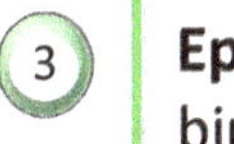

3 **Epidiolex (CBD)** has low affinity for the cannabinoid receptors (CB1,2) but binds to other receptors including **serotonin 5-HT1A receptors** and **increases γ-aminobutyric acid (GABA) affinity** for its receptor.

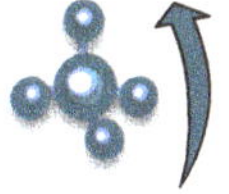

4 **CBD increases the effectiveness of serotonin** and modulates **GABA activity to decrease** anxiety and depression.

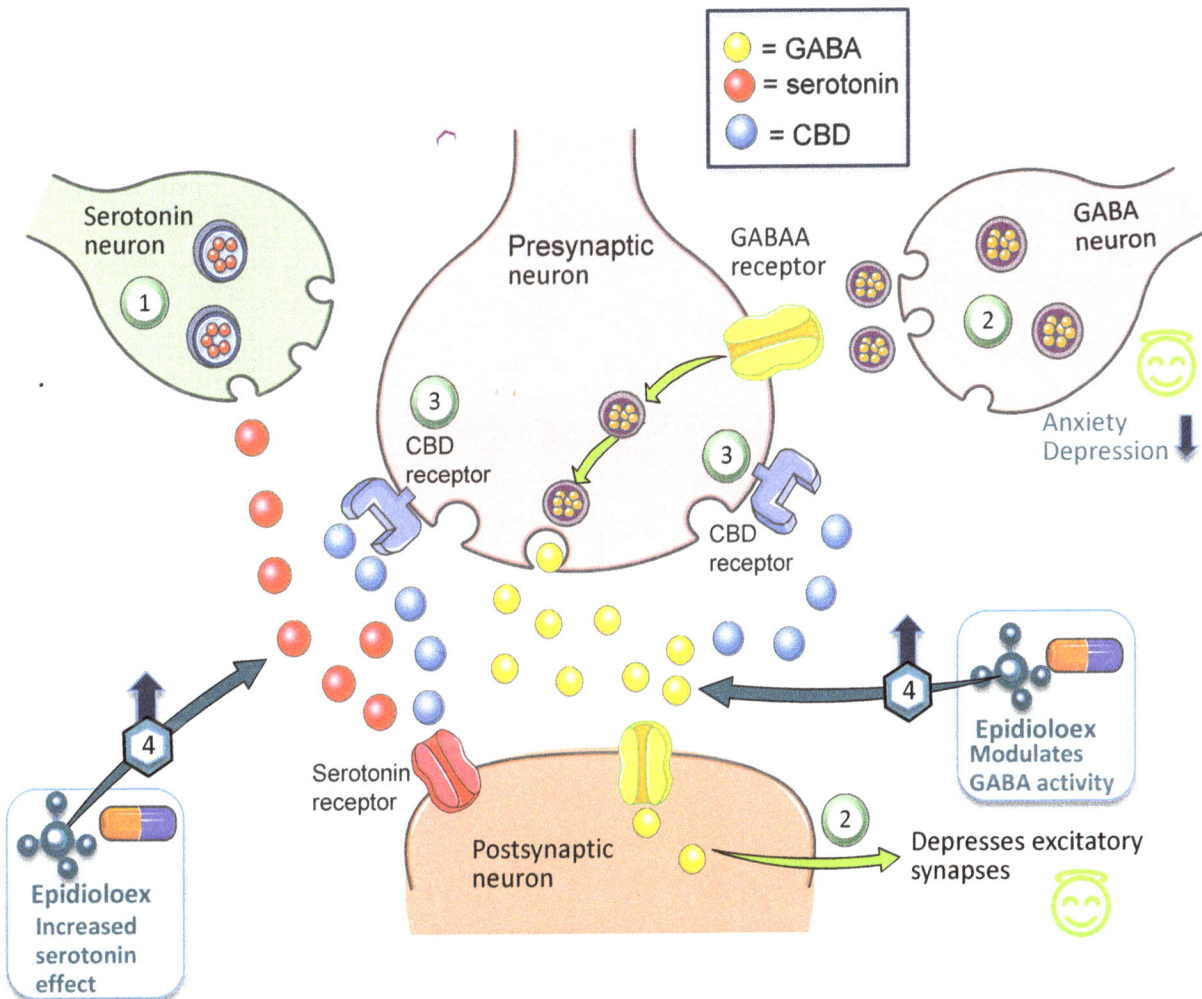

= GABA
= serotonin
= CBD

Serotonin neuron
1
Presynaptic neuron
GABAA receptor
GABA neuron
2
3
CBD receptor
3
CBD receptor
Anxiety
Depression
4
Epidioloex Modulates GABA activity
4
Serotonin receptor
Postsynaptic neuron
2
Depresses excitatory synapses
Epidioloex Increased serotonin effect

The disease: Fabry disease

Fabry disease is an inherited disorder due to **mutations in the GLA gene,** located on the X chromosome, which codes for the enzyme α-GalA and breaks down the glycolipid GB3. Misfolded α-galactosidease A (α-GalA) is decomposed in the cell and leads to **accumulation of Gb3 in blood vessels** with symptoms including skin and kidney damage, heart attack, and stroke.

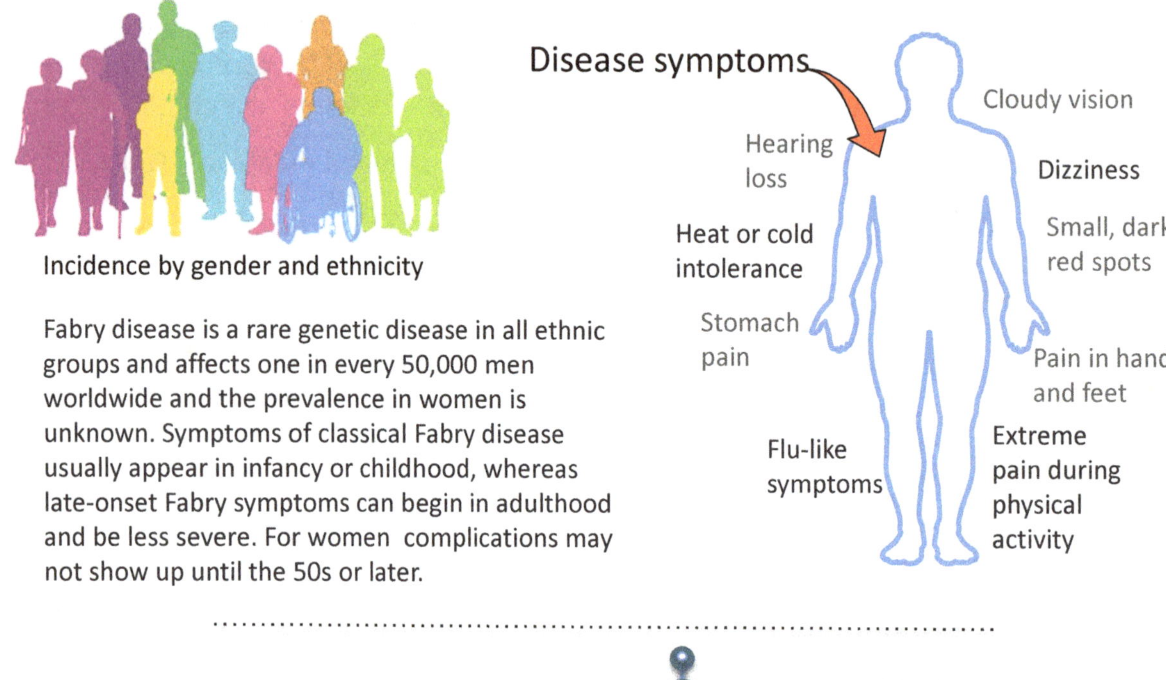

Incidence by gender and ethnicity

Fabry disease is a rare genetic disease in all ethnic groups and affects one in every 50,000 men worldwide and the prevalence in women is unknown. Symptoms of classical Fabry disease usually appear in infancy or childhood, whereas late-onset Fabry symptoms can begin in adulthood and be less severe. For women complications may not show up until the 50s or later.

The medicine

Migalastat: Galafold, FDA Approval 2020

Fabry disease occurs from a **mutation** on the X chromosome of the gene responsible for making **alpha-galactosidase enzyme.** Hemizygous males with a single copy of the gene (no α-galactosidase A activity) may display all signs of the disease, whereas heterozygous females may have mild symptoms.

Migalastat binds to faulty α-GalA enzyme and **promotes a shift in folding** to generate a functional enzyme.

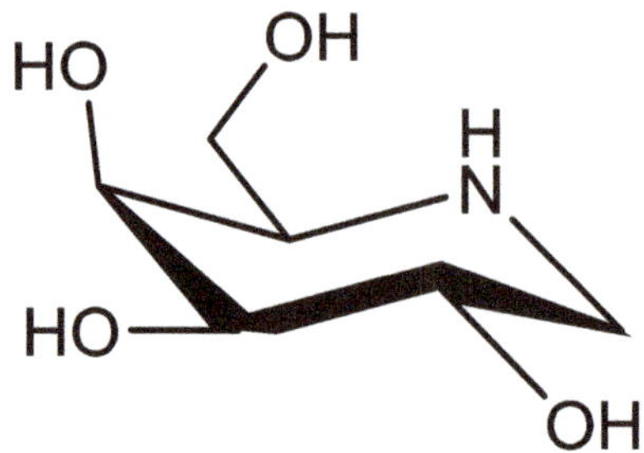

Small molecule drugs: Fabry disease, Migalastat

Action of Migalastat on cell and disease biology

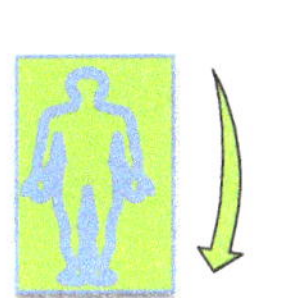

1 **Glycolipids such as GP3** are components of cellular membranes with a hydrophobic lipid tail and hydrophilic sugar groups.

2 **α-Galactosidase A** (α-GalA, coded by the GLA gene) catalyzes the removal of terminal α-galactose groups from GB3.

3 **Lysosome** functions as the waste **disposal system** and storage diseases are due to enzyme deficiencies with build-up of toxic materials in the cell.

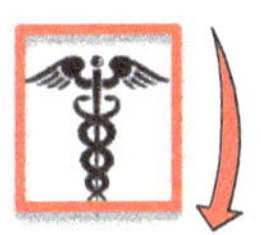

4 The largest number of mutations in the GLA gene (over 300) are **missense mutations** with single amino acid changes (~40%) resulting in **misfolding** and loss of activity of the α-GalA enzyme.

5 Glycolipid **GB3 accumulates** in blood vessels and other tissues resulting in enlarged cells in a wide range of organs and tissues and resulting problems including cardiac, renal, and skin disease.

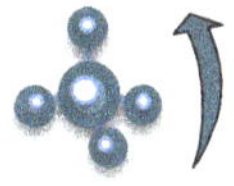

6 **Migalastat** binds to α-GalA to **shift the folding behavior of** misfolded mutants toward the active 3D shape.

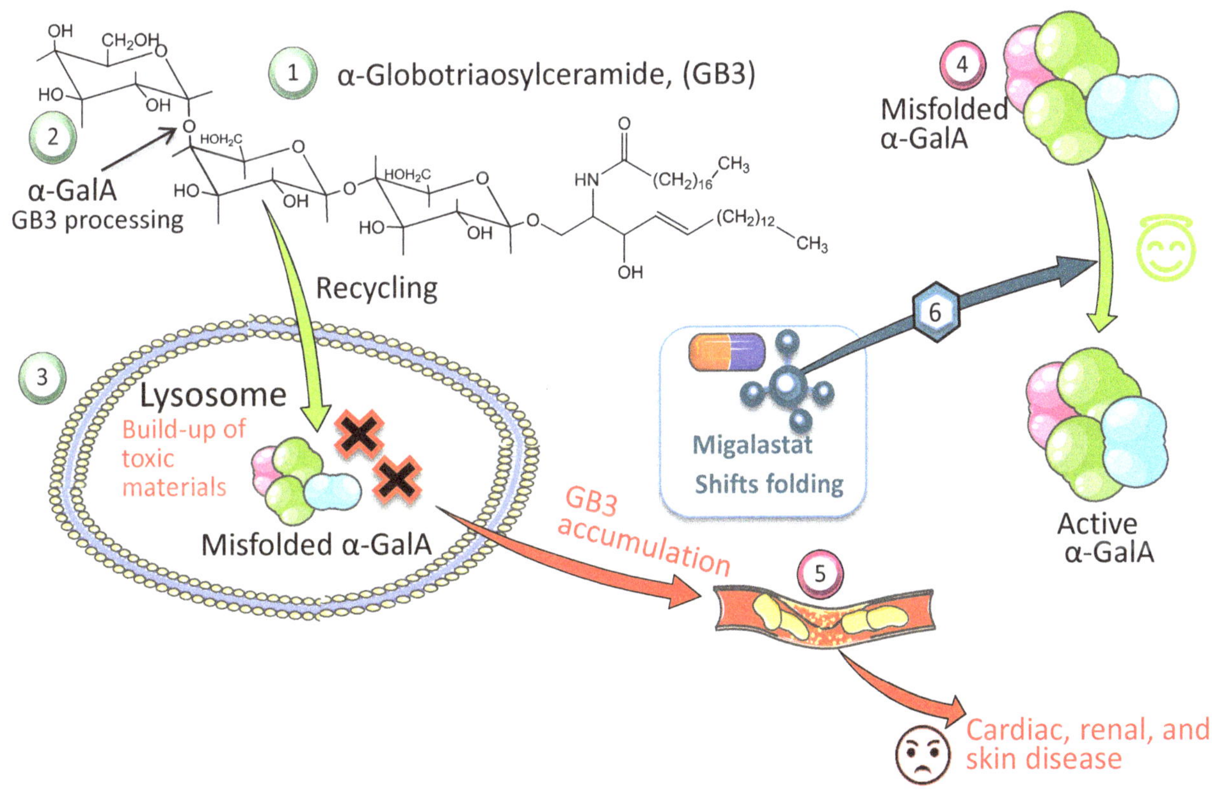

Small-molecule drugs: Fabry disease, Migalastat

The disease: Breast cancer

A serious type of breast cancer with the genetic profile—human epidermal growth factor receptor 2 (HER2)-negative, **abnormal**-inherited **BRCA gene** (5%–10% of all breast cancers), and the cancer has spread to other parts of the body (locally advanced or metastatic).

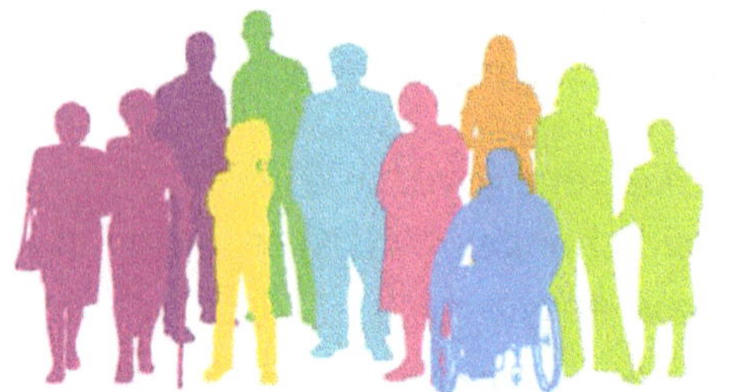

Incidence by gender and ethnicity

Non-Hispanic women have the highest overall incidence rate for breast cancer in the United States, whereas Native American women have the lowest rate. The lowest mortality rates for breast cancer are found in China and Japan (6%–7%), whereas Europe and North America have a rate of around 20%–25%.

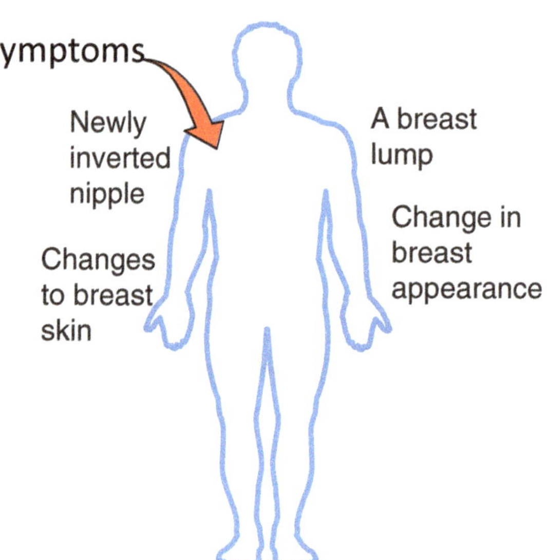

The medicine

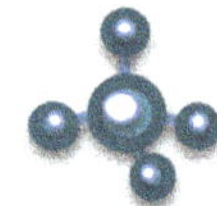

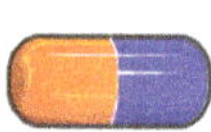

Talazoparib: Talzenna, FDA Approval 2018

Talazoparib is for the treatment of patients with a BRCA-mutated HER2-negative breast cancer that is locally advanced or metastasized. Talzenna is an **inhibitor of the poly adenosine diphosphate (ADP) ribose polymerase** (PARP) enzyme, which is involved in DNA repair.

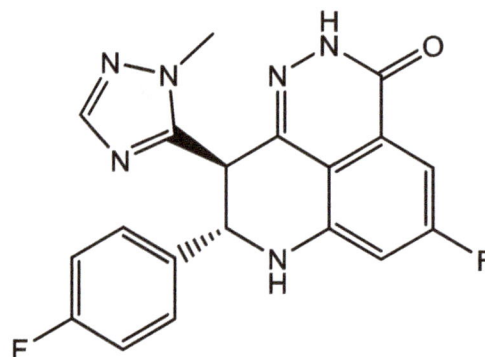

Small-molecule drugs: Breast cancer, Talazoparib

Action of Talazoparib virus on cell and disease biology

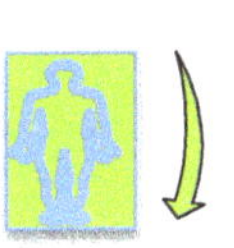

1 **DNA breaks** can be caused by irradiation, chemical agents, ultraviolet light.

2 **PolyADP-ribose** is made from the addition of ADP-ribose groups and nuclear proteins to form **PARP**, a polyvalent, highly charged complex.

3 **PARP detects a DNA break**, binds to the DNA, assembles the repair complex.

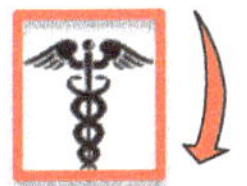
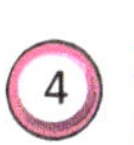

4 **BRCA mutation** is an inactivating mutations of the tumor suppressor gene, cancer cells then dependent on PARP1 for DNA repair.

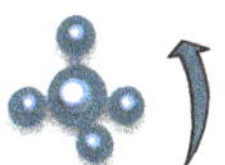

5 **Talazoparib** binds to the NAD$^+$ binding site and **traps the PARP complex** and thus inhibits DNA repair.

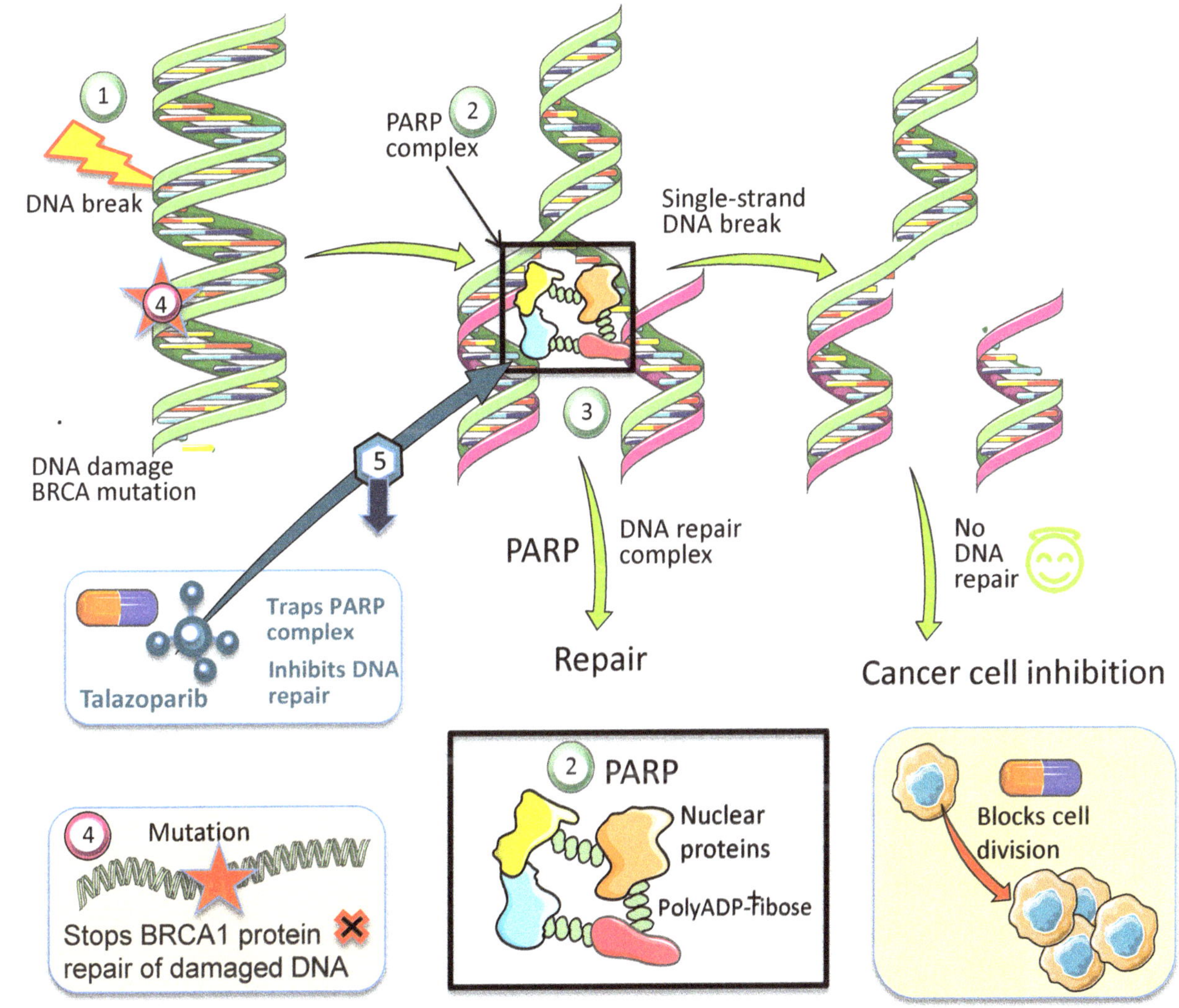

1
DNA break
4
DNA damage
BRCA mutation
PARP complex 2
Single-strand DNA break
3
5
Talazoparib
Traps PARP complex
Inhibits DNA repair
PARP
DNA repair complex
Repair
No DNA repair
Cancer cell inhibition
4 Mutation
Stops BRCA1 protein repair of damaged DNA
2 PARP
Nuclear proteins
PolyADP-ribose
Blocks cell division

Small-molecule drugs: Breast cancer, Talazoparib

The disease: Metastatic breast cancer

Advanced or metastatic breast cancer (mBC) is hormone receptor (HR)-positive, human epidermal growth factor receptor 2 (HER2)-negative and has a **mutation in phosphatidylinositol 3-kinase** (PI3K). The cancer has spread to other parts of the body, which includes the lungs, liver, bones, or brain.

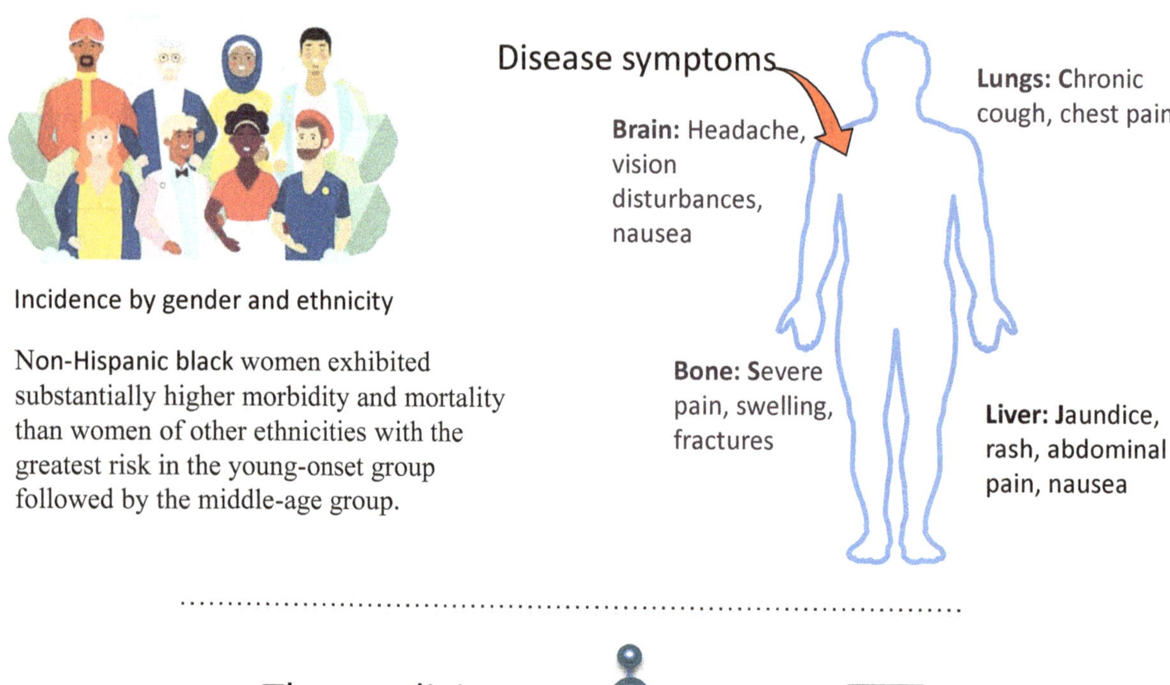

Incidence by gender and ethnicity

Non-Hispanic black women exhibited substantially higher morbidity and mortality than women of other ethnicities with the greatest risk in the young-onset group followed by the middle-age group.

The medicine

Alpelisib: Piqray, FDA Approval 2019

Alpelisib is a small-molecule PI3K inhibitor that **selectively inhibits the catalytic unit of PI3K.** Alpelisib is used to treat breast cancer that has spread to nearby tissues or other parts of the body in women who have already gone through menopause and for male patients.

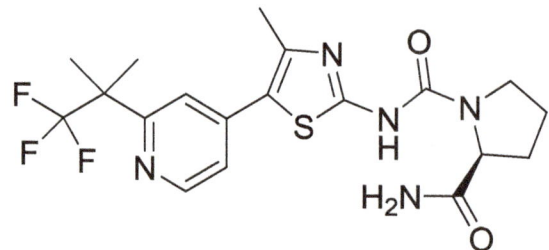

Action of Alpelisib on cell and disease biology

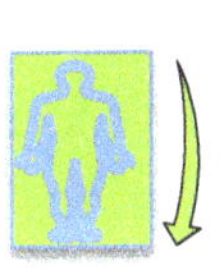

1. The PI3K (**phosphatidylinositol 3-kinase**) and Akt (protein kinase B) or PI3K/AKT signaling pathway regulates cell survival and proliferation.

2. **Activating mutations** of the PI3K catalytic unit with hyperactivation of the signaling pathways, proliferation of cells, and metastatic tumor development.

3. **Protrusions** are formed by **metastatic tumor cells** and degrade the **extracellular matrix** basement membrane by release of proteases.

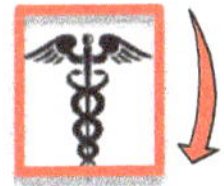

4. **Aberrant activation** of the PI3K/AKT pathway is observed in metastatic breast cancer in the lung, brain, liver, and bone.

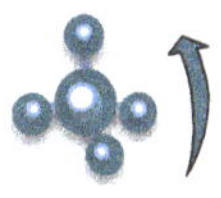

5. **Alpelisib** blocks the **catalytic unit of PI3**K, which is mutated in breast cancer, to cause cell death, inhibit the proliferation of malignant cells.

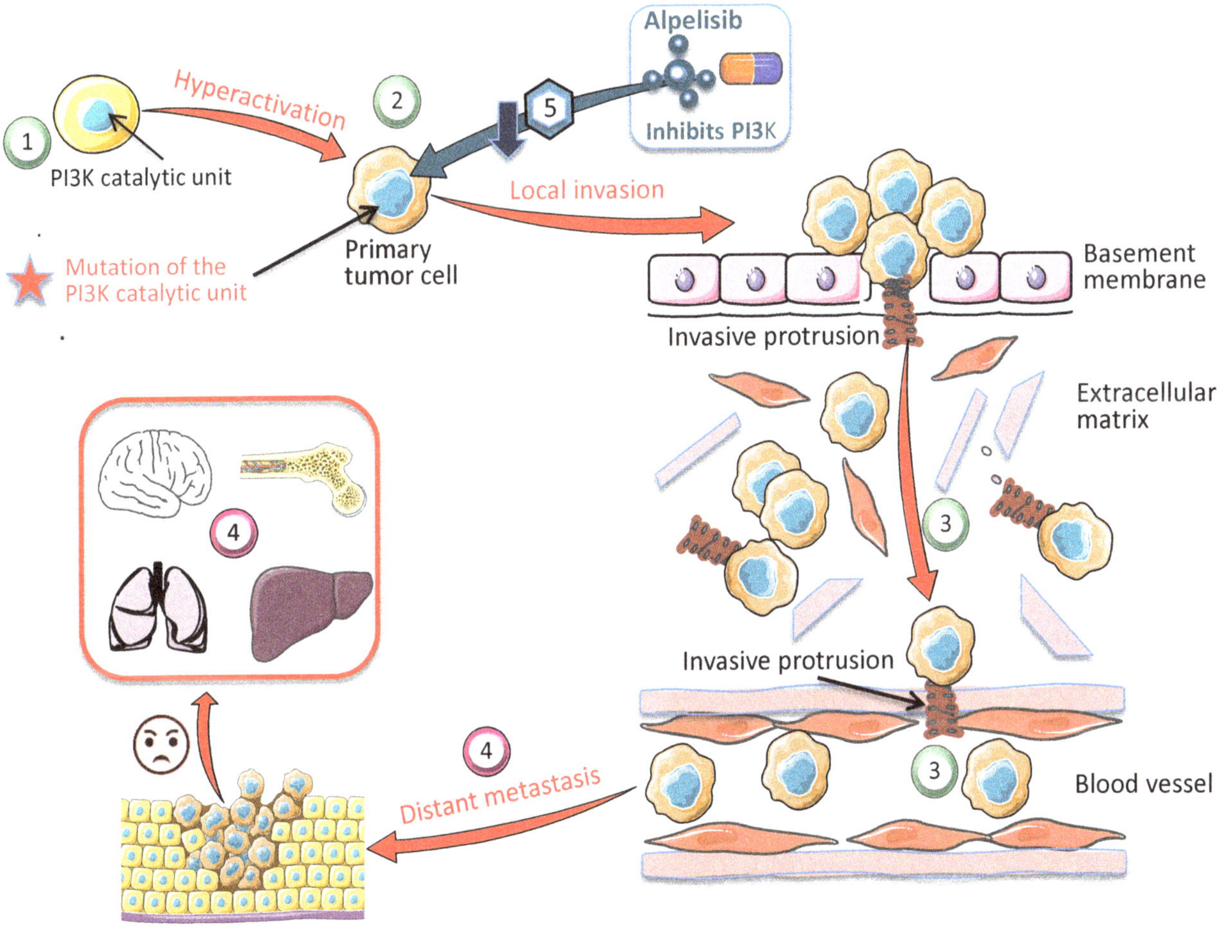

Alpelisib
Inhibits PI3K
1
PI3K catalytic unit
Hyperactivation
2
5
Mutation of the PI3K catalytic unit
Primary tumor cell
Local invasion
Basement membrane
Invasive protrusion
Extracellular matrix
3
4
Invasive protrusion
3
Blood vessel
4
Distant metastasis

Small-molecule drugs: Metastatic breast cancer, Alpelisib

The disease: Amyloid cardiomyopathy

Transthyretin-mediated amyloid cardiomyopathy (ATTR-CM), which is a rare and fatal condition, which is a **hereditary disease** caused by either a mutation or aging associated **destabilization of transthyretin (TTR).** TTR is a plasma protein that transports thyroxine and retinol in serum and cerebrospinal fluid. The destabilization of this transport protein results in **heart failure**, which is caused by the deposition of **fibrils in the heart**.

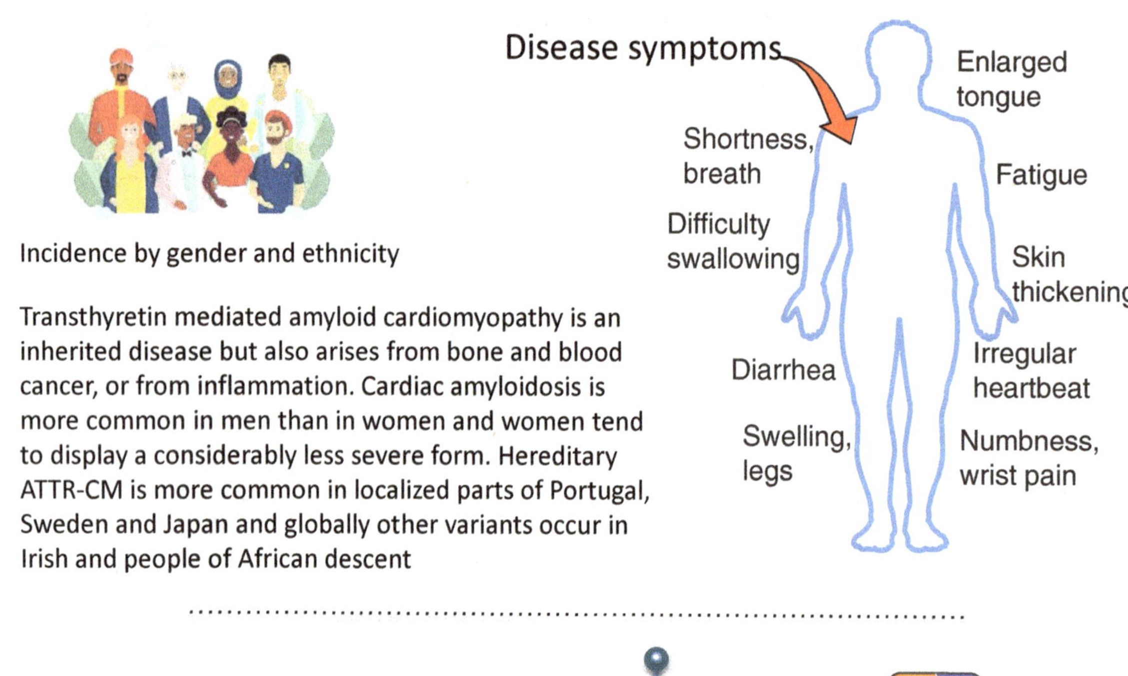

Incidence by gender and ethnicity

Transthyretin mediated amyloid cardiomyopathy is an inherited disease but also arises from bone and blood cancer, or from inflammation. Cardiac amyloidosis is more common in men than in women and women tend to display a considerably less severe form. Hereditary ATTR-CM is more common in localized parts of Portugal, Sweden and Japan and globally other variants occur in Irish and people of African descent

The medicine

Tafamidis; Vyndamax, FDA Approval 2019

Tafamidis **is a transthyretin (TTR) stabilizer** that selectively binds tightly to transthyretin and stabilizes the tetramer, slowing monomer formation with misfolding that generates amyloid.

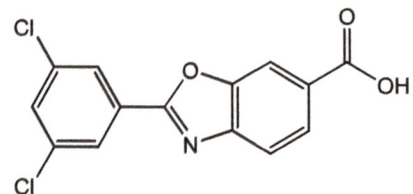

Action of Tafamidis on cell and disease biology

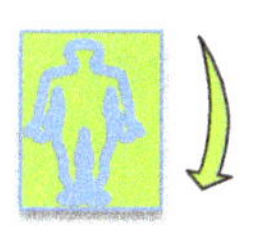
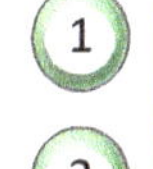

1 **Cardiomyopathy** results from single point **mutations** in the coding region of the TTR gene which **destabilizes** the structure of **monomer.**

2 **Aggregation** of misfolded protein can give rise to amorphous aggregates and results in **amyloid inclusion bodies.**

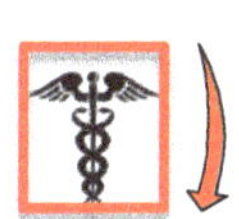
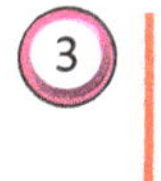

3 Amyloid buildup causes the **heart muscle to stiffen** resulting in an abnormal heartbeat (arrhythmia)**.**

TTR binding to amyloid protein may **prevent plaque accumulation** in the early stages of Alzheimer's disease.

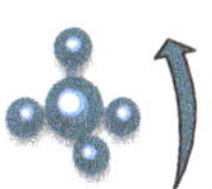

4 **Tafamidis** binds with high affinity and selectivity to **TTR** to **stabilize the tetramer.**

Tafamidis slows monomer formation, misfolding, and formation of fibrils and then amyloid formation.

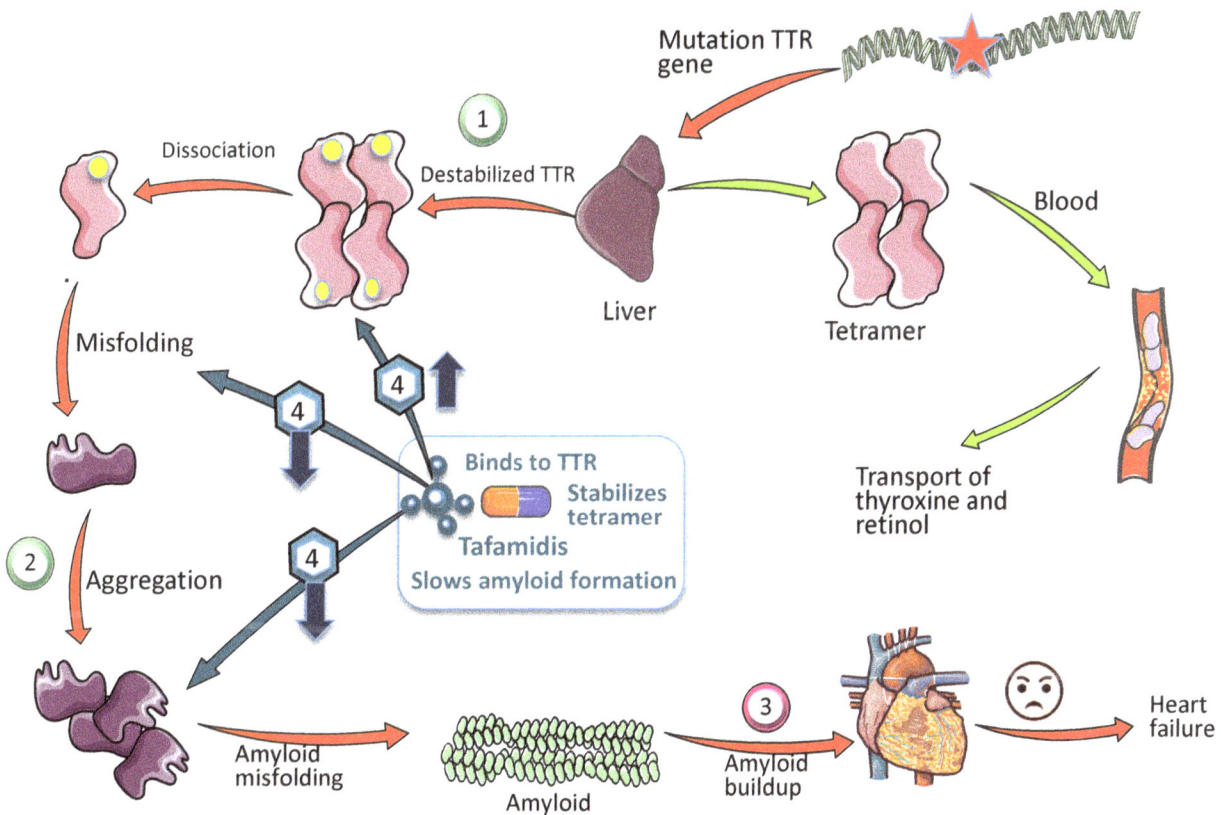

Mutation TTR gene

1

Dissociation

Destabilized TTR

Liver

Tetramer

Blood

Misfolding

4

4

4

Binds to TTR

Stabilizes tetramer

Tafamidis

Slows amyloid formation

Transport of thyroxine and retinol

2

Aggregation

4

Amyloid misfolding

Amyloid

3

Amyloid buildup

Heart failure

The disease: Hutchinson–Gilford (progeroid) syndrome

Hutchinson–Gilford (progeroid) syndrome (HGPS) is associated with premature aging and a severe failure to thrive, where patients live to late teen age. HGPS is one of the most severe disorders among laminopathies, which are a group of rare genetic disorders caused by **mutations in nuclear lamina** and defects of the nuclear envelope.

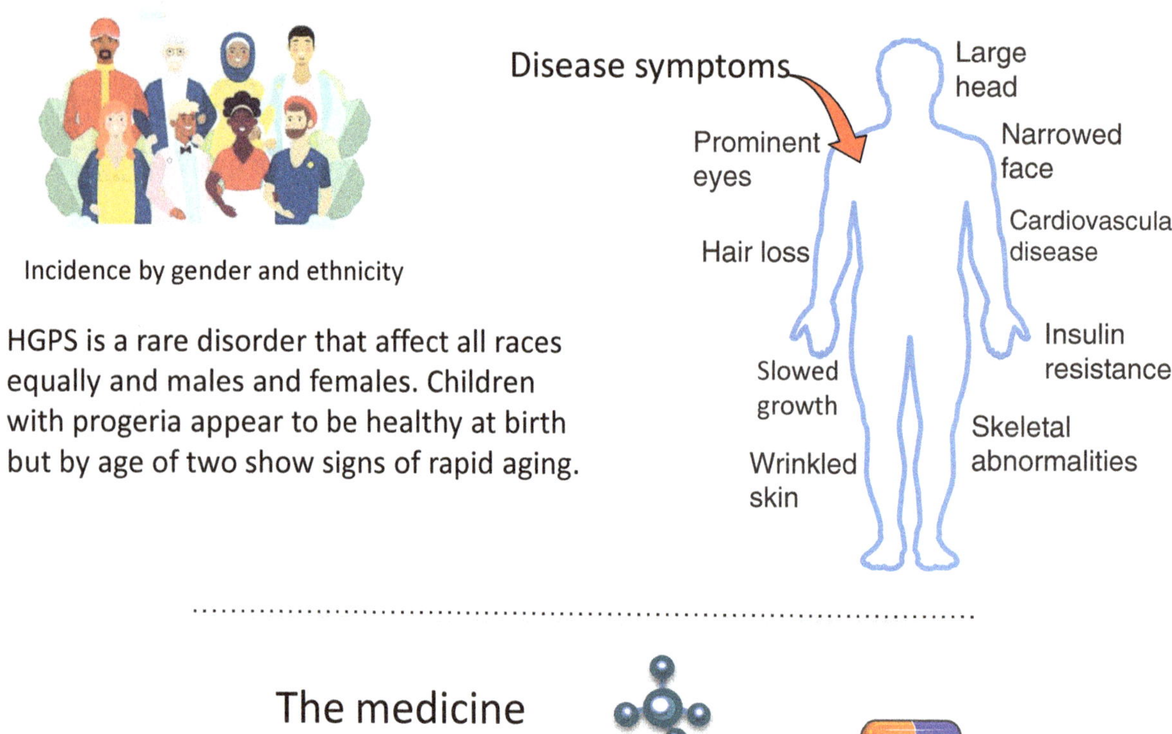

Incidence by gender and ethnicity

HGPS is a rare disorder that affect all races equally and males and females. Children with progeria appear to be healthy at birth but by age of two show signs of rapid aging.

The medicine

Lonafarnib; Zokinvy, FDA Approval 2020

Lonafarnib is a farnesyltransferase inhibitor, which reduces the farnesylation of progerin and inhibits localization to the nuclear membrane. Improves symptoms in Hutchinson–Gilford progeria syndrome and other processing-deficient progeroid laminopathies.

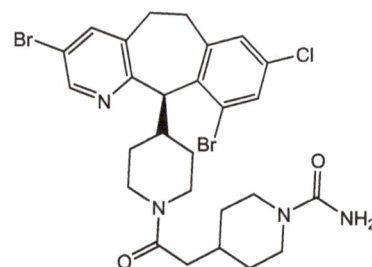

Br, N, Cl, Br, N, O, N, O, NH_2

Action of Lonafarnib on cell and disease biology

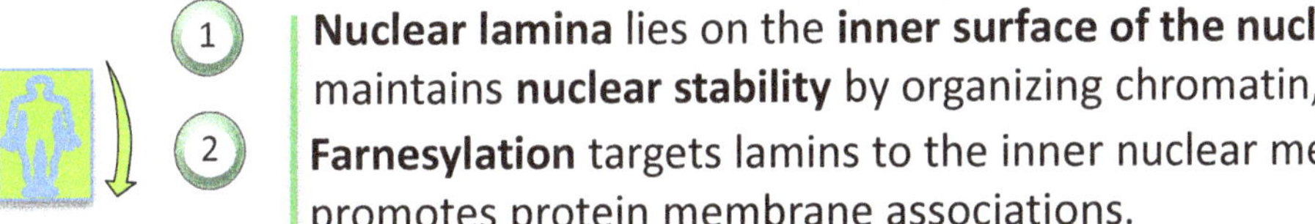

1 **Nuclear lamina** lies on the **inner surface of the nuclear membrane** and maintains **nuclear stability** by organizing chromatin, nuclear complexes.

2 **Farnesylation** targets lamins to the inner nuclear membrane and promotes protein membrane associations.

3 HGPS is a result of a **mutation** in the **lamina gene**, a change in gene splicing, which results in synthesis of progerin (lacking 50 amino acids).

4 In HGPS, **progerin accumulates** in the inner nuclear membrane with profound **alterations in shape of nucleus**, resulting in **DNA repair defects**, chromosome instability, disrupted gene expression, and DNA replication.

5 **Lonafarnib** is an **inhibitor of protein farnesyltransferase** and of progerin farnesylation and subsequent insertion into the nuclear membrane.

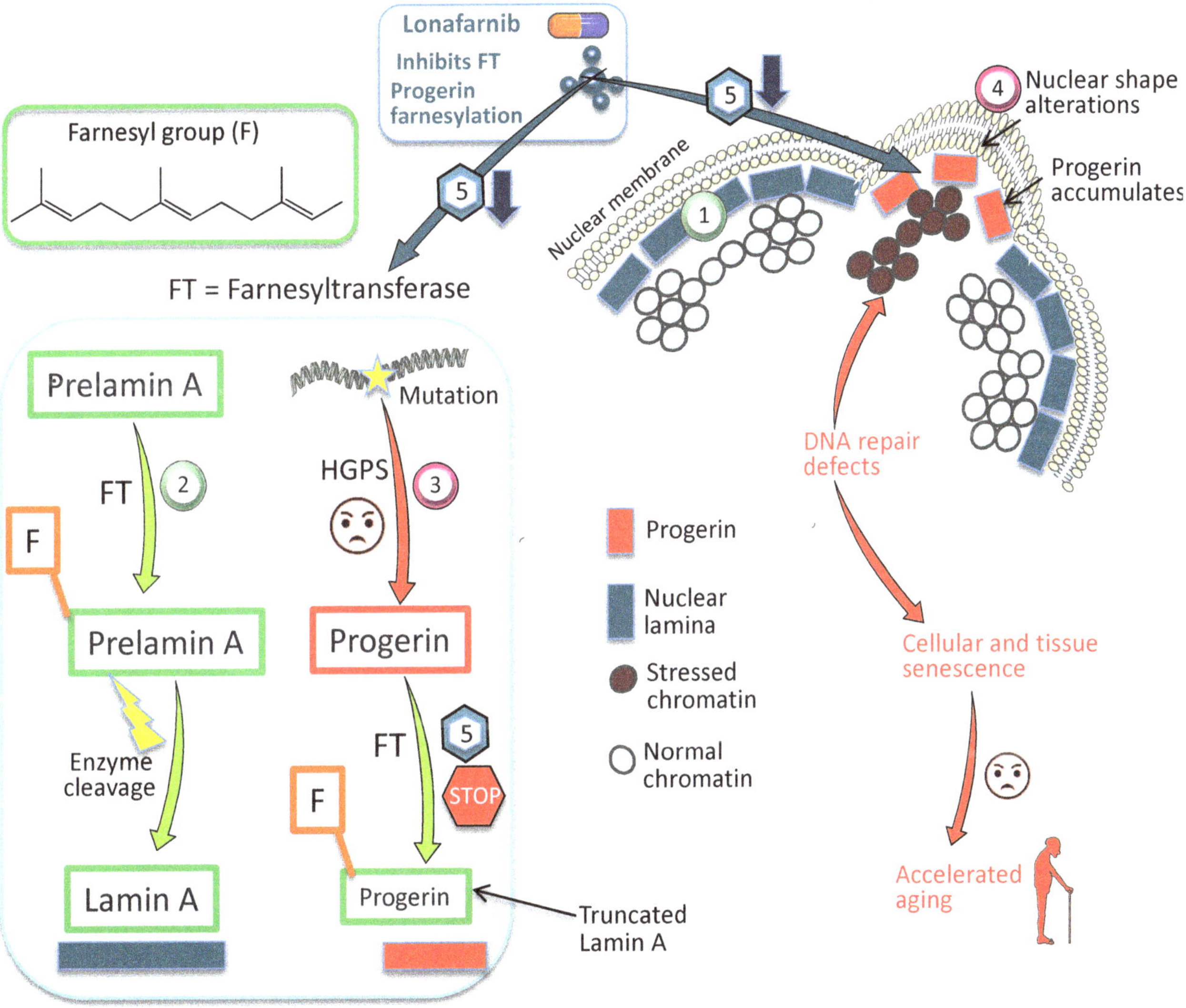

Lonafarnib
Inhibits FT
Progerin farnesylation
Farnesyl group (F)
FT = Farnesyltransferase
Nuclear membrane
Nuclear shape alterations
Progerin accumulates
Prelamin A
FT
F
Prelamin A
Enzyme cleavage
Lamin A
Mutation
HGPS
Progerin
FT
STOP
F
Progerin
Truncated Lamin A
Progerin
Nuclear lamina
Stressed chromatin
Normal chromatin
DNA repair defects
Cellular and tissue senescence
Accelerated aging

Blastic plasmacytoid dendritic cell neoplasm (BPDCN) is a rare and aggressive blood cancer of the bone marrow caused by the overexpression of dendritic cells that can affect other organs such as the lymph nodes, spleen, central nervous system with skin lesions, as well as a low red and white blood cell and platelet counts.

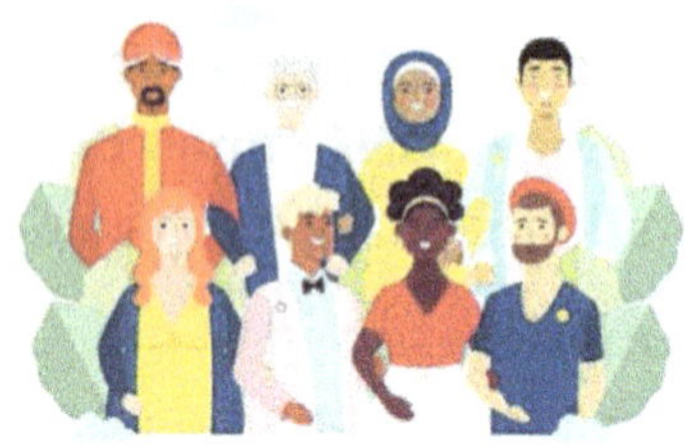

Incidence by gender and ethnicity

BPDCN occurs in all ethnic groups and is a disease of the middle-aged (median age in the mid-60s), with approximately 75% of cases occurring in men. Pediatric cases have been described in children as young as 8 months of age.

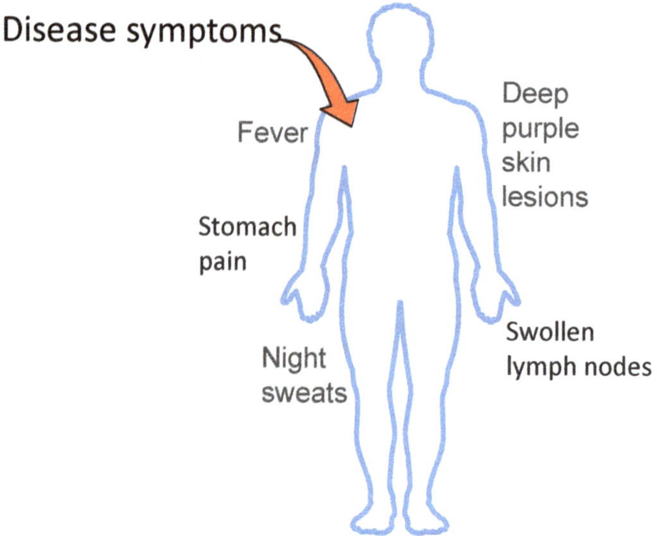

The medicine

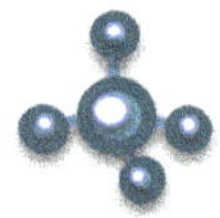

Tagraxofusp; Elzonris, FDA Approval 2018

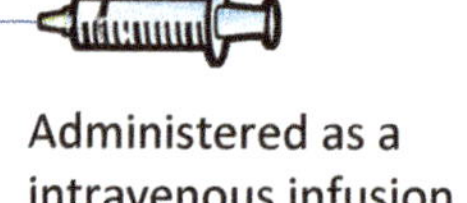

Administered as a intravenous infusion

Tagraxofusp is a cytotoxin targeting the interleukin-3 receptor for the treatment of BPDCN. Tagraxofusp is a recombinant fusion protein produced in *Escherichia coli*, which consists of interleukin-3 (IL-3) fused via a His-Met linker to diphtheria toxin catalytic and translocation domains.

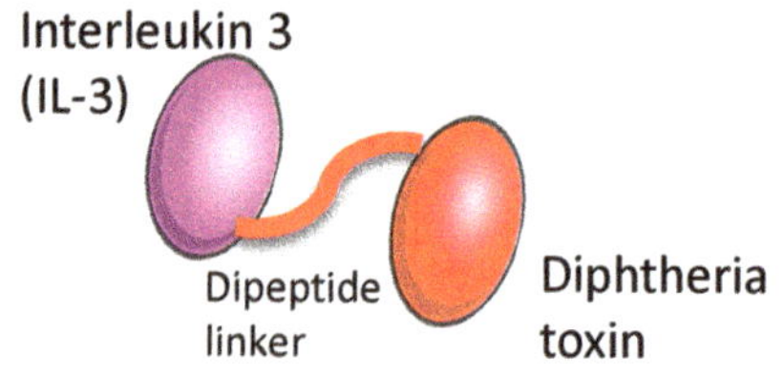

Action of Tagraxofusp on cell and disease biology

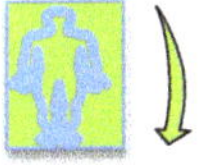  **Plasmacytoid dendritic cells (pDCs) are the** T-cell counterpart to plasma B cells but secrete lymphokines such as interleukin (IL)-3, a **signaling protein.**

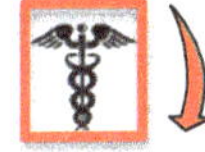 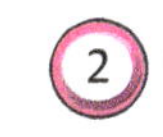 **Blastic plasmacytoid dendritic cell neoplasm** features nonactivated pDCs with elevated blood levels of proinflammatory white blood cells (eosinophils).

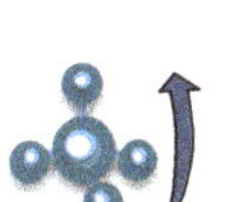  **Tagraxofusp is a targeted cytotoxin** for **plasmacytoid dendritic cells** with high levels of IL-3 receptor.

 **Tagraxofusp binds to IL-3 receptor,** internalized, **diphtheria toxin (DT) shuttled to the cytosol**.

 **Catalytic domain** of diphtheria toxin **inactivates elongation factor** (EF-2),inhibits protein synthesis with **cell death** (apoptosis).

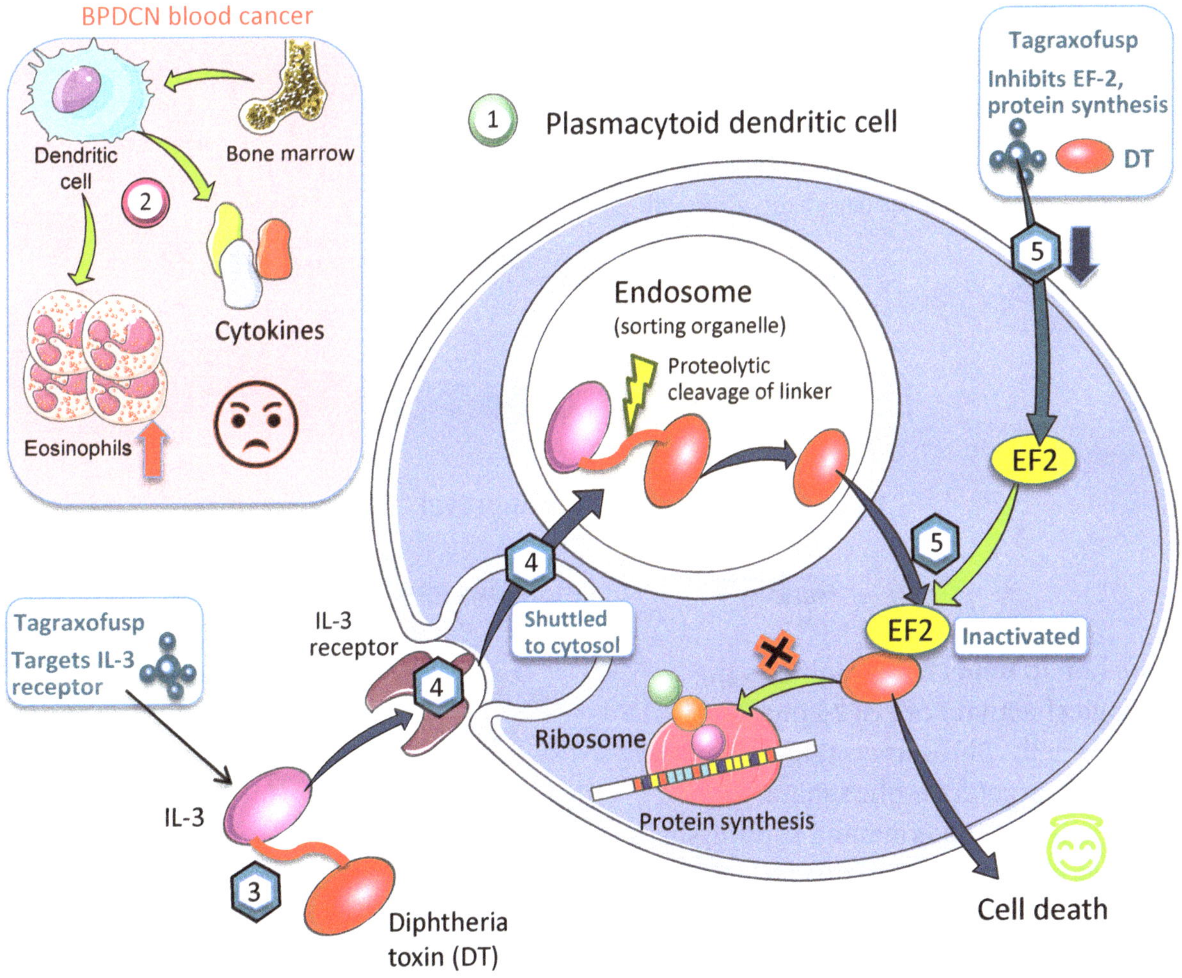

BPDCN blood cancer
Dendritic cell
Bone marrow
2
Cytokines
Eosinophils
1 Plasmacytoid dendritic cell
Tagraxofusp
Inhibits EF-2, protein synthesis
DT
5
Endosome
(sorting organelle)
Proteolytic cleavage of linker
EF2
5
4
Shuttled to cytosol
EF2 Inactivated
Tagraxofusp
Targets IL-3 receptor
IL-3 receptor
4
Ribosome
Protein synthesis
IL-3
3
Diphtheria toxin (DT)
Cell death

Small-molecule drugs: Blastic plasmacytoid dendritic cell neoplasm, Tagraxofusp

The disease: X-linked hypophosphatemia

X-linked hypophosphatemia (XLH) is a **rare, inherited form of rickets**, which leads to low levels of blood phosphorous and impaired bone growth. Rickets is the softening and weakening of bones in children, due to a prolonged vitamin D deficiency. Rare inherited problems can cause rickets due to mutations in the **XLH gene**, which **increase the activity of fibroblast growth factor 23** (FGF23) and reduces blood phosphate levels.

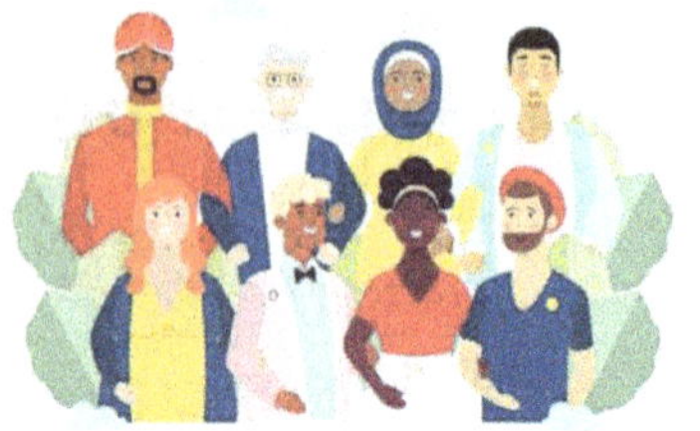

Incidence by gender and ethnicity

XLH is an X-linked dominant disorder with a case rate estimate of ~1 case per 20,000 live births. Males are affected by X-linked recessive disorders more frequently than females and females are more mildly affected. No genetic influences on XLH expression in patients have been observed.

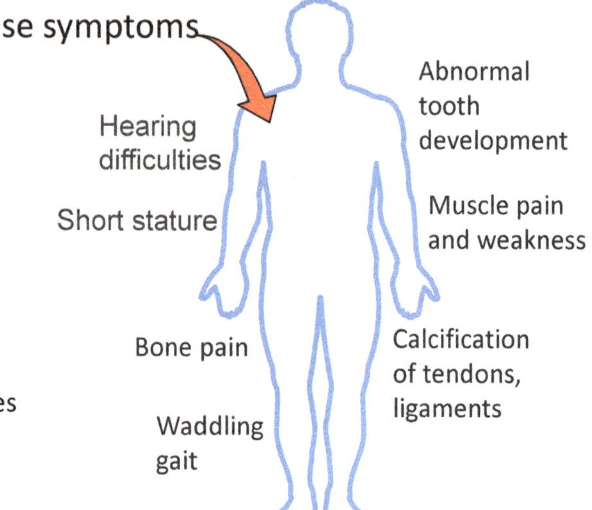

The medicine

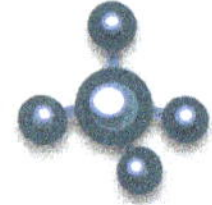

Burosumab; Crysvita, FDA Approval 2018

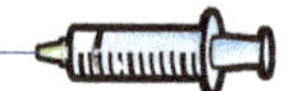

Subcutaneous injection

Burosumab **binds to and inhibits the biological activity of FGF23** produced in bone cells. Burosumab targets the kidney to accelerate phosphate excretion into the urine and suppresses vitamin D synthesis, thereby reducing blood phosphate levels.

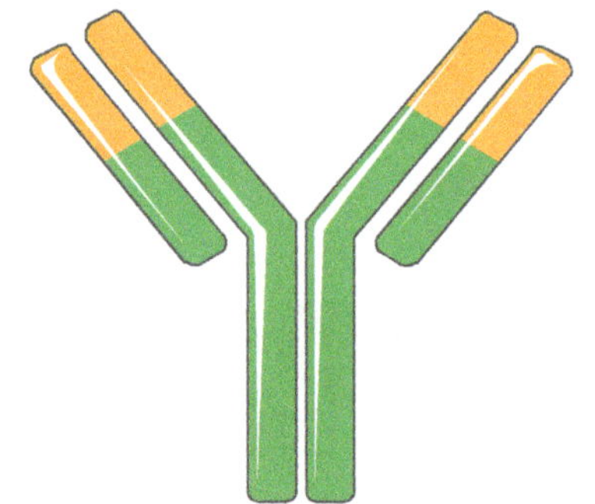

Antibody drugs: X-linked hypophosphatemia, Burosumab

Action of Burosumab on cell and disease biology

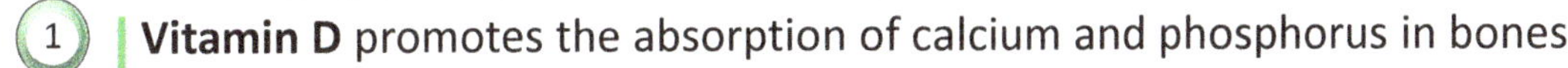

1. **Vitamin D** promotes the absorption of calcium and phosphorus in bones.
2. **Phosphate levels** are controlled by the kidneys, excess phosphate is excreted in urine and reabsorbed when more is needed.
3. **FGF23** suppresses the phosphate transporters in the kidney and **reduces phosphate reabsorption** in the proximal tubule.
4. **FGF23** is **produced** by osteoblasts/osteocytes, osteoblasts synthesize bone matrix, osteocytes (from osteoblasts) resorb bone.

5. **Burosumab inhibits FGF23** activity and increases the renal production of 1-α hydroxylase.

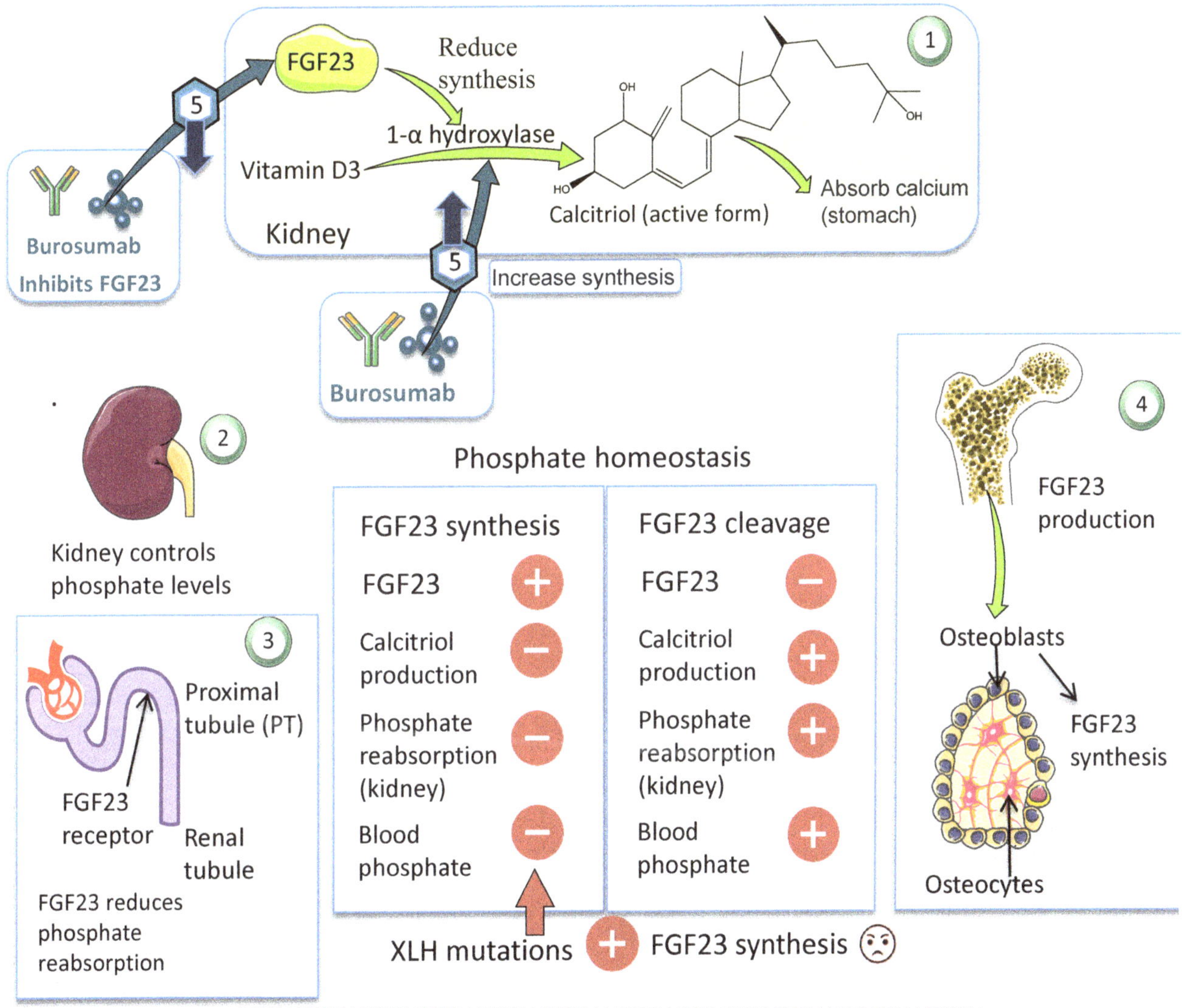

FGF23
5
Reduce synthesis
1-α hydroxylase
Vitamin D3
OH
OH
HO
Calcitriol (active form)
Absorb calcium (stomach)
1
Kidney
Burosumab
Inhibits FGF23
5
Increase synthesis
Burosumab

2
Kidney controls phosphate levels

3
Proximal tubule (PT)
FGF23 receptor
Renal tubule
FGF23 reduces phosphate reabsorption

Phosphate homeostasis

FGF23 synthesis		FGF23 cleavage	
FGF23	+	FGF23	−
Calcitriol production	−	Calcitriol production	+
Phosphate reabsorption (kidney)	−	Phosphate reabsorption (kidney)	+
Blood phosphate	−	Blood phosphate	+

XLH mutations + FGF23 synthesis ☹

4
FGF23 production
Osteoblasts
FGF23 synthesis
Osteocytes

The disease: Primary hemophagocytic lymphohistiocytosis

Primary hemophagocytic lymphohistiocytosis (HLH) is a rare inherited immune system disorder in which the body makes too many **activated immune cells** (macrophages and lymphocytes) that triggers aberrant activation of the immune system with a dramatic **increase** in levels of **gamma interferon** (IFNγ). HLH has been associated with autoimmune conditions such as systemic lupus erythematosus (SLE).

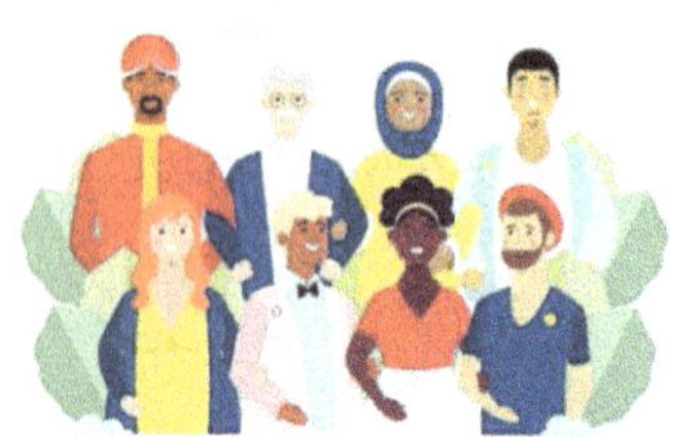

Incidence by gender and ethnicity

HLH primarily affects young infants and children. For the autosomal-recessive (two copies of the abnormal gene), there are an equal number of diagnosed males and females. In addition, there are X-linked forms of FHL, which affects only males. Secondary HLH is typically diagnosed in older patients with no family history of this disease. It may be associated with vaccinations, viral infections, and autoimmune disorders.

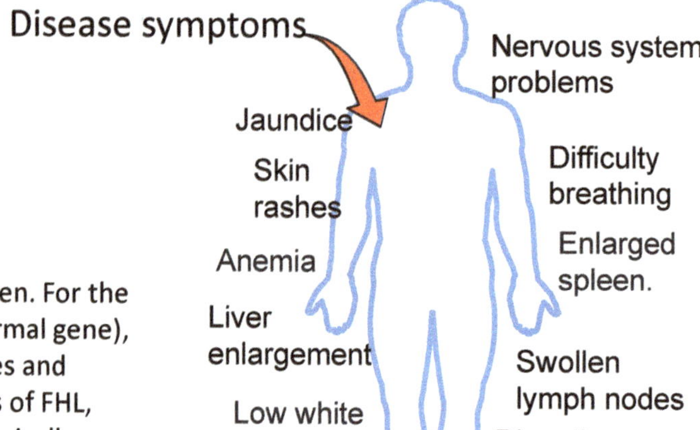

The medicine

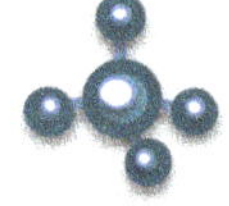

Emapalumab; Gamifant, FDA Approval 2018

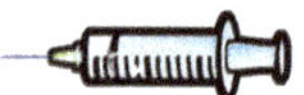

Administered as an intravenous infusion

Emapalumab is a fully human monoclonal antibody, which is a potent inhibitor of IFNγ. It can **bind and neutralize IFN-γ**, preventing it from inducing pathological effects. Emapalumab is indicated for the treatment of patients with refractory, recurrent, or progressive disease or intolerance to conventional HLH therapy.

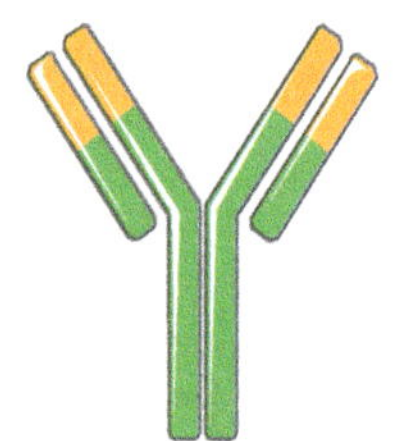

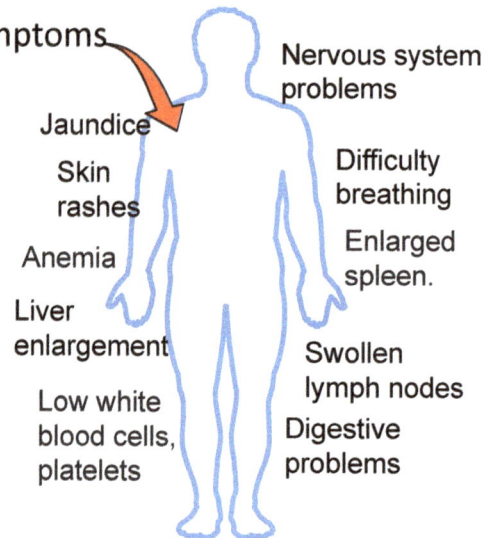

Action of Emapalumab on cell and disease biology

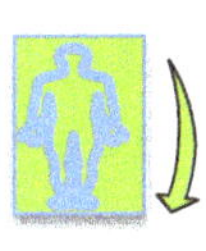

Interferon-gamma (IFNγ) activates macrophages, natural killer cells, and neutrophils to regulate immune functions.

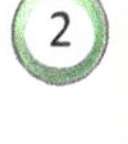

IFNγ is **produced by natural killer T** (NKT) cell and enhances NK cell cytotoxicity and proliferation during infections.

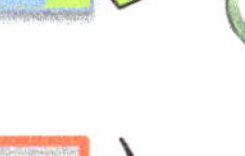
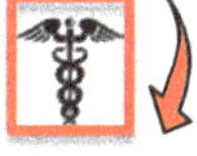
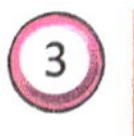

Systemic lupus Erythematosus **(SLE) is an autoimmune disease** with immune system attacks on multiple organs.

Emapalumab is a monoclonal **antibody** that binds to hypersecreted **interferon gamma** (IFNγ) and neutralizes it.

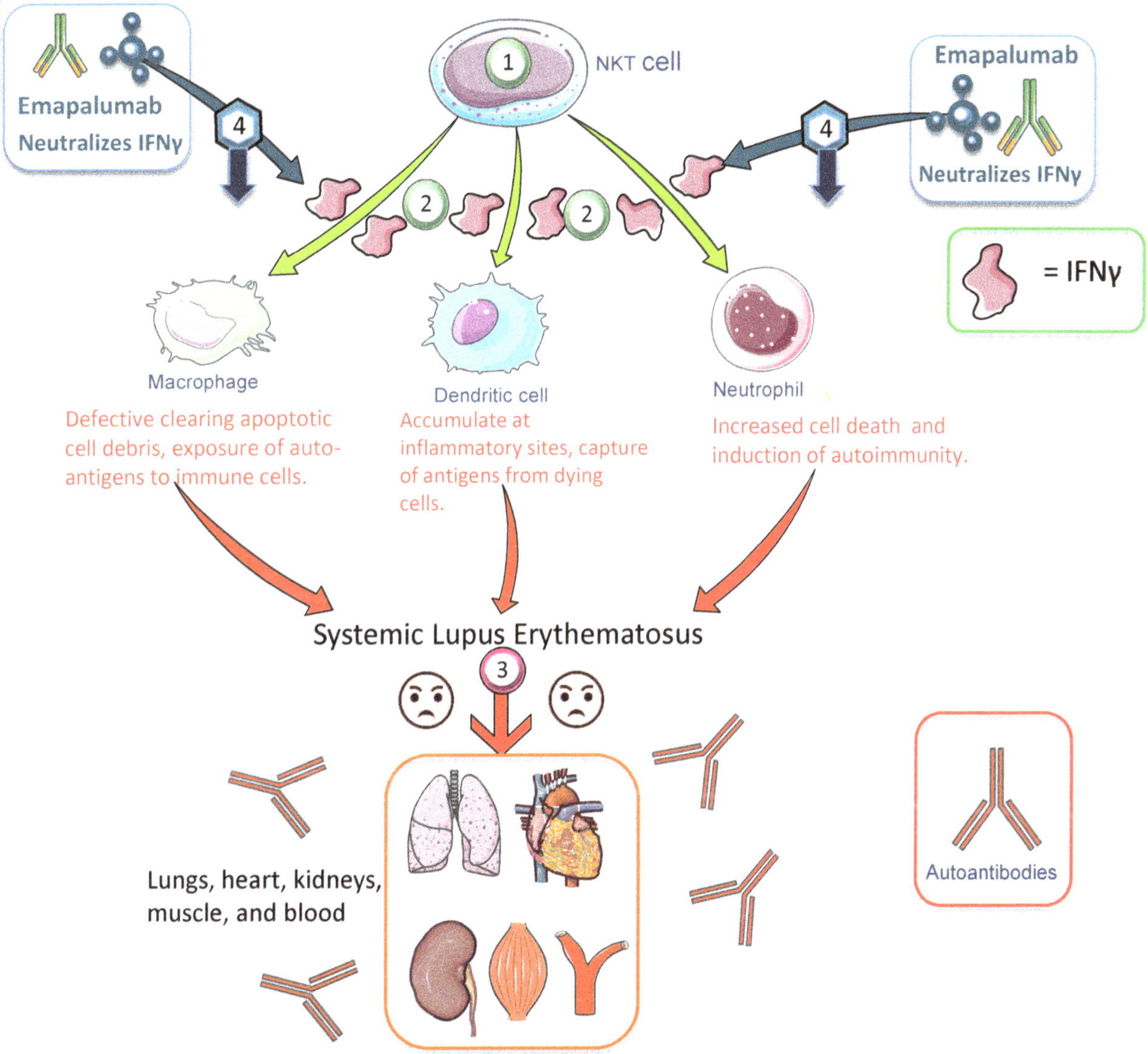

Emapalumab
Neutralizes IFNγ

NKT cell

Emapalumab
Neutralizes IFNγ

= IFNγ

Macrophage
Defective clearing apoptotic cell debris, exposure of auto-antigens to immune cells.

Dendritic cell
Accumulate at inflammatory sites, capture of antigens from dying cells.

Neutrophil
Increased cell death and induction of autoimmunity.

Systemic Lupus Erythematosus

Lungs, heart, kidneys, muscle, and blood

Autoantibodies

The disease: Hereditary angioedema

Types I and II **hereditary angioedema** (HAE) is a rare and serious genetic disease, which results in recurrent episodes of angioedema **(severe swelling)** in the stomach, limbs, face, and throat. The disease is caused by a mutation in the SERPING1 gene that makes the C1 inhibitor protein.

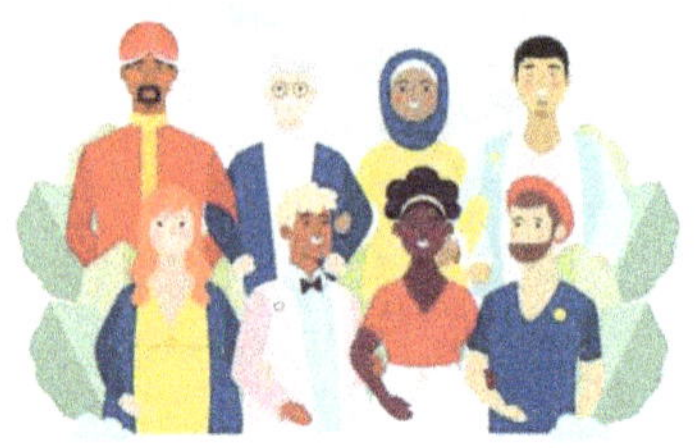

Incidence by gender and ethnicity

HAE with C1-inhibitor deficiency is inherited as a dominant trait (50% of offspring) for both genders. Clinical severity is similar in both sexes but worsens during pregnancy and estrogen administration. Acquired angioedema is rarer, affecting older persons with other conditions such as malignancies. There is no ethnic bias.

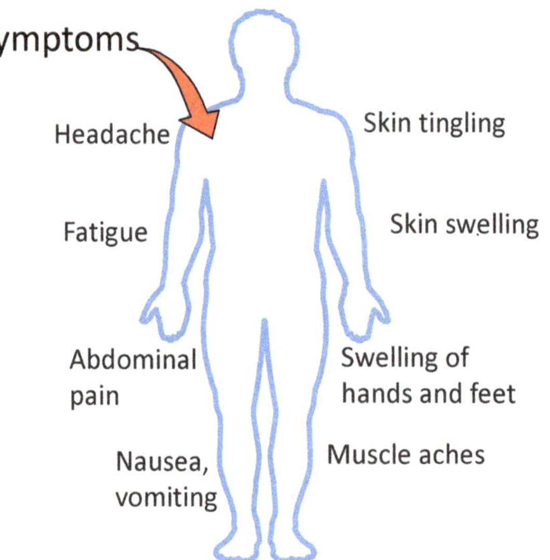

The medicine

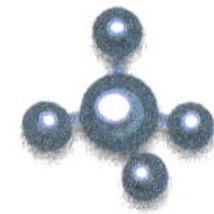

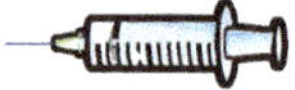

Subcutaneous injection directly under the skin

Lanadelumab;Takhzyro, FDA Approval 2018

Lanadelumab is a fully humanized IgG1 monoclonal antibody, which binds to and **inhibits plasma kallikrein** to control excess bradykinin generation in patients with HAE and prevent swelling attacks.

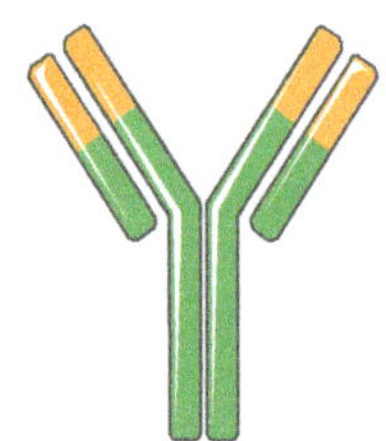

Action of Lanadelumab on cell and disease biology

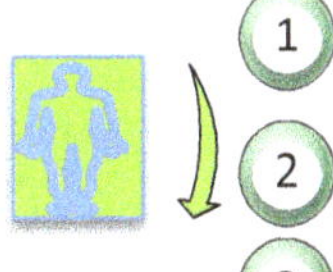

1 High-molecular-weight kininogen (HMWK) initiates blood coagulation and bradykinin formation. **Kallikrein cleaves HMWK** to generate bradykinin

2 **C1 inhibitor** (complement system blocker) inhibits and clears plasma kallikrein.

3 **Bradykinin triggers blood vessels to open** and become more permeable.

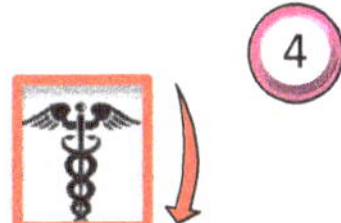

4 **Hereditary angioedema,** HAE (mutated C1 inhibitor) results in **increased** plasma **kallikrein** activity and bradykinin levels, which promotes inflammation by **increasing the permeability of blood vessel** walls, allowing fluids to leak into body tissues with resulting swelling and pain.

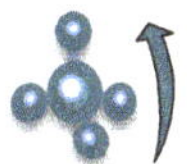

5 **Lanadelumab inhibits** the proteolytic activity of **kallikrein** to block bradykinin formation which is increased in HAE.

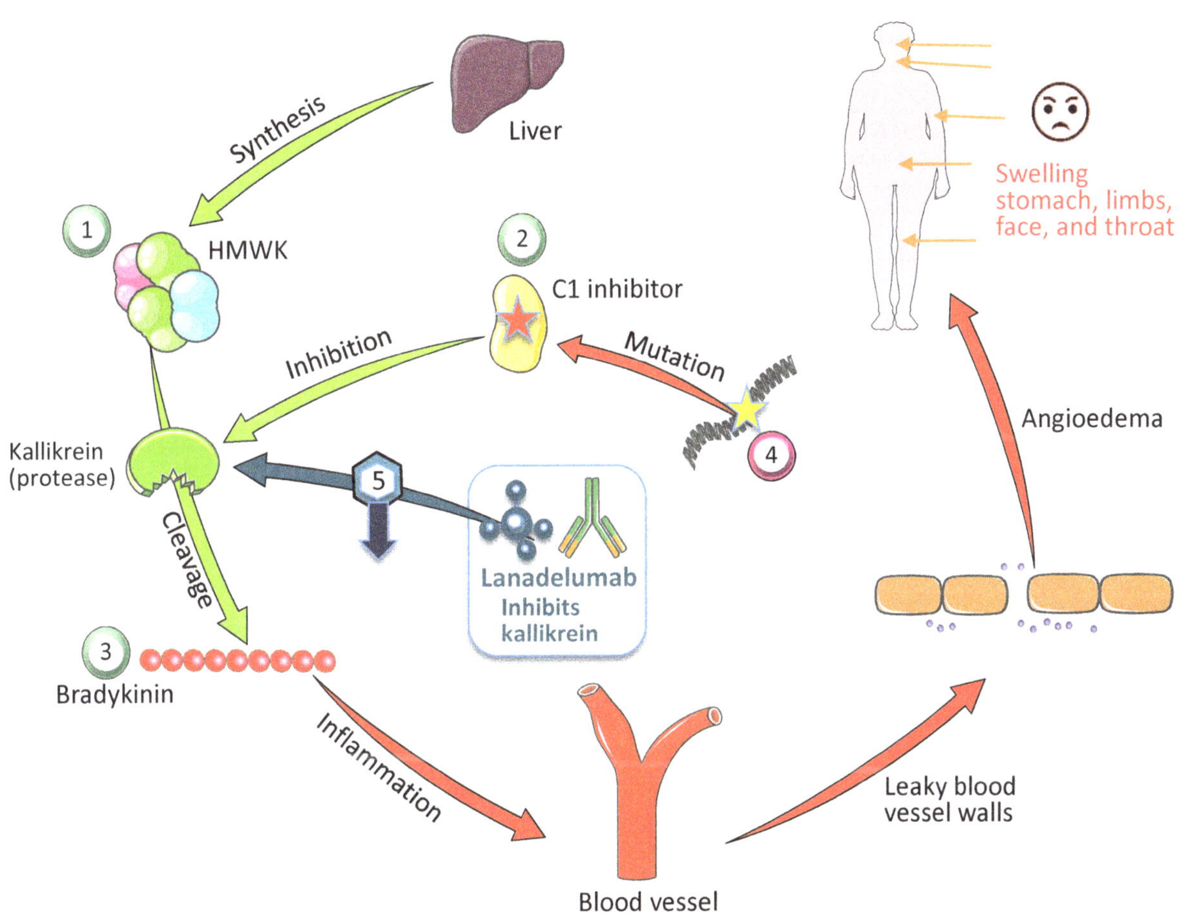

The disease: Osteoporosis

Osteoporosis is a disease in which the density and **quality of bone is reduced** with increased risk of fracture. The leading cause of osteoporosis is a **lack of estrogen** in women, particularly in menopause, accompanied by lower estrogen levels.

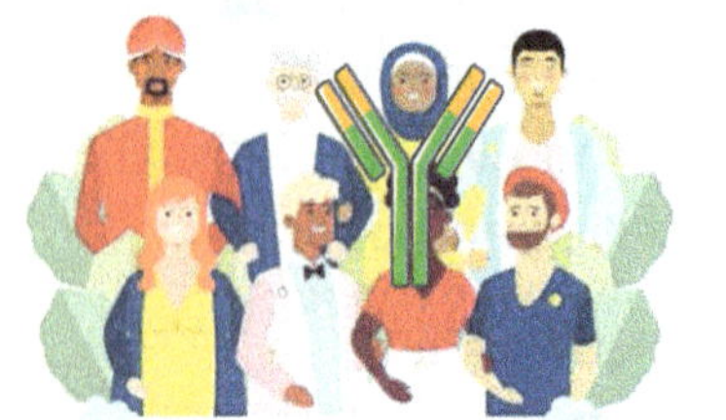

Incidence by gender and ethnicity

Due to hormone changes at menopause, the prevalence of osteoporosis and the risk of fracture are higher in women than in men. Even though women fracture more often, men tend to have worse outcomes after fractures. In older women, bone loss may be due to estrogen deficiency. Non-Hispanic white and Asian women over 50 years old have a greater level of osteoporosis (20%), compared with non-Hispanic black women (5%–10%) and Hispanic women (15%) of the same age.

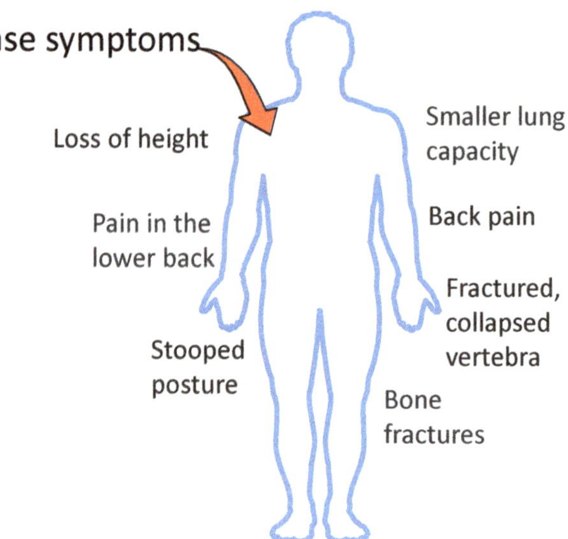

The medicine

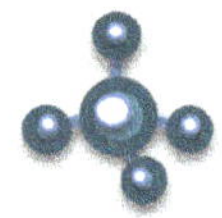

Romosozumab , Evenity, FDA Approval 2020

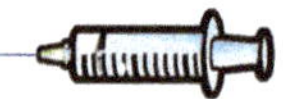

Subcutaneous injection directly under the skin

Romosozumab **blocks** the effects of the protein **sclerostin** with **increasing new bone formation** and strength and decreasing bone readsorption.

Romosozumab is used **to treat osteoporosis** in postmenopausal women with low bone density with a high risk of bone fracture who cannot use other osteoporosis medications.

Action of Romosozumab on cell and disease biology

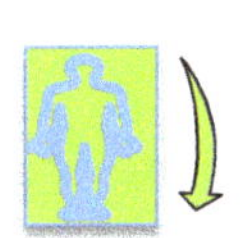
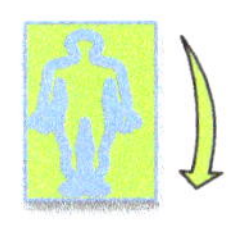

1 **Calcium** is the major component of the bone providing **skeletal strength** and structure by utilizing calcium from the bloodstream.

2 **Sclerostin** is primarily expressed in osteocytes in bone and binds to receptors on the cell surface of osteoblasts to **inhibit bone** formation.

Osteoblasts synthesize **bone matrix** and coordinate the mineralization of the skeleton especially during new bone formation and remodeling.

Osteoclasts degrade bone to initiate normal bone remodeling.

Osteocytes (from osteoblasts), 90% of bone cells, are **mechanosensors** that detect skeletal loading/unloading to initiate the bone remodeling cycle.

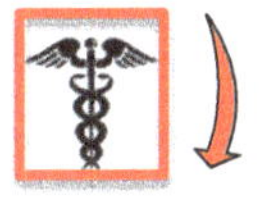

3 **Osteoporosis** is linked to **estrogen deficiency** and menopause accelerates bone loss with up to 20% loss.

4 Estrogen deficiency decreases intestinal calcium resorption, increases kidney calcium excretion, and has direct effects on bone estrogen receptors

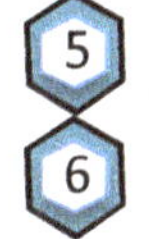
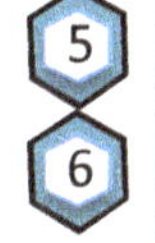

5 **Romosozumab** binds and **inhibits sclerostin** to decrease bone resorption.

6 Romosozumab **increases bone formation** by activating lining cells to bone-forming osteoblasts, increasing osteoblast activity and bone structure.

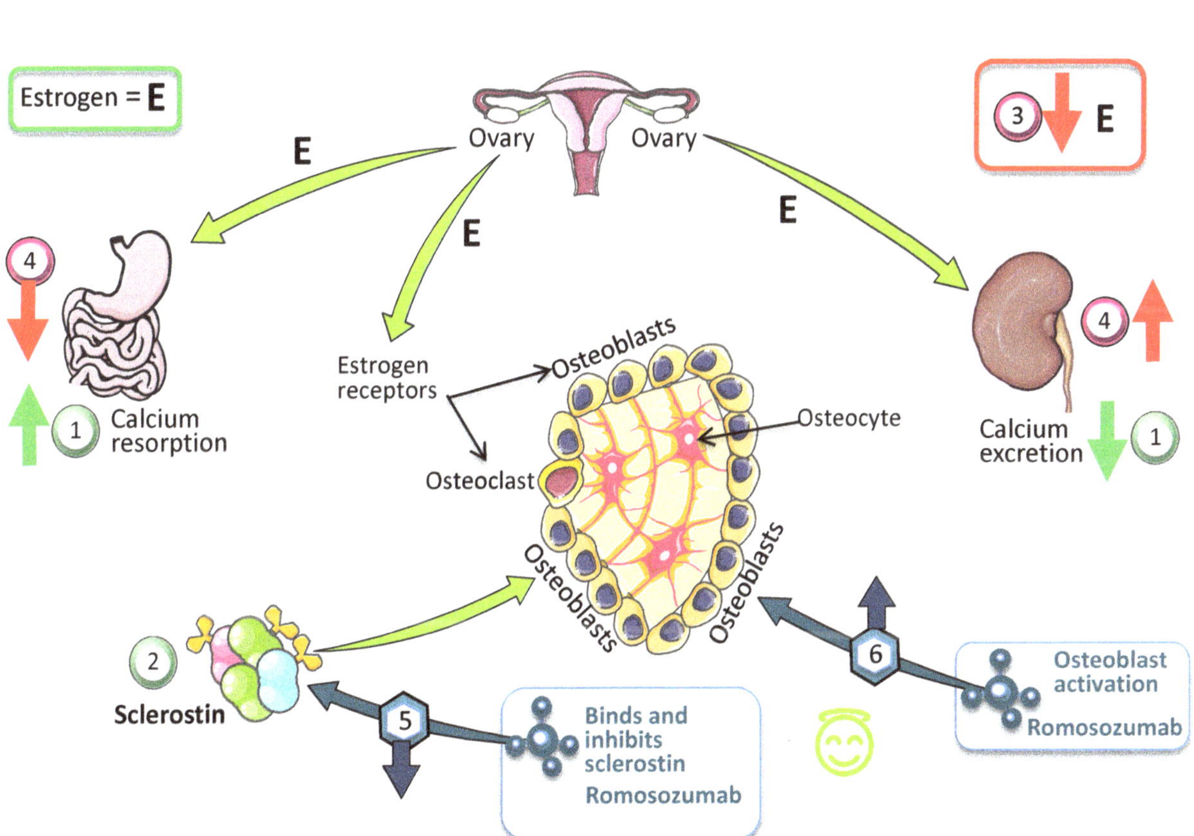

The disease: Neuroblastoma

Neuroblastoma is a **childhood cancer** that is diagnosed at a median age of about 17 months (7%–10% of childhood cancers). The patient group for this treatment is for **relapsed or refractory high-risk neuroblastoma** in the bone or bone marrow who have demonstrated a partial response, or stable disease to prior therapy.

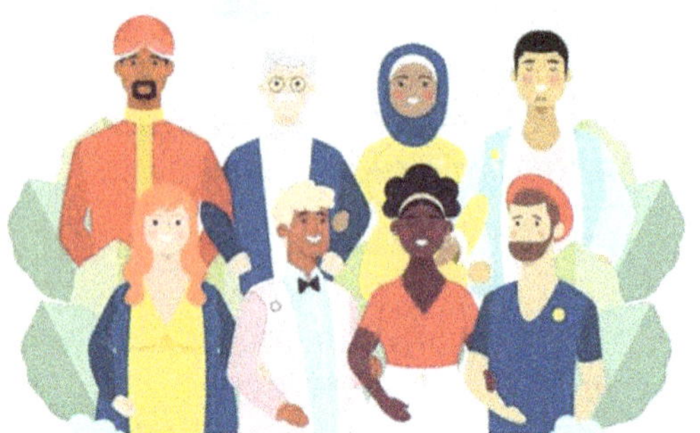

Incidence by gender and ethnicity

Neuroblastoma incidence higher in males than females (1.3 to 1). No environmental factors have been found, rarely more than 1 member of a family is affected and is most common in infants and very young children. Black, Asian, and Native American children have a more high-risk neuroblastoma compared to white children.

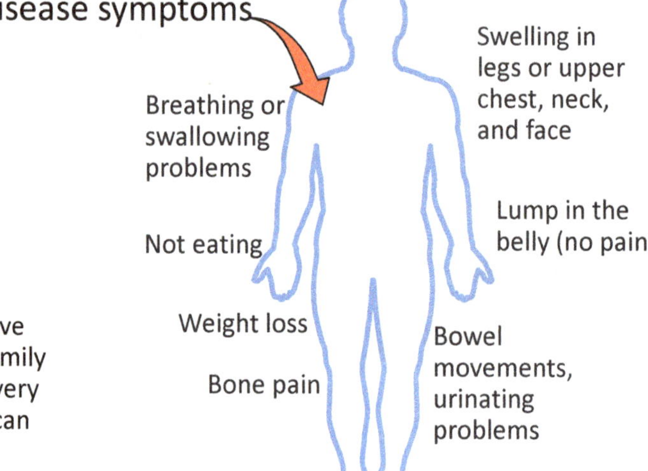

The medicine

Naxitamab; Danyleza, FDA Approval 2020

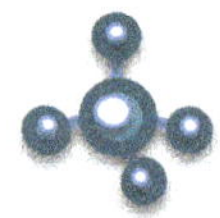

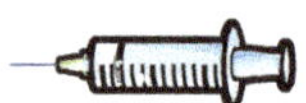

Administered as an intravenous infusion

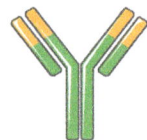

Naxitamab is a humanized, monoclonal antibody that **targets the ganglioside GD2**, which is highly expressed in neural epithelial cells and is used to prevent relapse in patients with neuroblastoma. It an immunotherapeutic approach for the eradication of residual neuroblastoma cells left at the completion of cytotoxic therapy.

Neuroblastoma develops from **immature nerve cells** but most commonly arises in areas where groups of nerve cells exist, the adrenal glands, other areas of the abdomen, the chest, neck, and near the spine.

Antibody drugs: Neuroblastoma, Naxitamab

Action of Naxitamab on cell and disease biology

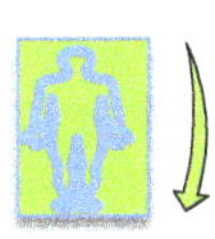

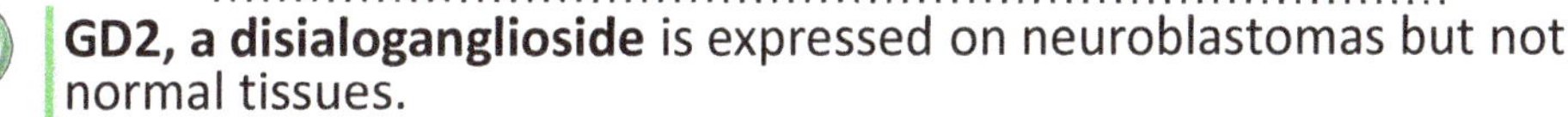

1 **GD2, a disialoganglioside** is expressed on neuroblastomas but not normal tissues.

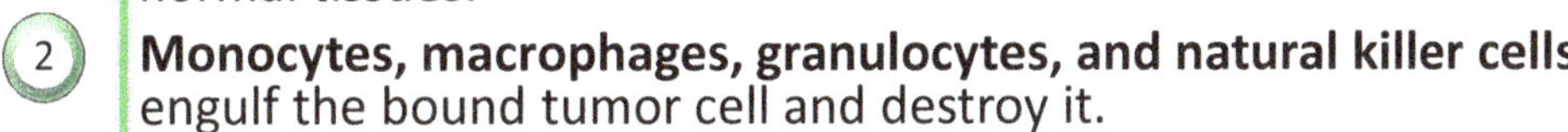

2 **Monocytes, macrophages, granulocytes, and natural killer cells** engulf the bound tumor cell and destroy it.

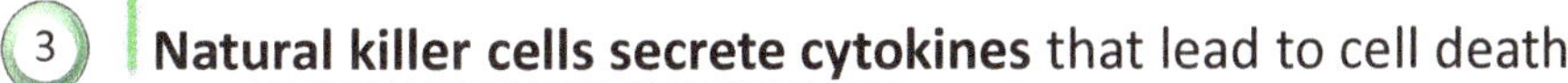

3 **Natural killer cells secrete cytokines** that lead to cell death.

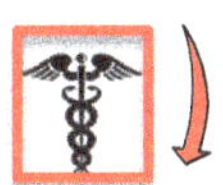

4 Neuroblastoma involves **abnormal neuroblasts** (stem cells) with a genetic **mutation** so the cells grow and divide uncontrollably, forming tumors.

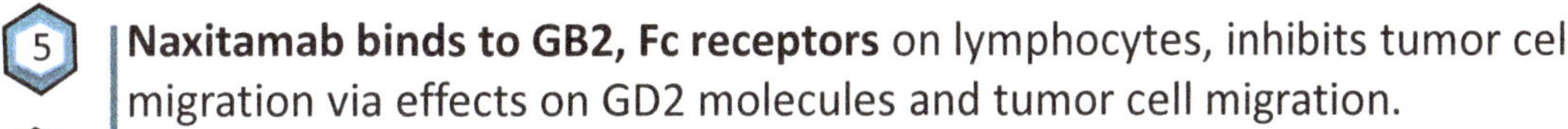

5 **Naxitamab binds to GB2, Fc receptors** on lymphocytes, inhibits tumor cell migration via effects on GD2 molecules and tumor cell migration.

6 Naxitamab **stimulates antibody-dependent cell-mediated cytotoxicity** (ADCC) against GD2-expressing tumor cells.

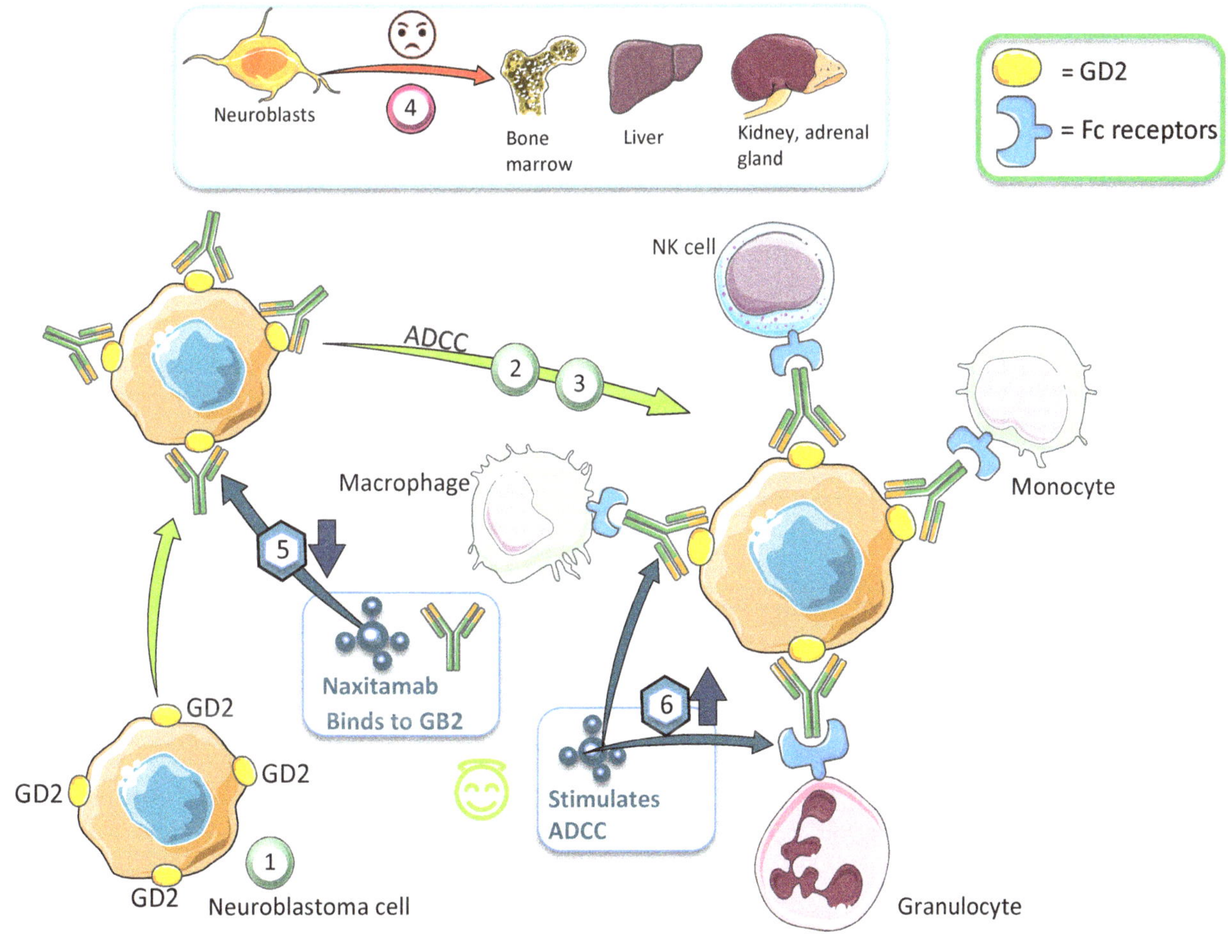

Neuroblasts
4
Bone marrow
Liver
Kidney, adrenal gland
= GD2
= Fc receptors
NK cell
ADCC
2
3
Monocyte
Macrophage
5
Naxitamab
Binds to GB2
6
Stimulates ADCC
GD2
GD2
GD2
GD2
1
Neuroblastoma cell
Granulocyte

Antibody drugs: Neuroblastoma, Naxitamab

The disease: Hemophilia A

Hemophilia A is caused by an inherited mutation in the coagulation factor VIII gene. Factor VIII binds to both factors IX and X, activating factor X and initiating blood clotting. A deficiency in the factor VIII protein can cause excessive internal and external bleeding.

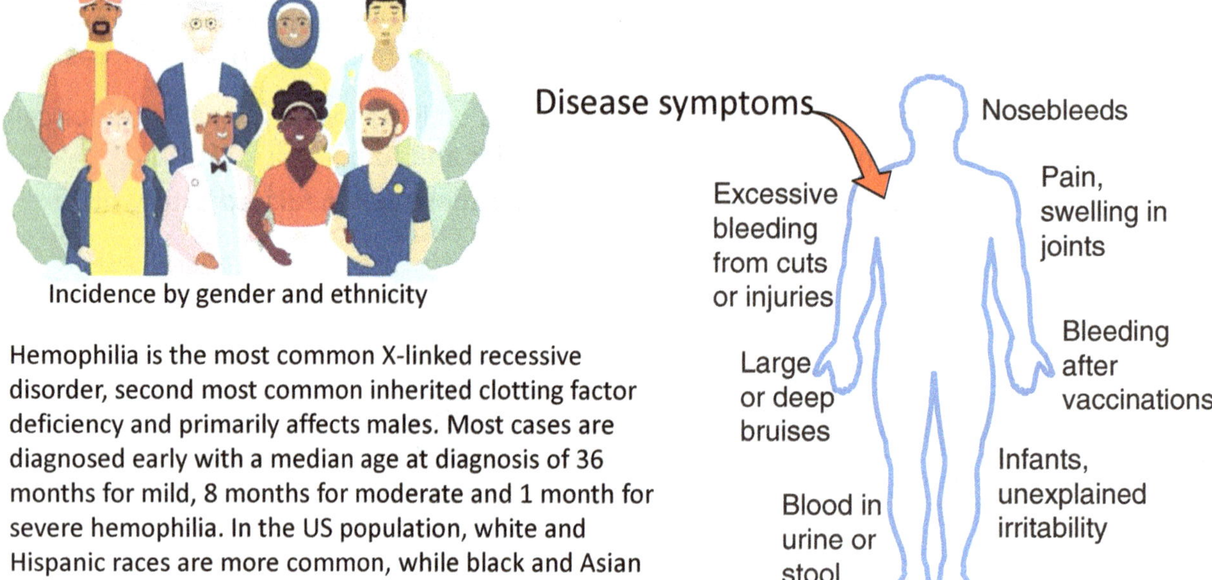

Incidence by gender and ethnicity

Hemophilia is the most common X-linked recessive disorder, second most common inherited clotting factor deficiency and primarily affects males. Most cases are diagnosed early with a median age at diagnosis of 36 months for mild, 8 months for moderate and 1 month for severe hemophilia. In the US population, white and Hispanic races are more common, while black and Asian cases are less common.

The medicine

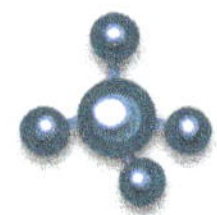

Emicizumab; Hemlibra, FDA Approval 2018

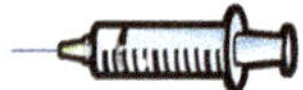

Subcutaneous injection directly under the skin

Emicizumab is a **bispecific antibody** designed to bind to two specific **targets factor IX and factor X,** thus mimicking the normal action of factor VIII. The binding helps **restore normal blood clotting** with less blood loss and reducing damage to internal tissues, muscles, and joints.

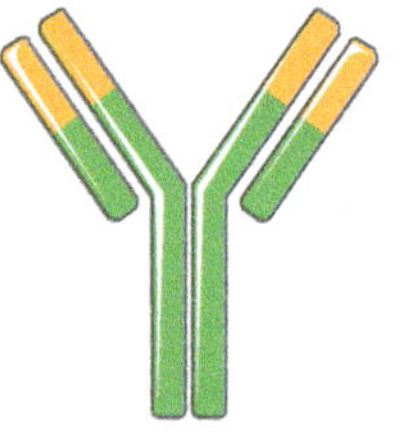

Monoclonal antibodies, Hemophilia A, Emicizumab

Action of Emicizumab on cell and disease biology

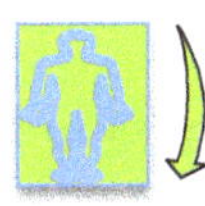

The **coagulation cascade** is a complex process using up to 10 different blood clotting factors in plasma to solidify blood at the site of an injury.

Factor VIII is a **cofactor for factor IXa** to form a complex that converts factor X to the activated form Xa.

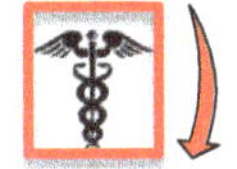

In **hemophilia,** the blood does not clot properly and leads to bleeding following injuries or surgery as well as spontaneous bleeding.

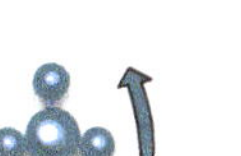

Bispecific monoclonal **antibodies** can recognize and bind simultaneously two different antigenic targets.

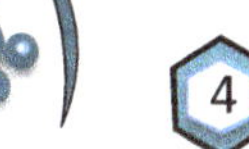

Emicizumab binds factors IXa and with activation of factor X, which mimics the actions of factor VIII.

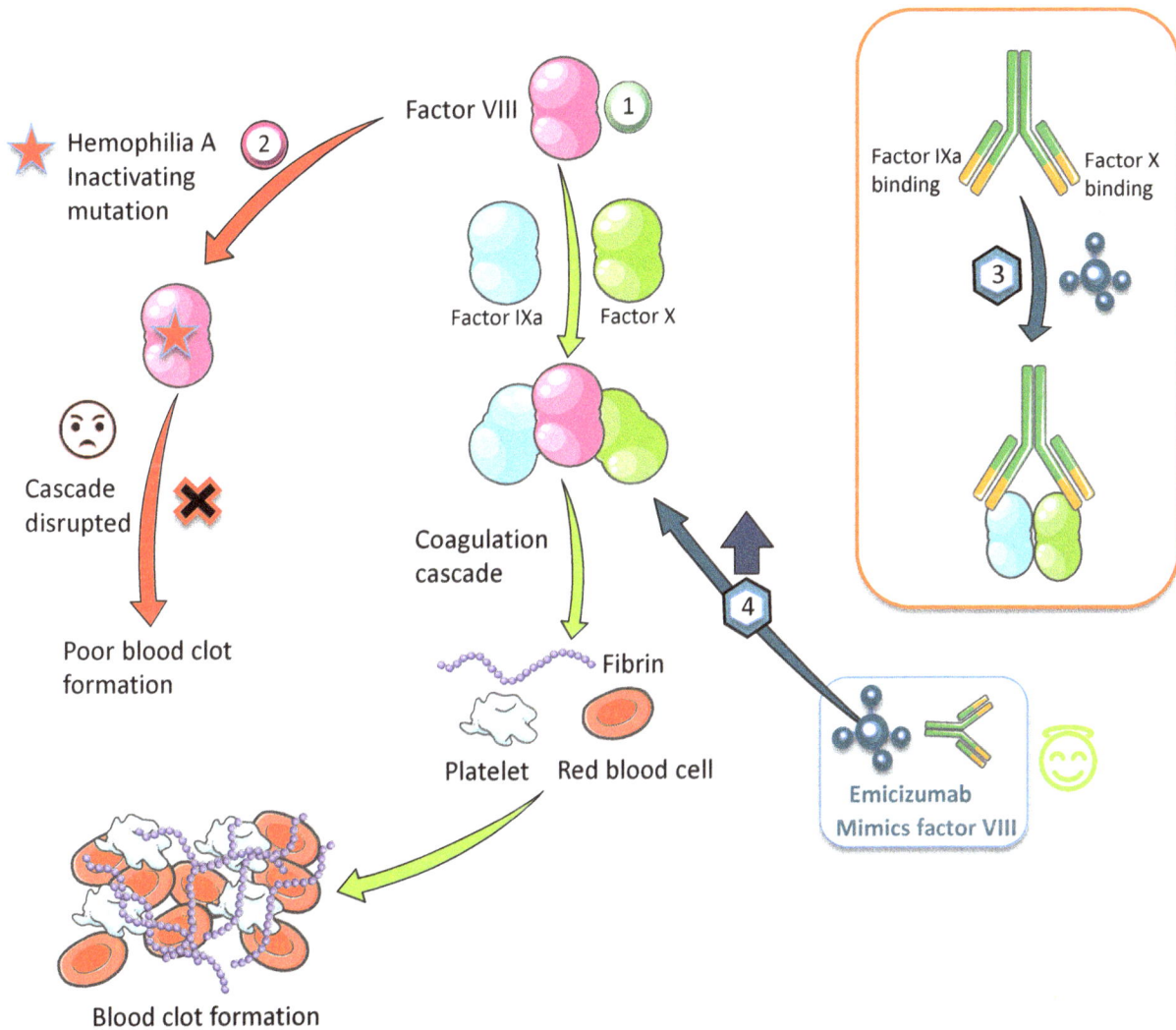

Factor VIII 1

Hemophilia A 2
Inactivating
mutation

Cascade
disrupted

Poor blood clot
formation

Factor IXa

Factor X

Coagulation
cascade

Fibrin

Platelet

Red blood cell

Blood clot formation

Factor IXa
binding

Factor X
binding

3

4

Emicizumab
Mimics factor VIII

Monoclonal antibodies, Hemophilia A, Emicizumab

The disease: Type 2 Diabetes

Type 2 diabetes, most common form of diabetes, occurring when the **pancreas makes insufficient insulin** or there is resistance to insulin action to keep blood sugar at normal levels. **Glucagon-like peptide (GLP-1)** is often found at **low levels** in type 2 diabetes patients.

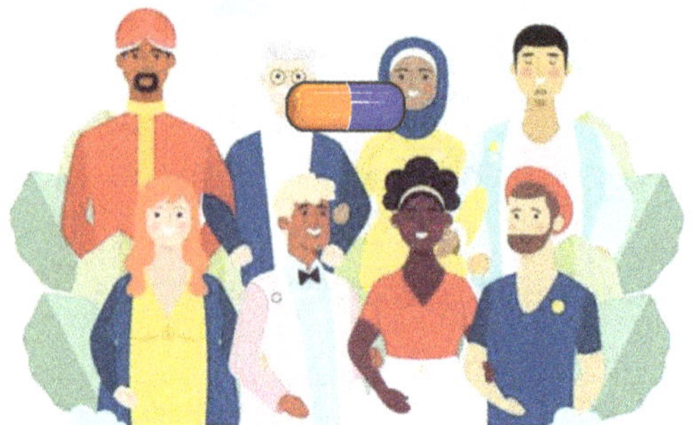

Incidence by gender and ethnicity

Men are twice as likely to develop diabetes than women (greatest at ages of 35–54) but women are more likely to have complications. Prevalence by ethnic group in the US is African Americans 13.2%, Hispanic 12.8%, Asians 9.0%, and non-Hispanic whites 7.6%. Asian Indians have the highest diabetes prevalence rate (14.2%), whereas Asian Americans from Korea and Japan have the lowest rates (4.0% and 4.9%).

Disease symptoms

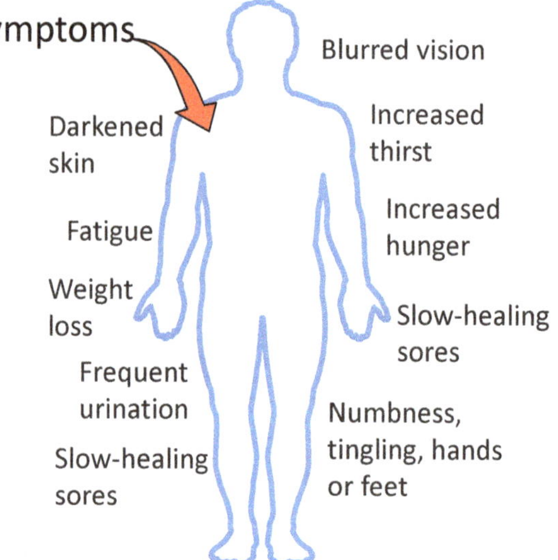

The medicine

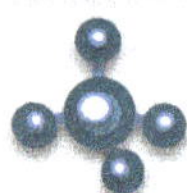

Semaglutide; Rybelsus, FDA Approval 2019

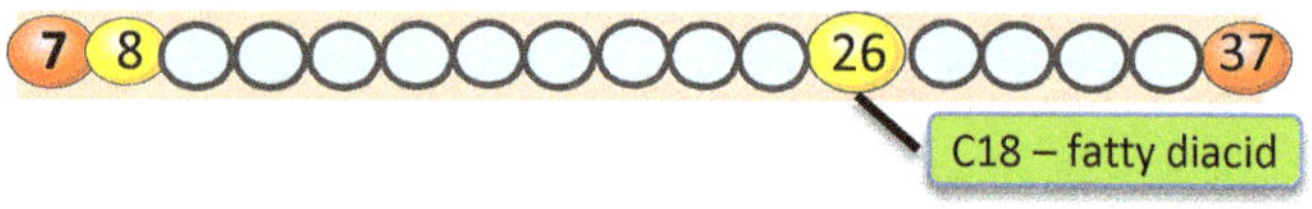

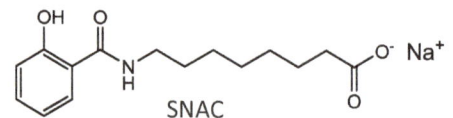

SNAC

Semaglutide is an oral glucagon-like peptide-1 (GLP-1) analog (Type 2 diabetes) that activates the GLP-1 receptor. Rybelsus reduces liver synthesis of glucose and assists pancreatic production of insulin.

The duration of action of semaglutide is increased by albumin binding (by a C18 fatty diacid and hydrophilic spacer at lysine 26) with reduced renal clearance. A substitution at position 8 **prevents protease degradation** increasing duration of action.

Oral peptide drugs are normally poorly absorbed (low permeability, GI tract), low pH instability and protease digestion**.**

Salcaprozate sodium (SNAC) is an absorption enhancer added used to enable once-daily oral administration. **SNAC promotes absorption of peptide drugs** across epithelial cells and protects against digestion.

Peptide drugs: Type 2 diabetes, Semaglutide

Action of Semaglutide on cell and disease biology

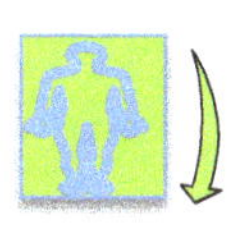

Glucagon-like peptide-1 receptor **(GLP-1)** is produced in the **intestine** (ileum and colon) and stimulates insulin release from the pancreas.

GLP-1 slows gastric emptying by **inhibiting glucagon release**, stimulating pancreatic β-cell proliferation and improving satiety.

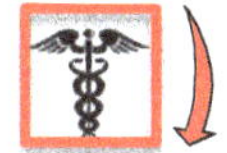

GLP-1 is **decreased** in **type 2 diabetes** and found in insufficient levels.

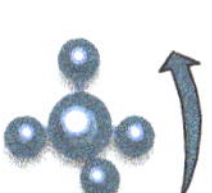

Semaglutide acts as a long-acting and selective **GLP-1 receptor activator** with binding and activation of the receptor.

Semaglutide slows digestion, reduces liver sugar synthesis, the pancreas produce more insulin when needed and **lowers glucagon secretion.**

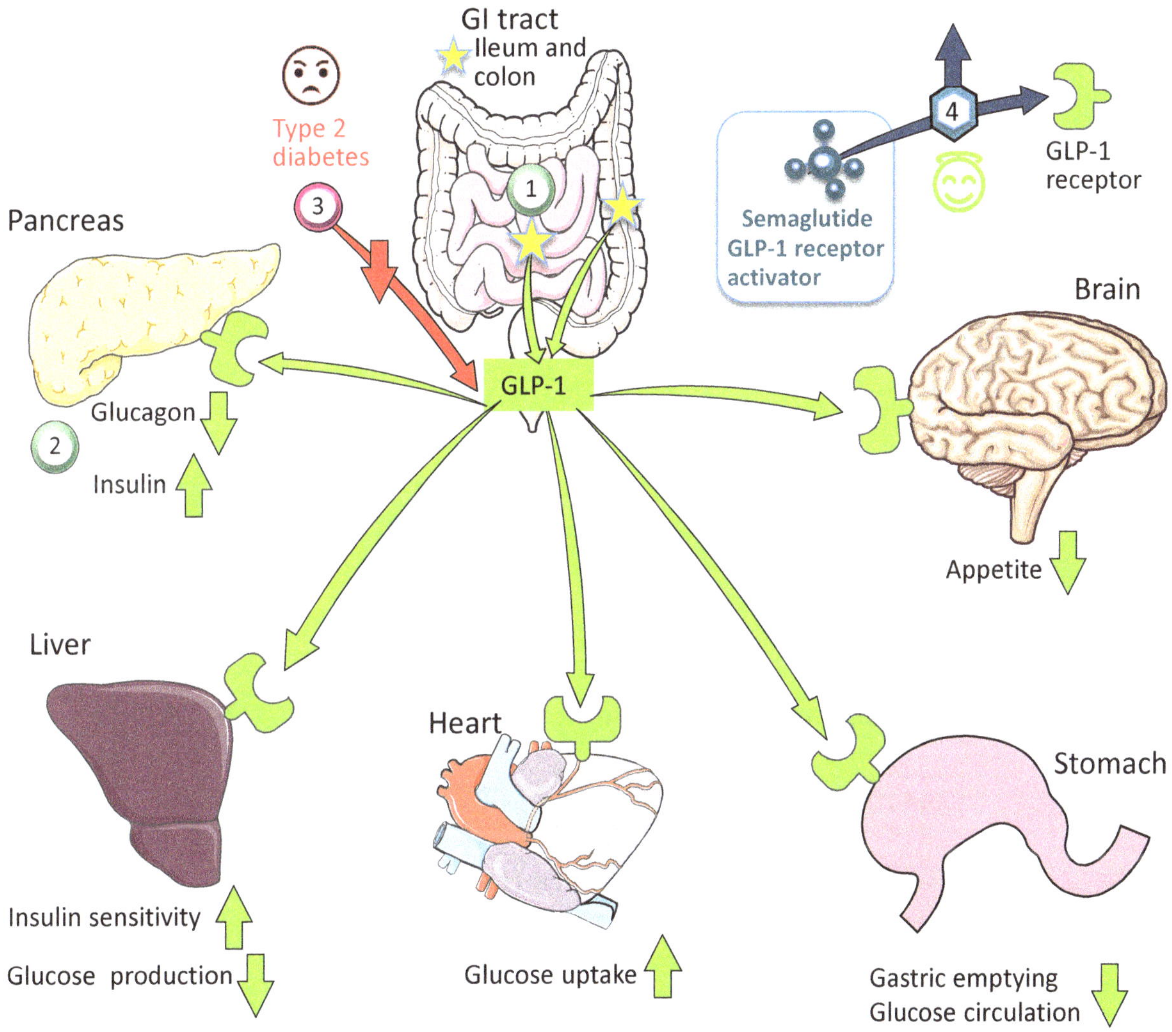

GI tract
Ileum and colon
1
Type 2 diabetes
3
4
GLP-1 receptor
Semaglutide GLP-1 receptor activator
Pancreas
GLP-1
Glucagon
2
Insulin
Brain
Appetite
Liver
Insulin sensitivity
Glucose production
Heart
Glucose uptake
Stomach
Gastric emptying
Glucose circulation

Peptide drugs: Type 2 diabetes, Semaglutide

The disease: Severe early-onset obesity

Severe early-onset obesity that is due to three **rare genetic conditions**: pro-opiomelanocortin (POMC) deficiency, PCSK1 enzyme deficiency, and leptin receptor (LEPR) deficiency that affect the melanocortin-4 receptor (MC4R) signaling pathway. **Symptoms include extreme hunger**, early-onset obesity, and adrenal insufficiency.

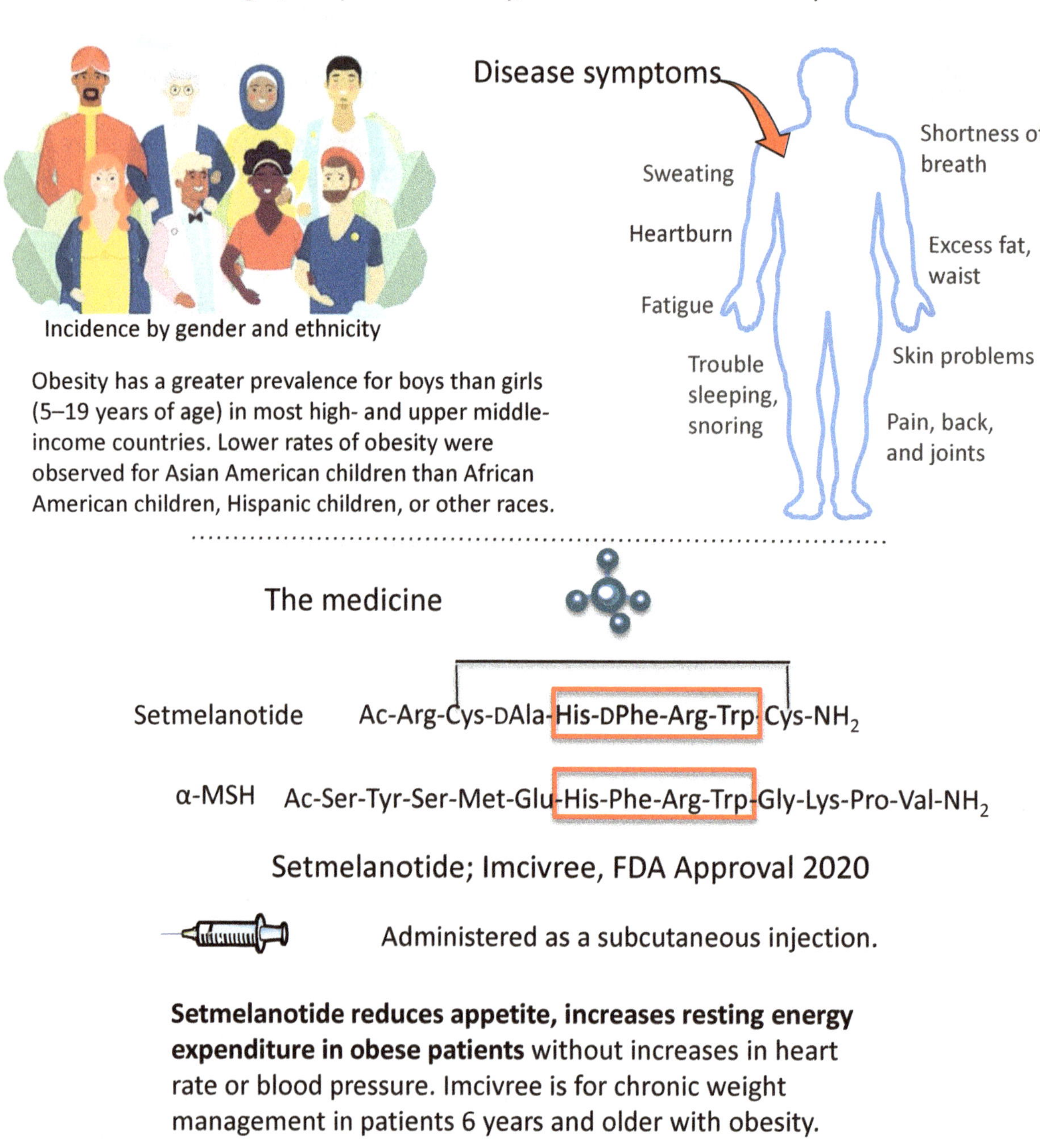

Incidence by gender and ethnicity
Obesity has a greater prevalence for boys than girls (5–19 years of age) in most high- and upper middle-income countries. Lower rates of obesity were observed for Asian American children than African American children, Hispanic children, or other races.
Disease symptoms
Sweating
Heartburn
Fatigue
Trouble sleeping, snoring
Shortness of breath
Excess fat, waist
Skin problems
Pain, back, and joints
The medicine
Setmelanotide Ac-Arg-Cys-DAla-His-DPhe-Arg-Trp-Cys-NH_2
α-MSH Ac-Ser-Tyr-Ser-Met-Glu-His-Phe-Arg-Trp-Gly-Lys-Pro-Val-NH_2

Setmelanotide; Imcivree, FDA Approval 2020

Administered as a subcutaneous injection.

Setmelanotide reduces appetite, increases resting energy expenditure in obese patients without increases in heart rate or blood pressure. Imcivree is for chronic weight management in patients 6 years and older with obesity.

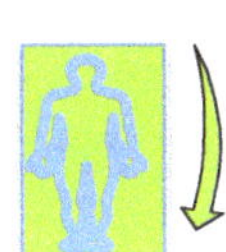
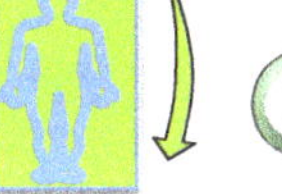

1 **α-melanocyte–stimulating hormone** (α-MSH) is an endogenous peptide hormone (neuropeptide), a powerful appetite suppressant through activation of the **Melanocortin 4 receptor** (MC4R).

2 MC4 receptors are located in the control centers of the **hypothalamus** and are involved in the regulation of appetite.

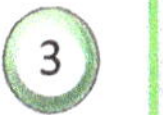

3 **Pro-opiomelanocortin** (POMC) in the hypothalamus is **regulated by leptin**. Protease cleavage of POMC **generates α-MSH**.

4 **Setmelanotide** binds to and activates **MC4 receptors** and results in **appetite suppression**.

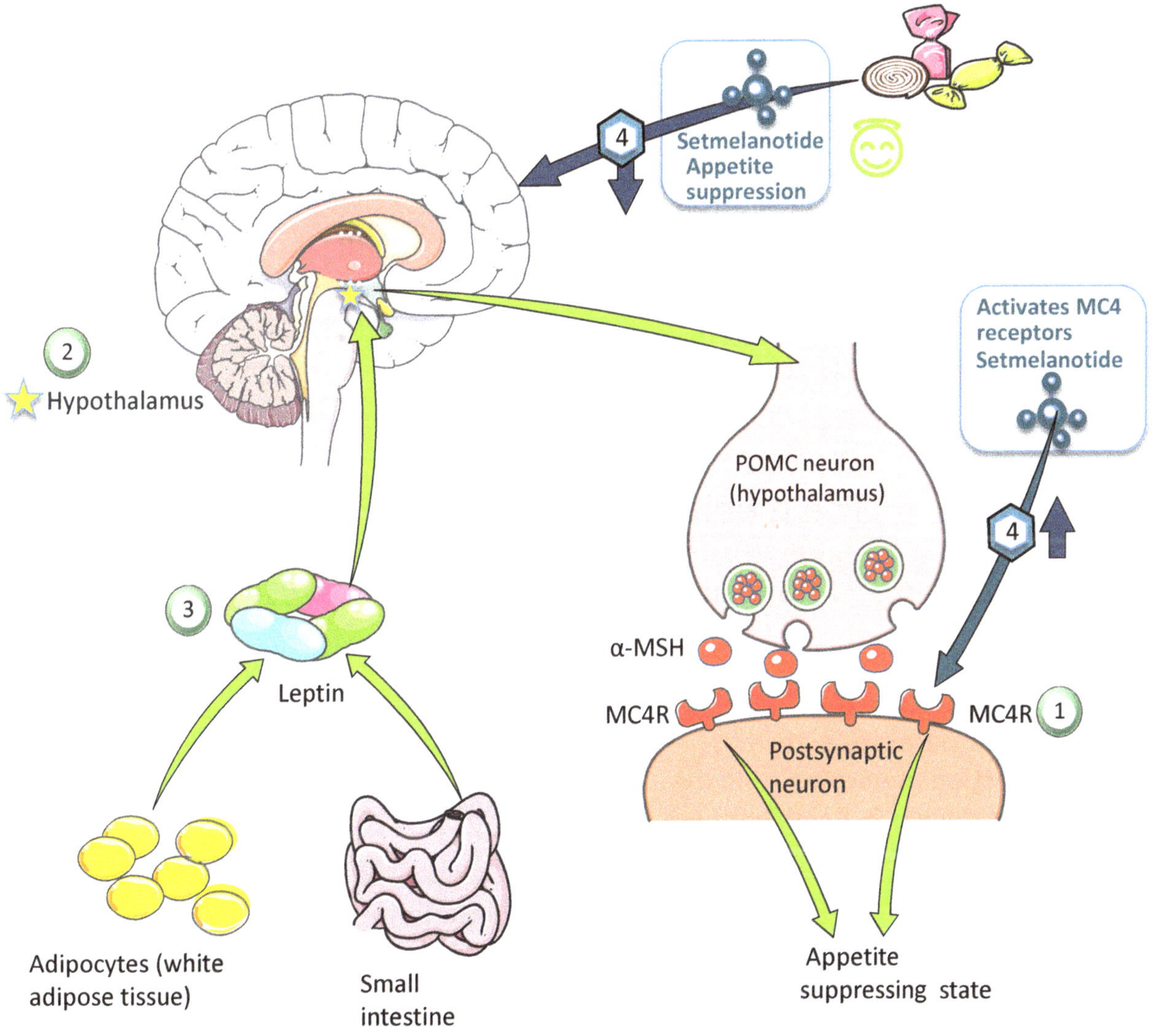

4 Setmelanotide Appetite suppression

2 Hypothalamus

Activates MC4 receptors Setmelanotide

POMC neuron (hypothalamus)

4

3 Leptin

α-MSH

MC4R

MC4R 1

Postsynaptic neuron

Adipocytes (white adipose tissue)

Small intestine

Appetite suppressing state

The disease: Acute hepatic porphyria

Acute hepatic porphyria is a genetic disorder resulting in the buildup of toxic porphyrin molecules (from heme production) with severe **abdominal neuropathic pain,** which can cause paralysis and respiratory failure. **The disease is** related to **ingestion of chemicals,** for example, barbiturates, hydantoins, alcohol, as well as fasting.

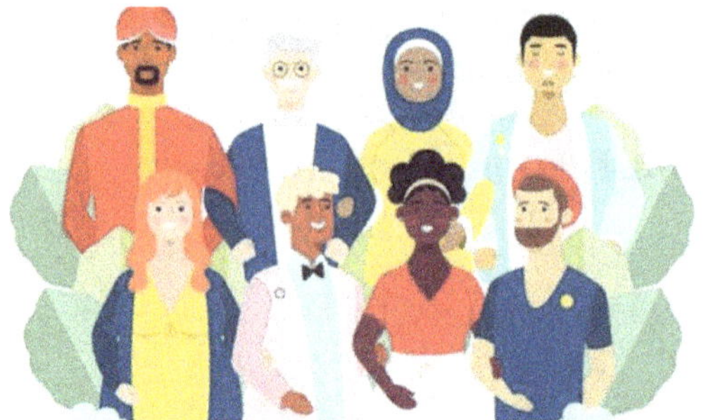

Incidence by gender and ethnicity

Porphyria is usually inherited, about 1 in 10,000 people of European ancestry have a mutation that cause the disease where one or both parents pass along the abnormal gene. The disease can occur in individuals of all ethnic backgrounds, although less common in African Americans. Acute hepatic porphyria has a higher incidence in females.

Disease symptoms

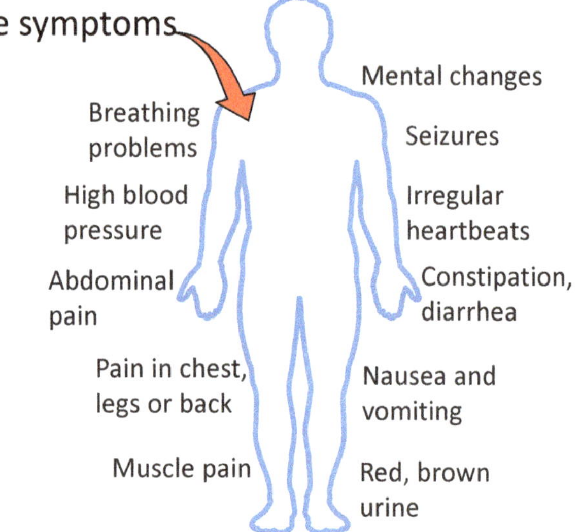

The medicine

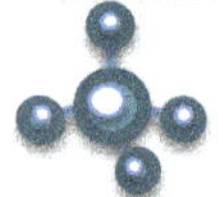

Givosiran; Givlaari, FDA Approval 2019

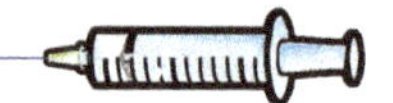

Administered as an intravenous infusion

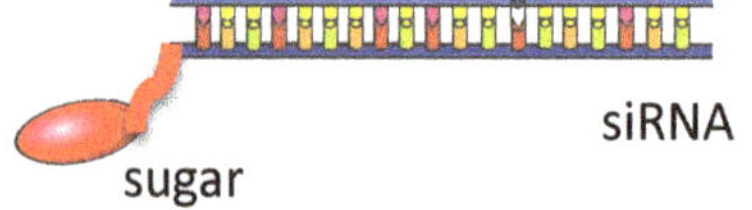

With **hepatic porphyrias**, there is **overproduction of porphyrins** in the liver due to defects in heme synthesis. **Givosiran** is an RNA interference medicine that **targets aminolevulinic acid synthase 1** (ALAS1), an enzyme that accumulates to toxic levels in the liver of people with acute hepatic porphyria.

Givosiran consists of a **double stranded small interfering RNA (ALAS1 siRNA)** with chemically modified nucleotides **conjugated to a sugar residue** (triantennary N-acetyl galactosamine) to facilitate delivery of the siRNA to the liver.

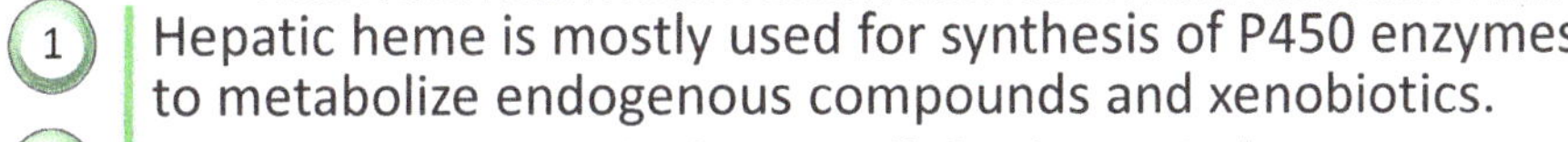

Action of Givosiran on cell and disease biology

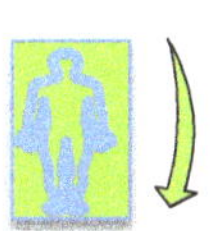

1 Hepatic heme is mostly used for synthesis of P450 enzymes to metabolize endogenous compounds and xenobiotics.

2 A critically **low level of intracellular heme** in hepatocytes triggers **overproduction of delta-aminolevulinic acid (ALAS1)**

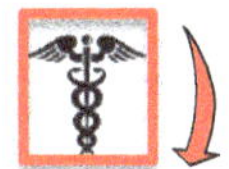

3 Abdominal neuropathic pain, is accompanied by overproduction of **neurotoxic** delta-aminolevulinic acid and porphobilinogen.

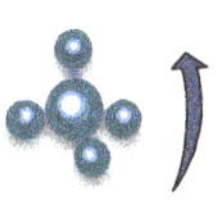

4 **Givosiran** forms an **RNA-silencing complex binding to ALAS1 mRNA** and reducing expression of the ALAS1.

Givosiran reduces build-up of liver ALAS1 mRNA and intermediates aminolevulinic acid and porphobilinogen circulating in blood.

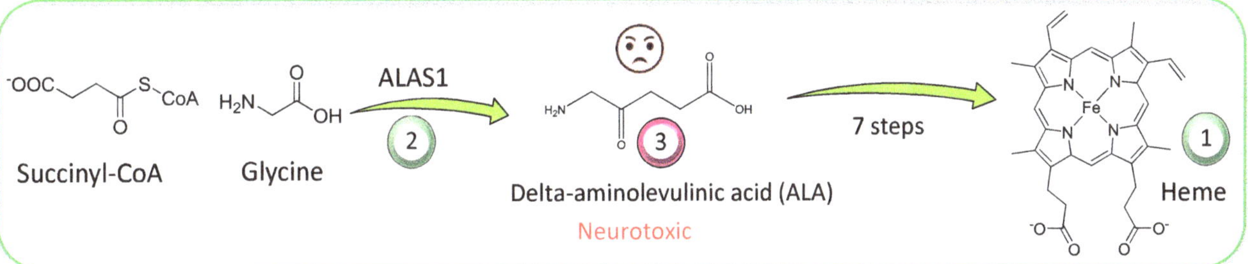

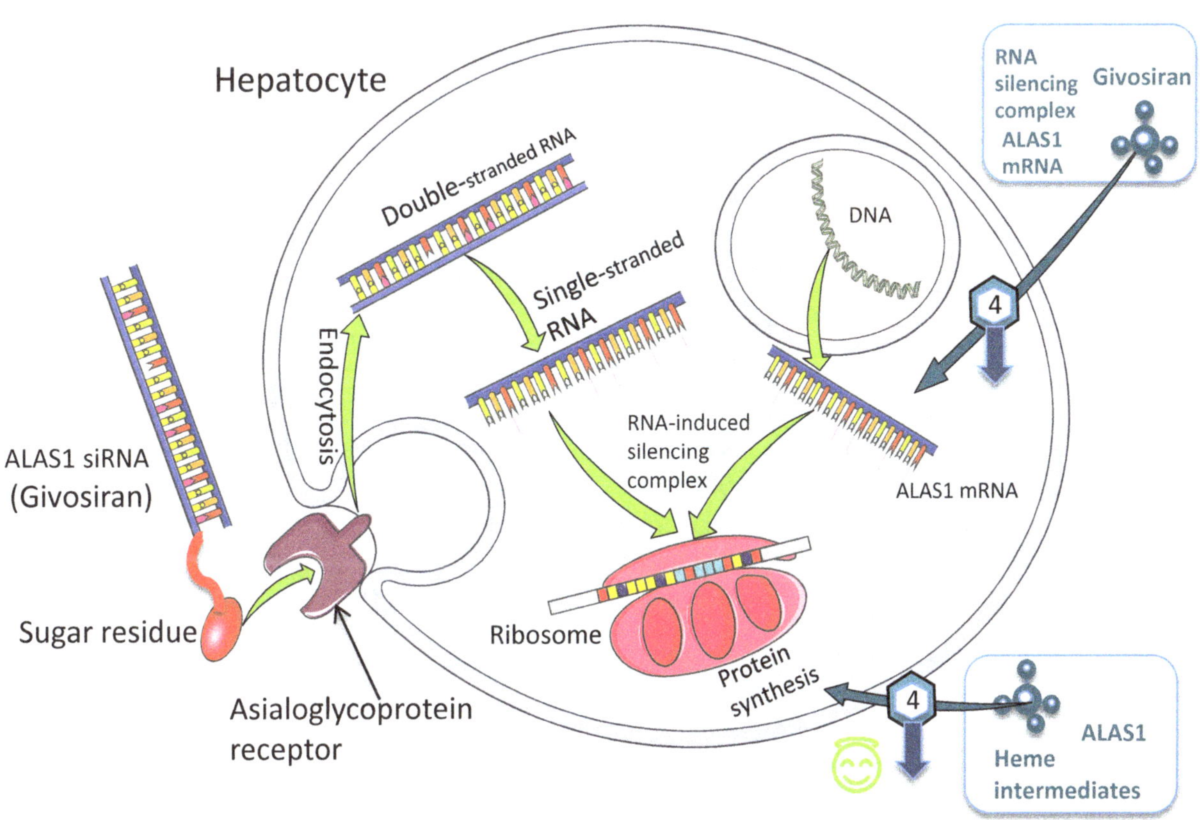

RNA drugs, small interfering RNA(siRNA): Hepatic porphyria, Givosiran

The disease: Duchenne muscular dystrophy

Duchenne muscular dystrophy (DMD) is caused by **mutations in the DMD gene** which encodes for the protein dystrophin. Without a functional dystrophin protein, DMD patients gradually lose their mobility as their muscles degenerate. The DMD gene is one of the **largest human genes** and codes for a protein of 3685 amino acid residues, which acts like a **shock absorber** during muscle contraction.

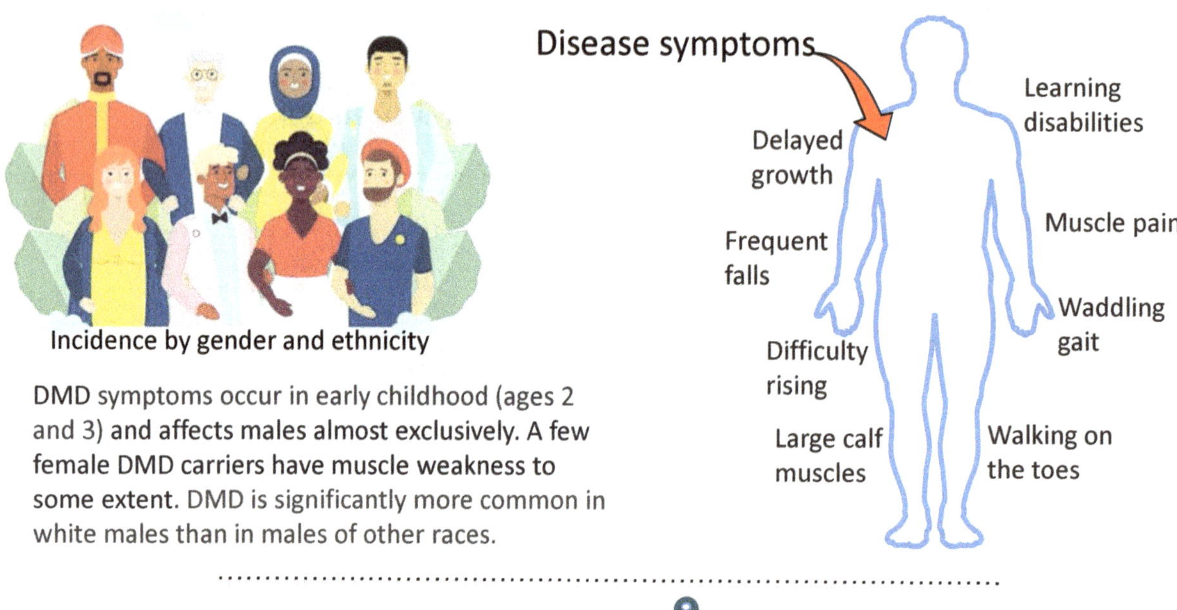

Incidence by gender and ethnicity

DMD symptoms occur in early childhood (ages 2 and 3) and affects males almost exclusively. A few female DMD carriers have muscle weakness to some extent. DMD is significantly more common in white males than in males of other races.

The medicine

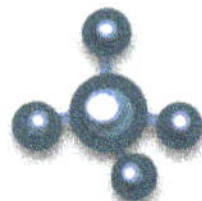

Golodirsen; Vyondys, FDA Approval 2019

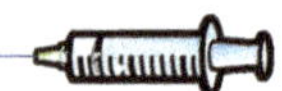

Administered as an intravenous infusion

Golodirsen is a **single-stranded antisense RNA,** which **increases dystrophin** production in muscular dystrophy. The synthetic RNA uses a PMO group which achieves long half-lives in vivo.

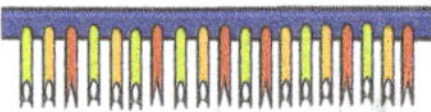

The **phosphorodiamidate morpholino (PMO)** structure uses a six-sided morpholine rings instead of five-sided ribose rings makes the antisense drug **resistant to nucleases**, electrically neutral, and maintains full binding to the complementary strand to **inhibit expression of a specific mRNA**.

RNA drugs, antisense RNA: Duchenne muscular dystrophy, Golodirsen

Action of Golodirsen on cell and disease biology

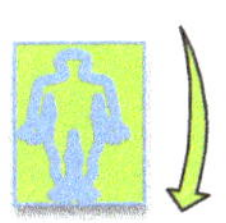

1 **Dystrophin** is a long protein with numerous redundant coils, which acts as a **shock absorber** during contraction. Without functional dystrophin to support muscle strength and stability, muscle fibers are easily damaged.

2 Dystrophin **links the cytoskeleton** of muscle fibers to the surrounding connective tissue (basal lamina).

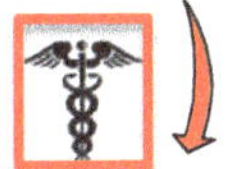

3 DMD gene **mutations terminate the dystrophin synthesis** and result in a short, dysfunctional protein.

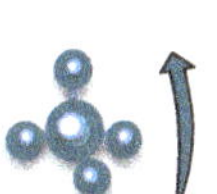

4 **Exon skipping** uses an **antisense sequence against the splice junctions** of exon 53, to cause cells to **"skip" over the faulty section** and exclusion from the mature mRNA**.**

5 **Golodirsen** binds to exon 53 and skips (excludes) this damaged part of a patient's genetic code. **Skipping of the exon 53** generates a shorter but still **functional Dystrophin.**

Exon skipping strategy

Golodirsen
Skip exon 53
4
DMD gene
Pre-mRNA
51 52 53 54 55
Mature mRNA
51 52 54 55
Protein coding exons
Golodirsen

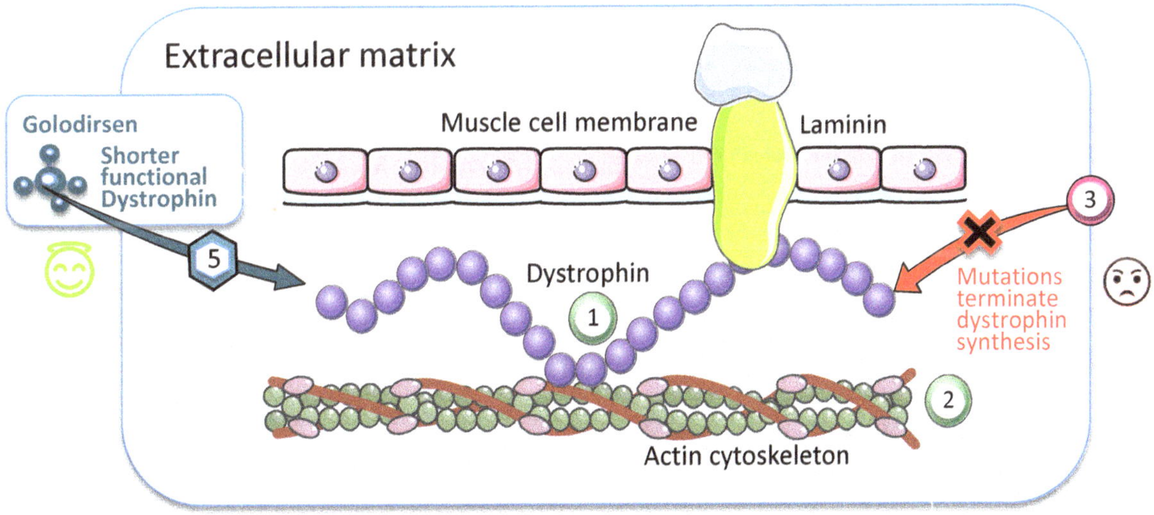

Extracellular matrix
Golodirsen
Shorter functional Dystrophin
5
Muscle cell membrane
Laminin
3
Dystrophin
1
Mutations terminate dystrophin synthesis
2
Actin cytoskeleton

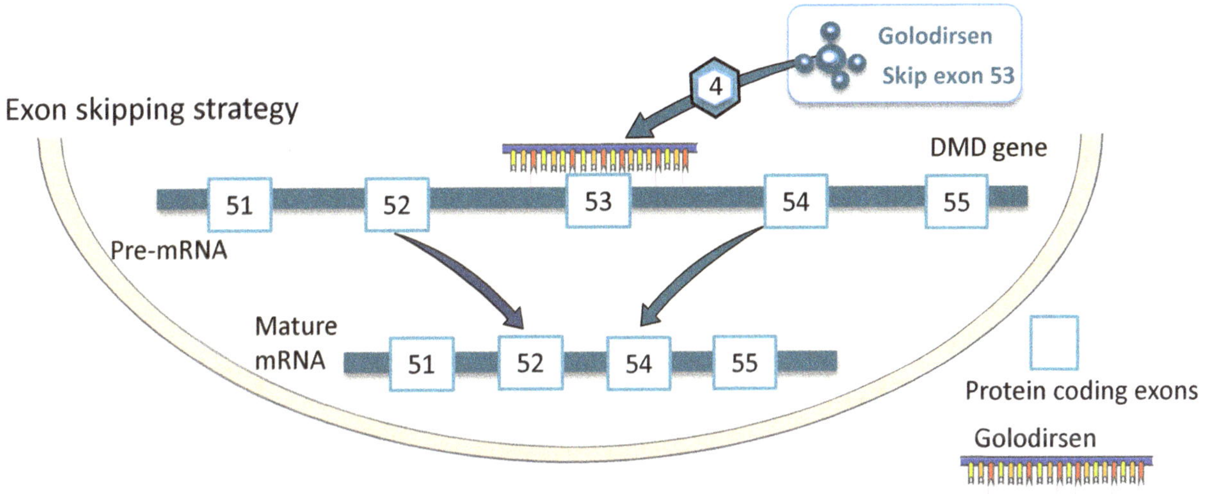

RNA drugs, antisense RNA: Duchenne muscular dystrophy, Golodirsen

The disease: Hereditary transthyretin (TTR) amyloidosis

Hereditary transthyretin (TTR) amyloidosis (ATTR) in adults is caused by **mutation of transthyretin (TTR)** with extracellular deposition of mutated and misfolded proteins as amyloid fibrils. This results in destruction of the peripheral nervous system which is connected to the heart, and/ or gastrointestinal tract and is life-threatening (median survival of 5 years) with neuropathic pain, muscle weakness, and impaired balance.

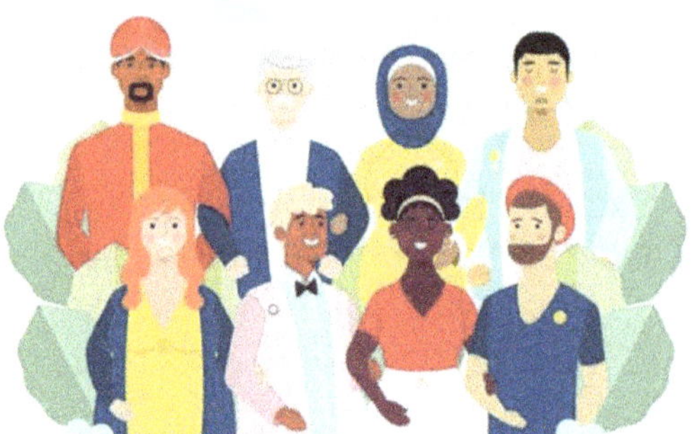

Incidence by gender and ethnicity

TTR amyloidosis is either hereditary (genetic mutation) or nonhereditary where transthyretin misfolds, forming amyloid. Age-related ATTR is predominately male, but disease prevalence increases with age and patients are likely to be female. In the United States, the hereditary form disproportionately afflicts black Americans.

Disease symptoms

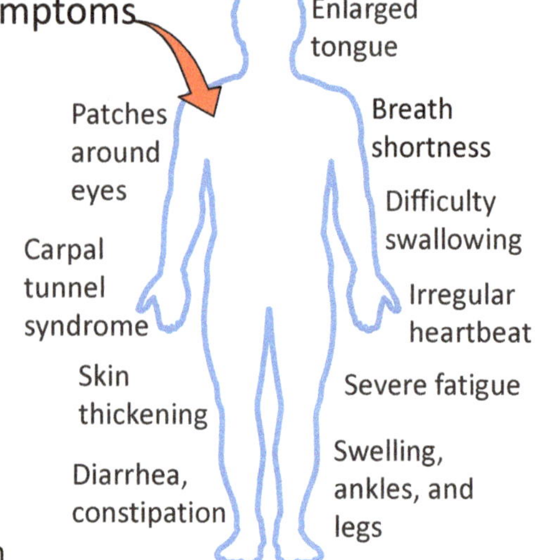

The medicine

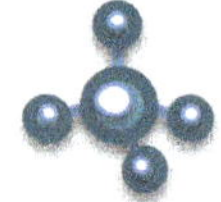

Patisiran; Onpattro, FDA Approval 2019

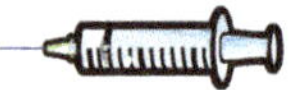

Administered as an intravenous infusion

Patisaran is a siRNA formulated as a lipid complex for delivery to hepatocytes. Patisiran **targets a sequence within the transthyretin (TTR) mRNA** that is conserved in both wild-type and TTR variants. **Patisaran decreases** hepatic production of mutant and wild-type **TTR**.

Small interfering RNA (siRNA) is a class of **double-stranded non coding RNA molecules**, 20–25 base pairs in length. The siRNA duplex unwinds in the cytoplasm and the antisense strand targets a disease related messenger RNA (mRNA).

Action of Patisiran on cell and disease biology

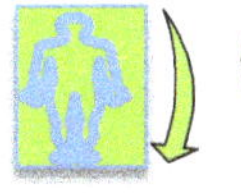

1 Transthyretin (TTR), produced in **the liver, transports vitamin A (retinol) and thyroxine**. Functional transthyretin consists of a four-protein unit (tetramer).

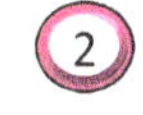

2 TTR protein deposits (**amyloid build up**, amyloidosis) occur in the peripheral nervous system (peripheral neuropathy) and the autonomic nervous system (effects blood pressure, heart rate, digestion).

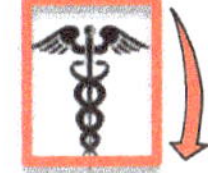

3 **Cardiac amyloidosis** is a serious and progressive infiltrative disease that is caused by the deposition of amyloid fibrils. As the deposits increase, the heart gets increasingly stiff and eventually the pumping function deteriorates.

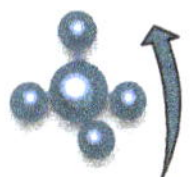

4 **Patisiran** degrades mutant and wild-type TTR mRNA by RNA interference, resulting in a reduction of serum TTR protein and tissue deposition.

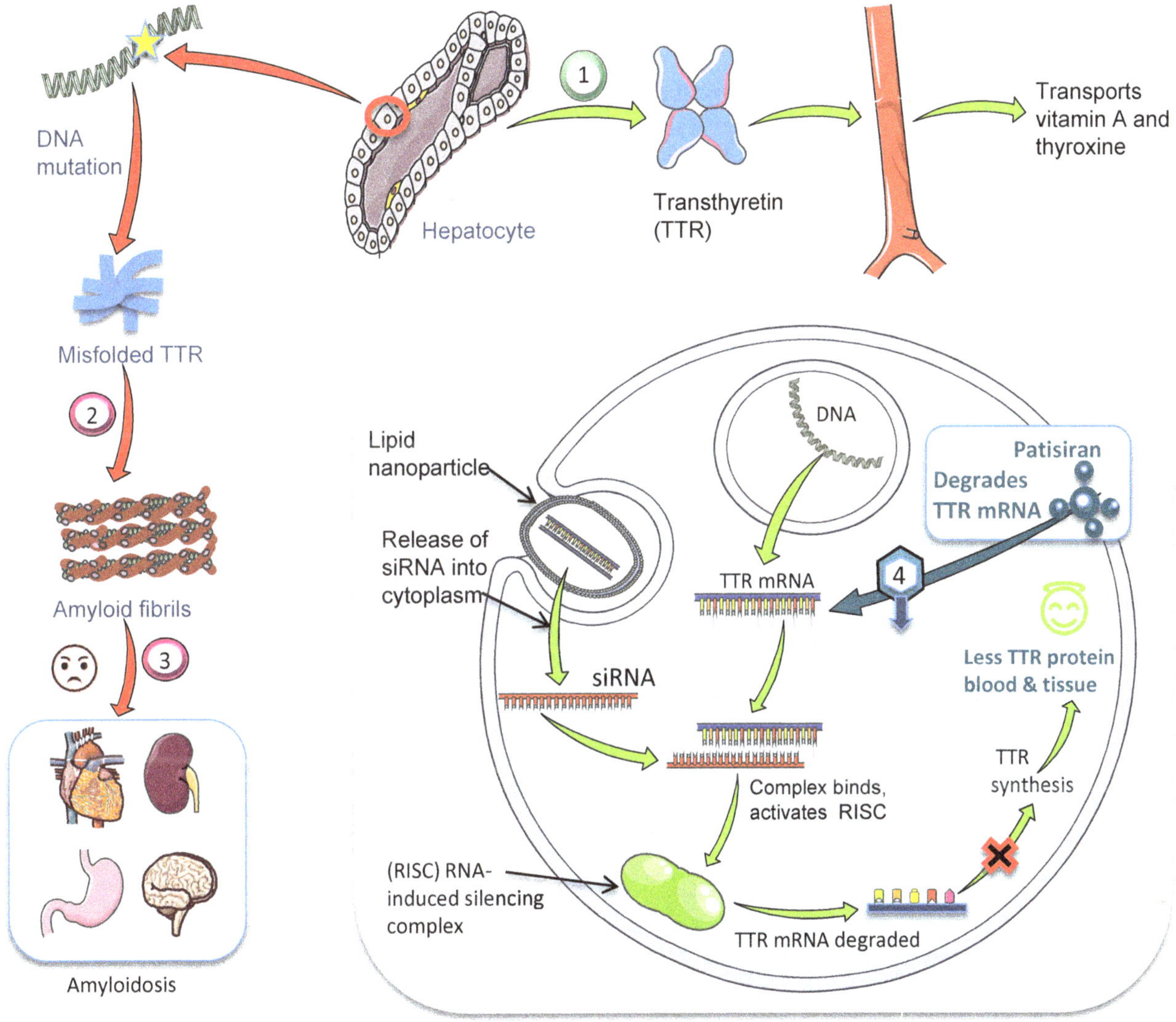

DNA mutation
Hepatocyte
1
Transthyretin (TTR)
Transports vitamin A and thyroxine
Misfolded TTR
2
Amyloid fibrils
3
Amyloidosis
Lipid nanoparticle
Release of siRNA into cytoplasm
DNA
Patisiran Degrades TTR mRNA
TTR mRNA
4
Less TTR protein blood & tissue
siRNA
TTR synthesis
Complex binds, activates RISC
(RISC) RNA-induced silencing complex
TTR mRNA degraded

RNA drugs, small interfering RNA(siRNA): Hereditary transthyretin amyloidosis, Patisiran

The disease: Primary hyperoxaluria type 1

Primary hyperoxaluria type 1 (PH1) is a a rare genetic disease caused by mutations in the gene AGT which codes for alanine-glyoxylate aminotransferase. Reduced activity of the enzyme impairs the conversion of glyoxylate into glycine with **accumulation of oxalate in the kidneys (as kidney stones) and urinary tract**.

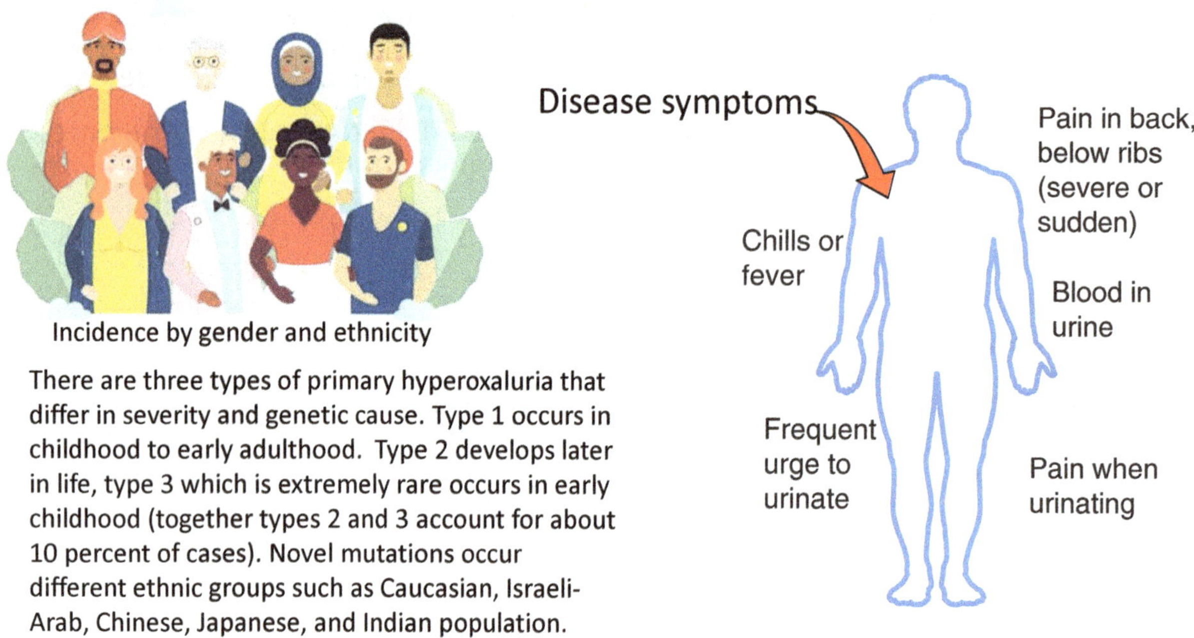

Incidence by gender and ethnicity

There are three types of primary hyperoxaluria that differ in severity and genetic cause. Type 1 occurs in childhood to early adulthood. Type 2 develops later in life, type 3 which is extremely rare occurs in early childhood (together types 2 and 3 account for about 10 percent of cases). Novel mutations occur different ethnic groups such as Caucasian, Israeli-Arab, Chinese, Japanese, and Indian population.

The medicine

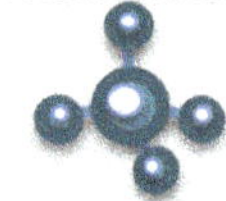

Lumasiran; Oxlumo, FDA Approval 2020

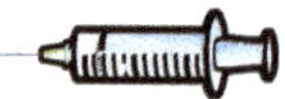

Administered as a subcutaneous injection.

Lumasiran is a **double-stranded small interfering ribonucleic acid (siRNA)** that **reduces** levels of the **glycolate oxidase** (GO) enzyme by targeting its messenger ribonucleic acid (mRNA).

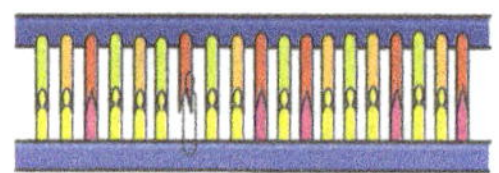

The blocking of GO production in hepatocytes **reduces of urinary oxalate levels**. As the GO enzyme is upstream of the **deficient alanine-glyoxylate aminotransferase**, the action of lumasiran is independent of the exact location of the gene mutation (175 mutations in the AGXT gene).

Action of Lumasiran on cell and disease biology

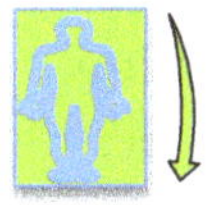

1 The glycolate oxidase gene is expressed primarily in liver and pancreas and the resulting GO enzyme oxidizes glycolate to glyoxalate.

2 **Glyoxylate** is converted **into oxalate**, an end product of metabolism and eliminated in urine.

3 Alanine-glyoxylate aminotransferase (**AGT**) catalyzes the formation of glycine from glyoxylate and **prevents oxalate** formation from glyoxylate.

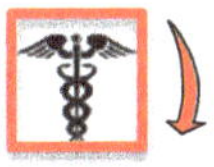

4 Mutations in gene AGXT and **insufficiency of AGT** results in excess glyoxylate converted to oxalate resulting in high blood levels of oxalate with massive **calcium oxalate deposition** throughout the entire body.

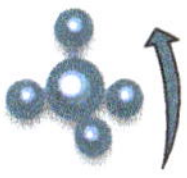

5 siRNA duplex of **Lumasiran** unwinds and the **antisense strand** specifically activates RNA-induced silencing complex (RISC), which **targets HAO1 mRNA** and **blocks GO** enzyme production.

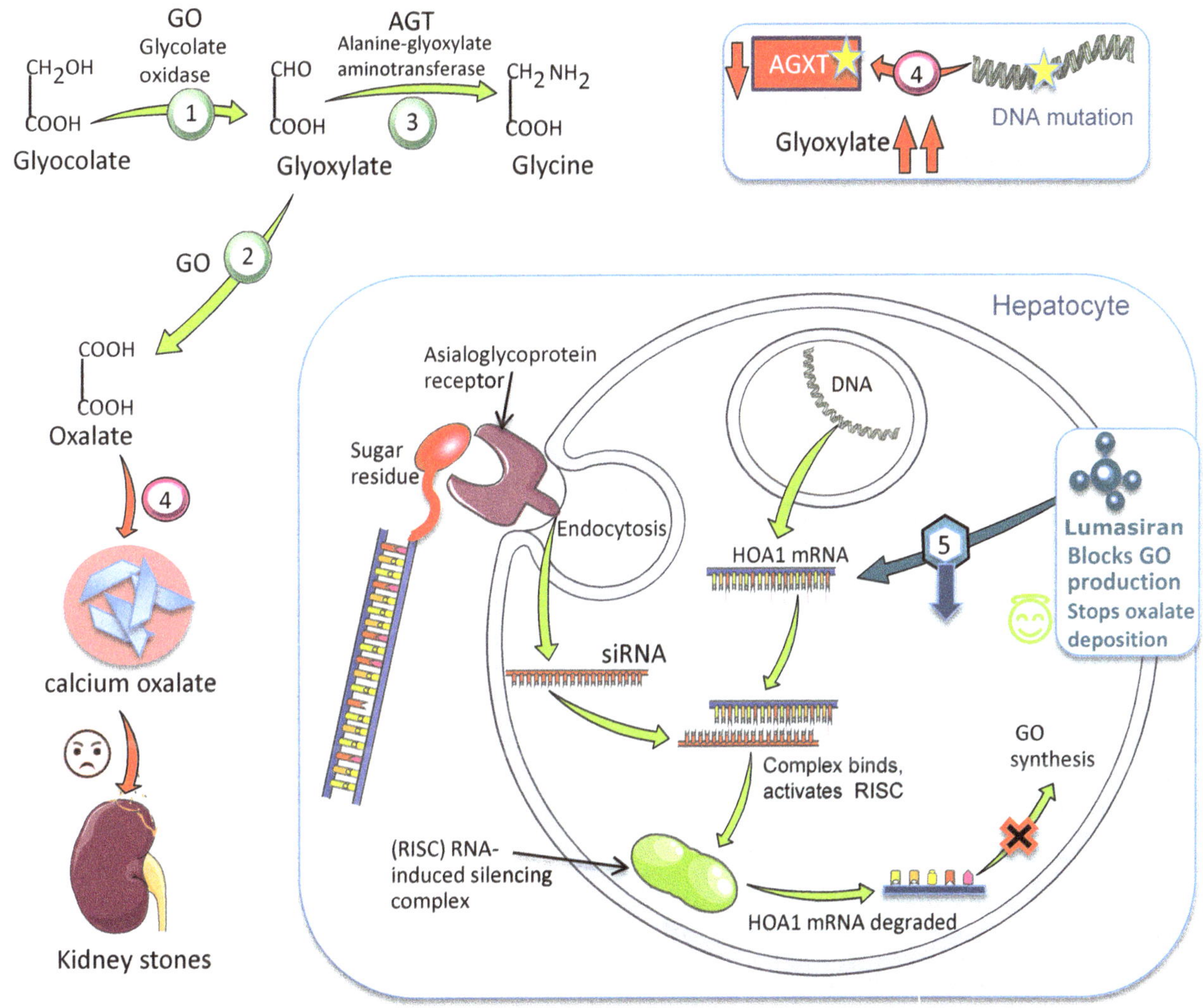

RNA drugs, small interfering RNA(siRNA): Primary hyperoxaluria type 1, Lumasiran

The disease: B-cell lymphoma

B-cell lymphoma is one of the two main types of **non-Hodgkin lymphoma** (NHL) including **large B-cell (LBCL) as well as follicular lymphoma (FL)**. It is a blood cancer that arises in lymph nodes from B lymphocytes.

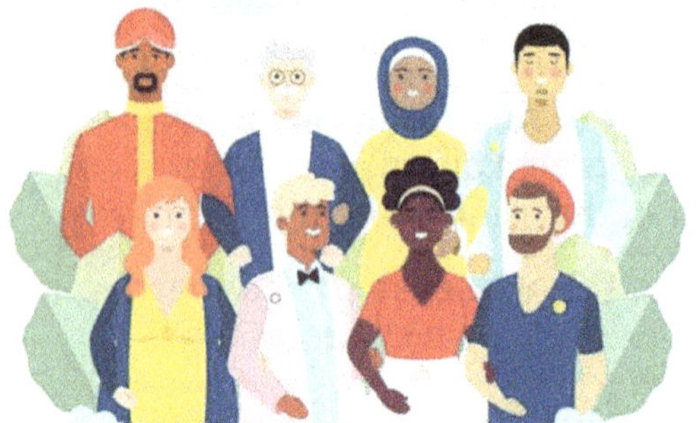

Incidence by gender and ethnicity

In male and female patients NHL mortality was higher for older patients (male patients 1.2 times more susceptible). In patients with age less than 60 years, males are 3.28 times more likely to die. In the United States, whites are more likely than African Americans and Asian Americans to develop NHL. Worldwide, non-Hodgkin lymphoma is more common in developed countries, with the United States and Europe having the highest rates.

Disease symptoms

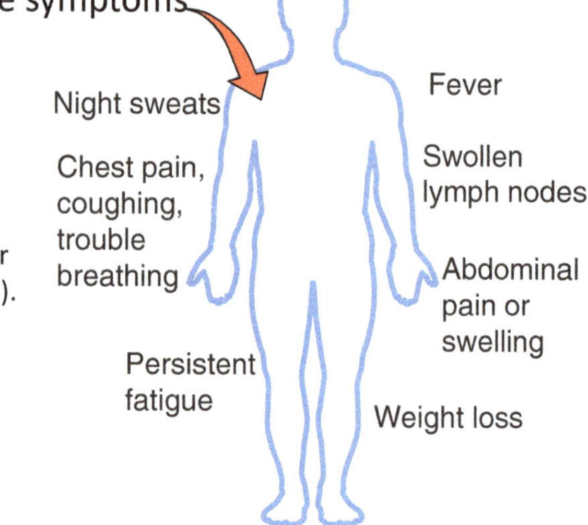

The medicine

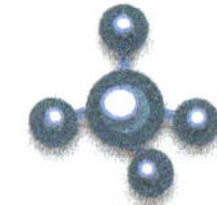

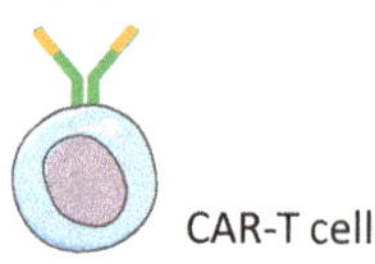

CAR-T cell

Axicabtagene ciloleucel; Yescarta, FDA Approval 2017

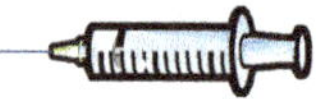

Administered as an intravenous (IV) infusion.

Yescarta, a **chimeric antigen receptor (CAR-T)** cell therapy for adult patients with relapsed LBCL. **Cell-based gene therapy** uses the **patient's T- cells**, modified to recognize the lymphoma cells, amplified, and then transferred intravenously to the patient via a single infusion. CAR T-cells are **activated, proliferate and attack the cancer cells.**

Lentiviral vectors stably integrate relatively large inserts, effectively deliver genetic material to both dividing and nondividing cells, maintain long-term stable expression in target cells, are nonpathogenic without an inflammatory response.

Cell and gene therapy: B-cell lymphoma, Yescarta

Action of Yescarta on cell and disease biology

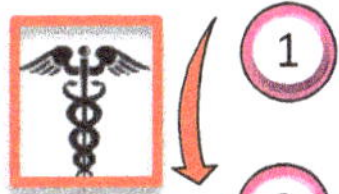

1 **Follicular lymphoma** (FL) is a type of NHL and grouped tumor cells can grow to form **nodules**.

2 Transformation of FL results in **more aggressive** diffuse large B-cell lymphoma (**DLBCL**) where cancer cells spread and destroy the lymph node structure.

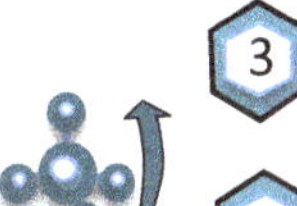

3 **CD19** (signaling regulator) is expressed on most B cell malignancies but not on blood stem cells, ideal for on-target treatment effects.

4 In **CAR-T cell therapy** T cells (CD4⁺ and CD8⁺) are removed from patients, genetically modified. **Chimeric antigen receptors** are inserted to produce chimeric antigen receptor T cells (CAR-T) that recognize and destroy lymphoma cells via surface antigens. The genetically engineered CAR-T cells are grown in the laboratory (billions) and are infused back into the patient.

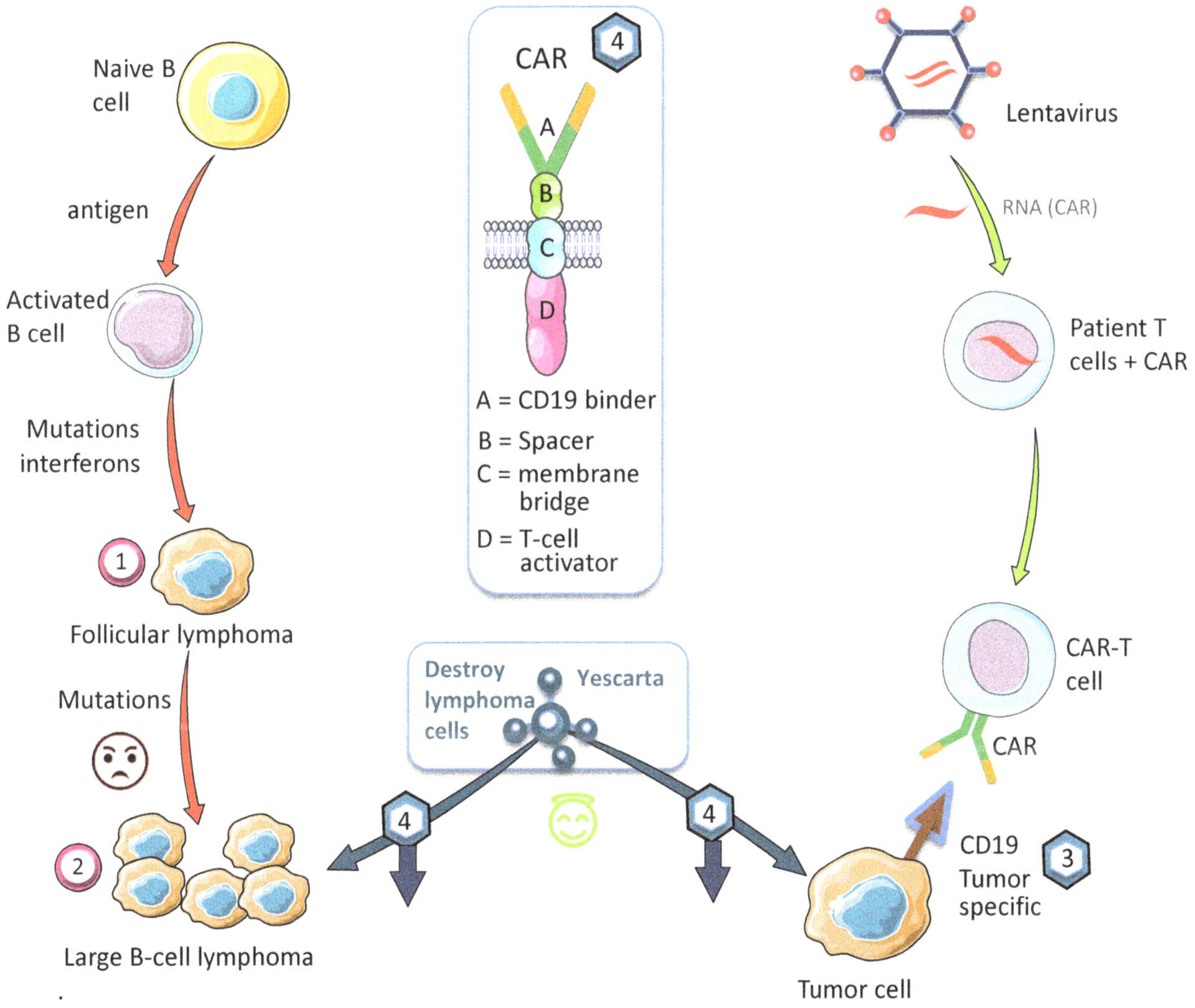

Naive B cell
antigen
Activated B cell
Mutations interferons
1 Follicular lymphoma
Mutations
2 Large B-cell lymphoma

CAR 4
A
B
C
D
A = CD19 binder
B = Spacer
C = membrane bridge
D = T-cell activator

Destroy lymphoma cells
Yescarta
4
4

Lentavirus
RNA (CAR)
Patient T cells + CAR
CAR-T cell
CAR
CD19 Tumor specific 3
Tumor cell

Cell and gene therapy: B-cell lymphoma, Yescarta

Spinal muscular atrophy (SMA) is caused by **deletion or mutations in the SMN gene,** which codes for the **survival motor neuron protein 1**. The mutation is characterized by the degeneration of α-motor neurons resulting in lower limb and proximal muscle weakness with associated paralysis.

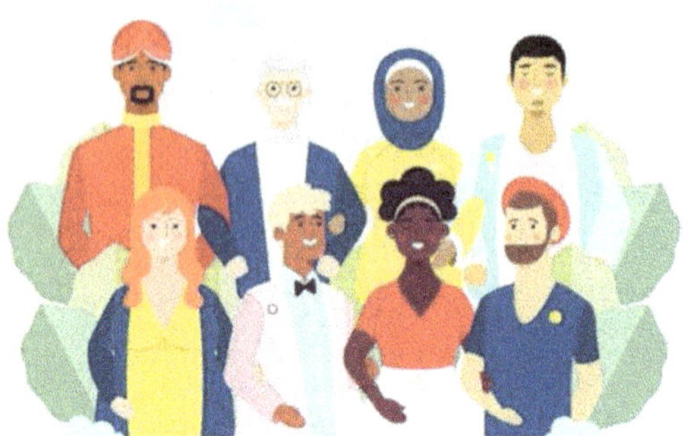

Incidence by gender and ethnicity

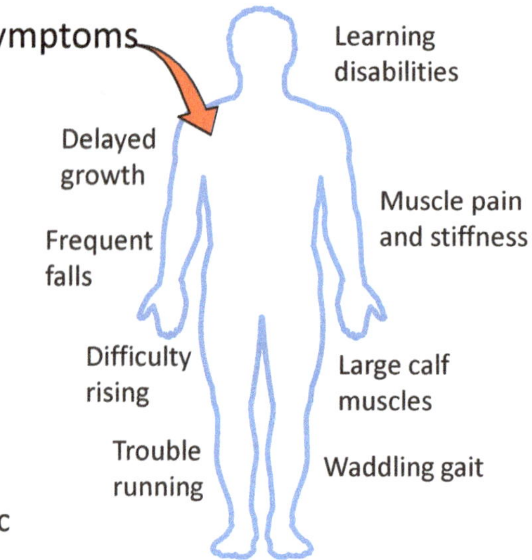

The clinical course of SMA is more severe in males but life expectancy is similar for both sexes. At 8 years or older, the incidence in females decreases. SMA is found in individuals of every race and ethnic background, but most common among Caucasians.

The medicine

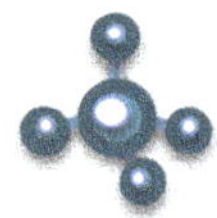

Onasemnogene abeparvovec-xioi, Zolgensma, FDA Approval 2019

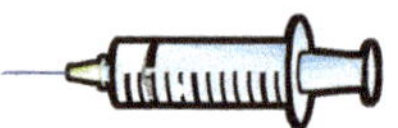

Delivered as **a single-dose intravenous infusion** into the bloodstream or injected into the spinal canal for gene delivery to specialized motor nerve cells.

Zolgensma consists of the human SMN gene contained inside a **AAV9 vector,** which is used to **deliver the SMN gene** to motor neuron cells throughout the body. The vector does not cause disease and is not integrated into the patient's DNA.

Adeno-associated virus serotype 9 **(AAV9) bypasses the blood–brain barrier**, which results in widespread access throughout the central nervous system and gene expression.

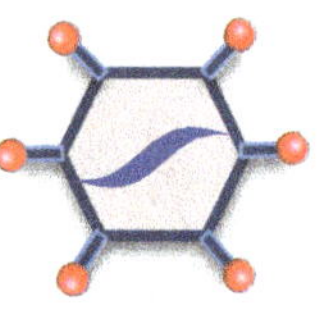

Action of Zolgensma on cell and disease biology

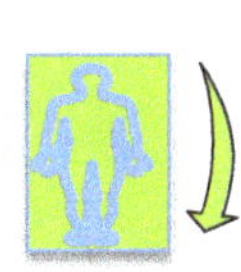
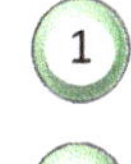

1 Adeno-associated virus 9 (AAV9) are small viruses (**single-stranded DNA)** and low genotoxicity in humans make it a leading gene therapy vector.

2 **SMN complex** regulates transcription and the **development of dendrites and axons** from nerve cells required for the transmission of impulses between neurons and from neurons to muscle cells.

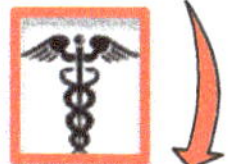

3 **Defects in the SMN complex** effects maintenance of motor neurons and signaling from the brain and spinal cord to contract skeletal muscles.

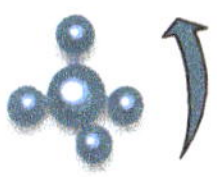

4 **Zolgensma** uses the **vector AA9 to deliver a functional SMN1 gene.** In the manufacturing process, the DNA of the virus is removed and replaced by the new SMN gene, which codes for the survival motor neuron protein.

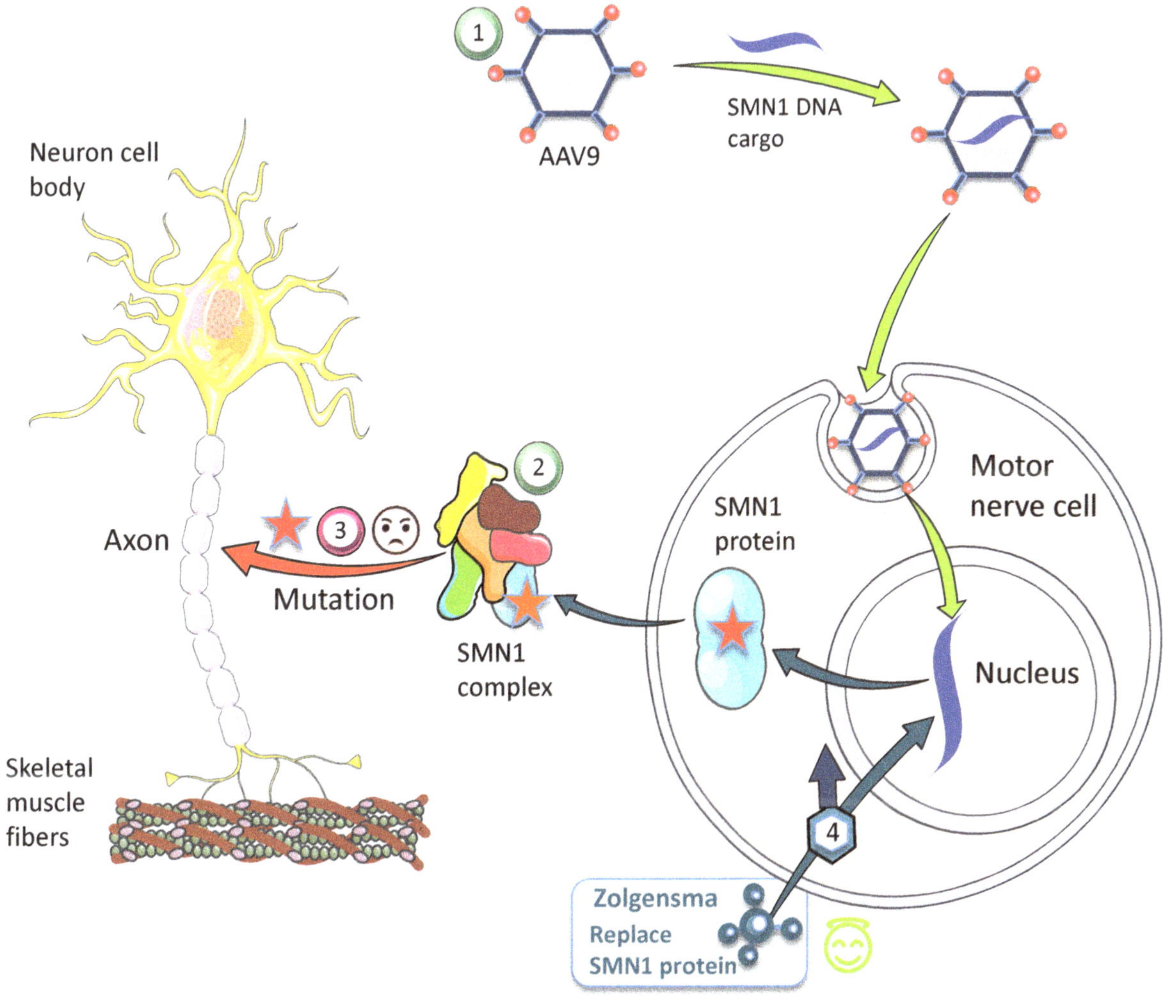

Chapter 7 Viruses, diseases, drugs, and vaccines

The Diversity of Viruses

<u>RNA Viruses</u>

The Influenza (flu) virus

Human immunodeficiency virus (HIV)

Ebola virus

SARS-CoV-2

<u>DNA Viruses</u>

Smallpox (variola) virus

Hepatitis B

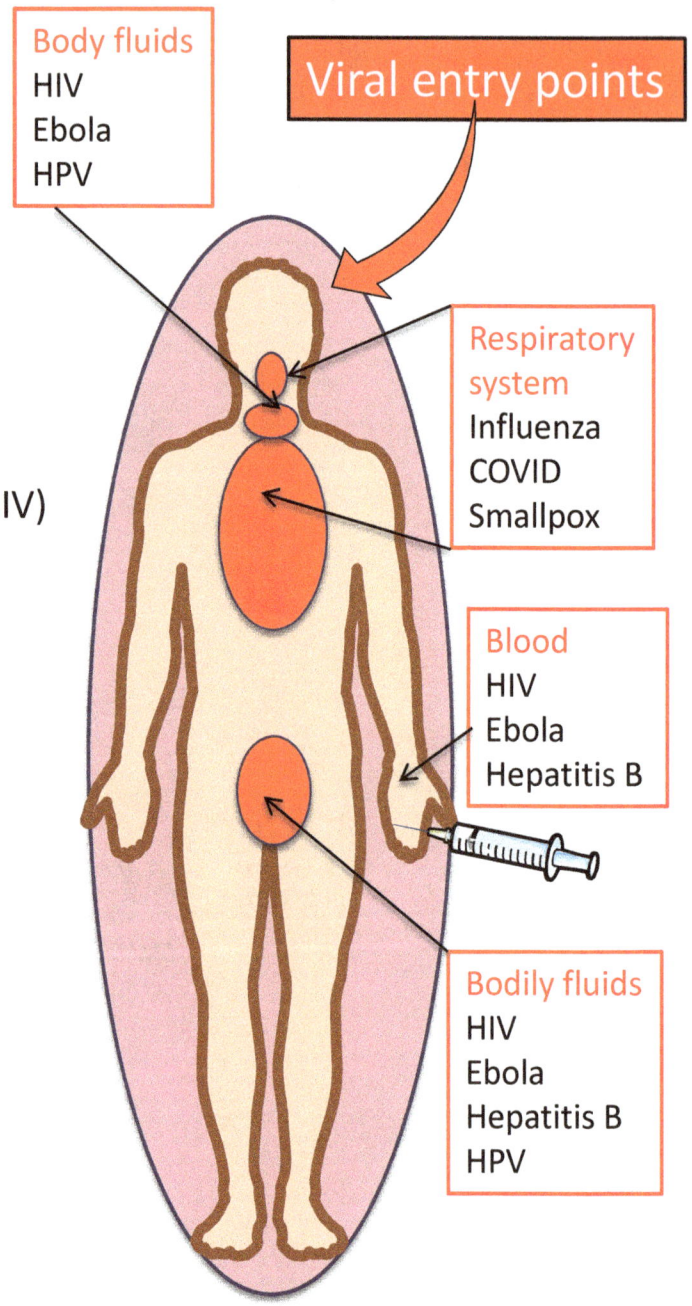

Human papillomavirus (HPV) virus

Selected drugs approved by the FDA for viral diseases.
√ = Drugs approved recently (2017–2021)

RNA viruses

a) Influenza
- Zanamivir D
- Oseltamivir D
- Baloxavir D
- Fluzone V

b) Human immunodeficiency virus
- Tenofovir D
- Darunavir D
- Dolutegravir D
- Enfuvirtide D

c) Ebola-19
- Inmazeb Ab (✓)
- Ervebo V (✓)

d) COVID-19
- Remdesivir D (✓)
- Molnupiravir, EUA (✓) D
- Nirmatrelvir, EUA (✓) D
- Belantamab, etesevimab, EUA(✓)Ab
- Casirivimab, imdevimab, EUA (✓)Ab
- BNT162b2, mRNA-1273, Ad26.COV2, EUA V (✓)

DNA viruses

- Smallpox
  - Tecovirimat D (✓)
  - ACAM2000 V
- Hepatitis B
  - Entecavir D
  - Recombivax, Engerix, Heplisav-B V (✓)
- Human papillomavirus
  - Gardasil-9 V

D = drug
Ab = antibody
V = vaccine

Chapter 7 Overview

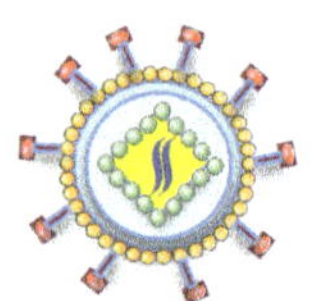

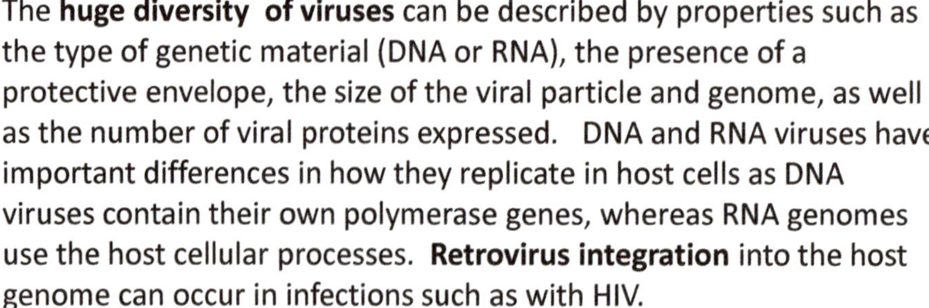

The **huge diversity of viruses** can be described by properties such as the type of genetic material (DNA or RNA), the presence of a protective envelope, the size of the viral particle and genome, as well as the number of viral proteins expressed. DNA and RNA viruses have important differences in how they replicate in host cells as DNA viruses contain their own polymerase genes, whereas RNA genomes use the host cellular processes. **Retrovirus integration** into the host genome can occur in infections such as with HIV.

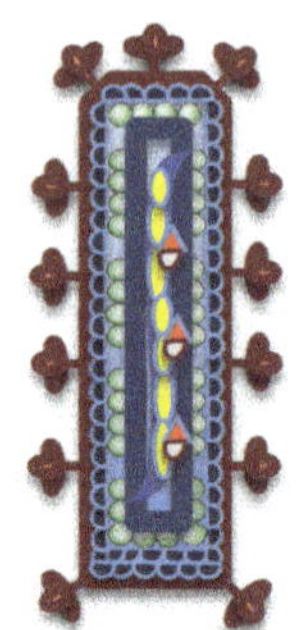

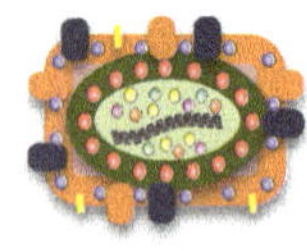

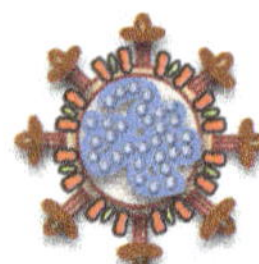

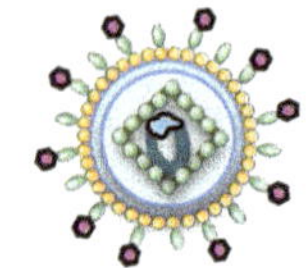

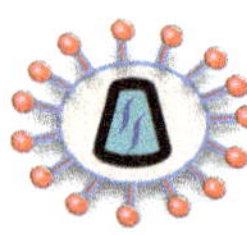

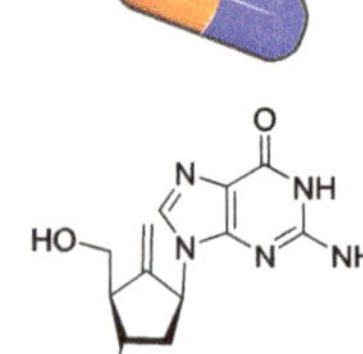

Antiviral drugs can target attachment of the virus to the host cell or its release, or block key enzymes responsible for production of viral building blocks or viral replication enzymes with minimal effect on the host cells. HIV is chosen as an important example of the development of drug therapies as the absence of an effective vaccine has resulted in a suite of different types of antiviral drugs. Other examples include drugs for influenza and hepatitis B, together with recent FDA approvals for the treatment of COVID-19 and smallpox. A recent development is the use of **neutralizing antibodies** for the inhibition of viral replication (Ebola, COVID-19).

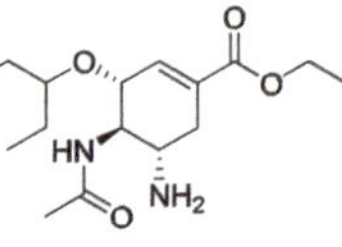

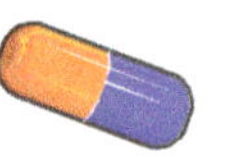

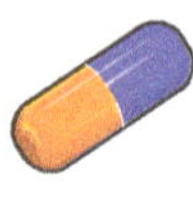

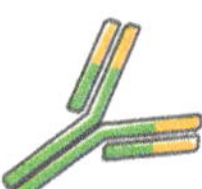

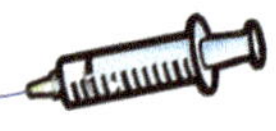

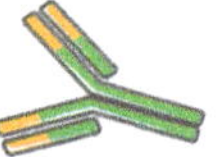

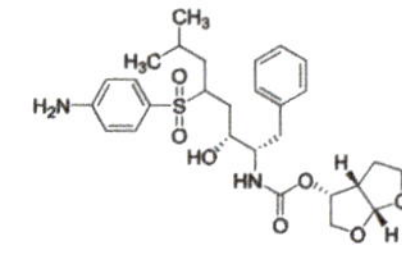

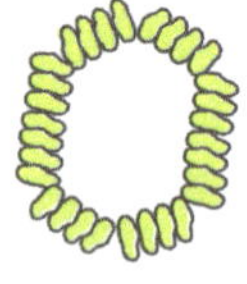

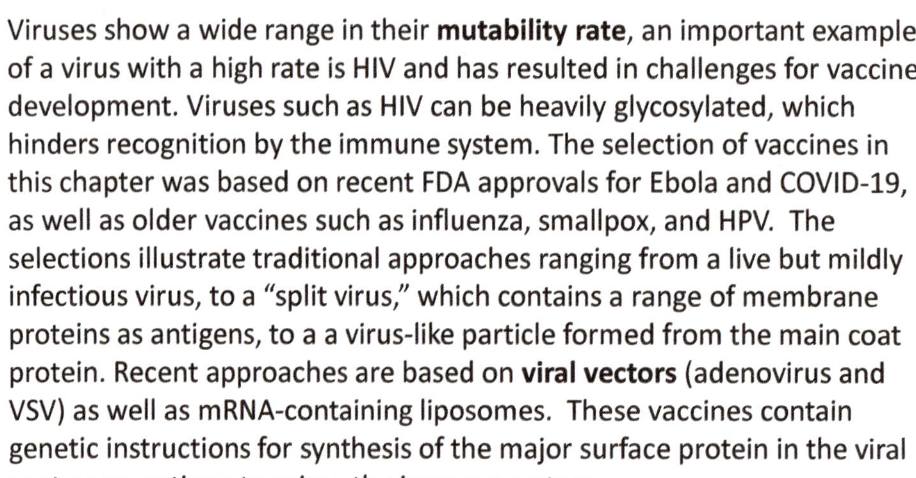

Viruses show a wide range in their **mutability rate**, an important example of a virus with a high rate is HIV and has resulted in challenges for vaccine development. Viruses such as HIV can be heavily glycosylated, which hinders recognition by the immune system. The selection of vaccines in this chapter was based on recent FDA approvals for Ebola and COVID-19, as well as older vaccines such as influenza, smallpox, and HPV. The selections illustrate traditional approaches ranging from a live but mildly infectious virus, to a "split virus," which contains a range of membrane proteins as antigens, to a a virus-like particle formed from the main coat protein. Recent approaches are based on **viral vectors** (adenovirus and VSV) as well as mRNA-containing liposomes. These vaccines contain genetic instructions for synthesis of the major surface protein in the viral coat as an antigen to prime the immune system.

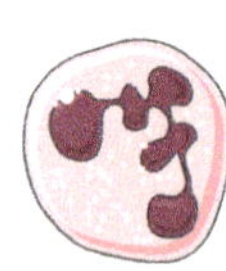

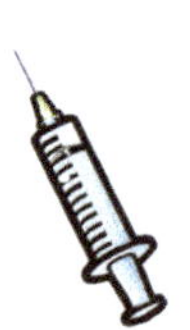

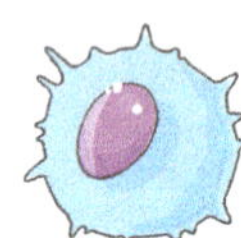

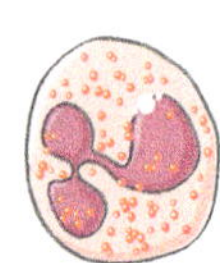

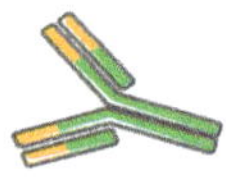

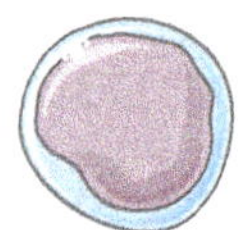

Introduction: Diversity of DNA and RNA viruses

Sources of diversity

Enveloped viruses are composed of an envelope and nucleocapsid and nucleic acid and are more sensitive to environmental conditions.

Nonenveloped viruses are composed of capsid protein and nucleic acid.

The **viral envelope (**derived from the host cell membranes) and capsid **protects genetic material** when traveling between host cells.

Virus size ranges from 20 to 500 nm.

Genome sizes ranges from 2 to 30 kb, which codes for ~3 to 12+ genes.

1. Lipid-protein envelope
2. Additional capsid
3. Different enzymes for replication
4. Viral genome is either single or double stranded RNA or DNA
5. **Glycoproteins** on the surface bind to host's cell membrane

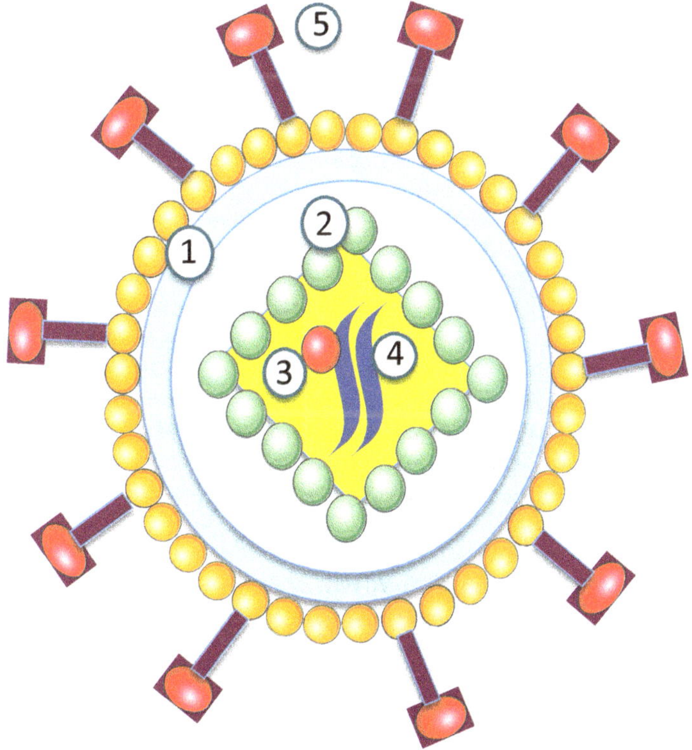

RNA viruses
- Astrovirus (diarrhea)
- Coronaviruses
- Coxsackie (hand, foot, mouth disease)
- Dengue virus
- Echovirus (meningitis)
- Ebola virus
- Human immunodeficiency virus
- Human T-cell leukemia virus
- Hepatitis A, C, and E viruses
- Measles virus
- Mumps virus
- Norovirus
- Parainfluenza virus
- Poliovirus
- Respiratory syncytial virus
- Rotavirus (gastroenteritis)
- Yellow fever virus
- West Nile virus
- Zika virus

DNA viruses.
- Adenovirus (respiratory, GI infections)
- BK virus (nephropathy)
- Cytomegalovirus (retinitis)
- Epstein–Barr virus (mononucleosis)
- Hepatitis B virus
- Herpes simplex virus-1 (cold sores)
- Herpes simplex virus-2 (genital herpes)
- Human herpes viruses 6 and 7 (roseola)
- Human herpes viruses 8 (Kaposi's sarcoma)
- JC virus (leukoencephalopathy
- Papillomavirus (cervical cancer)
- Parvovirus B19 (Fifth disease)
- Variola virus (smallpox)
- Varicella–Zoster virus (chickenpox and shingles)

Introduction: The complexity of RNA and DNA viruses

RNA viruses

Replication of the RNA genome

Single-stranded RNA viruses have **2 possible genomes**
- Sense or "plus" (+) strand
- Nonsense or "minus" (−) strand

RNA (+strand) acts as a mRNA and is immediately translated but **RNA (−strand) must be copied** to the complementary +−sense mRNA by a viral RNA-dependent RNA-polymerase (RdRp).

RNA viruses replicate their genomes by **two unique pathways**
- RNA-dependent RNA synthesis
- Retroviruses use RNA-dependent DNA synthesis (reverse transcription)

Double-stranded RNA viruses contain RNA synthesizing enzymes to generate single-stranded RNA (+−sense) genomes in the host cell.

A retrovirus inserts a copy of its genome into the infected host cell DNA with changes in the host genome.
If integration occurs in germline cells, the changes can be passed onto subsequent generations.

Viral mutations

Reverse transcriptase (RT) enzymes, which copy RNA into DNA have a **low-fidelity proofreading function** to check for any resulting errors. This is a major mechanism for generating genetic variation within retroviral populations. For example, the great diversity of HIV-1 stems from its high rate of spontaneous mutation.

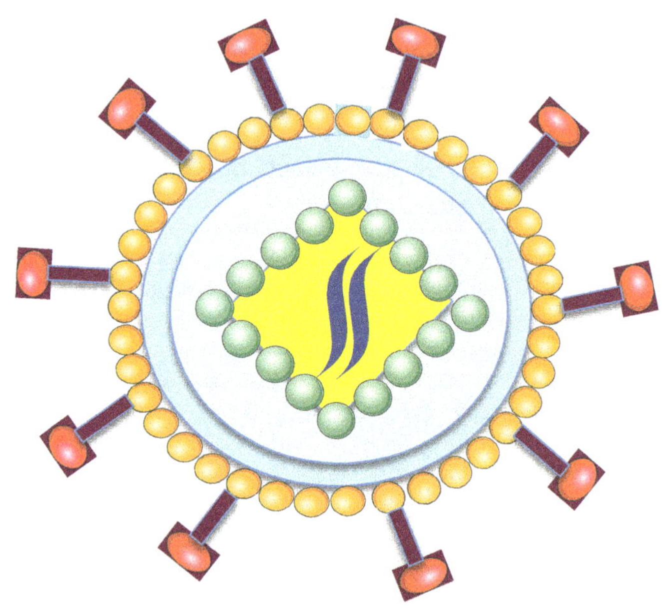

The high mutation rates of RNA viruses results in enhanced virulence, ability to emerge in novel hosts, and escape vaccine-induced immunity. These genetic changes are passed on to the viral progeny in successive infection cycles.

Human cancer cases are associated with RNA viruses
- Important examples include HTLV-1 (adult T-cell leukemia [ATL]) and hepatitis C virus.
- Associated diseases are adult T-cell leukemia and hepatocellular carcinoma.

The properties of RNA viruses

Influenza (flu) virus

Influenza A is a spherical virus (80–120 nm) with a negative-sense, **single-stranded RNA genome** (13.6 kb) of eight segments coding for 11 different proteins. The genome is replicated in the nucleus of infected cells by **viral RNA polymerase** to produce positive sense full-length complementary RNA, which serves as templates for new viral RNA.

Hemagglutinin has a role in both **attachment of the virus** and then fusion with the host cell membrane.

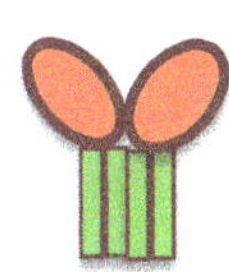

Hemagglutinin binds to epithelial cells present in the human respiratory tract. The targets are surface receptors with sialic acid attached to the outermost ends of polysaccharide chains.

Neuraminidase removes sialic acid from surface glycoprotein receptors on the host cell, releasing mature virus particles.

Negative-sense, single-stranded, segmented RNA.

NP **nucleoprotein** encapsulates viral RNA genome.

RNA polymerase (PB1, PB2, PA).

M2 ion channel equilibrates viral membrane pH during cell entry.

M1 matrix protein.

NEP (NS2) protein **exports viral RNA to host nucleus.**

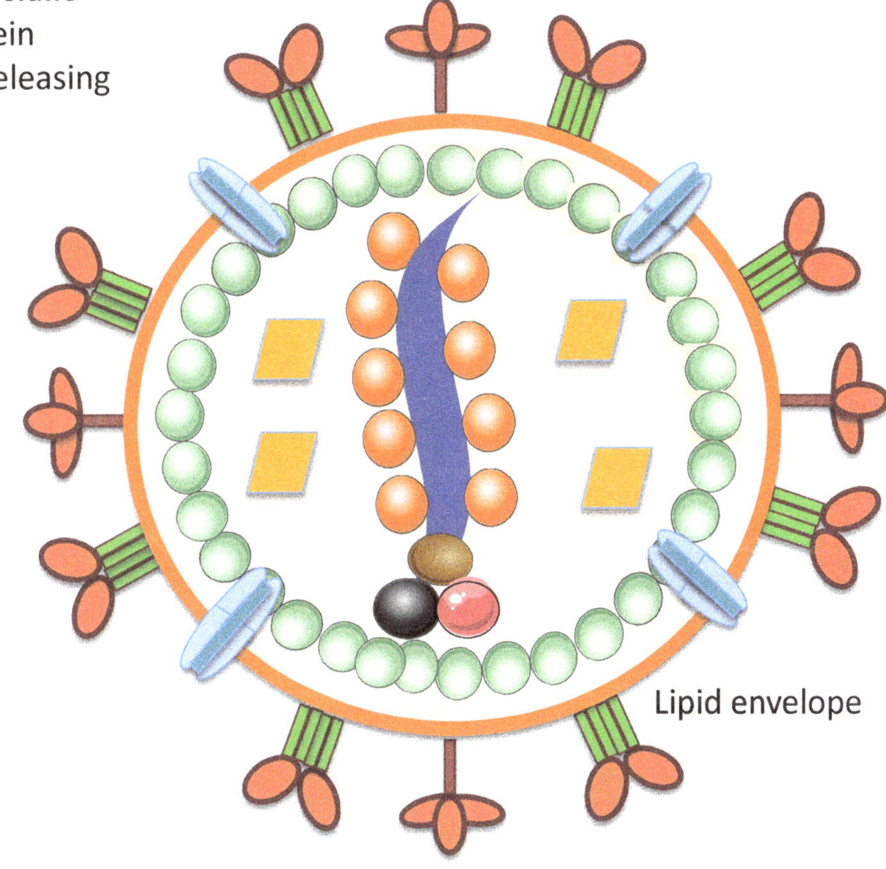

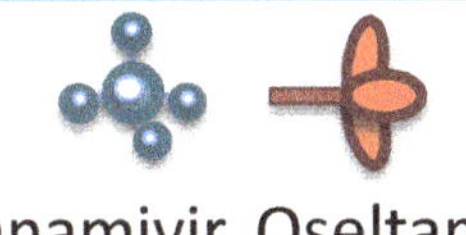

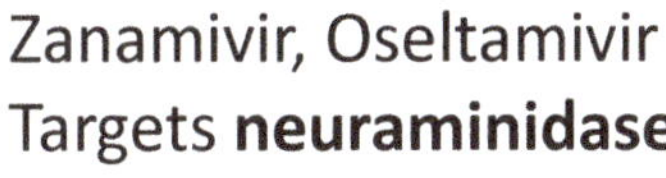

Zanamivir, Oseltamivir Targets **neuraminidase**

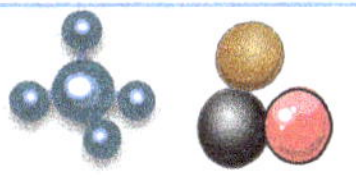

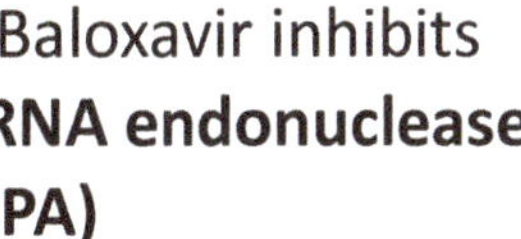

Baloxavir inhibits **RNA endonuclease (PA)**

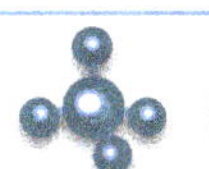

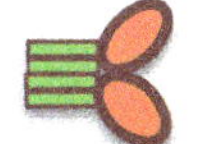

Influenza vaccine major antigen, **hemagglutinin**

RNA viruses: Description of the influenza virus

The disease: Influenza

Influenza is an acute viral infection of epithelial cells in the respiratory tract (nose, throat, lungs) with sudden onset of high fever, cough, and inflammation of the upper respiratory tree and trachea.

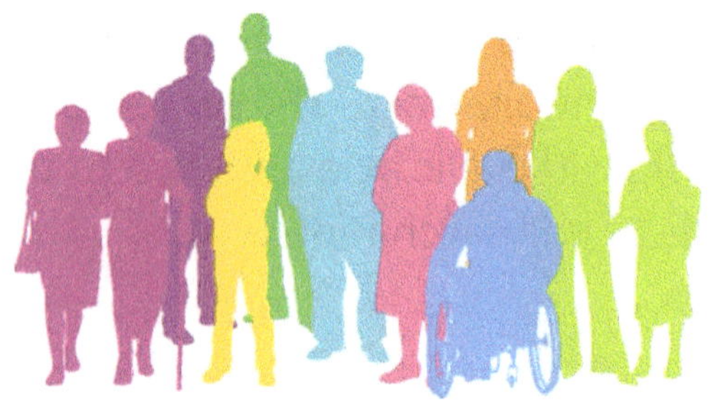

Incidence by gender and ethnicity

The highest influenza hospitalization rates were as follows: non-Latino Black, American Indian or Alaska Native people, Latino people, and non-Latino white people. Children younger than 18 are more than twice as likely to develop a symptomatic flu infection than adults 65 and older.

Disease symptoms

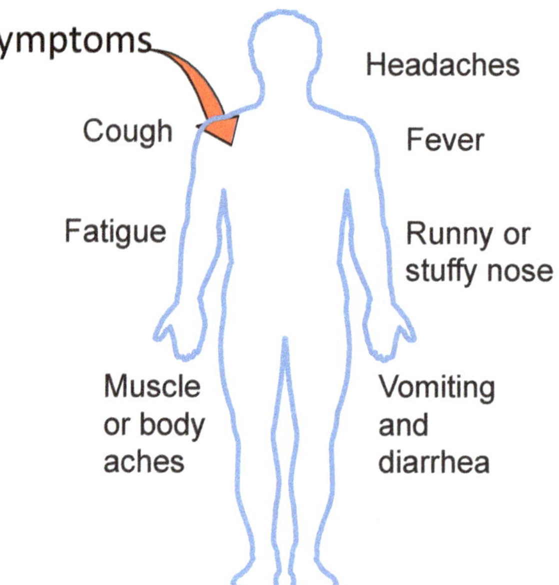

The medicine

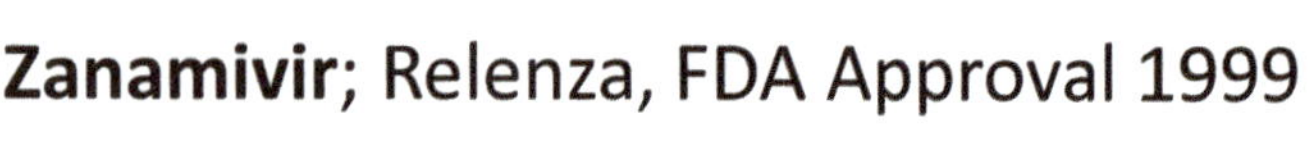

Zanamivir; Relenza, FDA Approval 1999

Oseltamivir; Tamiflu, FDA Approval 1999

Zanamivir and Oseltamivir are oral anti-viral medicines for **treatment over 5 days of acute uncomplicated illness due to influenza A and B virus** for patients who have been symptomatic for no more than 2 days. The medicines inhibit influenza virus neuraminidase, which blocks the influenza virus escape the host cell and infect other cells.

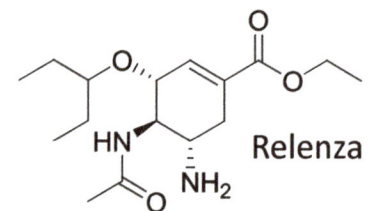

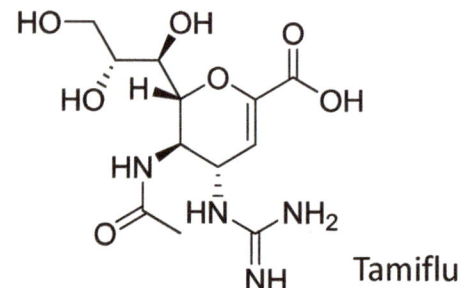

Relenza

Tamiflu

Influenza treatment: Neuraminidase inhibition, Zanamivir, Oseltamivir.

Action of Zanamivir and Oseltamivir on cell and disease biology

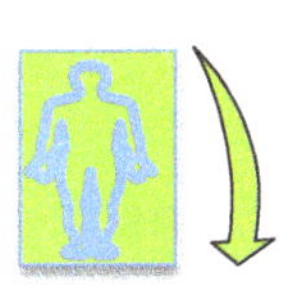

① **Epithelial cells** of the lung located at the surface interface serve many important functions including **barrier protection.**

② The surface of epithelial cells contain glycoconjugates (membrane proteins and lipids) with sialic acids on the outermost ends.

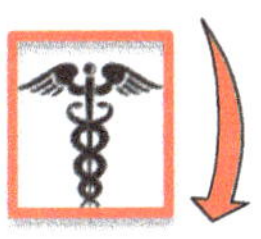

③-⑤ **Viral binding via hemagglutinin** onto sialic acid—glycoproteins present on the targeted cell surfaces.

⑥ **Viral particle released from cell surface (budding)** by cleavage of receptor sialic acid on cellular surface by the viral neuraminidase.

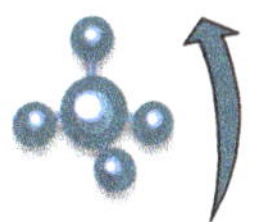

⑦ **Zanamivir and Oseltamivir inhibit influenza virus neuraminidase**, which renders the virus unable to escape the host cell and infect other cells.

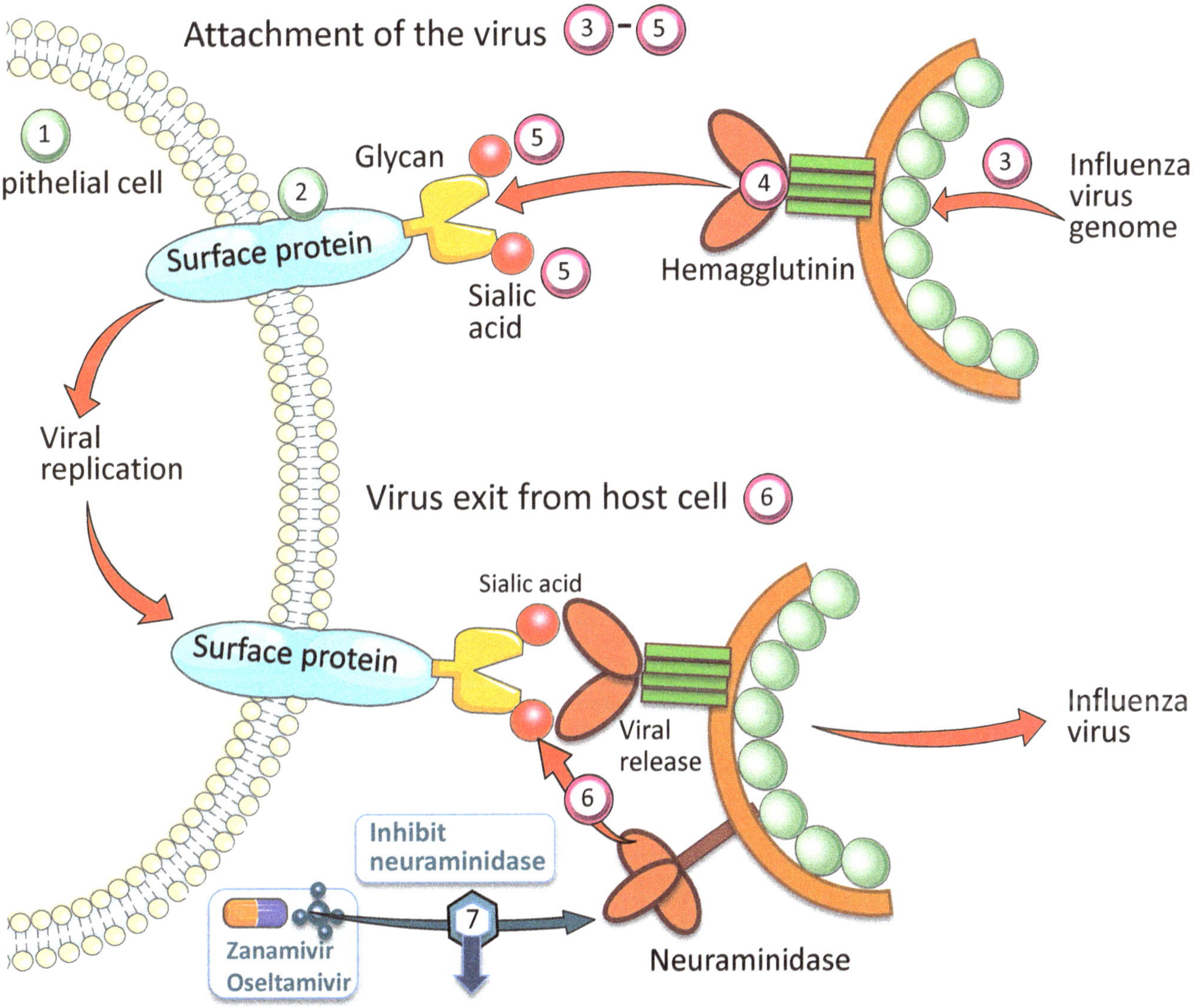

Attachment of the virus ③-⑤

① Epithelial cell

② Surface protein

Glycan ⑤

Sialic acid ⑤

④ Hemagglutinin

③ Influenza virus genome

Viral replication

Virus exit from host cell ⑥

Surface protein

Sialic acid

Viral release

Influenza virus

⑥

Inhibit neuraminidase

Zanamivir Oseltamivir

⑦

Neuraminidase

Influenza treatment: Neuraminidase inhibition, Zanamivir, Oseltamivir.

The disease: Influenza

Acute, uncomplicated influenza for patients who have been symptomatic for no more than 48 hours and who are at high risk of developing flu-related complications.

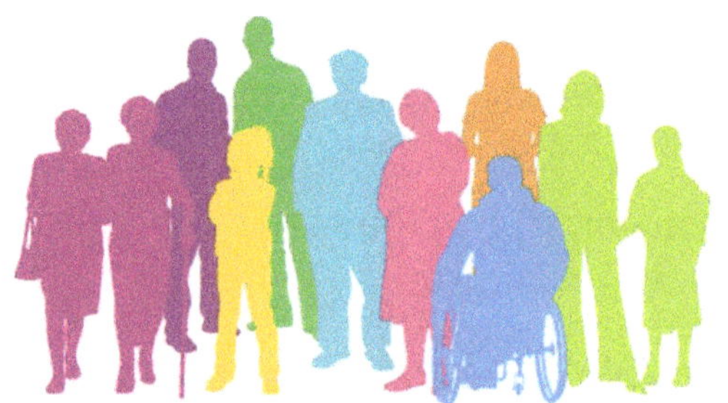

Incidence by gender and ethnicity

People had the highest influenza hospitalization rates were in the following order: non-Latino Black, American Indian or Alaska Native people, Latino people, and non-Latino white people. Children younger than 18 are more than twice as likely to develop a symptomatic flu infection than adults 65 and older.

Disease symptoms

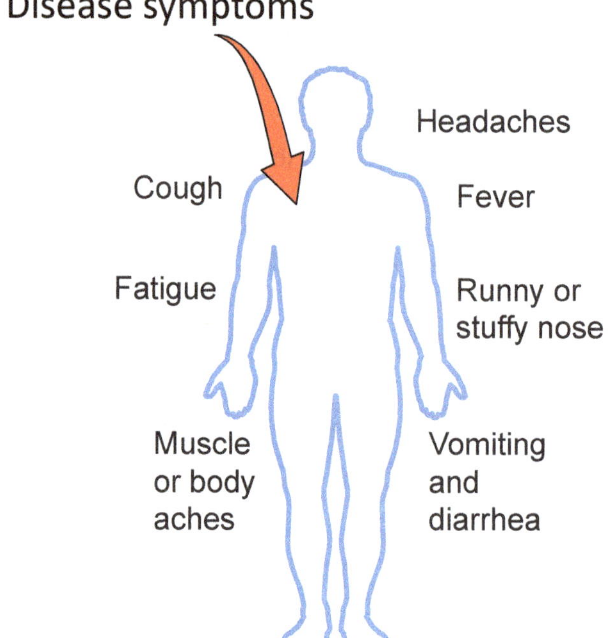

The medicine

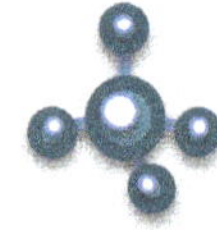

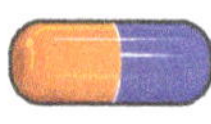

Baloxavir; Xofluza, FDA Approval 2018

Baloxavir is a one-dose oral medicine that **inhibits influenza virus mRNA synthesis in the nucleus of the host cell**. Proteins needed for the construction of new influenza virions cannot be synthesized in the presence of the drug.

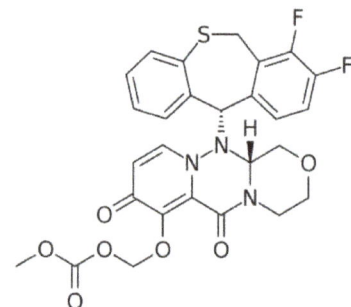

Influenza treatment: Inhibition of influenza viral RNA translation, Baloxavir

Action of Baloxavir on cell and disease biology

1 Influenza virus genome is a negative antisense strand RNA, which is divided into eight viral RNA segments including a "cap" removing endonuclease.

2 The minus strand is noncoding and must be copied with RNA polymerase to produce a translatable **positive sense viral mRNA**.

3 The **cap structure** on mRNA protects from degradation by cellular nucleases and prevents recognition by host immunity mechanisms.

4 The **viral mRNA** is translated into proteins necessary for production of new **viral proteins** by the host ribosomes.

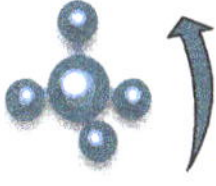

Baloxavir selectively **inhibits RNA endonuclease**.

1 Negative strand viral RNA

Cytoplasm

Nucleus

Nuclear pore

2

Noncoding viral RNA

RNA polymerase

Positive sense viral RNA with cap

3 Cap-dependent endonuclease

Baloxavir Inhibits RNA endonuclease

5

Positive sense viral RNA

4

Viral protein synthesis in cytoplasm

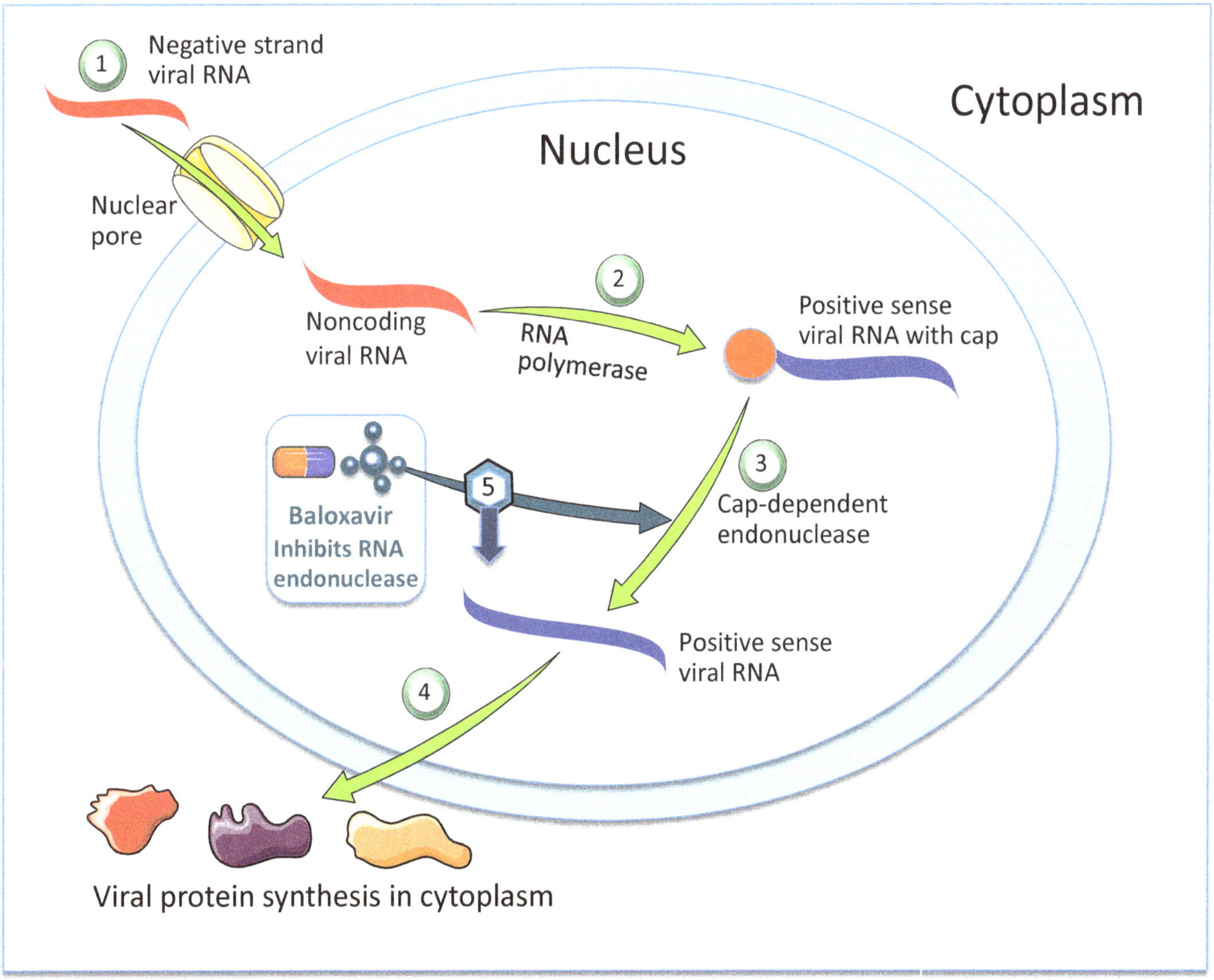

Influenza treatment: Inhibition of influenza viral RNA translation, Baloxavir

The disease: Influenza

Influenza is an acute disease with **infection of epithelial cells** in the respiratory tract with sudden onset of high fever, cough, and inflammation of the upper respiratory tree and trachea.

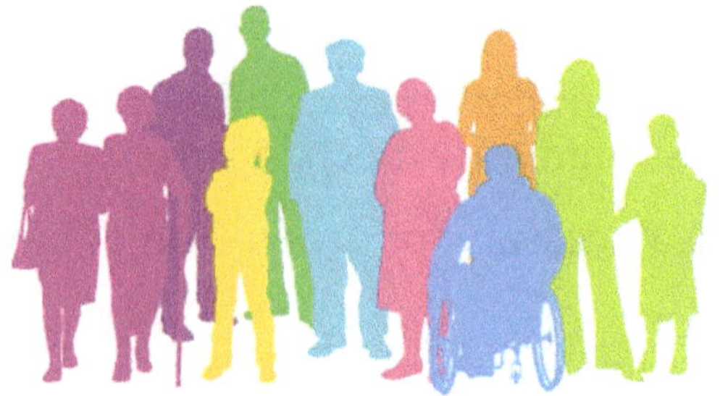

Incidence by gender and ethnicity

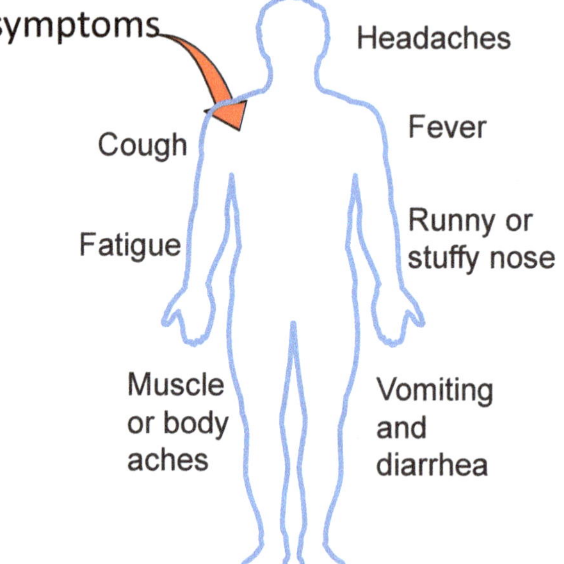

People had the highest influenza hospitalization rates were in the following order: non-Latino Black, American Indian or Alaska Native people, Latino people, and non-Latino white people. Children younger than 18 are more than twice as likely to develop a symptomatic flu infection than adults 65 and older.

The medicine

Fluzone; FDA Approval 2019

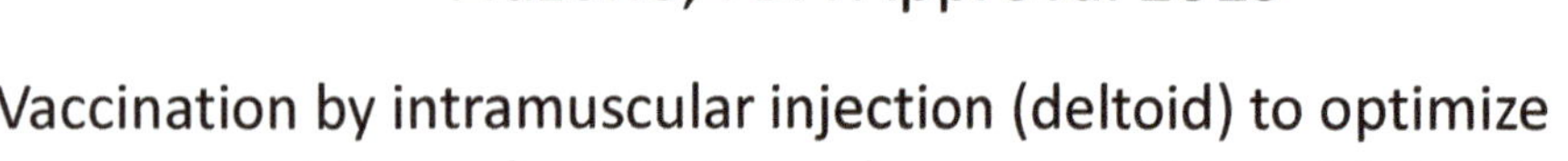

Vaccination by intramuscular injection (deltoid) to optimize immunogenicity and minimizes adverse reactions at injection site.

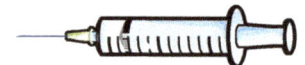

Fluzone high-dose quadrivalent is a vaccine against influenza A and B strains. The 4 strains selected by the World Health Organization for the 2020–2021 influenza season are based on the antigenic properties of the viral hemagglutinin (Type A—H1N1 and H3N2-like lineages and Type B—Victoria and Yamagata-like lineages).

The egg derived virus is disrupted with a nonionic surfactant to produce a **"split virus**" that contains membrane fragments with hemagglutinin antigen (HA) and neuraminidase **(**NA) but with removal of the viral RNA and is then concentrated.

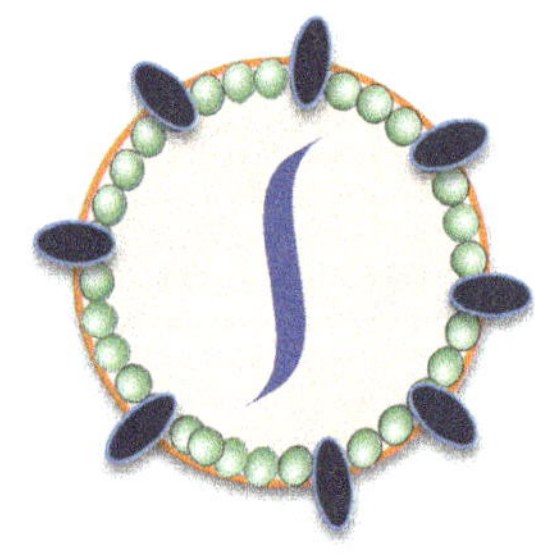

Influenza treatment: Vaccination with a split virus preparation, Fluzone

Action of Fluzone on cell and disease biology

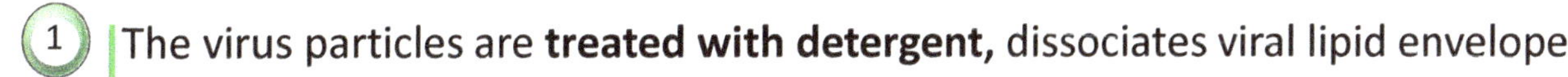

1. The virus particles are **treated with detergent,** dissociates viral lipid envelope.
2. **Viral hemagglutinin (HA)** is the major influenza antigenic protein.
3. HA binds to antigen presenting cells (APCs) via surface sialic acid.
4. **MHC II presents HA fragments** to helper T-cells, which recognize influenza virus antigens, whereas antibodies target surface-exposed viral proteins.

5. **Fluzone is a split virus vaccine** that produces a humoral immune response, promote cytokine release, B cell proliferation, and **antibody production**.
6. **Antibodies target HA** to neutralize virus and prevent infection and disease.

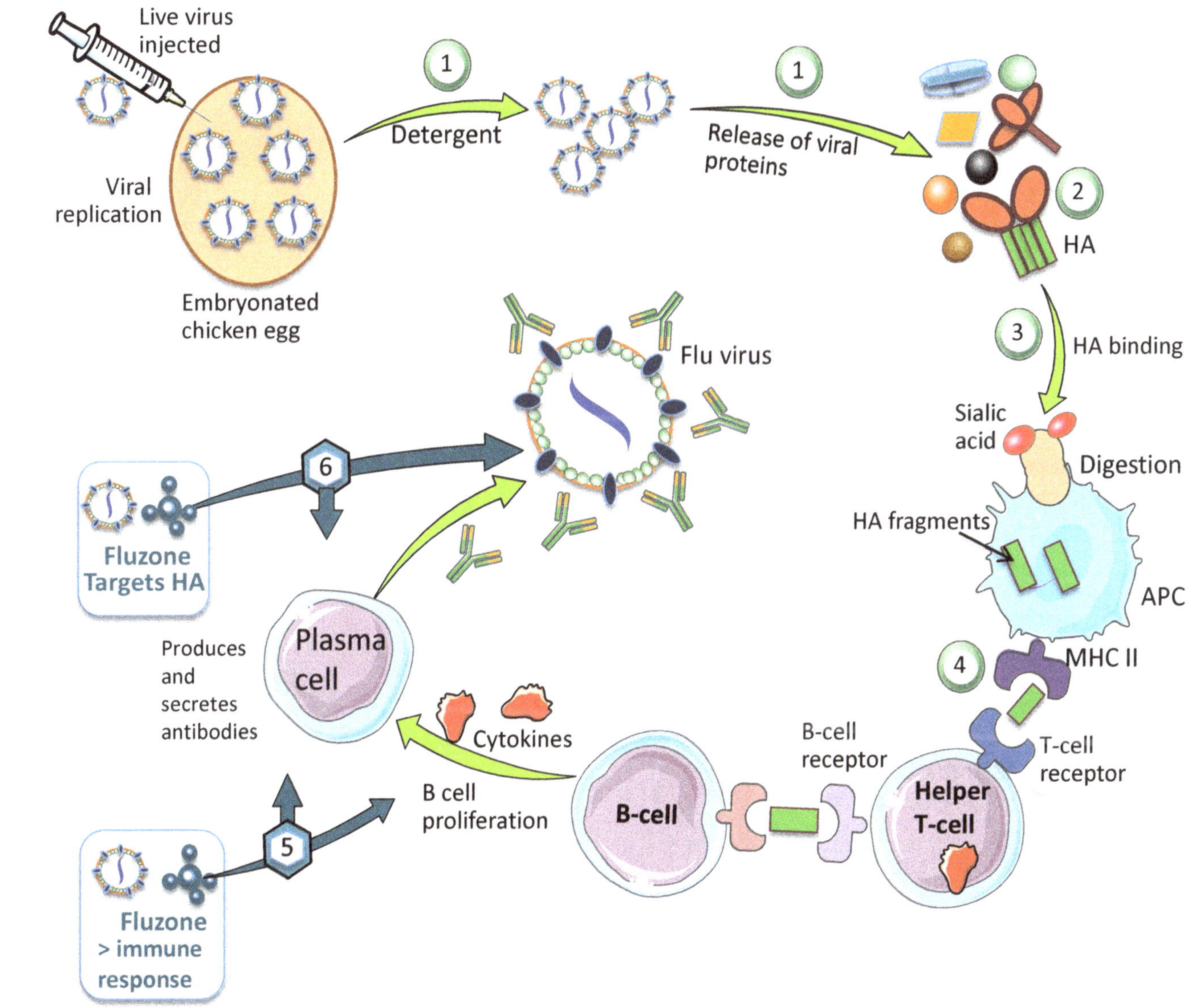

Influenza treatment: Vaccination with a split virus preparation, Fluzone

Human immunodeficiency virus (HIV)

Acquired immunodeficiency syndrome (AIDS) is a chronic, potentially life-threatening condition caused by the human immunodeficiency virus (HIV) with the resulting severe damage to the immune system and inability to fight infection and disease.

The virus is spherical (120 nm) and composed of a capsid core containing two folded helices of **RNA genetic material** (9.6 kb) surrounded by a protein envelope. The HIV-1 genome encodes nine open reading frames which code for 15 viral proteins.

The viral RNA genome is **reverse transcribed** into double-stranded DNA. The viral DNA is then integrated into the cellular DNA of CD4$^+$ cells.

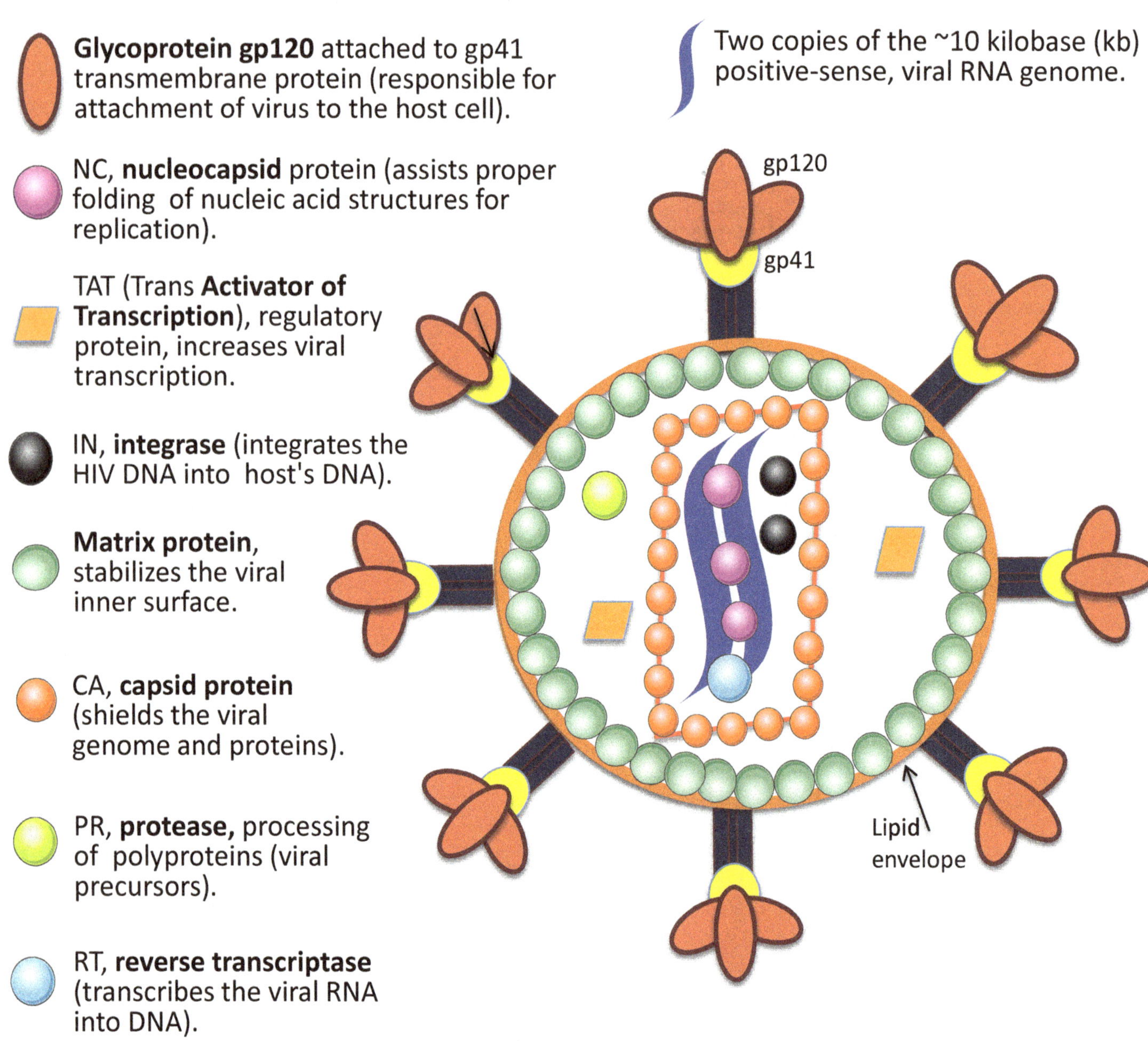

Glycoprotein gp120 attached to gp41 transmembrane protein (responsible for attachment of virus to the host cell).
Two copies of the ~10 kilobase (kb) positive-sense, viral RNA genome.
NC, nucleocapsid protein (assists proper folding of nucleic acid structures for replication).
TAT (Trans Activator of Transcription), regulatory protein, increases viral transcription.
IN, integrase (integrates the HIV DNA into host's DNA).
Matrix protein, stabilizes the viral inner surface.
CA, capsid protein (shields the viral genome and proteins).
PR, protease, processing of polyproteins (viral precursors).
RT, reverse transcriptase (transcribes the viral RNA into DNA).
gp120
gp41
Lipid envelope

RNA viruses: Structure of the HIV virus

Acquired immunodeficiency syndrome (AIDS) pathogenesis results in a progressive depletion of $CD4^{+}$ T-cell populations and is accompanied by impairment of cellular immunity and increasing susceptibility to opportunistic infections.

HIV is classified as a **retrovirus**, which uses reverse transcriptase to copy its RNA genome into DNA.

1. HIV infects human immune cells to replicate.
2. Adsorption and uncoating of viral RNA.
3. Transcribes viral RNA into DNA.
4. Viral DNA imported, **integrated** into host DNA.

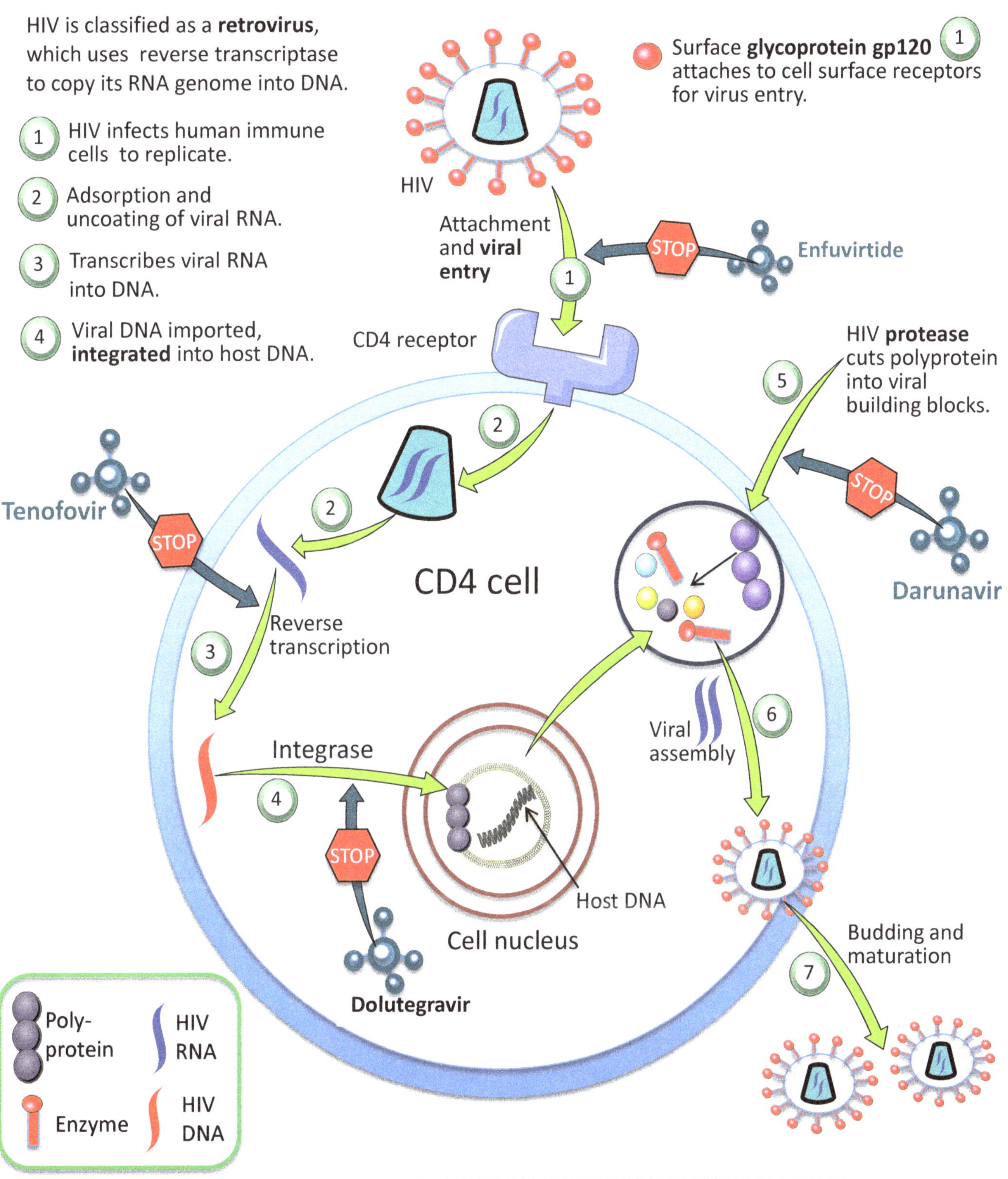

RNA viruses: HIV infection of immune cells

The disease: Acquired immunodeficiency syndrome (AIDS)

Acquired immunodeficiency syndrome (AIDS) is a chronic, sexually transmitted infection caused by the human immunodeficiency virus (HIV).

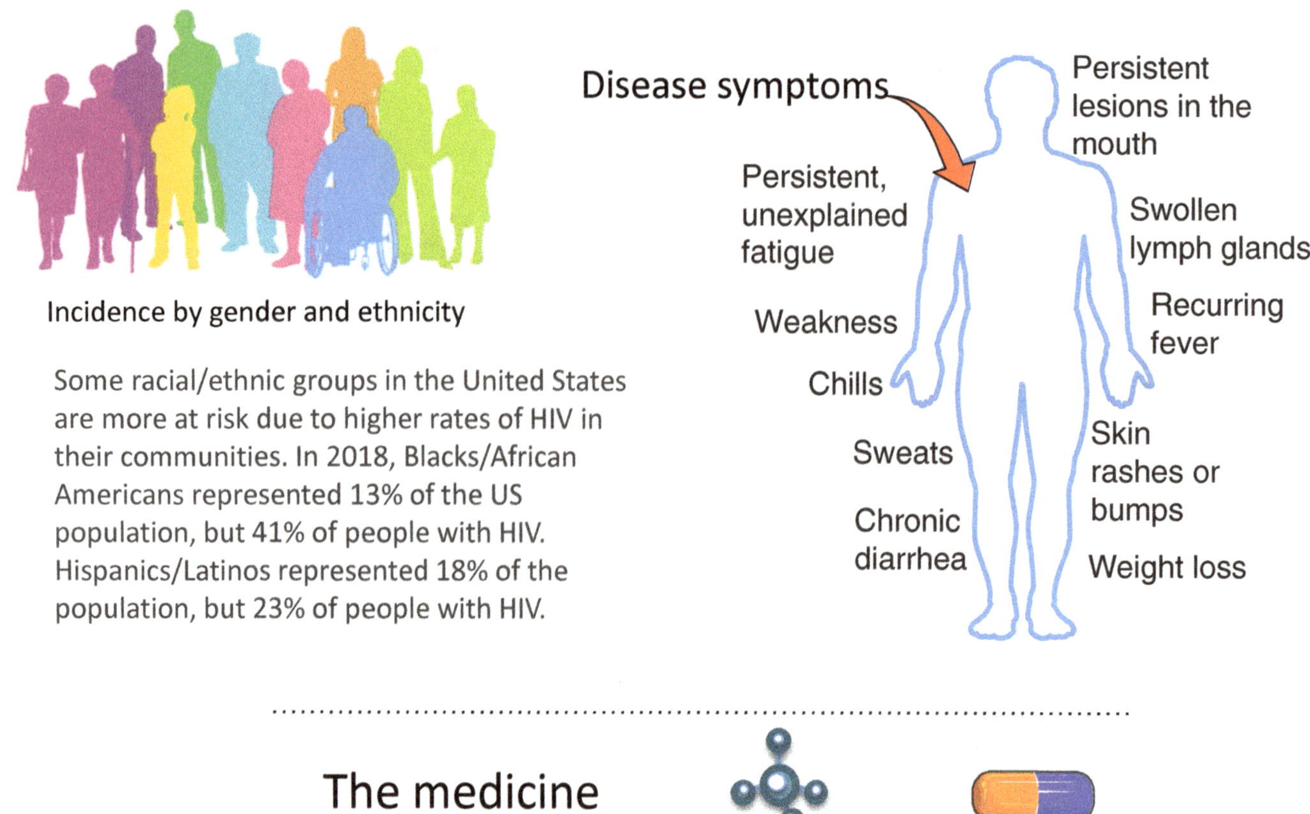

Incidence by gender and ethnicity

Some racial/ethnic groups in the United States are more at risk due to higher rates of HIV in their communities. In 2018, Blacks/African Americans represented 13% of the US population, but 41% of people with HIV. Hispanics/Latinos represented 18% of the population, but 23% of people with HIV.

The medicine

Tenofovir disoproxil; Viread , FDA Approval 2001

Tenofovir is a **nucleotide reverse transcriptase inhibitor**, which decreases HIV levels in the blood, reduces damage to the immune system and the risk of AIDS-related illnesses.

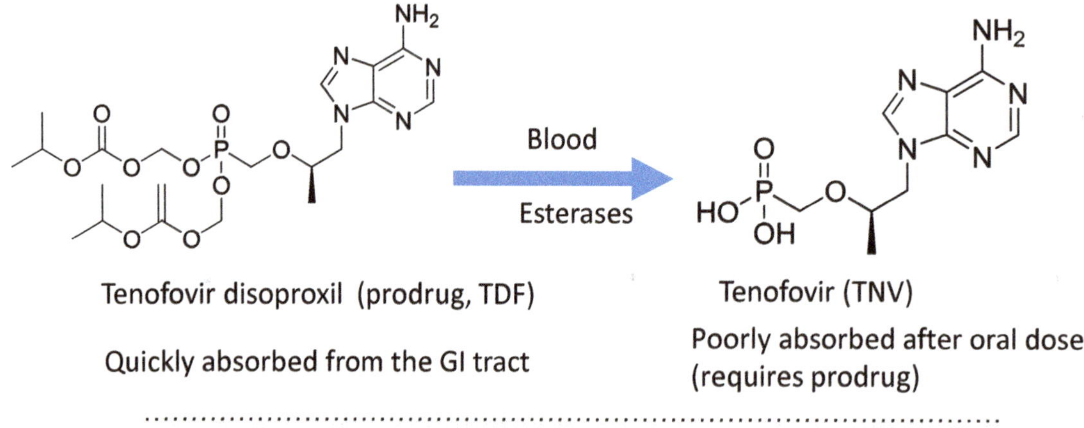

Tenofovir disoproxil (prodrug, TDF)

Quickly absorbed from the GI tract

Tenofovir (TNV)

Poorly absorbed after oral dose (requires prodrug)

AIDS: Inhibition of HIV reverse transcription, Tenofovir disoproxil

Action of Tenofovir on cell and disease biology

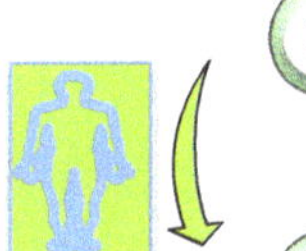

1 **HIV reverse transcriptase** (DNA polymerase) converts single-stranded viral RNA genome into double-stranded DNA (dsDNA) to integrate into host genome.

2 The four common deoxyribonucleotides present in deoxyribonucleic acid, DNA, are deoxyadenosine (dA), deoxyguanosine (dG), deoxythymidine (dT), and deoxycytosine (dC).

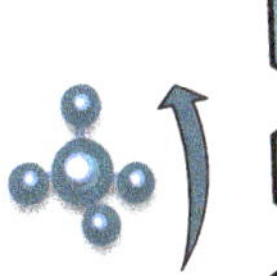

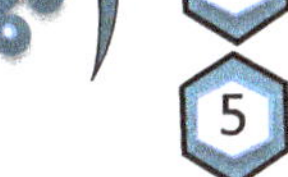

3 **Prodrug TDF** is rapidly converted by serum esterases to Tenofovir (TNV).

4 Tenofovir is **phosphorylated** by host nucleotide kinases to TDP.

5 **TDP inhibits reverse transcriptase** via viral DNA chain termination by competing with dATP, which prevents viral replication.

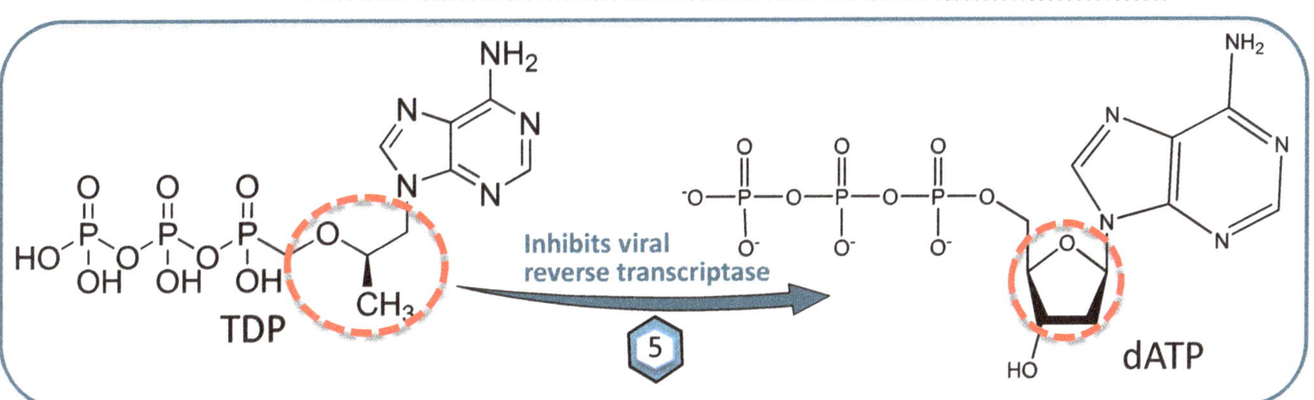

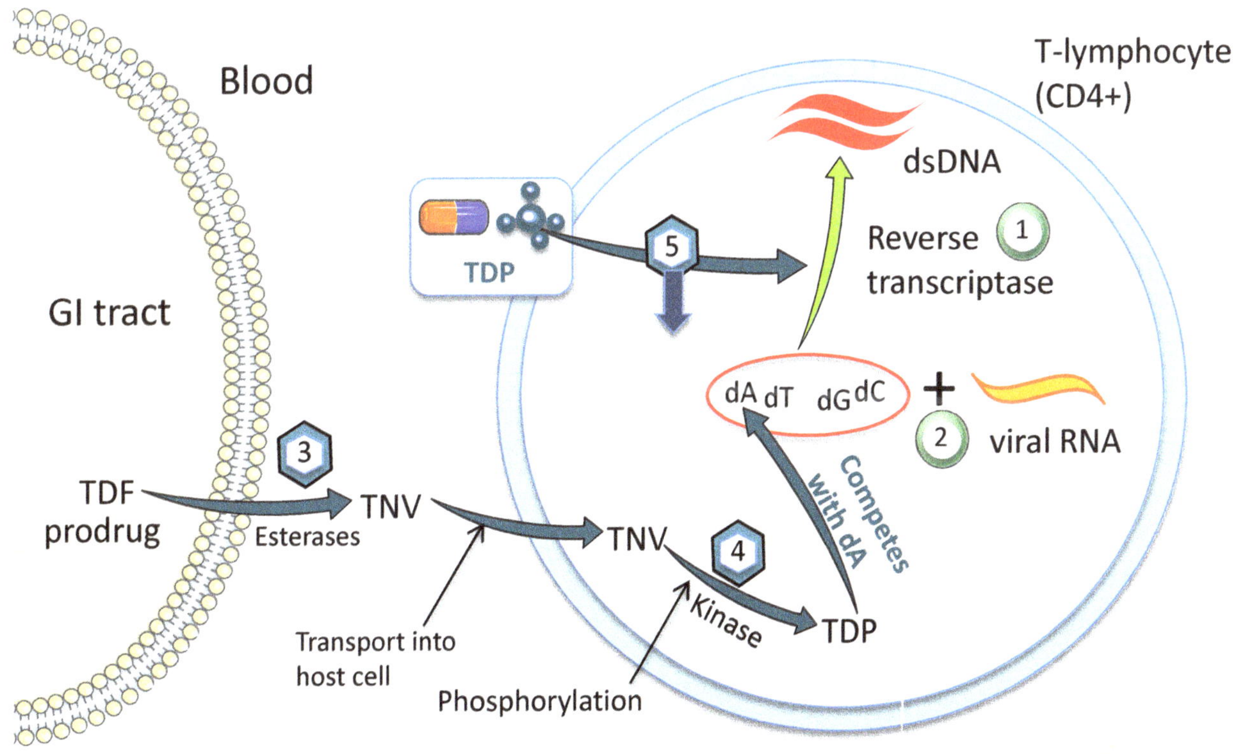

AIDS: Inhibition of HIV reverse transcription, Tenofovir disoproxil

The disease: Acquired immunodeficiency syndrome (AIDS)

Acquired immunodeficiency syndrome (AIDS) is a chronic, sexually transmitted infection caused by the human immunodeficiency virus (HIV).

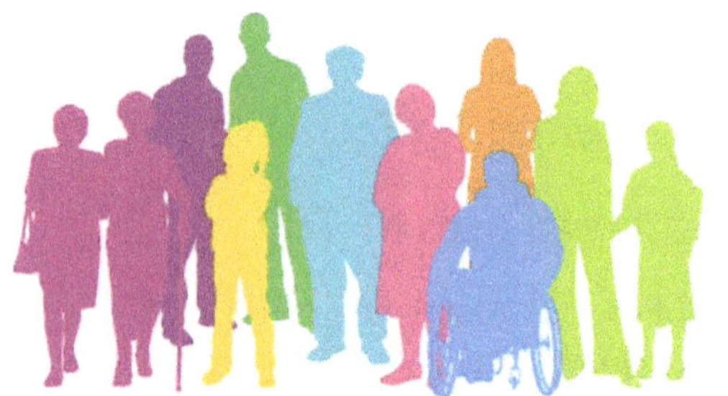

Incidence by gender and ethnicity

Some racial/ethnic groups in the United States are more at risk due to higher rates of HIV in their communities. In 2018, Blacks/African Americans represented 13% of the US population, but 41% of people with HIV. Hispanics/Latinos represented 18% of the population, but 23% of people with HIV.

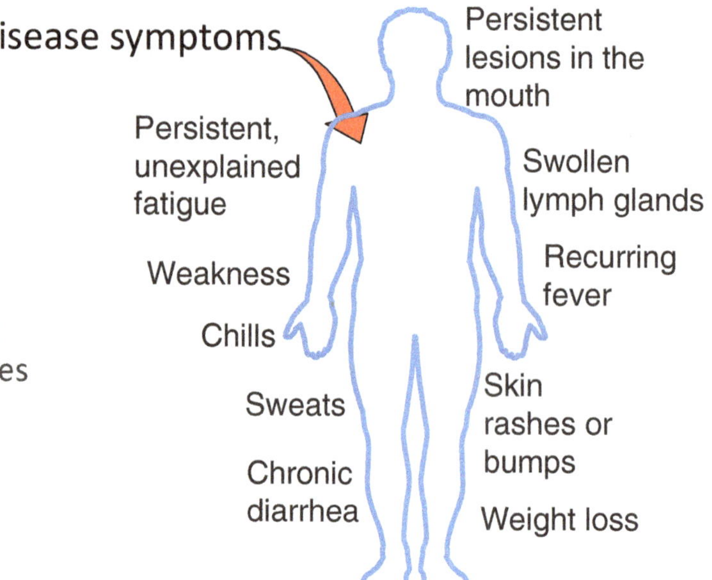

The medicine

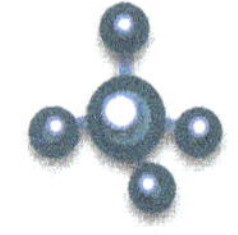

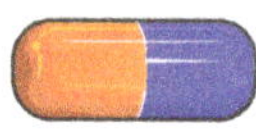

Darunavir; Prezista, FDA Approval 2006

Darunavir is a **protease inhibitor** used with other HIV protease inhibitor drugs to slow HIV replication and decreases the amount of virus in the blood with delayed damage to the immune system. As a second-generation protease inhibitor, darunavir is designed to combat resistance to standard HIV therapy.

AIDS: Inhibition of HIV protease polyprotein cleavage, Darunavir.

Action of Darunavir on cell and disease biology

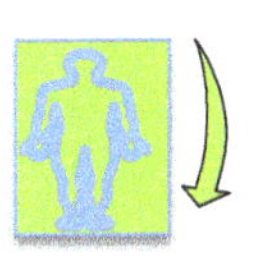
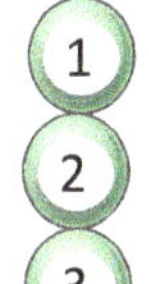

1 2 3 The HIV genome encodes 15 viral proteins, which are synthesized as **polyproteins,** which on **cleavage** with **HIV protease** produce proteins for virion interior (Gag), viral enzymes (Pol), or glycoproteins of the virus envelope (env).

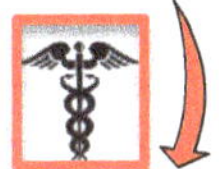

4 During HIV infection, the immature **polyprotein is cleaved** by **HIV protease** to form the viral proteins needed to form immature viral particles.

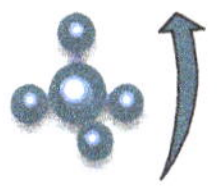

5 Darunavir is an **inhibitor of HIV-1 protease**, which blocks the polyprotein from binding to the enzyme active site and thus prevents viral replication.

Gag Pol Env

HIV protease

Polyprotein

Darunavir
Inhibit HIV-1 protease

Gag 1
Core proteins
Matrix
Capsid

Pol 2
Reverse transcriptase
RNAse H
Integrase

Env 3
Envelope protein
gp120
gp41

HIV particle

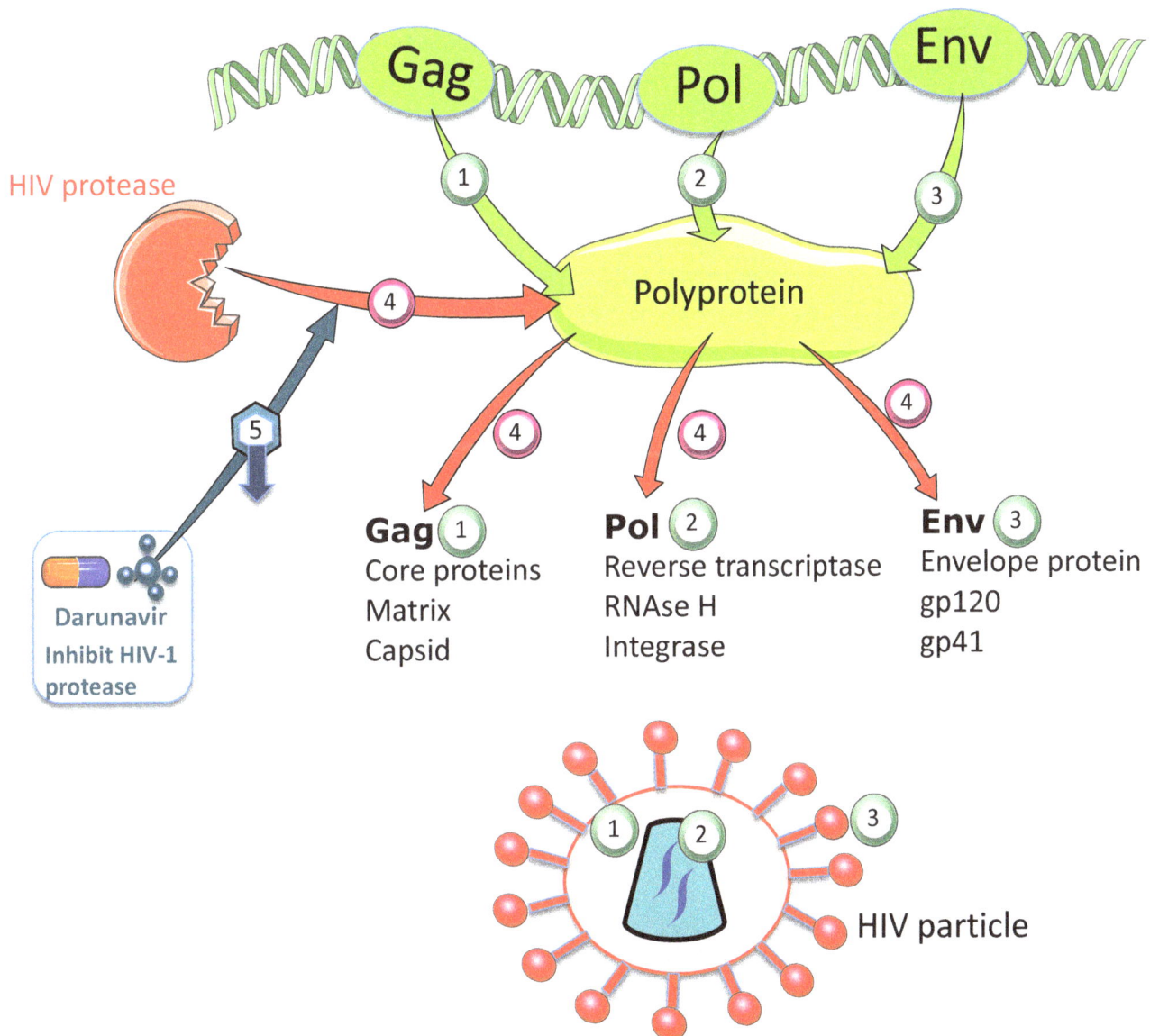

AIDS: Inhibition of HIV protease polyprotein cleavage, Darunavir.

The disease: Acquired immunodeficiency syndrome (AIDS)

Acquired immunodeficiency syndrome (AIDS) is a chronic, sexually transmitted infection caused by the human immunodeficiency virus (HIV).

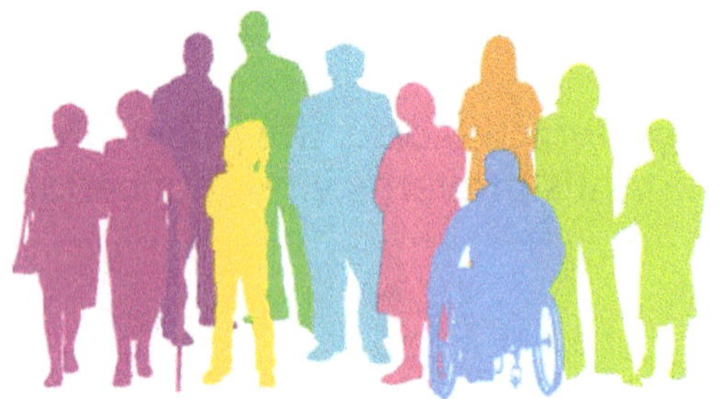

Incidence by gender and ethnicity

Some racial/ethnic groups in the United States are more at risk due to higher rates of HIV in their communities. In 2018, Blacks/African Americans represented 13% of the US population, but 41% of people with HIV. Hispanics/Latinos represented 18% of the population, but 23% of people with HIV.

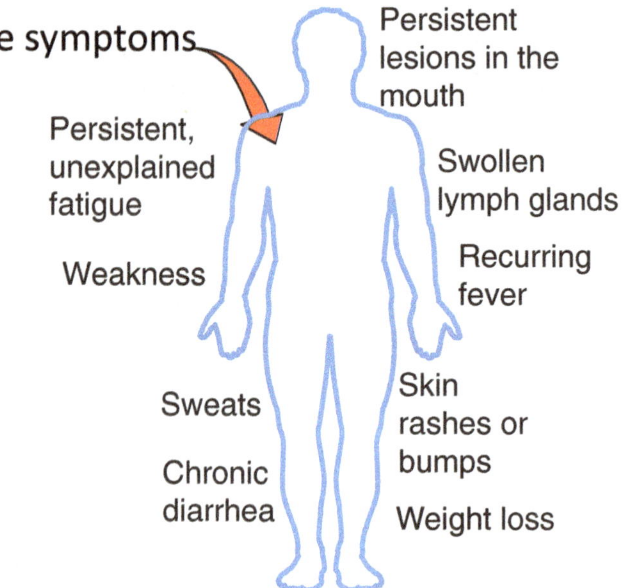

The medicine

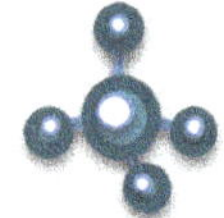

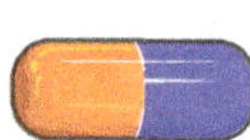

Dolutegravir; Tivicay, FDA Approval 2006

Dolutegravir inhibits HIV's integrase action and blocks the strand transfer step for integration of the viral genome into the host cell and integration into human cells. Due to the uniqueness of the drug action, the treatment has low toxicity. Dolutegravir plus rilpivirine (similar to tenofir) is the first complete two drug treatment of HIV.

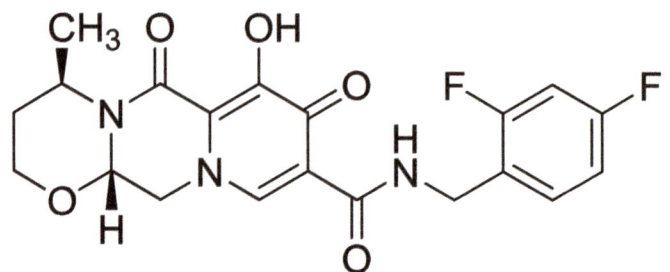

AIDS: Inhibition of HIV integrase, Dolutegravir

Action of Dolutegravir on cell and disease biology

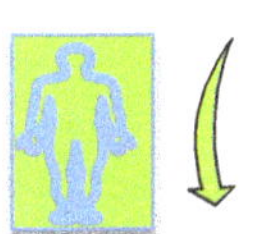

1. In the cytoplasm, viral RNA **is reverse-transcribed to viral DNA.**

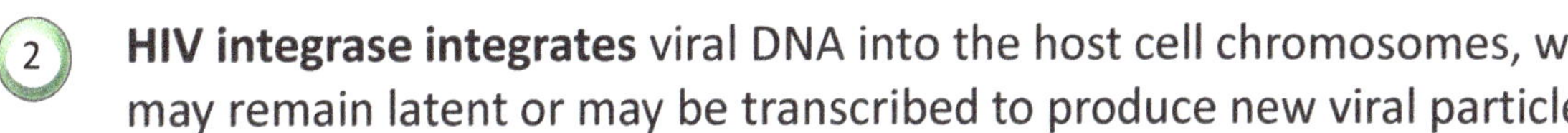

2. **HIV integrase integrates** viral DNA into the host cell chromosomes, which may remain latent or may be transcribed to produce new viral particles.

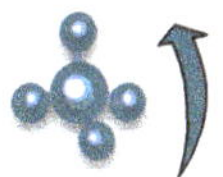

3. Dolutegravir inhibits HIV integrase by binding to the active site and thus blocking the enzyme's ability to catalyze the strand transfer step.

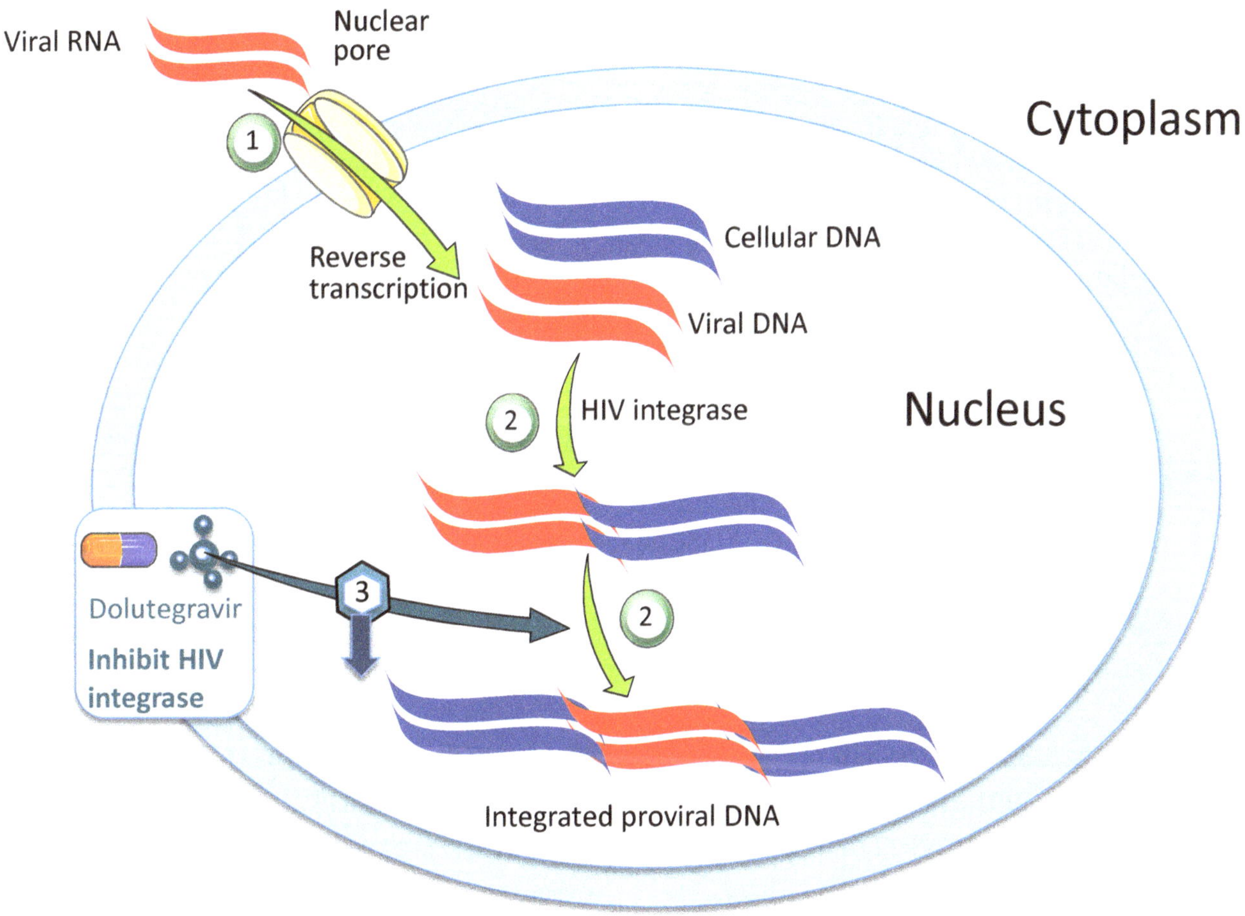

Viral RNA
Nuclear pore
Cytoplasm
1
Reverse transcription
Cellular DNA
Viral DNA
2
HIV integrase
Nucleus
Dolutegravir
Inhibit HIV integrase
3
2
Integrated proviral DNA

AIDS: Inhibition of HIV integrase, Dolutegravir

The disease: Acquired immunodeficiency syndrome (AIDS)

Acquired immunodeficiency syndrome (AIDS) is a chronic, sexually transmitted infection caused by the human immunodeficiency virus (HIV).

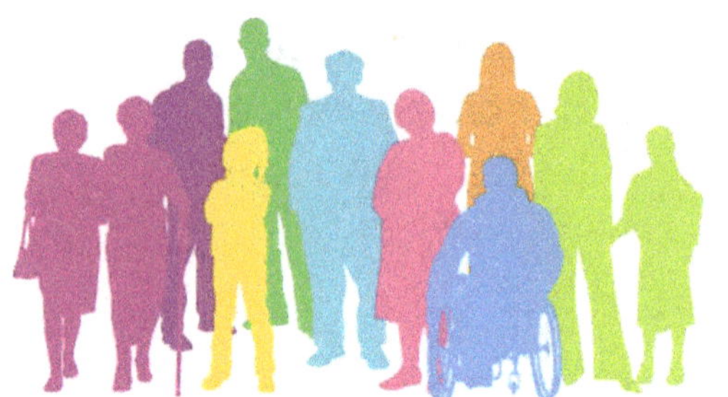

Incidence by gender and ethnicity

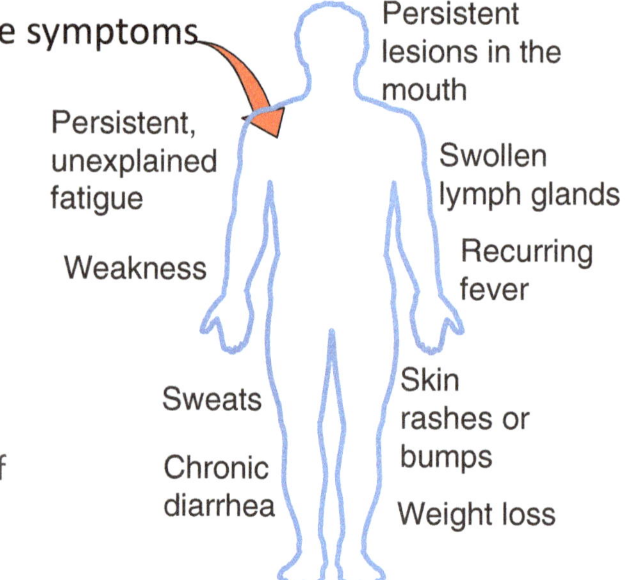

Some racial/ethnic groups in the United States are more at risk due to higher rates of HIV in their communities. In 2018, Blacks/African Americans represented 13% of the US population, but 41% of people with HIV. Hispanics/Latinos represented 18% of the population, but 23% of people with HIV.

The medicine

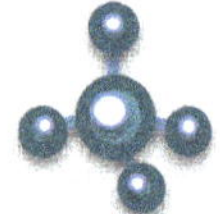

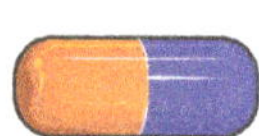

Enfuvirtide; Fuzeon, FDA Approval 2003

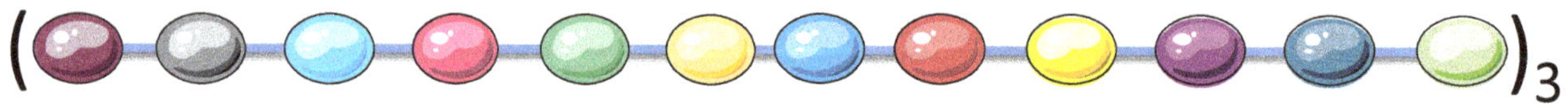

Enfuvirtide is a 36 amino acid synthetic peptide that is first in a novel class of antiretroviral drugs called **HIV fusion inhibitors**. This drug is used with other HIV medications to decrease the amount of HIV resident in the patient's system.

Enfuvirtide is based on the sequence of the HR-2 region of gp41 and **interferes with** the conformational changes required for **membrane fusion.**

AIDS: Inhibition of fusion of HIV genetic material into target cell, Enfuvirtide

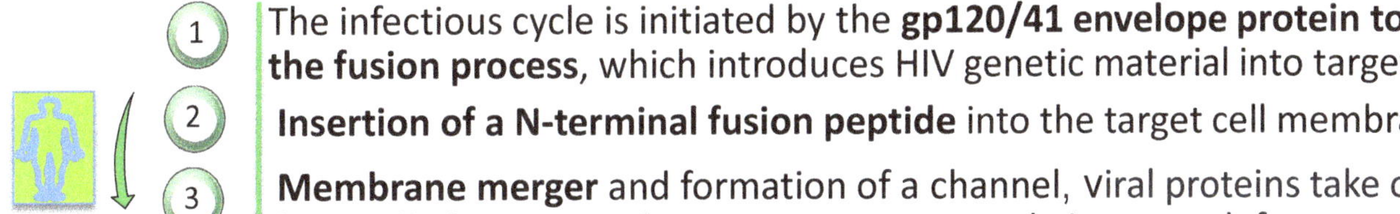

1 The infectious cycle is initiated by the **gp120/41 envelope protein to start the fusion process**, which introduces HIV genetic material into target cells.

2 **Insertion of a N-terminal fusion peptide** into the target cell membrane.

3 **Membrane merger** and formation of a channel, viral proteins take over host cell plasma membrane receptors to evade immune defense systems.

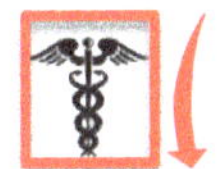

4 HIV-1 activates signaling pathways from the plasma membrane to **initiate viral replication.**

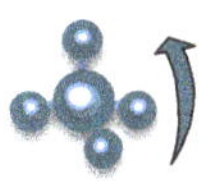

5 **Enfuvirtide** binds to HR1 motif of GP41 fusion peptide, **inhibits the membrane fusion process** and entry of HIV genetic material.

Step 1
Virus attack

T-lymphocyte
(CD4+)

gp120/41

HIV

CD4

1 Binds CD4 receptor

4 Viral replication

Activate signaling pathways

2

Enfuvirtide
5 Inhibits GP41 membrane fusion

Entry of viral RNA

3 HR1

Insertion GP41 fusion peptide

Step 2
Virus entry

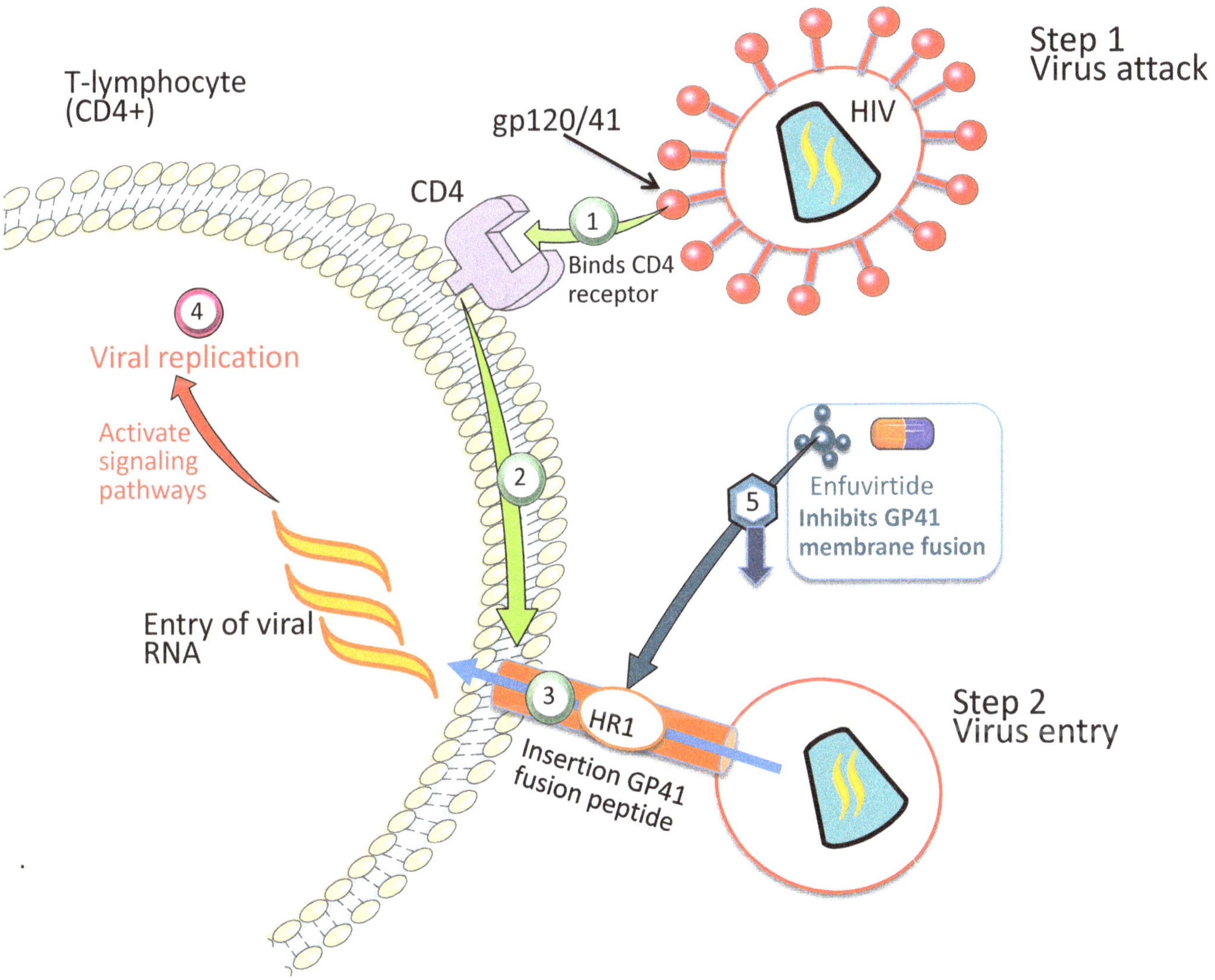

AIDS: Inhibition of fusion of HIV genetic material into target cell, Enfuvirtide

Ebola virus (ZEBOV)

ZEBOV **infects most types of cells**. However, **macrophages and dendritic cells** allow a strong replication and **spread of the virus** through the lymph and blood circulatory system to reach lymph nodes, liver, and spleen and then other tissues.

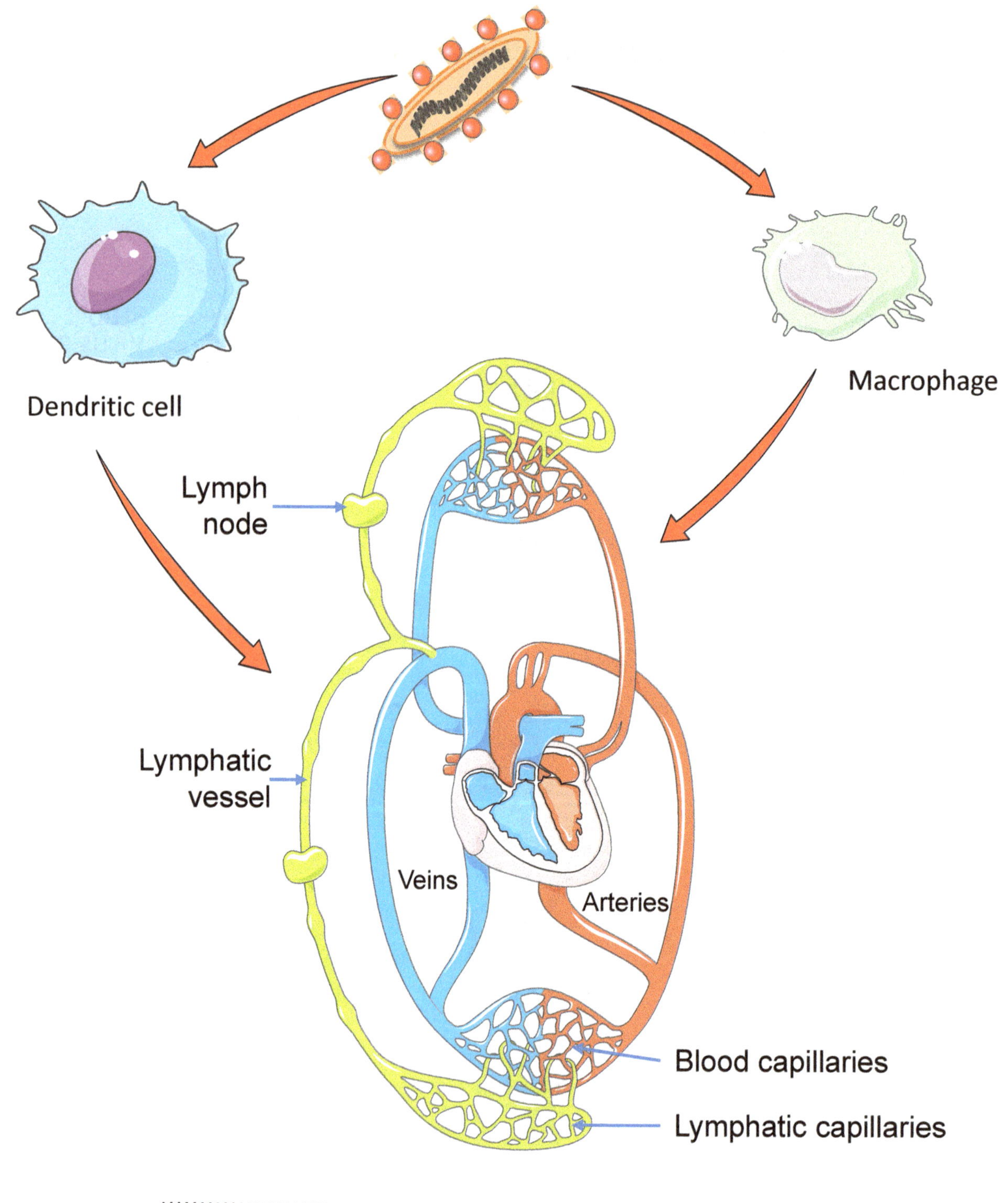

Ebola virus (ZEBOV)

The nucleocapsid (nucleoproteins, nucleic acid) contains the **single-stranded RNA genome** of ZEBOV (19k nucleotides, codes for seven viral proteins). The **multi-functionality** of Ebola's viral proteins allows the virus to have a minimal set of proteins and a compact structure.

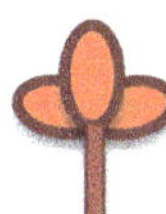

GP1,2 surface glycoprotein, virus attachment and host cell membrane fusion.

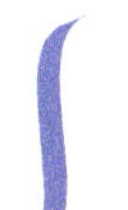

RNA nonsegmented, negative-stranded.

NP (**nucleoprotein**) coats the RNA, for virus particle formation and replication.

VP35 protein, **viral polymerase** complex, inhibits host immunity.

L (large) protein, part of **RNA polymerase** complex with NP and VP30 and VP35.

VP30, phosphoprotein, initiation of **transcription**.

VP24 **matrix protein** for virion assembly, budding, viral transcription, and replication.

VP40 **matrix protein.**

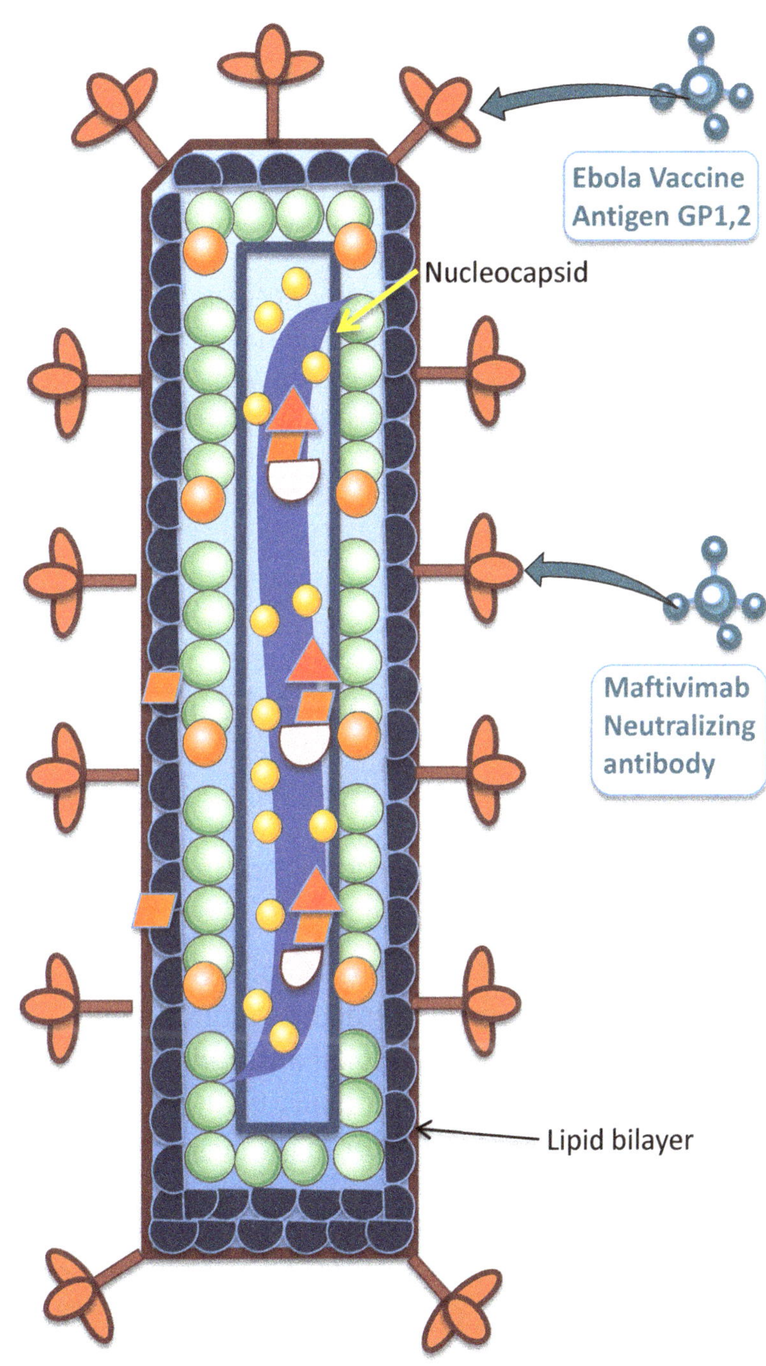

RNA viruses: Description of the Ebola virus

The disease: Ebola virus disease

Ebola is a rare but deadly virus that causes fever, body aches, diarrhea, and reduces blood-clotting associated with **severe internal and external bleeding**. When the virus spreads through the body, it damages the immune system and organs. Zaire ebolavirus infection or Ebola virus disease (EBOV) was previously known as Ebola haemorrhagic fever.

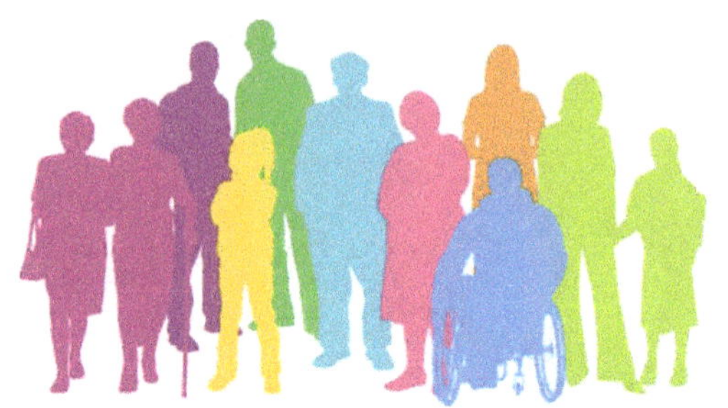

Incidence by gender and ethnicity

Up to 75% of Ebola cases and 60% of fatalities were women in Guinea, Liberia, and Sierra Leone. Women more vulnerable to infection with African women's role in caretaking, performing funeral rites, and cross-border trading. Children and the elderly with weaker immune systems were more likely to die after infection.

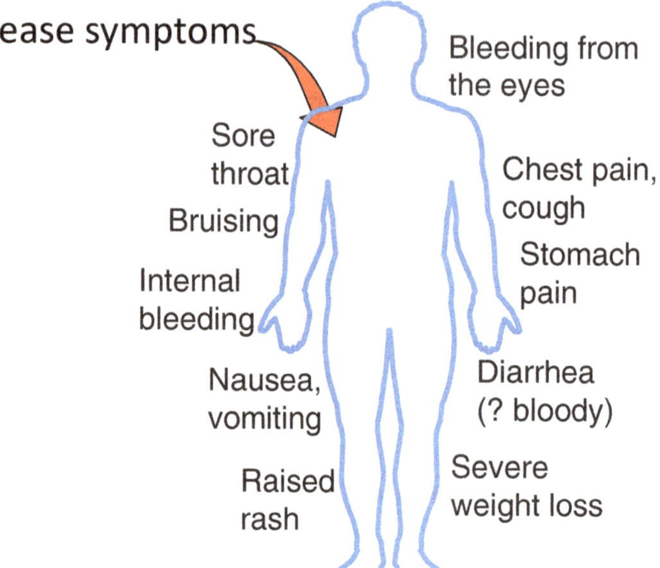

The medicine

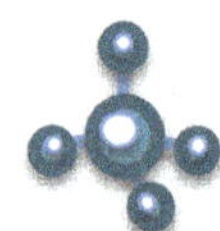

Atoltivimab, Maftivimab, Odesivimab; Inmazeb, FDA Approval 2020

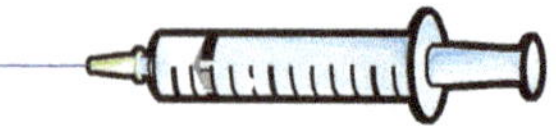

Administered as an intravenous (IV) infusion.

Inmazeb is a mixture of three glycoprotein-directed recombinant human monoclonal **antibodies** atoltivimab, maftivimab, and odesivimab that is administered intravenously.

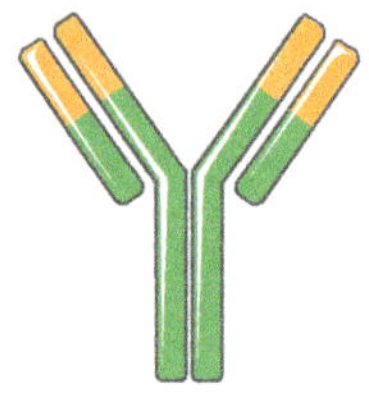

Inmazeb treats Ebola viral (EBOV) infection and binds to different and nonoverlapping epitopes on the **EBOV surface glycoprotein**, blocking interactions between viral and host cell membranes, preventing viral entry into the cell.

Ebola viral disease: Antibody cocktail for blocking infection, Inmazeb

Action of Inmazeb on cell and disease biology

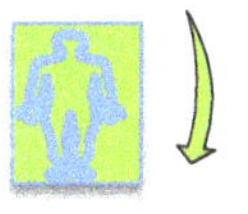

1 **Macrophages** are the initial target of viral infection with cell death.

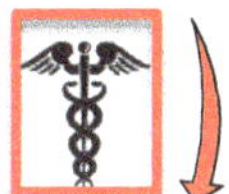

2 **EBOV surface glycoprotein GP1,2** promotes entry of virus into the host cells and evasion of the immune system.

3 GP1,2 appears on the surface of EBOV-infected cells and is targeted by neutralizing and **cytotoxic (Fc-mediated) antibodies** to combat EBOV infection and target infected cells.

4 **Breakdown of endothelial cells** leading to blood vessel injury with multiorgan failure and septic shock.

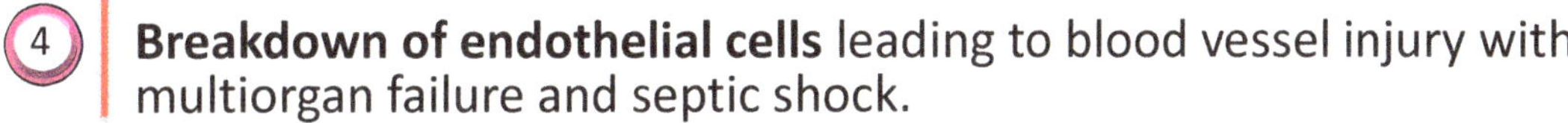

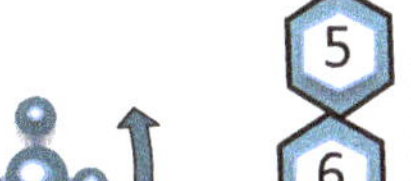

5 **Maftivimab binds** to the soluble form of **EBOV GP1,2**.

6 **Atoltivimab** provides protective and Fc-dependent antibody activity.

7 **Odesivimab** (Fc region) recruits other immune cells to target EBOV and infected cells with surface viral antigens.

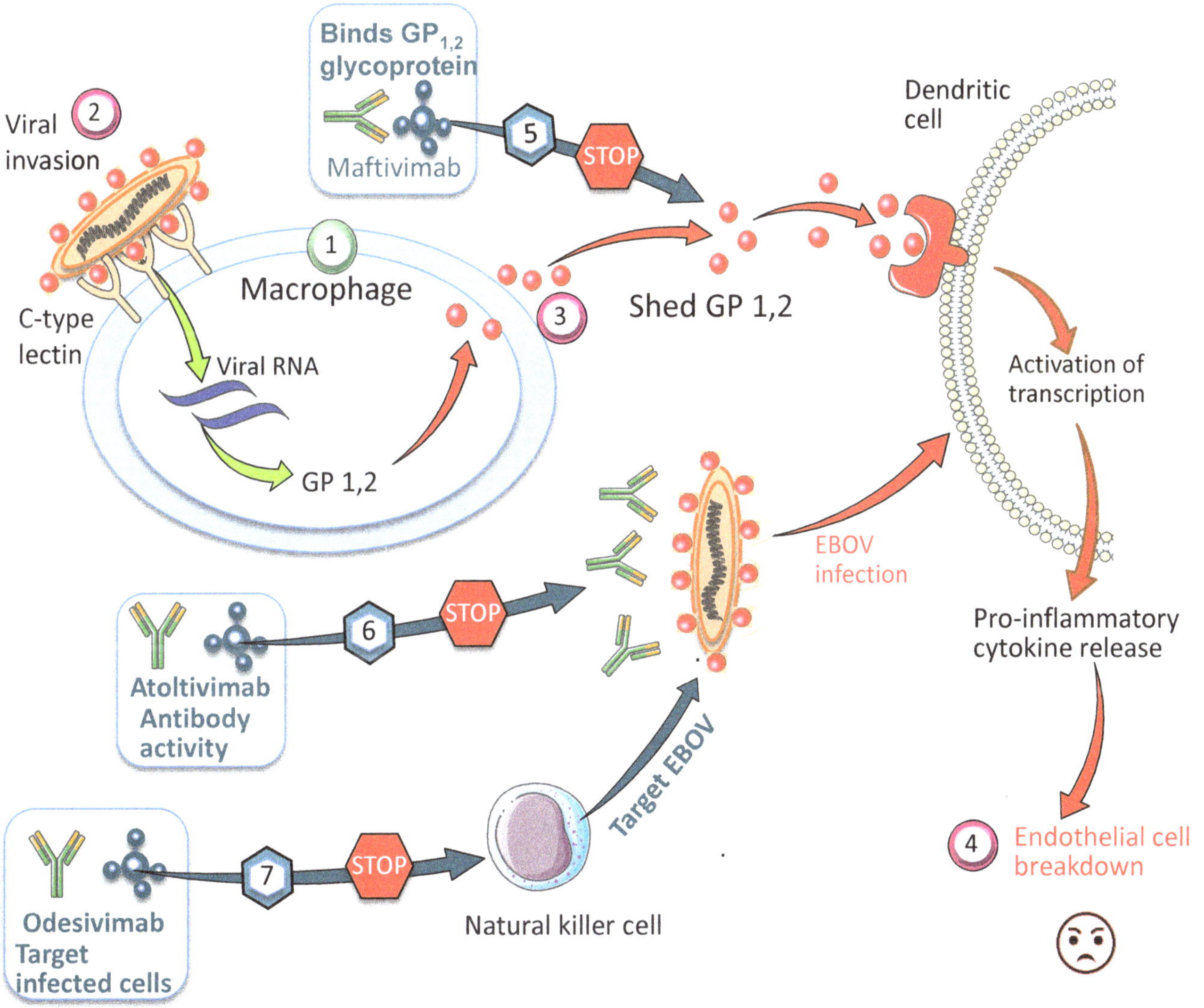

Binds $GP_{1,2}$ glycoprotein
Maftivimab
5
STOP
Dendritic cell
Viral invasion 2
C-type lectin
1 Macrophage
Viral RNA
GP 1,2
3
Shed GP 1,2
Activation of transcription
EBOV infection
Pro-inflammatory cytokine release
Atoltivimab Antibody activity
6
STOP
Target EBOV
Odesivimab Target infected cells
7
STOP
Natural killer cell
4 Endothelial cell breakdown

The disease: Ebola virus disease

Ebola is a rare but deadly virus that causes fever, body aches, diarrhea, and reduces blood-clotting associated with severe internal and external bleeding. When the virus spreads through the body, it damages the immune system and organs. Zaire ebolavirus infection or Ebola virus disease (EBOV) was previously known as Ebola haemorrhagic fever.

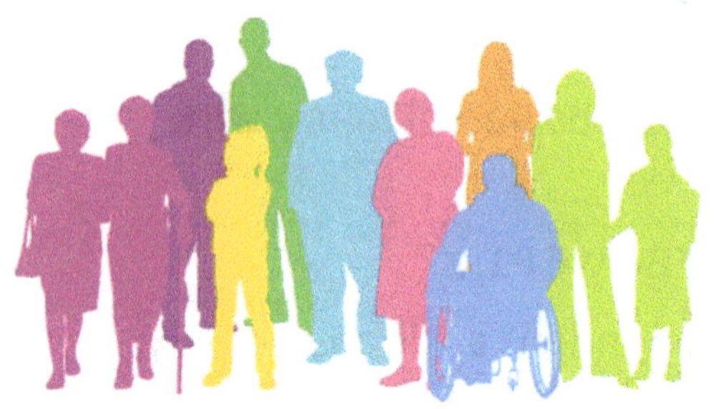

Incidence by gender and ethnicity

Up to 75% of Ebola cases and 60% of fatalities were women in Guinea, Liberia, and Sierra Leone. Women more vulnerable to infection as African women's role in caretaking, performing funeral rites, and cross-border trading. Children and the elderly with weaker immune systems were more likely to die after infection.

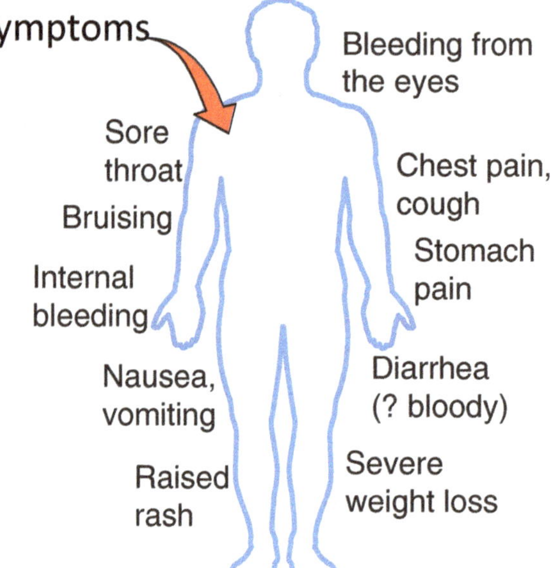

The medicine

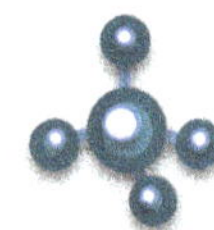

Ebola Zaire Vaccine; Ervebo, FDA Approval 2019

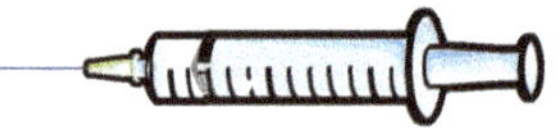

Vaccination by intramuscular injection (deltoid muscle)

Ervebo consists of a live **attenuated recombinant Vesicular Stomatitis Virus (rVSV)** in which the gene encoding the envelope has been replaced by one encoding the Zaire **Ebola** virus (ZEBOV) **surface glycoprotein**. Ervebo is a vaccine for adults for disease caused by the Zaire ebolavirus and induces strong, protective immune responses after a single dose.

Chimeric vesicular stomatitis virus (VSV). Wild-type VSV can infect humans with no or mild illness.

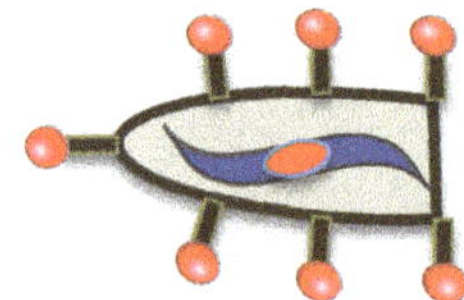

In rVSV-EBOV VSV envelope glycoprotein is replaced with ZBOV glycoprotein 1,2 (GP1,2).

Ebola viral disease: Vaccination with Ebola surface glycoprotein, Ervebo

Action of Ervebo on cell and disease biology

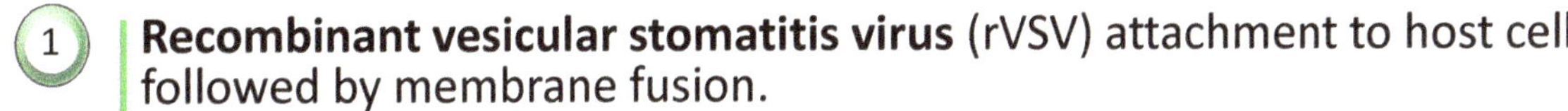

1. **Recombinant vesicular stomatitis virus** (rVSV) attachment to host cell followed by membrane fusion.
2. Release of viral mRNA containing gene coding for the Zaire Ebola virus **surface glycoprotein GP1,2**, which is the sole viral envelope protein.
3. Truncated versions, soluble GP (sGP), small soluble GP (ssGP), are produced.
4. **Antigen presenting cell** (APC) presents GP1,2 fragments to B- and T-cells to generate an adaptive immune response.
5. Natural killer cells are selectively cytotoxic to virus-infected cells and B-cells produce virus specific antibodies.
6. Ervebo **vaccine triggers an an adaptive immune response** against GP1,2 which protects against future Ebola infections.

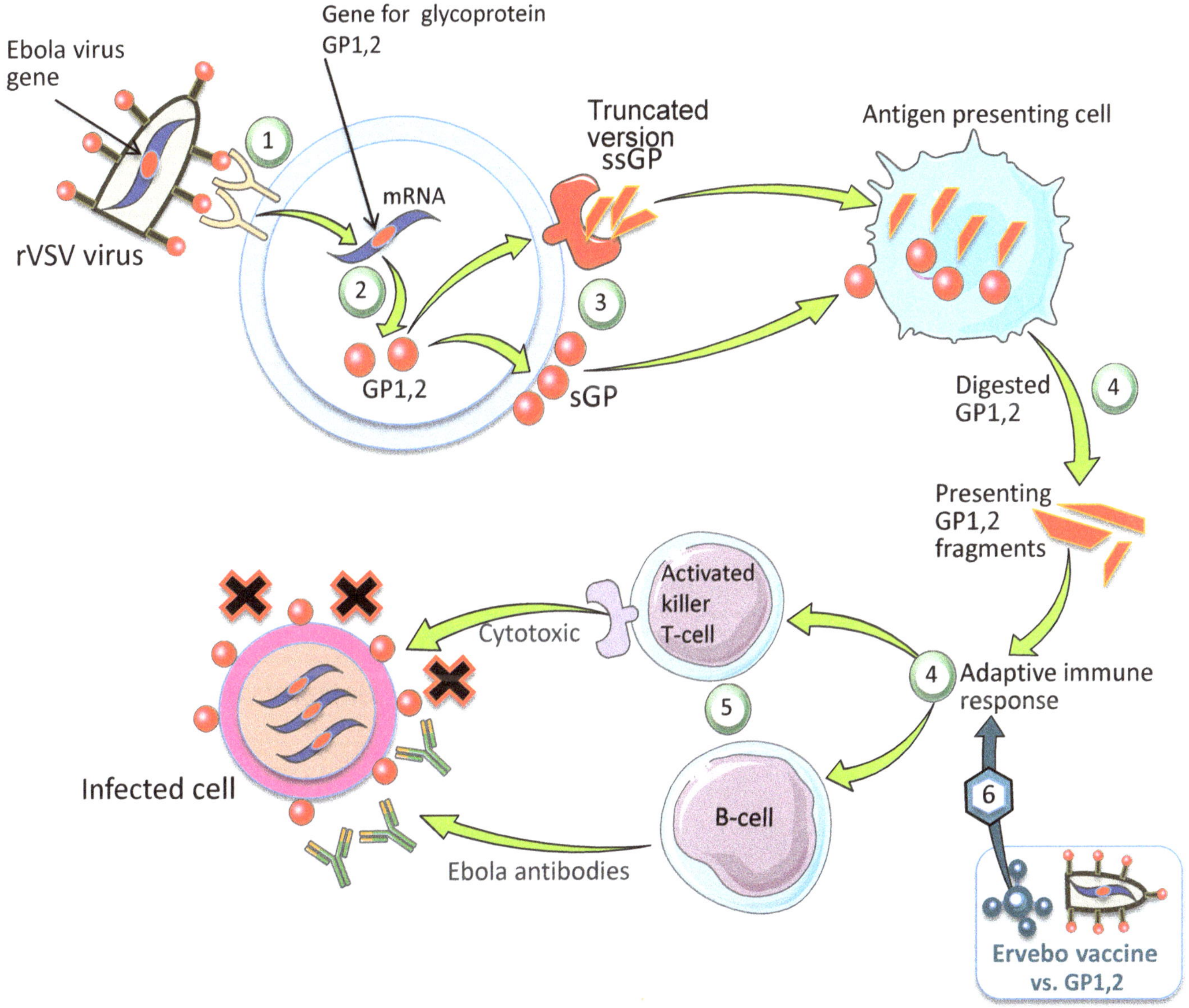

Ebola viral disease: Vaccination with Ebola surface glycoprotein, Ervebo

SARS-CoV-2 (severe acute respiratory syndrome coronavirus 2)

Coronavirus SARS-CoV-2 causes coronavirus disease 2019 (COVID-19), which is a contagious disease caused by infection through aerosols of the **upper or lower respiratory tract** with a wide range of symptoms, ranging from mild to severe illness.

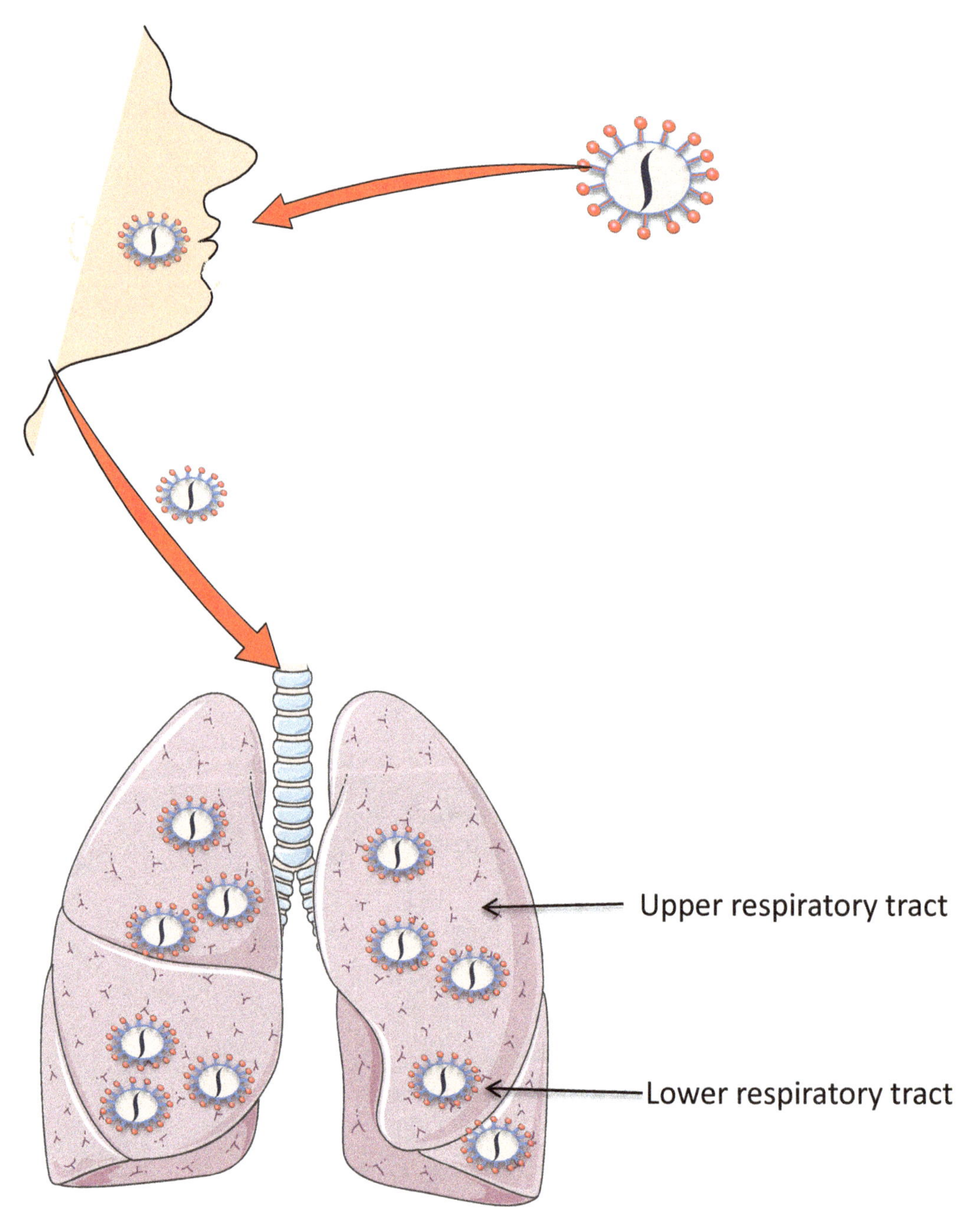

SARS-CoV-2 (severe acute respiratory syndrome coronavirus 2)

SARS-CoV-2 is a spherical virus (100 nm) has the **largest genome (30 kb)** of the RNA virus family with a single-stranded **positive-sense RNA**, which codes for four structural proteins (S, E, M, and N) and 16 nonstructural proteins (nsp1–16) that are involved in viral RNA transcription and replication.

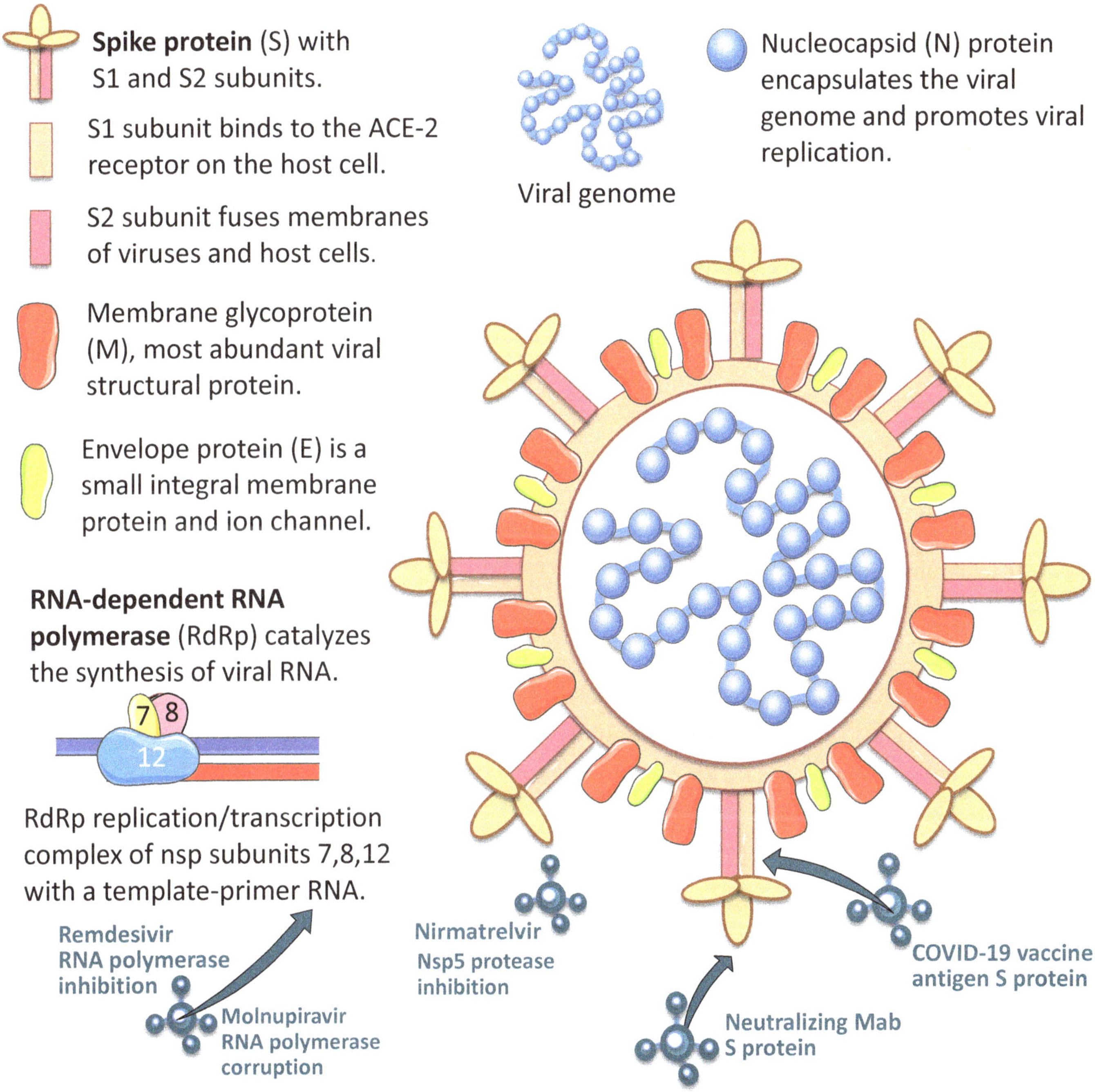

Spike protein (S) with S1 and S2 subunits.

S1 subunit binds to the ACE-2 receptor on the host cell.

S2 subunit fuses membranes of viruses and host cells.

Membrane glycoprotein (M), most abundant viral structural protein.

Envelope protein (E) is a small integral membrane protein and ion channel.

RNA-dependent RNA polymerase (RdRp) catalyzes the synthesis of viral RNA.

7 8

12

RdRp replication/transcription complex of nsp subunits 7,8,12 with a template-primer RNA.

Viral genome

Nucleocapsid (N) protein encapsulates the viral genome and promotes viral replication.

Remdesivir
RNA polymerase
inhibition

Molnupiravir
RNA polymerase
corruption

Nirmatrelvir
Nsp5 protease
inhibition

Neutralizing Mab
S protein

COVID-19 vaccine
antigen S protein

RNA viruses: Description of Coronavirus SARS-CoV-2

The disease: Severe acute respiratory syndrome coronavirus 2

COVID-19 (caused by the coronavirus SARS-CoV-2) is a contagious disease caused by infection through aerosols of the upper or lower respiratory tract and people with COVID-19 have reported a wide range of symptoms, ranging from mild symptoms to severe illness.

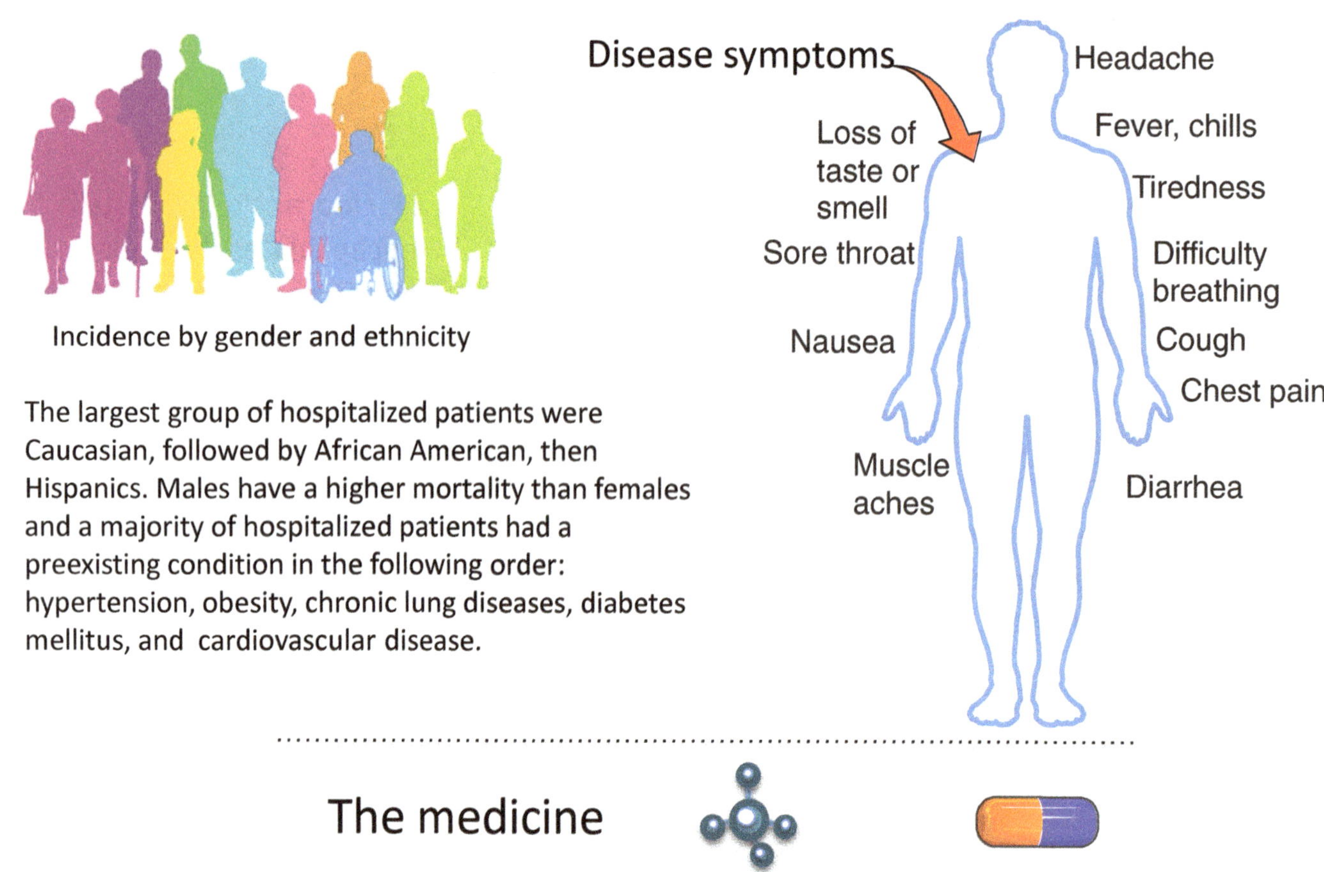

Incidence by gender and ethnicity

The largest group of hospitalized patients were Caucasian, followed by African American, then Hispanics. Males have a higher mortality than females and a majority of hospitalized patients had a preexisting condition in the following order: hypertension, obesity, chronic lung diseases, diabetes mellitus, and cardiovascular disease.

The medicine

Remdesivir ; Veklury, FDA Approval 2020

Remdesivir is a nucleotide analogue prodrug that perturbs viral replication by inhibiting RNA-dependent RNA polymerase and is used for the treatment of severe COVID-19.

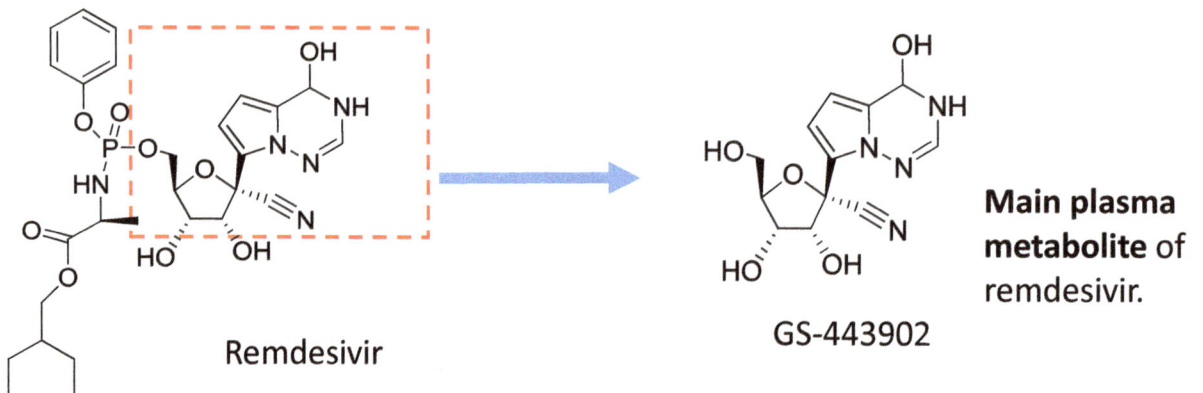

Remdesivir

GS-443902

Main plasma metabolite of remdesivir.

COVID-19 : Inhibition of RNA polymerase, Remdesivir

Action of Remdesivir on cell and disease biology

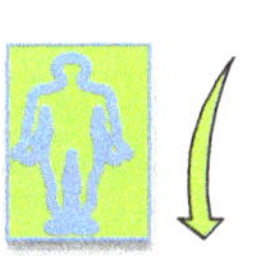

1. SARS-CoV-2 **enters into cells** by binding to the human **ACE2 receptor**.
2. Viral uncoating followed by release of viral RNA.
3. RNA-Dependent RNA Polymerase catalyzes the synthesis of viral RNA.

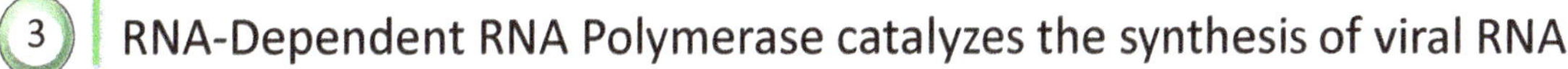

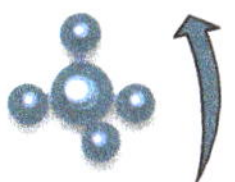

4. RTP **blocks viral RNA-dependent RNA polymerase**, decreasing viral RNA production.
5. **Remdesivir** works as a delayed chain terminator that results in premature termination of RNA replication.

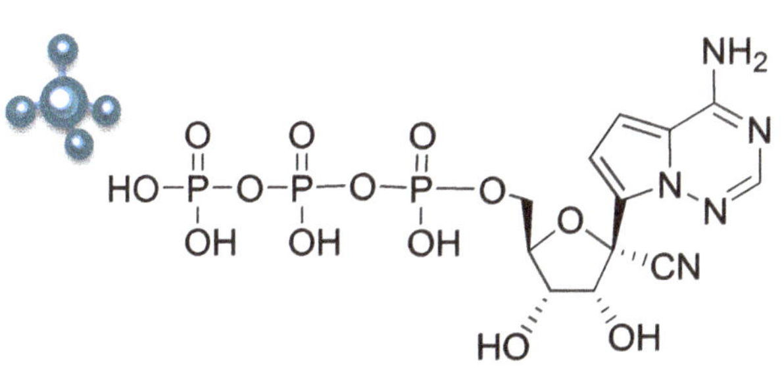

Remdesivir triphosphate (RTP, analog of ATP)

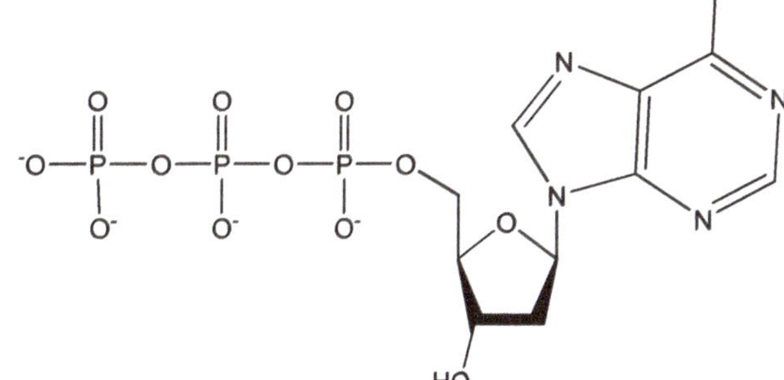

Adenosine nucleoside triphosphate (ATP)

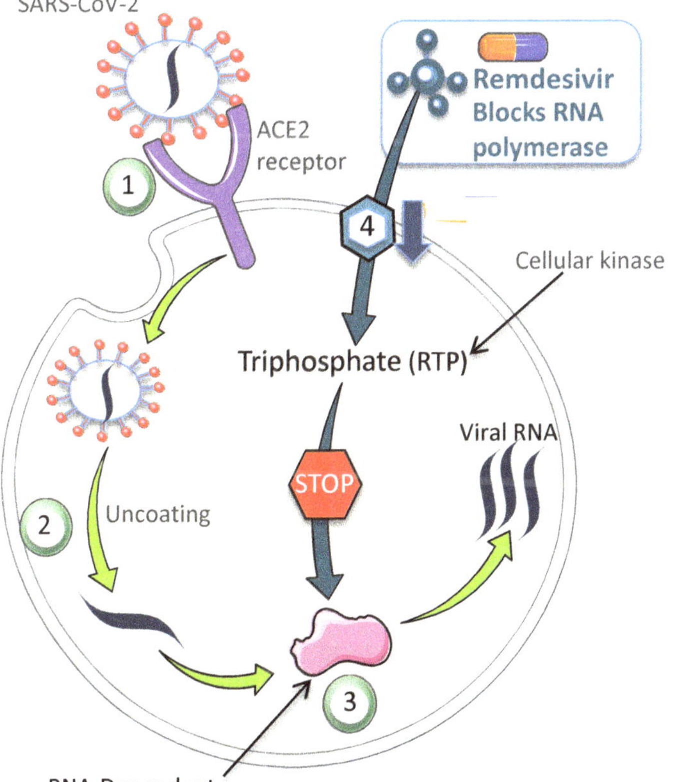

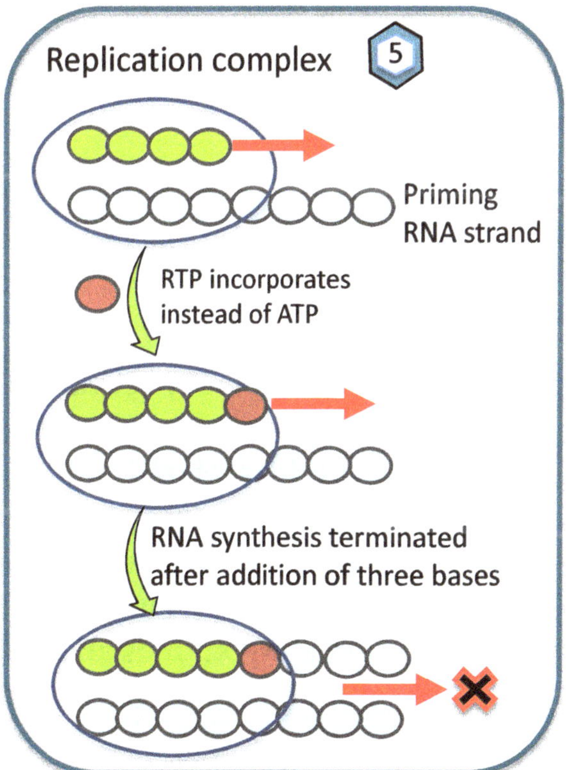

COVID-19: Inhibition of RNA polymerase, Remdesivir

The disease: Severe acute respiratory syndrome coronavirus 2

COVID-19 (caused by the coronavirus SARS-CoV-2) is a contagious disease caused by infection through aerosols of the upper or lower respiratory tract and people with COVID-19 have reported a wide range of symptoms, ranging from mild symptoms to severe illness.

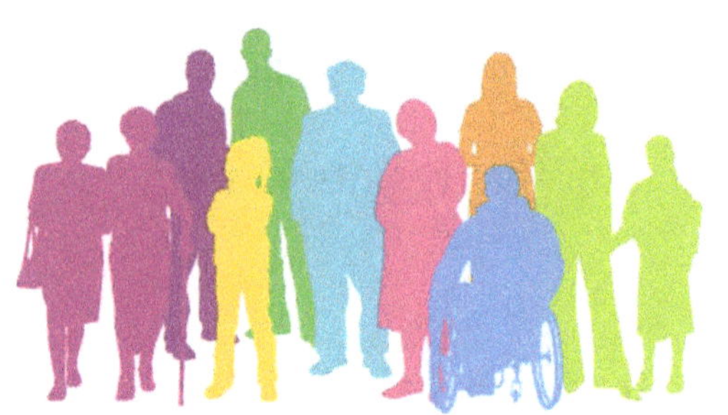

Incidence by gender and ethnicity

The largest group of hospitalized patients were Caucasian, followed by African American, then Hispanics. Males have a higher mortality than females and a majority of hospitalized patients had a pre-existing condition in the following order: hypertension, obesity, chronic lung diseases, diabetes mellitus, and cardiovascular disease.

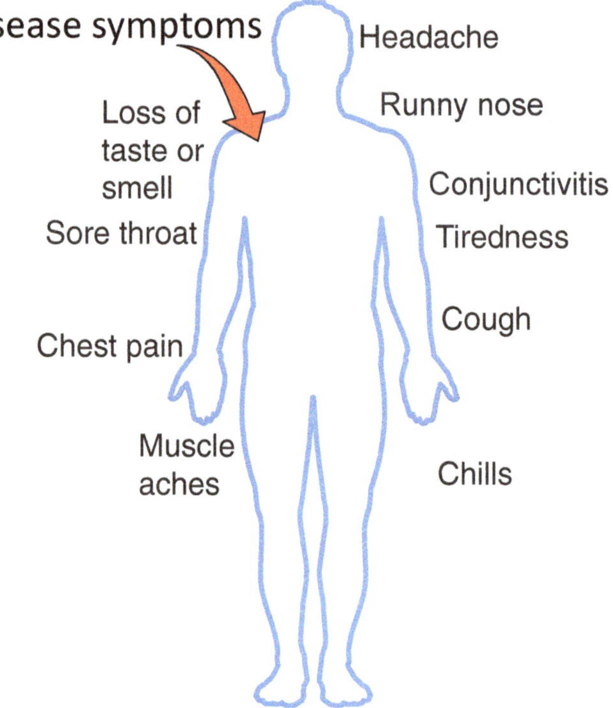

The medicine

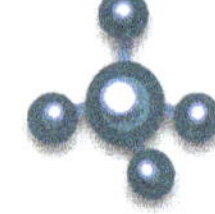

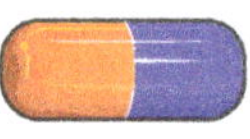

Molnupiravir, FDA EUA 2021

EUA = emergency use authorization

Molnupiravir is an orally active **inhibitor of COVID-19, which acts during the viral replication cycle catalyzed by RNA-directed RNA polymerase.** Molnupiravir causes **extensive mutations of the viral genome via incorporation of a cytidine analog (NHC-TP) into new viral RNA strands and inhibits viral reproduction.** Molnupiravir is for treatment of adults with mild-to-moderate COVID-19.

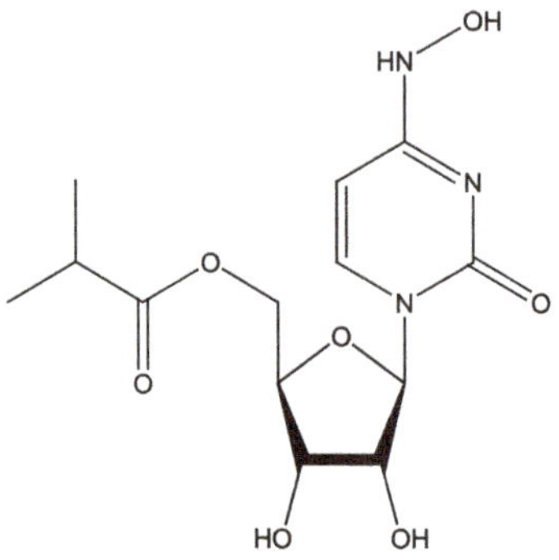

COVID-19 : Corruption of RNA polymerase, Molnupiravir

Action of Molnupiravir on cell and disease biology

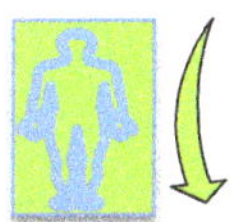

1 RNA-dependent RNA polymerase catalyzes the synthesis of viral RNA.

2 **Molnupiravir** is rapidly converted by serum esterases and then host cell kinases to Molnupiravir triphosphate (NHC-TP), which is a **CTP analog**.

NHC-TP escapes the virus proofreading exonuclease enzymes without repair of the mutated RNA products.

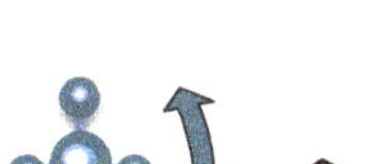

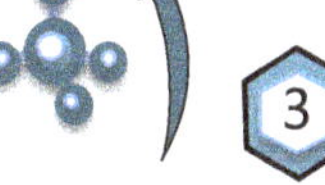

3 **Mutated RNA** with NHC residues causes further errors with rounds of replication by RNA polymerase where NHC is copied either as C or U.

4 As the modified residues accumulate the increasingly mutated RNA results in a collapse of the viral population.

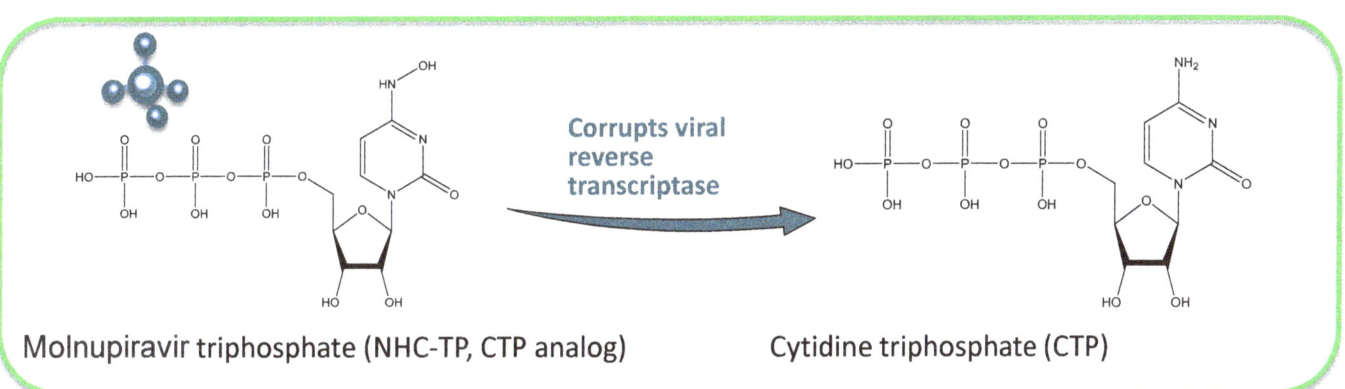

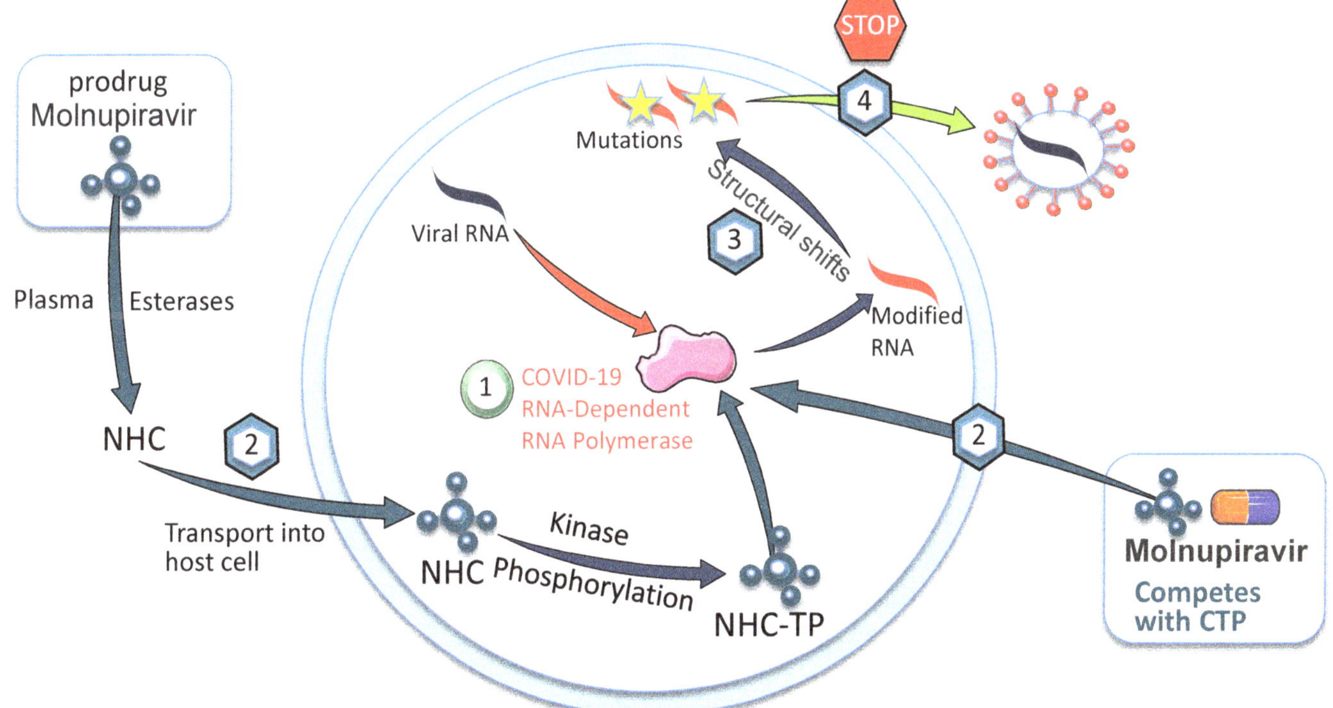

COVID-19: Corruption of RNA polymerase, Molnupiravir

The disease: Severe acute respiratory syndrome coronavirus 2

COVID-19 (caused by the coronavirus SARS-CoV-2) is a contagious disease caused by infection through aerosols of the upper or lower respiratory tract and people with COVID-19 have reported a wide range of symptoms, ranging from mild symptoms to severe illness.

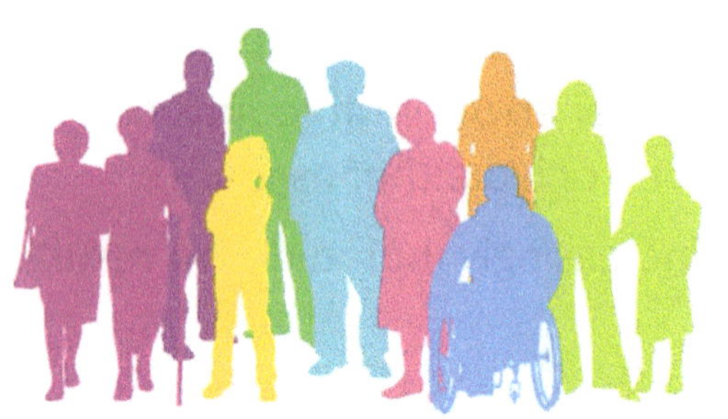

Incidence by gender and ethnicity

The largest group of hospitalized patients were Caucasian, followed by African American, then Hispanics. Males have a higher mortality than females and a majority of hospitalized patients had a pre-existing condition in the following order: hypertension, obesity, chronic lung diseases, diabetes mellitus, and cardiovascular disease.

Early disease symptoms

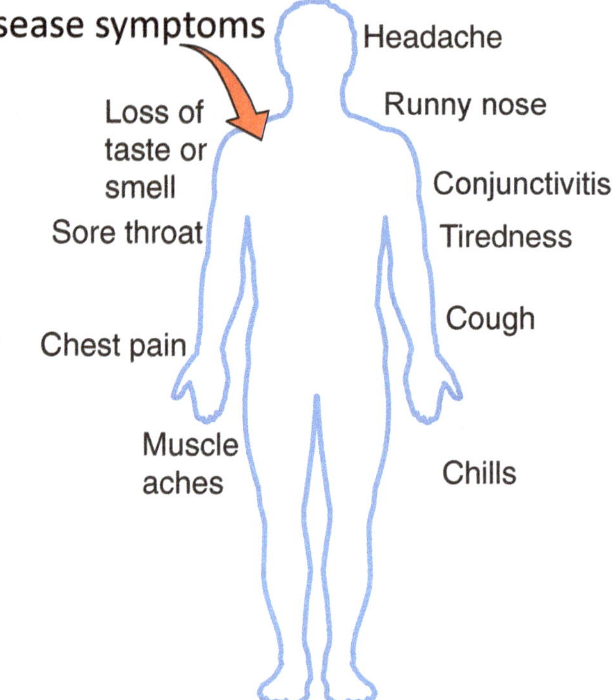

The medicine

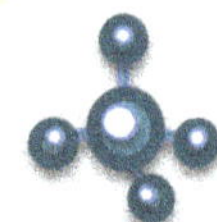

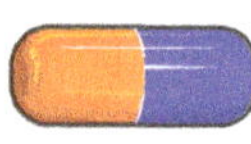

Nirmatrelvir, Ritonavir ; Paxlovid, FDA EUA 2021

EUA = emergency use authorization

Paxlovid is an orally active **inhibitor of 3CLpro** (MPro), which is combined with **ritonavir** (inhibits the cytochrome P450 3A family of monooxygenases) to **slow the metabolism** and increase the half-life of Paxlovid, which achieves higher concentrations to help combat the virus. Paxlovid is prescribed for high-risk patients and should be taken within five days of symptom onset and a diagnosis of COVID-19.

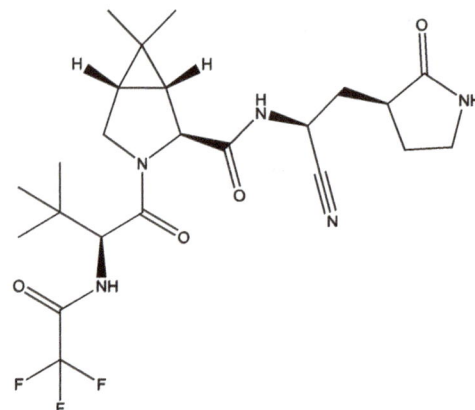

COVID-19 : Inhibition of protease, Nirmatrelvir

Action of Nirmatrelvir on cell and disease biology

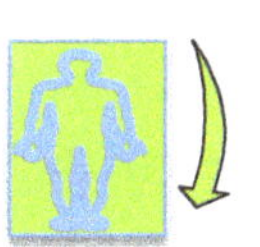

1 Coronavirus **gene ORF1ab** contains overlapping open reading frames (ORF1a and ORF1b) that code for **polyproteins pp1a and pp1ab**.
Production of the longer (PP1ab) or shorter protein (PP1a) depends on a ribosomal frameshifting event.

2 Polyproteins are **processed by proteases**, **3CLpro or Mpro** (11 cleavage sites) and a papain-like protease, Plpro (3 cleavage sites) to generate 16 nonstructural proteins, including polymerase RdRp.

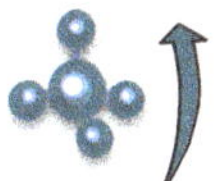

3 **Nirmatrelvir** is an **inhibitor of MPro protease** which blocks the polyprotein from binding to the enzyme active site and thus prevents viral replication.

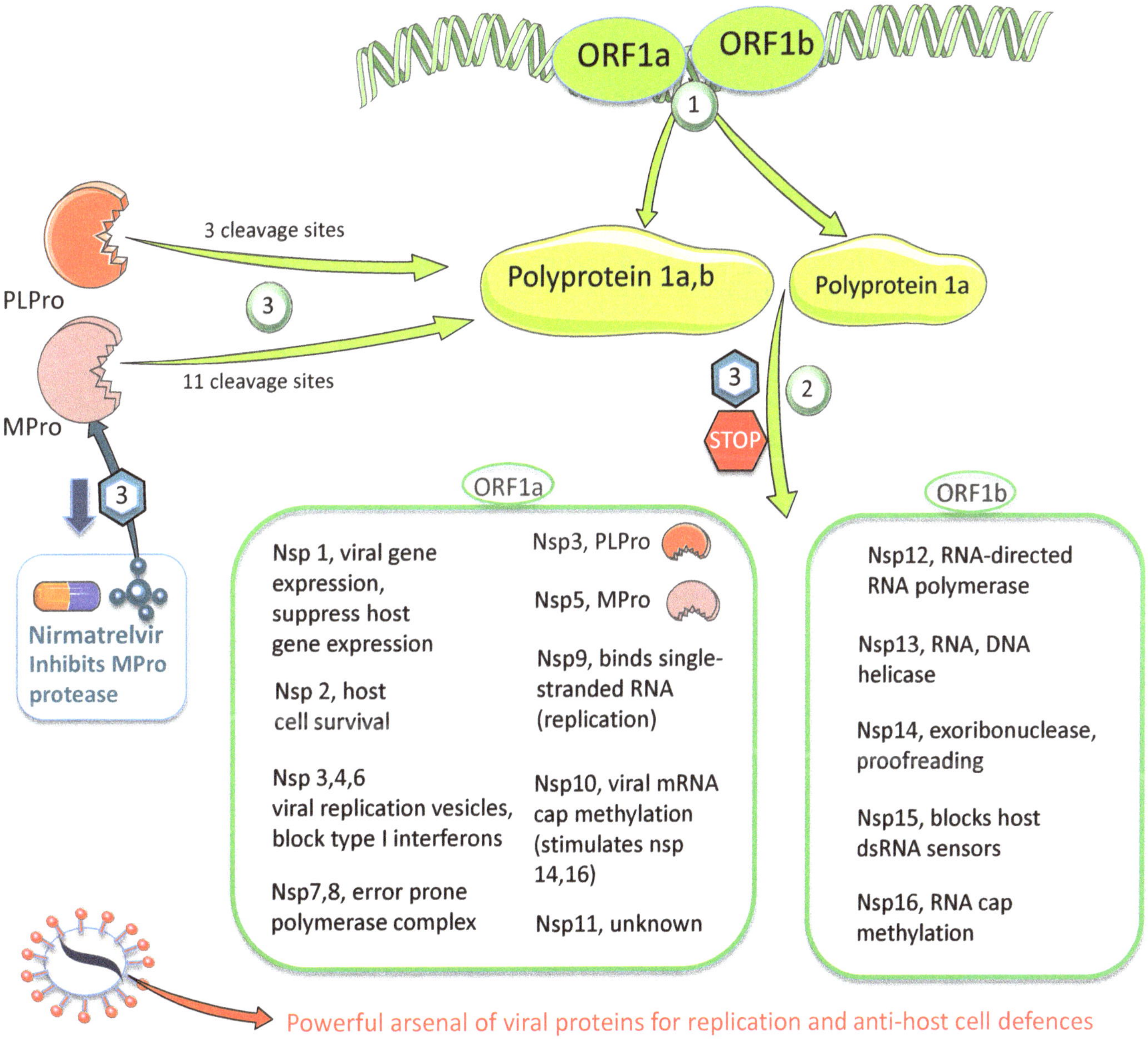

COVID-19 : Inhibition of protease, Nirmatrelvir

The disease: Severe acute respiratory syndrome coronavirus 2

COVID-19 (caused by the coronavirus SARS-CoV-2) is a contagious disease caused by infection through aerosols of the upper or lower respiratory tract results with a wide range of symptoms.

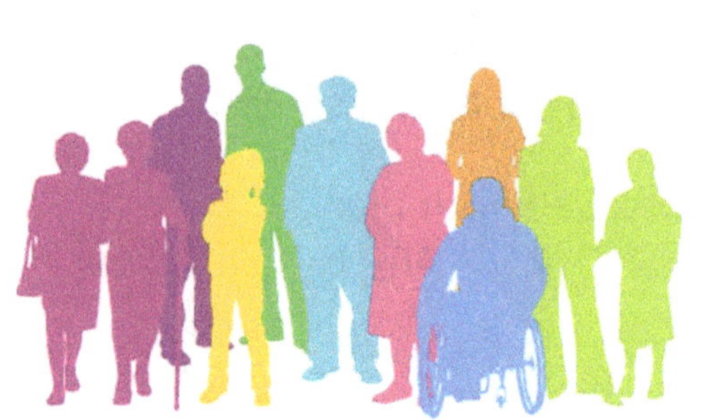

Incidence by gender and ethnicity

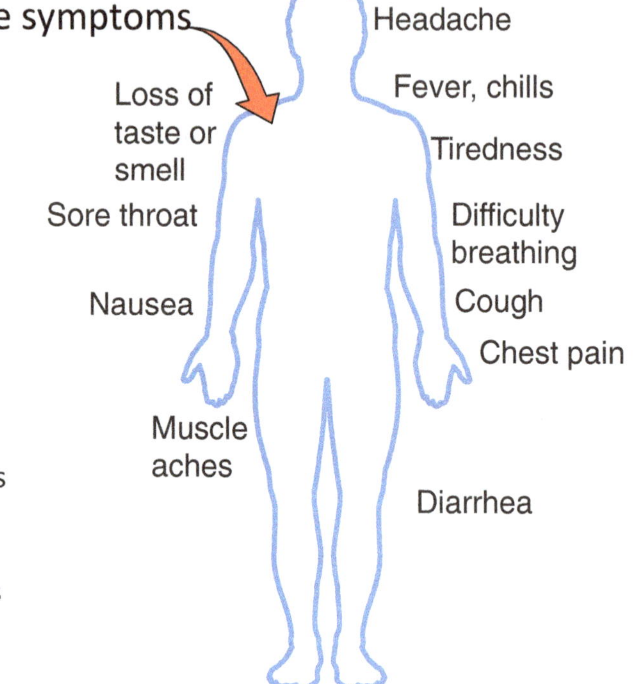

The largest group of hospitalized patients were Caucasian, followed by African American, then Hispanics. Males have a higher mortality than females and a majority of hospitalized patients had a pre-existing condition in the following order: hypertension, obesity, chronic lung diseases, diabetes mellitus, and cardiovascular disease.

The medicine

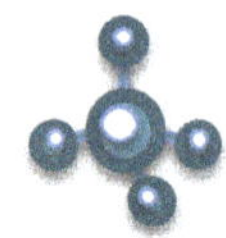

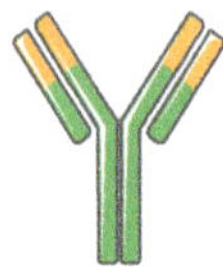

Bamlanivimab, etesevimab; LY-CoV555, LY-CoV016, FDA EUA 2021

Casirivimab, imdevimab; REGEN-COV, FDA EUA 2020

EUA = emergency use authorization

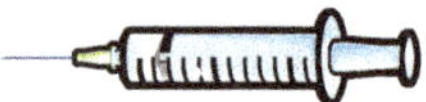

Administered as an intravenous (IV) infusion.

Antibody binding to the SARS-CoV-2 **receptor-binding domain (RBD) blocks attachment of the virus to the human ACE2 receptor**. The combination of multiple antibodies is intended to prevent mutational escape of the virus and development of viral resistance.

Bamlanivimab and etesevimab are humanized recombinant monoclonal antibodies, which bind to distinct but overlapping sites on the RBD of the spike protein. Bamlanivimab is a monoclonal antibody, which was derived from a COVID-1 patient.

Casirivimab and imdevimab bind to nonoverlapping epitopes of the RBD of SARS-CoV-2 (no competition of binding). The antibodies were derived from humanized mice as well as blood samples from patients who have recovered from COVID-19.

Action of neutralizing antibodies on cell and disease biology

1 **SARS-CoV-2 spike protein** is responsible for viral attachment, fusion and entry into target cell via two binding domains (S1 and S2).

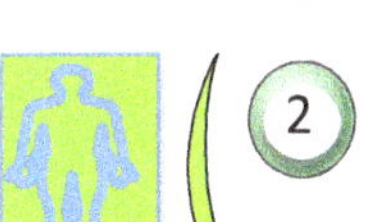

2 The **receptor binding domain** (RBD) of the spike protein binds to angiotensin-converting enzyme 2 **(ACE2) receptors** located in the lungs, kidneys, heart, arteries, and cerebral cortex.

3 The **spike structure** exists either in a **closed form** where the RBD is hidden from the host immune system or an **open form** for ACE2 binding.

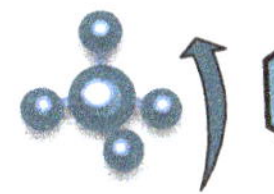

4 **Neutralizing** antibodies **bind to RBD** and block attachment of the virus to the human ACE2 receptor.

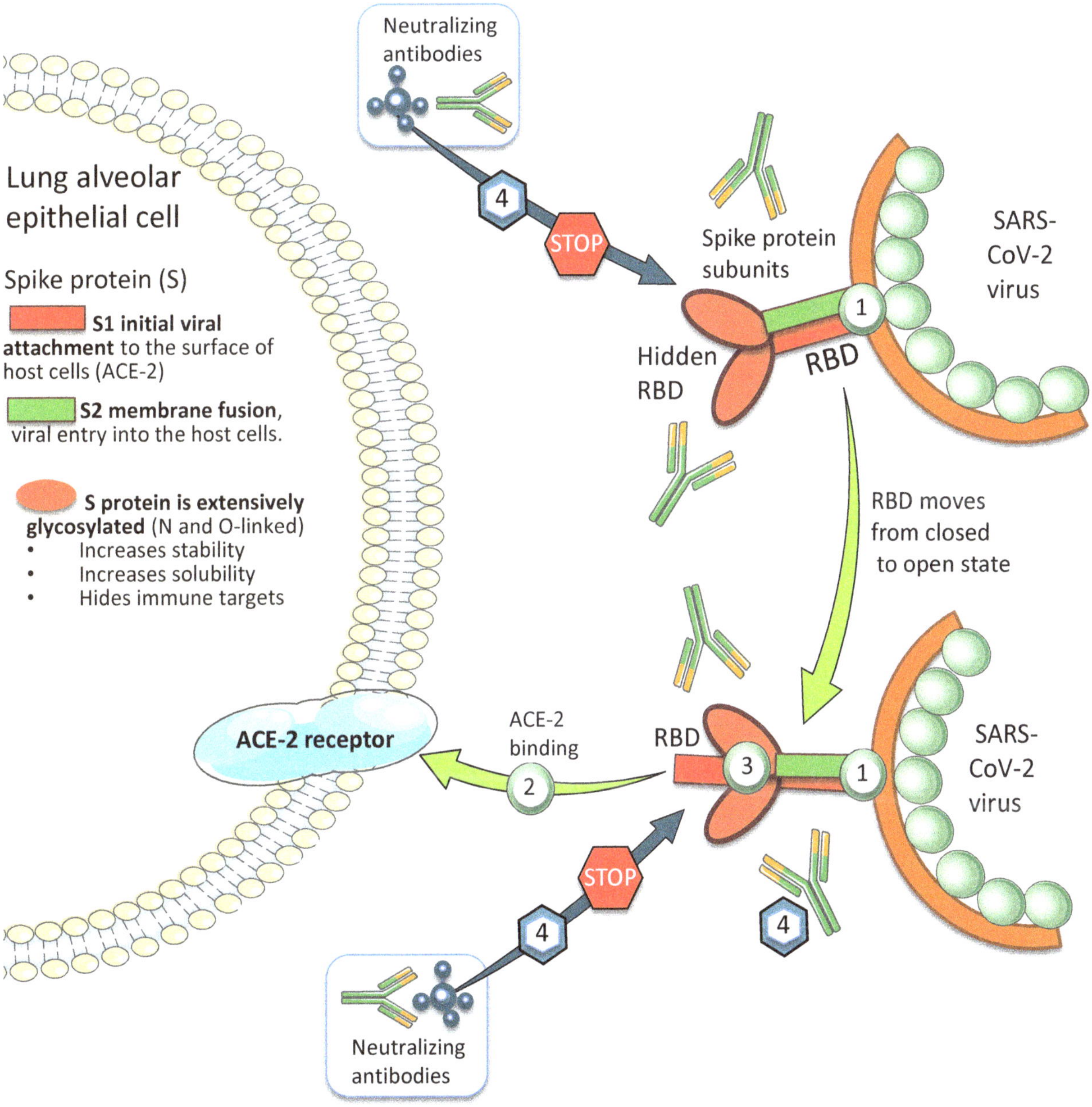

Neutralizing antibodies

Lung alveolar epithelial cell

Spike protein (S)

S1 initial viral attachment to the surface of host cells (ACE-2)

S2 membrane fusion, viral entry into the host cells.

S protein is extensively glycosylated (N and O-linked)

- Increases stability
- Increases solubility
- Hides immune targets

4 STOP

Spike protein subunits

SARS-CoV-2 virus

1

Hidden RBD

RBD

RBD moves from closed to open state

ACE-2 receptor

ACE-2 binding

2

RBD

3

1

SARS-CoV-2 virus

STOP 4

4

Neutralizing antibodies

COVID-19 : Neutralizing antibodies (LY-CoV555, LY-CoV016, REGEN-COV)

The disease: severe acute respiratory syndrome coronavirus 2

COVID-19 (caused by the coronavirus SARS-CoV-2) is a contagious disease caused by **infection through aerosols** of the upper or lower respiratory tract results with a wide range of symptoms.

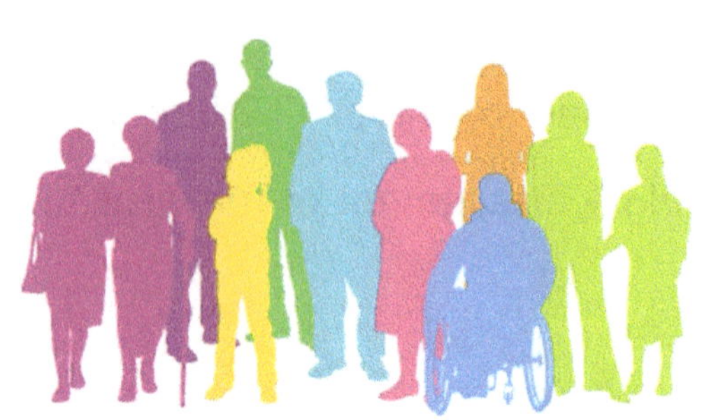

Incidence by gender and ethnicity

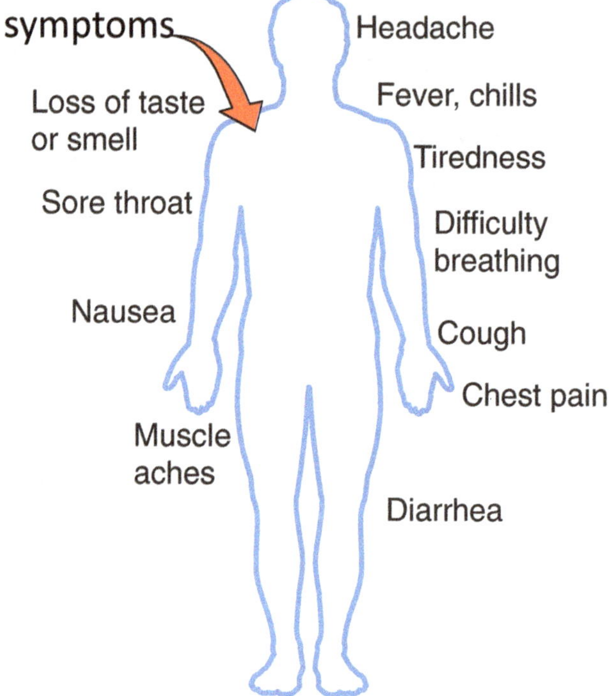

The largest group of hospitalized patients were Caucasian, followed by African American, then Hispanics. Males have a higher mortality than females and a majority of hospitalized patients had a pre-existing condition in the following order: hypertension, obesity, chronic lung diseases, diabetes mellitus, and cardiovascular disease.

The medicine

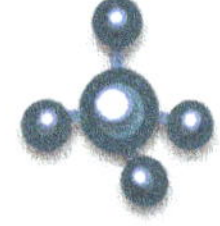
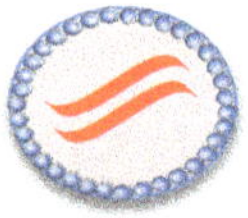
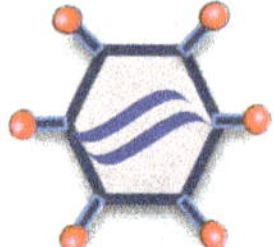

BNT162b2; Comirnaty, Pfizer-BioNTech, FDA EUA 2020

mRNA-1273, Moderna, FDA EUA 2020

Ad26.COV2, Janssen, FDA EUA 2020

EUA = emergency use authorization

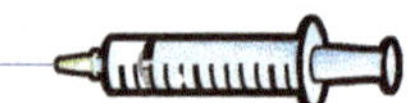

Injection site: deltoid muscle in the upper arm.

BNT**162b2 and mRNA-1273** contain synthetic **chemically modified messenger RNA** (mRNA) that encodes the SARS-CoV-2 spike (S) protein. The modifications include two stabilizing mutations (prolines) and a cap on the mRNA which enhances its translational efficiency.

Ad26.COV2.S, is a recombinant, **replication-incompetent adenovirus serotype 26** (Ad26). The viral genome encodes for a full-length and stabilized SARS-CoV-2 spike protein, which will reside in the host nucleus but does not integrate into host genome.

COVID-19 : Vaccines, Comirnaty, Moderna, Janssen

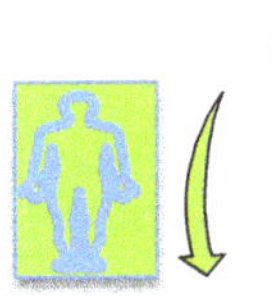

1. **Dendritic cells** (injection site) migrate to the lymph nodes and interact with T cells and B cells to initiate the adaptive immune response.
2. **Helper T cells** selectively activate antigen specific B-cells to generate plasma cells, which produce high-affinity antibodies.
3. A **killer T cell** recognizes the viral antigen on the surface of a virus-infected cell, killing the cell and preventing the infection.

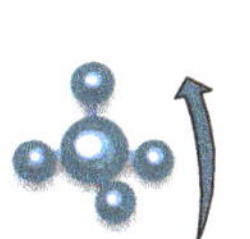

4. **Lipid nanoparticles** contain positively charged lipids (bind mRNA), pegylated lipids, phospholipids and cholesterol.
5. Replication-incompetent **adenovirus type 26** containing the DNA for the SARS-CoV-2 spike protein (stabilized conformation).

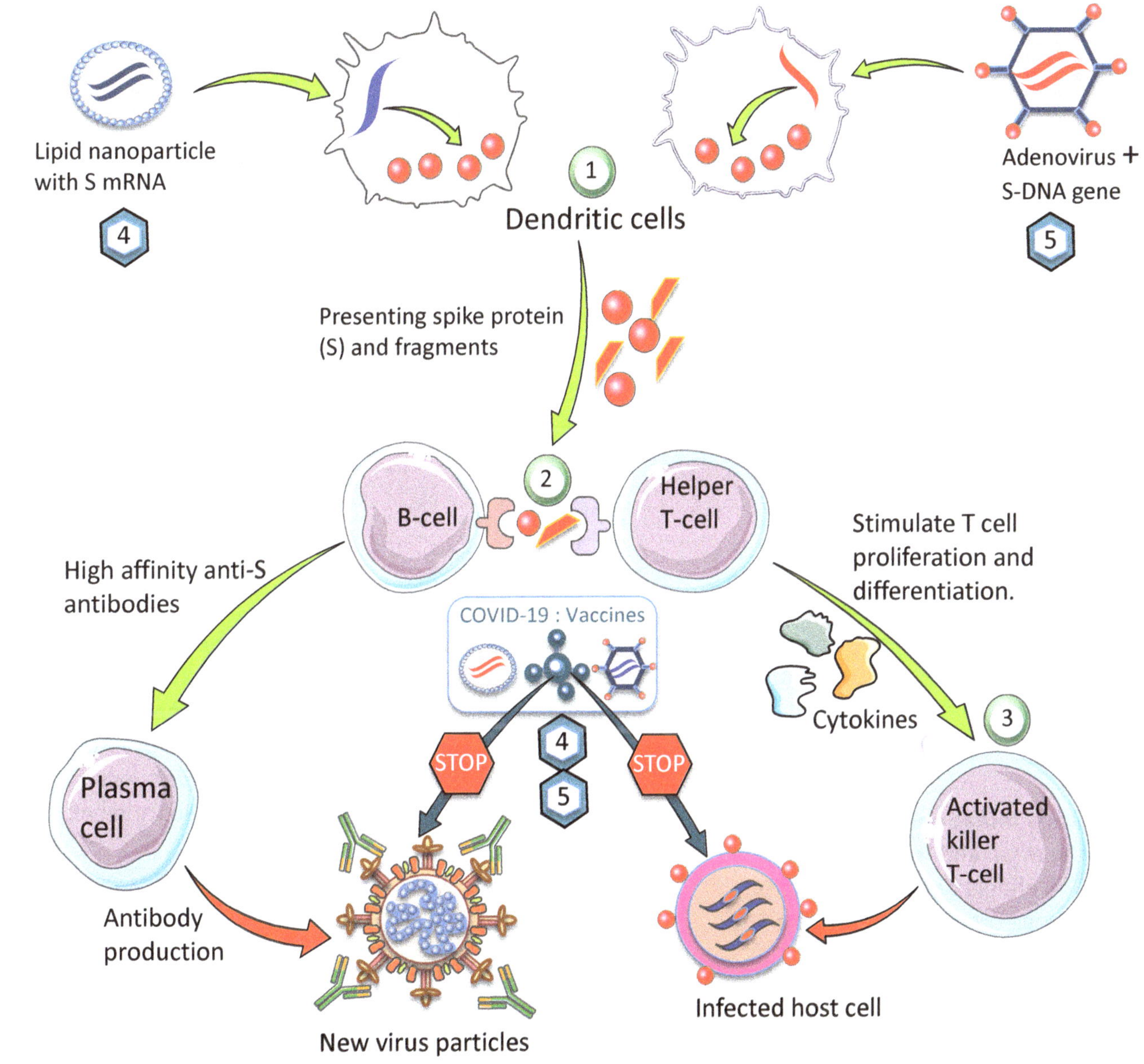

Lipid nanoparticle with S mRNA
4
1
Dendritic cells
Adenovirus + S-DNA gene
5
Presenting spike protein (S) and fragments
2
B-cell
Helper T-cell
High affinity anti-S antibodies
Stimulate T cell proliferation and differentiation.
COVID-19 : Vaccines
Cytokines
3
STOP
4
5
STOP
Plasma cell
Activated killer T-cell
Antibody production
New virus particles
Infected host cell

COVID-19 : Vaccines, Comirnaty, Moderna, Janssen

DNA Viruses

Gene expression in DNA viruses

- **Early genes** provide the proteins needed for DNA replication (stage 1) followed by genes for DNA synthesis.
- **Late genes** with expression of structural proteins needed to package DNA and form virus particles.

Human cancer is associated with DNA viruses

- **Important examples** include human papillomavirus, hepatitis B virus, Epstein–Barr virus and herpes viruses 8.
- **Associated diseases** are gastric, hepatocellular carcinomas, cervical cancers, and Kaposi's sarcoma.

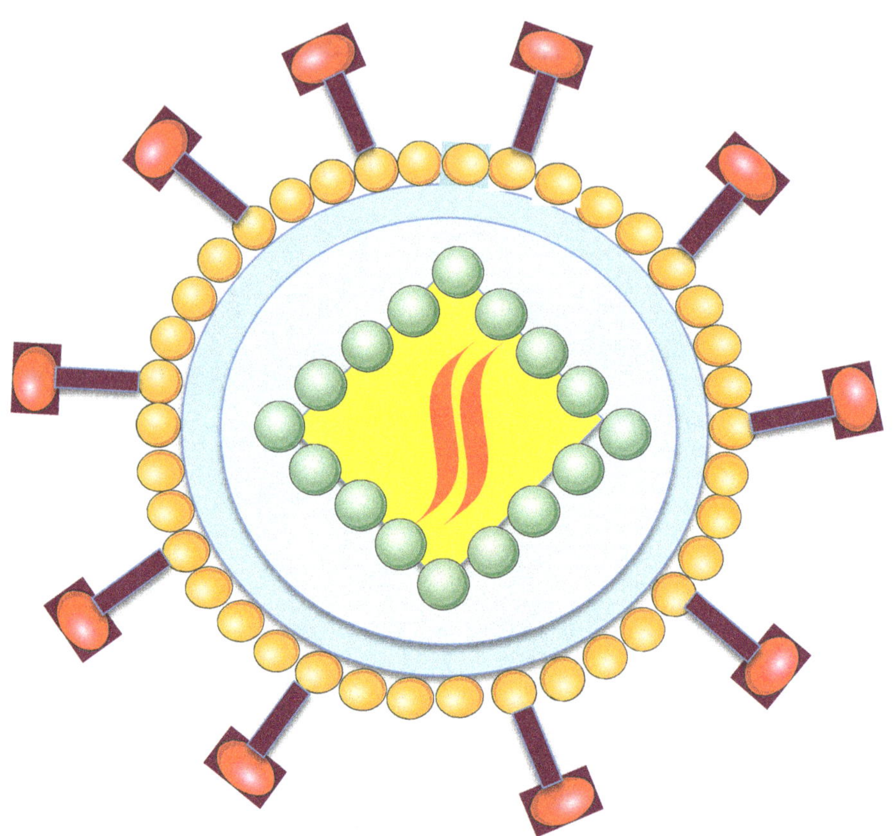

Large DNA viruses have double-stranded DNA (larger than10kb).
Small DNA viruses with single- or double-stranded circular DNA or replication through an RNA intermediate.

Spontaneous mutations have different rates in the small and large virus groups. The effects of these unrepaired genetic change are **passed on to the viral progeny** in successive infection cycles.

Oncogenic DNA viruses use a variety processes to disrupt cellular machinery and cause the infected cells to acquire the properties of cancer.

- Express virus cancer causing genes (oncogenes)
- Modify many cellular genes by changing expression patterns, or inactivation, or by targeting for degradation
- Disabling major tumor suppressor proteins and cell death
- Continued and increased proliferation of the host cell.
- Induce cellular genomic instability
- Inhibition of DNA damage repair
- Immunosuppression

The properties of DNA viruses

Smallpox (variola) virus

Smallpox is an acute, contagious disease caused by the variola virus and exists in two forms, **variola major and minor**. The more common major form causes increased severe disease with higher mortality (up to 30%). The minor form is less common and not as severe (mortality 1%). The two forms have a highly similar DNA sequence and the variable mortality may be due to gene expression differences.

A **poxvirus** is a brick-shaped virus (350 by 270 nm) with a **very large genome** (130–360 kb) consisting of single, linear double-stranded DNA coding for over 150 genes. DNA replication occurs in the cytoplasm of the host cell but using viral enzymes.

Members of the **poxvirus family** include **variola virus**, the causative agent of smallpox and the **vaccinia virus,** which is antigenically very similar to smallpox virus.

Smallpox (variola virus) is a poxvirus with a **genome** of a single, linear, double-stranded DNA (186kb) that codes for about 200 proteins.

1 Outer membrane

2 Core membrane

3 The outer surface of the virus consists of lipids and proteins

4 The core contains 10 enzymes that regulate gene expression and 100 nucleoproteins involved in DNA transcription

Membrane surface proteins facilitate attachment by binding to heparin or laminin on the host cell surface

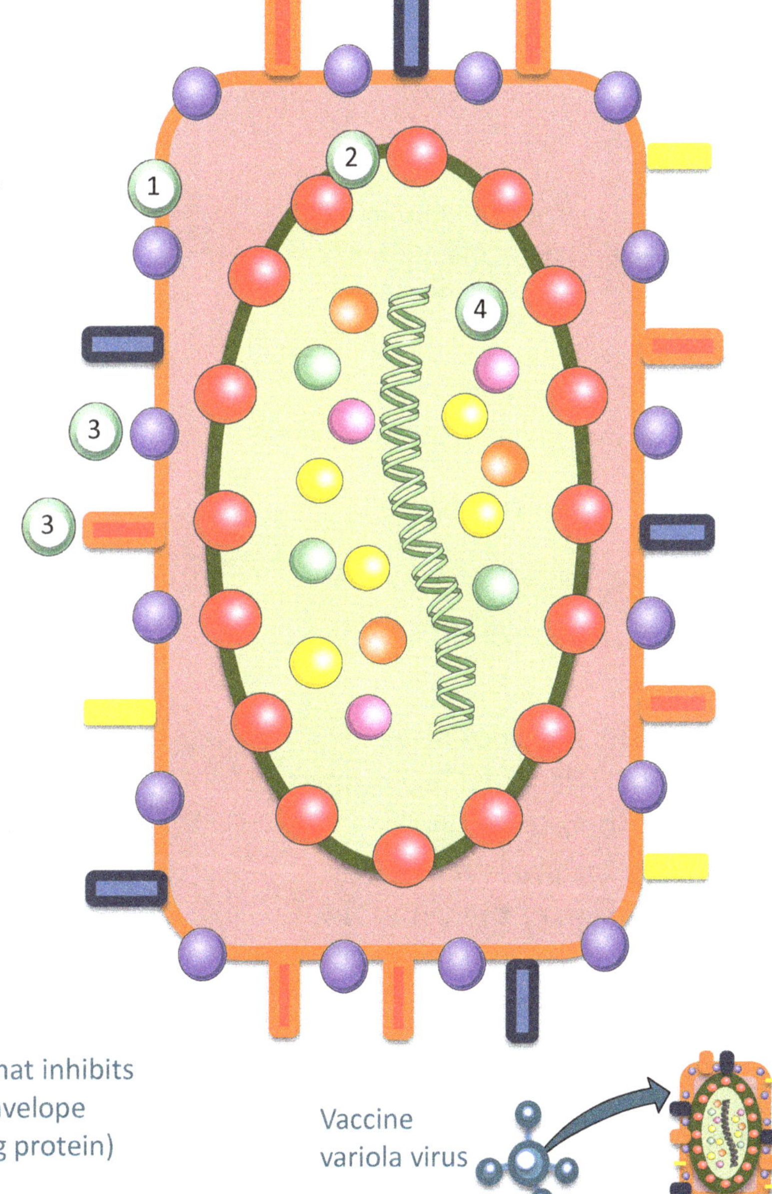

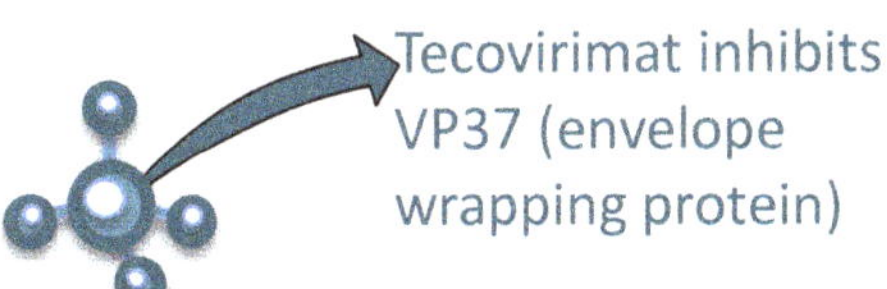

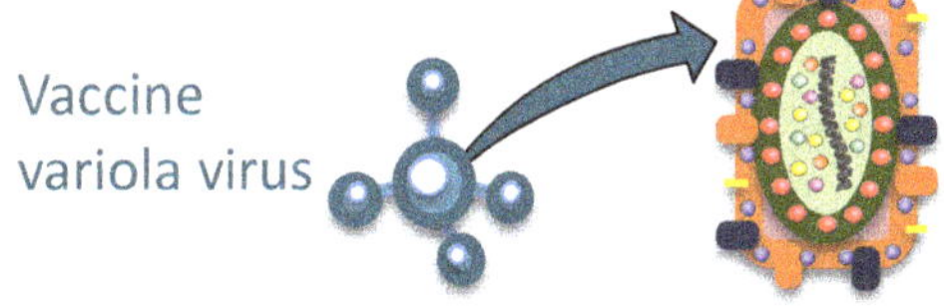

DNA viruses, description of the smallpox virus

The disease: Smallpox

Smallpox is caused by the variola virus, which causes fever with complications of encephalitis and blindness. Infection occurs in the respiratory mucosa or skin to invade nearby lymph nodes and the bloodstream to attack bone, spleen, and skin cells (blisters).

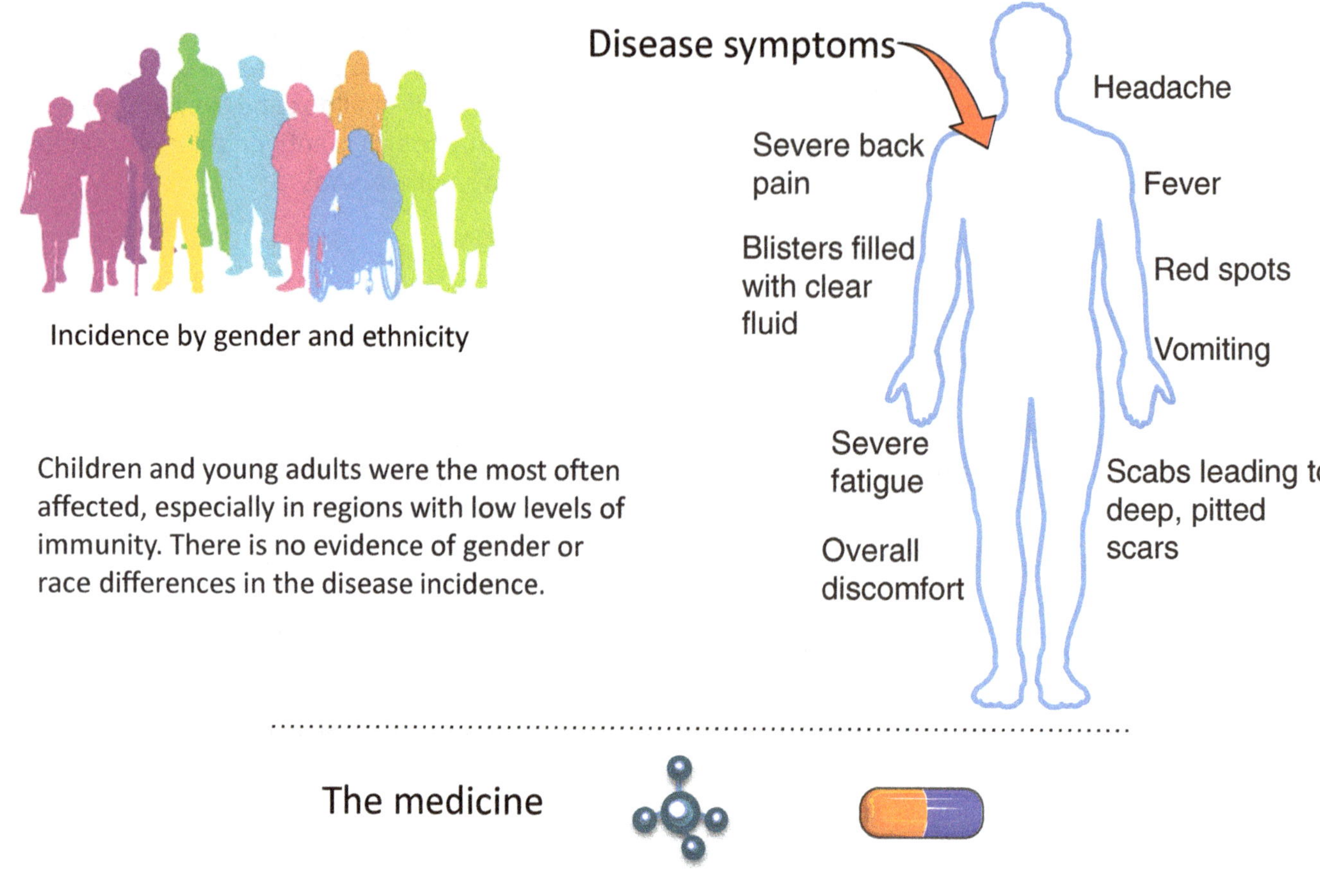

Incidence by gender and ethnicity

Children and young adults were the most often affected, especially in regions with low levels of immunity. There is no evidence of gender or race differences in the disease incidence.

The medicine

Tecovirimat; Tpoxx, FDA Approval 2018

Tecovirimat treats smallpox disease caused by the variola virus. Tecovirimat **inhibits** the orthopoxvirus VP37 **envelope wrapping protein** to block cellular transmission of the virus. This inhibition prevents dissemination of the virus in the host. Tecovirimat was approved under the US FDA's Animal Rule (based on efficacy in relevant animal models).

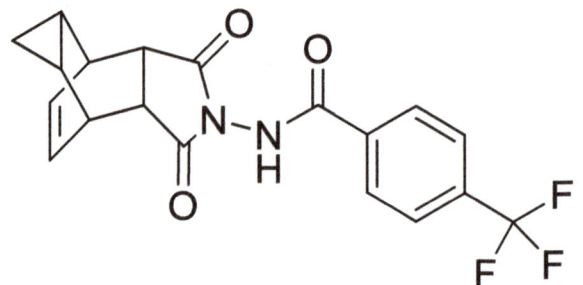

Smallpox viruses : Inhibition of viral wrapping, Tecovirimat

Action of Tecovirimat on cell and disease biology

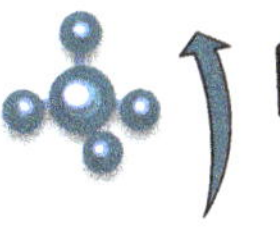

1 **Viral attachment** to the **cell surfaces**, membrane fusion, entry of the viral core into the cytoplasm, and expression of **early genes** needed for DNA replication.

2 To assemble the enveloped virus the DNA genome is encased in a protein core and an outer lipoprotein membrane, which is nucleated by the **envelope wrapping protein VP37.**

3 The **wrapping process** occurs in the **Golgi apparatus** followed by virus transfer to the cell-surface membrane.

4 **Tecovirimat inhibits the VP37 protein** from interacting with intracellular transport components and prevents the wrapping of viral membrane structures and production of enveloped virus.

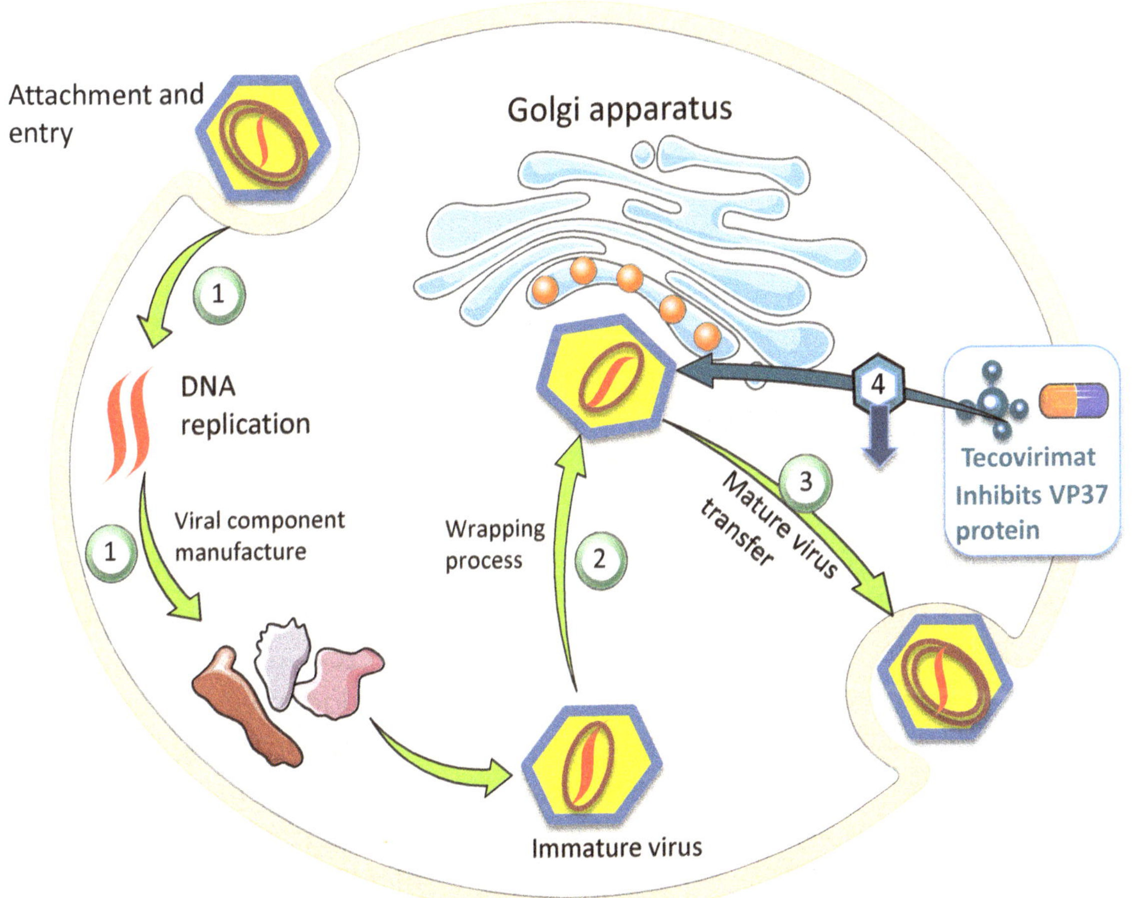

Smallpox viruses : Inhibition of viral wrapping, Tecovirimat

The disease: Smallpox

Smallpox is caused by the variola virus, which causes fever with complications of encephalitis and blindness. Infection occurs in the respiratory mucosa or skin to invade nearby lymph nodes and the bloodstream to attack bone, spleen and skin cells (blisters).

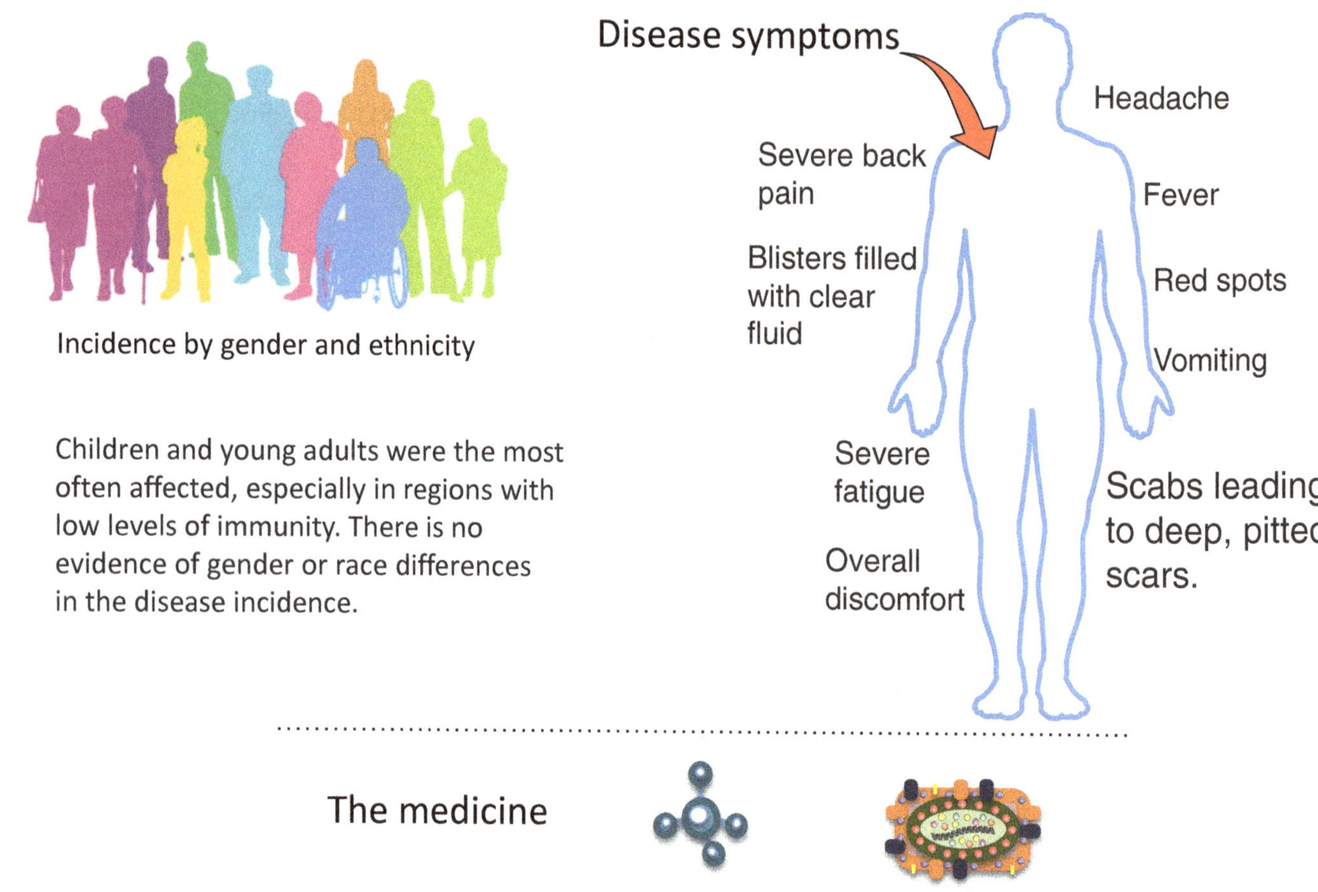

Incidence by gender and ethnicity

Children and young adults were the most often affected, especially in regions with low levels of immunity. There is no evidence of gender or race differences in the disease incidence.

The medicine

Smallpox (Vaccinia) Vaccine, Live; ACAM2000, FDA Approval 2007

The vaccine ACAM2000 involves active immunization with live vaccinia virus, which is a poxvirus similar to smallpox but causes mild infection such as rash and fever. The vaccine is administered to persons determined to be at high risk for smallpox infection as part of US emergency preparedness.

A droplet of ACAM2000 is administered through a needle-puncture of the skin. The injection of virus causes a **localized infection and stimulates the immune system** to protect against smallpox infection.

Smallpox viruses: Vaccination, ACAM2000

Action of ACAM2000 on cell and disease biology

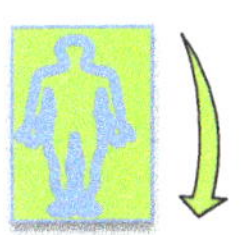

1 ACAM2000 is made from the less harmful poxvirus **vaccinia virus** and not from a killed or weakened virus like many other vaccines.

ACAM2000 is made by **culture in Vero cells** (monkey kidney epithelial cells). Cellular debris and genomic material are removed.

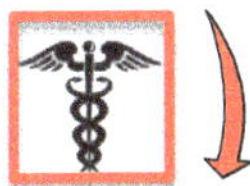

2 From the infected lungs the virus spreads via the bloodstream and results in **skin lesions, enlargement of liver and kidneys, and edema of brain**.

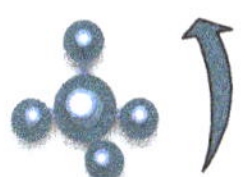

3 **ACAM2000** produces antibodies that protect against smallpox infection and helper T-cells stimulate interferon production to block viral replication.

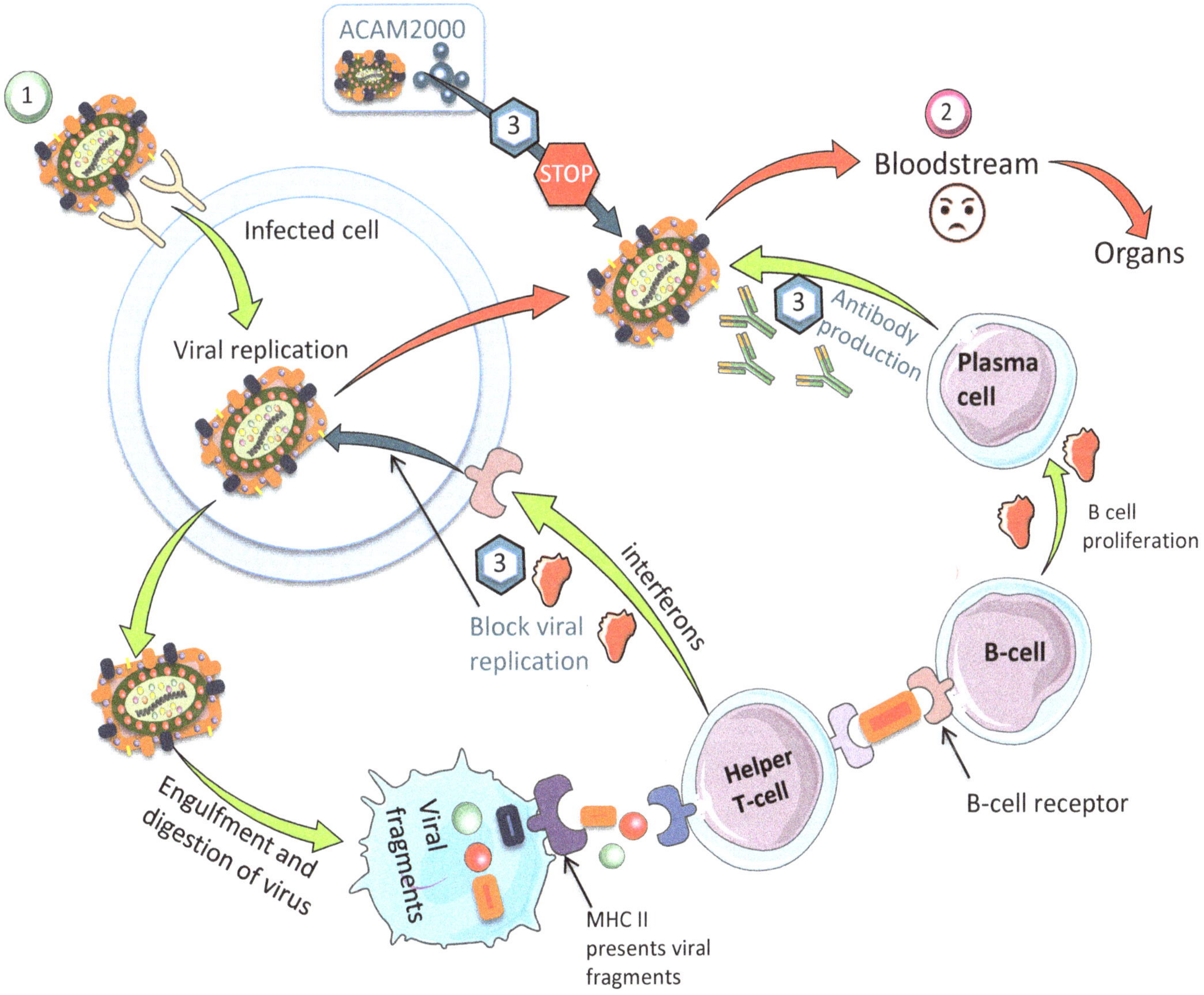

Hepatitis B (HBV)

Hepatitis means inflammation of the liver and is most often caused by viral hepatitis. In the United States, a total of about 3,000 cases of acute hepatitis B are reported annually.

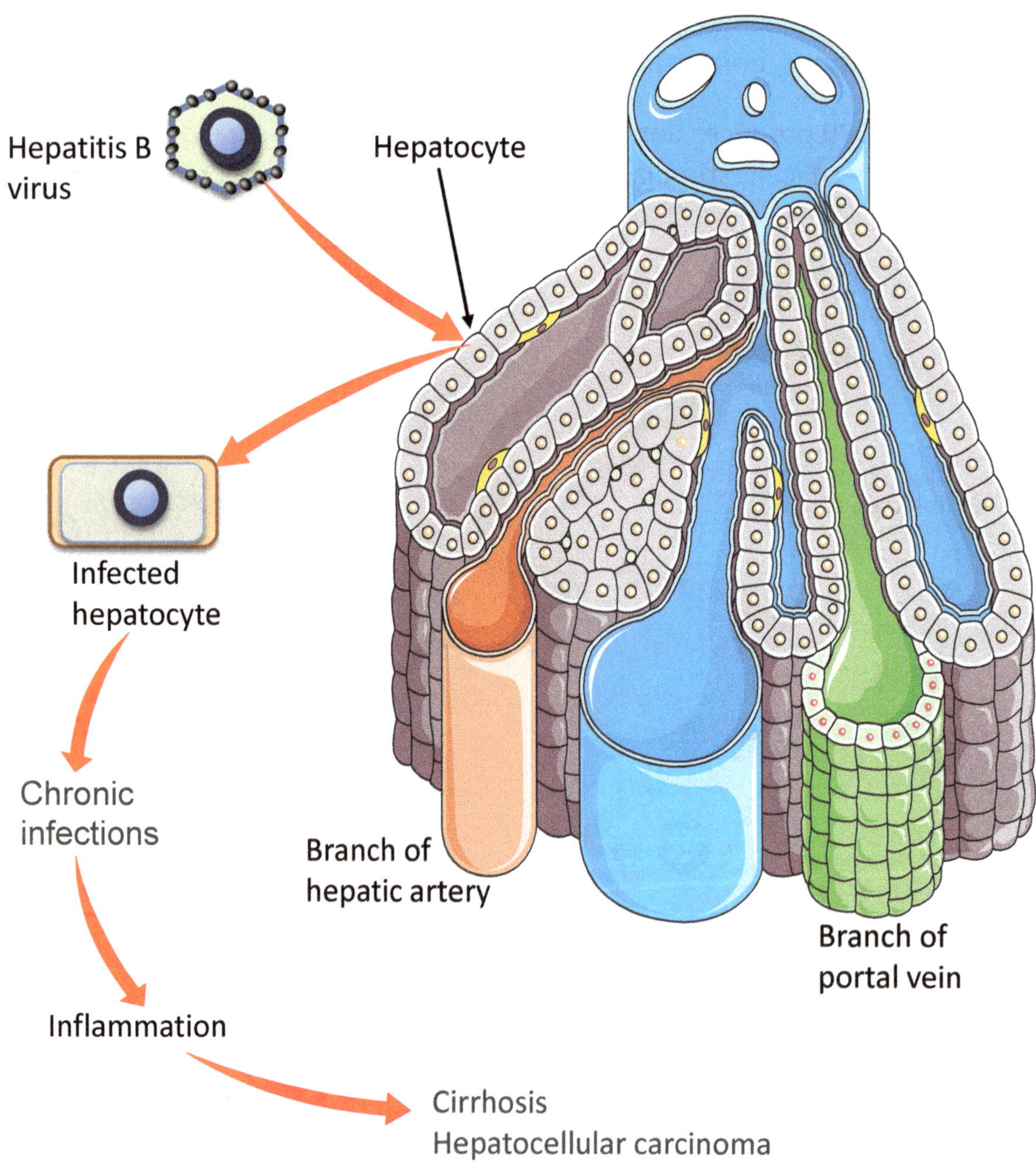

DNA viruses: Description of the hepatitis B virus (HBV)

Hepatitis B (HBV)

Hepatitis B is a spherical virus (42 nm) with a capsid containing a circular double-stranded DNA (3.2 and 1.8 kb) with four open reading frames which code for the proteins of DNA polymerase, HBsAg, HBcAg, and HBx.

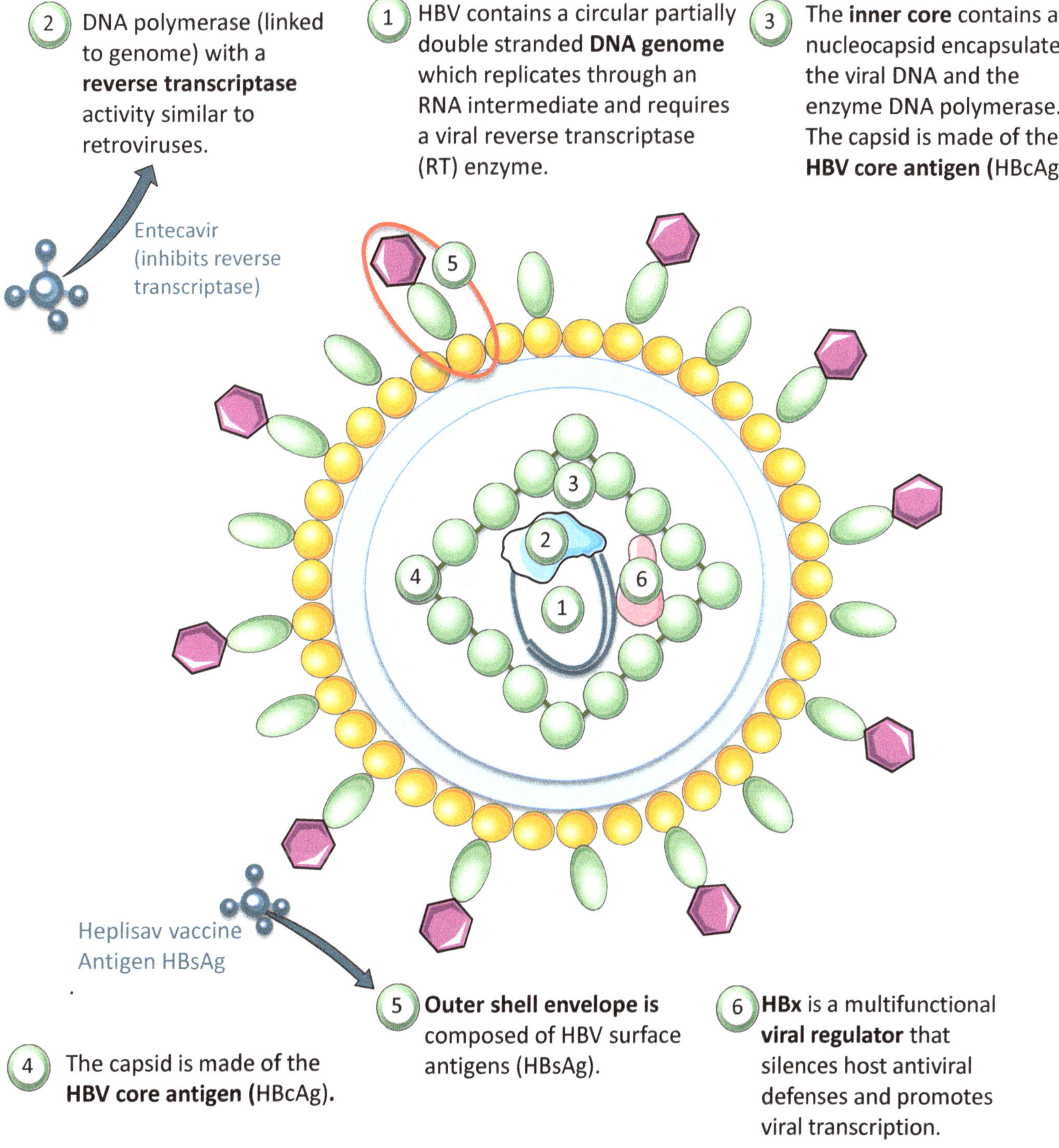

2 DNA polymerase (linked to genome) with a reverse transcriptase activity similar to retroviruses.
1 HBV contains a circular partially double stranded DNA genome which replicates through an RNA intermediate and requires a viral reverse transcriptase (RT) enzyme.
3 The inner core contains a nucleocapsid encapsulates the viral DNA and the enzyme DNA polymerase. The capsid is made of the HBV core antigen (HBcAg).
Entecavir (inhibits reverse transcriptase)
5
3
2
4
6
1
Heplisav vaccine Antigen HBsAg
5 Outer shell envelope is composed of HBV surface antigens (HBsAg).
6 HBx is a multifunctional viral regulator that silences host antiviral defenses and promotes viral transcription.
4 The capsid is made of the HBV core antigen (HBcAg).

DNA viruses: Description of the hepatitis B virus (HBV)

The disease: Hepatitis B

Hepatitis B is a liver infection caused by the hepatitis B virus (HBV), which can progress to "chronic" health problems including liver damage, cirrhosis, and liver cancer.

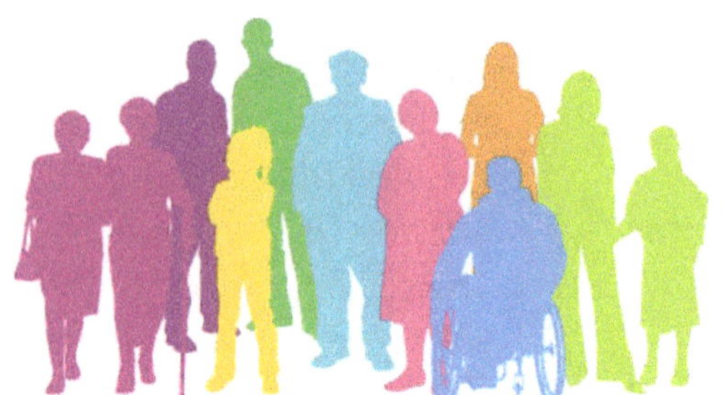

Incidence by gender and ethnicity

The prevalence of HBV infection and hepatocellular carcinoma is higher among men compared with women and female HBV carriers have lower viral loads than male carriers. HBV infection is highest among non-Hispanic Asian adults, followed by non-Hispanic black adults.

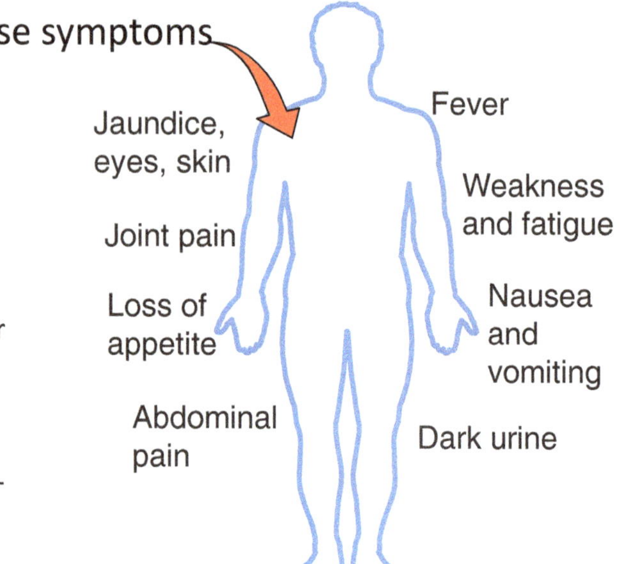

The medicine

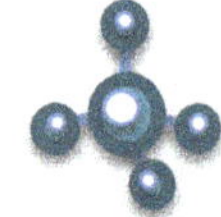

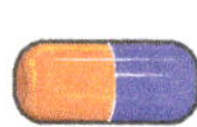

Entecavir, Baraclude; FDA Approval 2003

Entecavir triphosphate is a DNA analog, which **inhibits HBV reverse transcriptase** which synthesizes the positive strand of HBV DNA.

Entecavir **blocks viral replication** in liver cells and reduces HBV levels and infection of new liver cells.

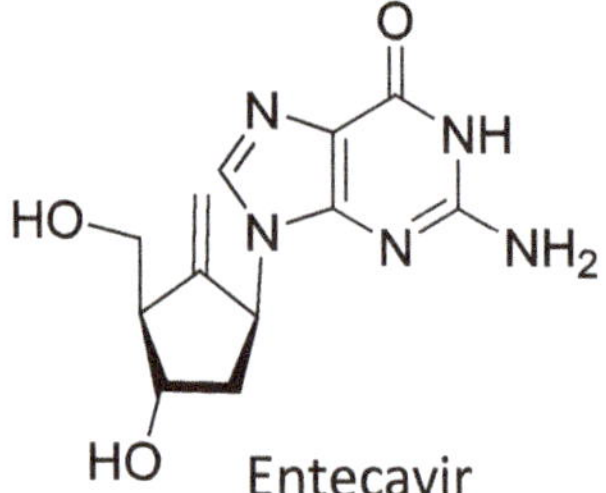

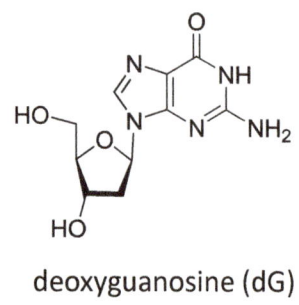

Entecavir

deoxyguanosine (dG)

Entecavir, a guanosine nucleoside analogue is phosphorylated to the active triphosphate form, which competes with the natural substrate dG.

Hepatitis B virus: Inhibition of reverse transcriptase, Entecavir

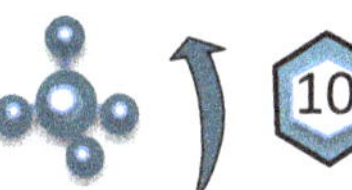

Steps of hepatitis B replication

1. Attachment of the virus to receptors
2. Cell entry and release of nucleocapsid (viral genome and protein coat)
3. Nuclear import of virus DNA
4. Synthesis of covalently closed circular DNA
5. Synthesis of RNA intermediate
6. Reverse transcriptase synthesizes HBV DNA genome.
7. Secretion of immature nucleocapsid to cytoplasm
8. Synthesis of mature nucleocapsid
9. Secretion of mature viron

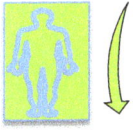

10 **Entecavir** is a guanine analogue that inhibits all three steps (4,5,6) in the viral replication process.

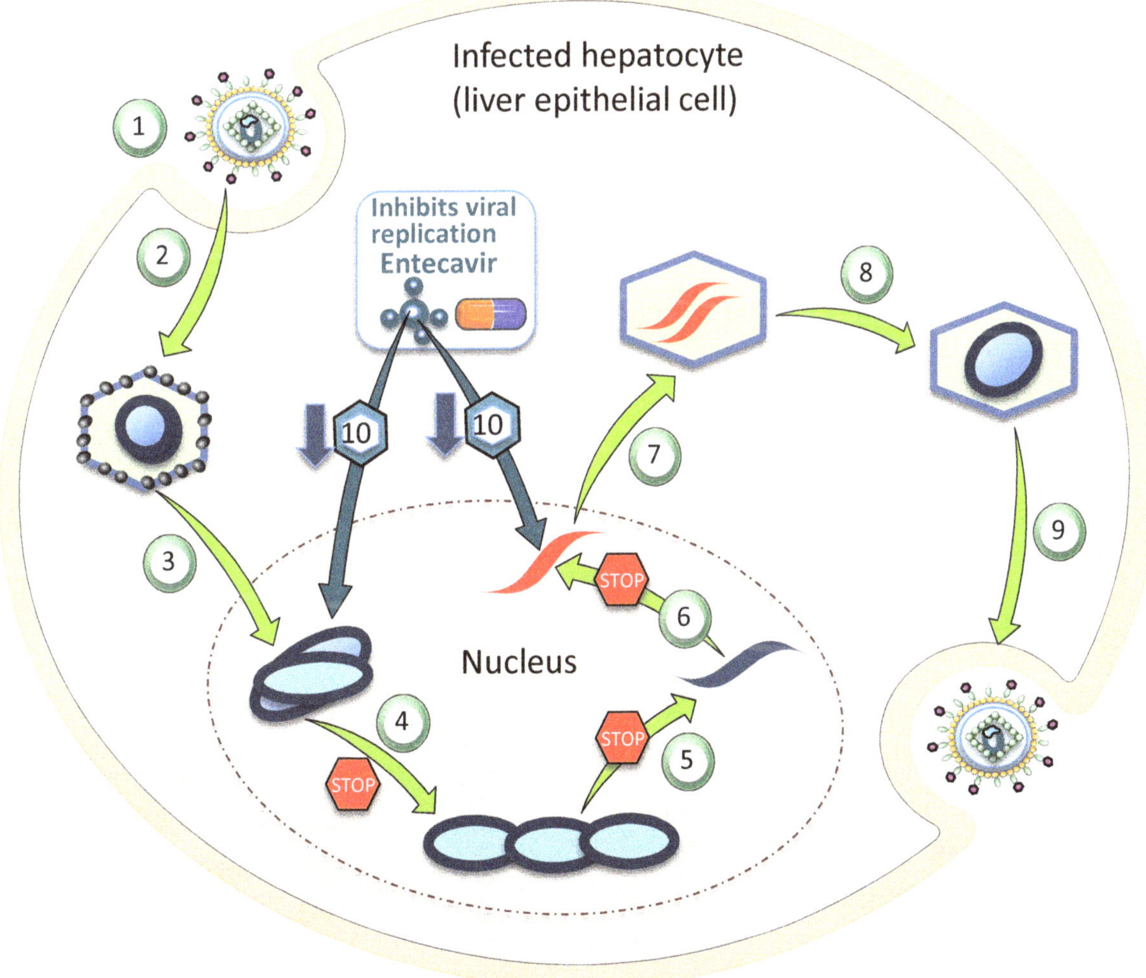

Hepatitis B virus: Inhibition of reverse transcriptase, Entecavir

The disease: Hepatitis B

Hepatitis B is a liver infection caused by the hepatitis B virus (HBV), which can progress to "chronic" health problems including liver damage, cirrhosis, and liver cancer.

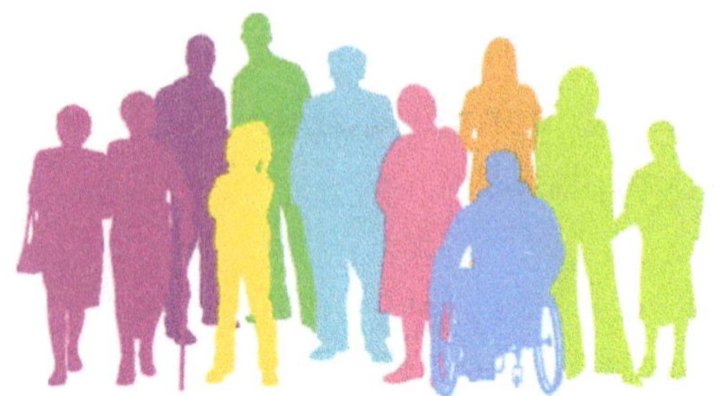

Incidence by gender and ethnicity

The prevalence of HBV infection and hepatocellular carcinoma is higher among men compared with women and female HBV carriers have lower viral loads than male carriers. HBV infection is highest among non-Hispanic Asian adults, followed by non-Hispanic black adults.

Disease symptoms

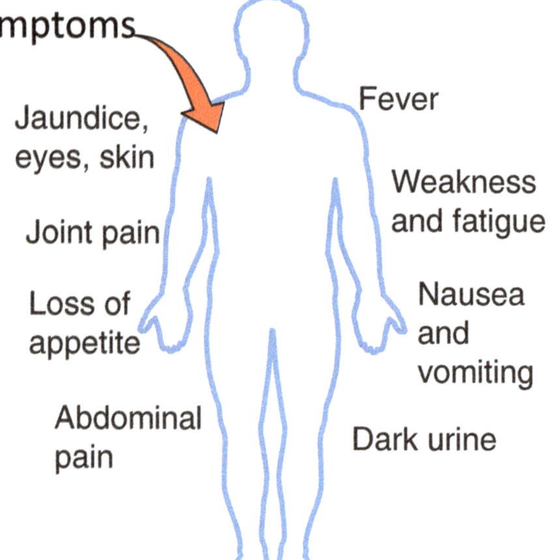

The medicine

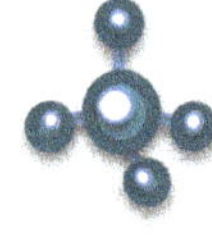

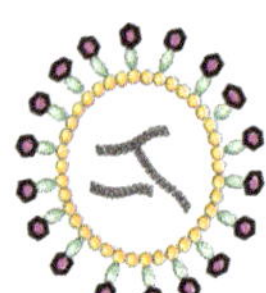

Recombivax, FDA Approval 1986 Engerix, FDA Approval 1989

Heplisav-B , FDA Approval 2020

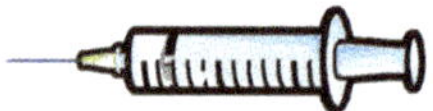

Vaccination by intramuscular injection into the deltoid muscle.

Recombivax, Engerix contain yeast expressed **hepatitis B surface antigen (HBsAg)** formulated as a suspension adsorbed on **aluminum hydroxide (adjuvant)** with an immunization schedule of three doses.

Heplisav is formulated from **recombinant HBsAg** made in yeast together with an **oligodeoxynucleotide (CpG 1018) adjuvant**. Heplisav requires only a two-dose schedule.

Hepatitis B virus: Vaccines, Recombivax, Engerix, Heplisav-B

Action of Hepatitis B vaccine on cell and disease biology

1. **Plasmid** initiates **yeast replication of** HBV surface antigen **(HBsAg)**, which then **self assembles** into repeated arrays (VLPs).
2. **Virus-like particles (VLPs)** are assemblies of HBsAg fragments without genetic material **and similar to viral structures**.
3. **VLP** promote **maturation** of **dendritic cells** and CpG adjuvant activates the **TLR9 receptor** with release of **cytokines**.
4. VLP peptides are loaded on major histocompatibility complex **(MHC) class I and class II proteins** to **activate CD4+ T cell** with B cell differentiation into antibody producing cells and activation of **helper T cells** with production of interferons to block HPV replication.

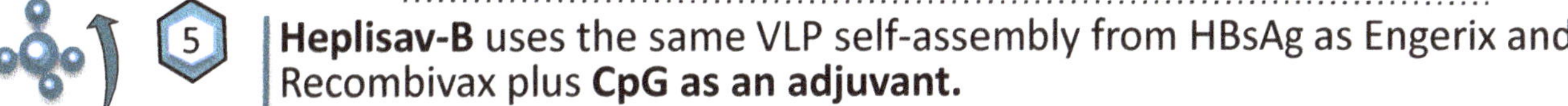

5. **Heplisav-B** uses the same VLP self-assembly from HBsAg as Engerix and Recombivax plus **CpG as an adjuvant.**

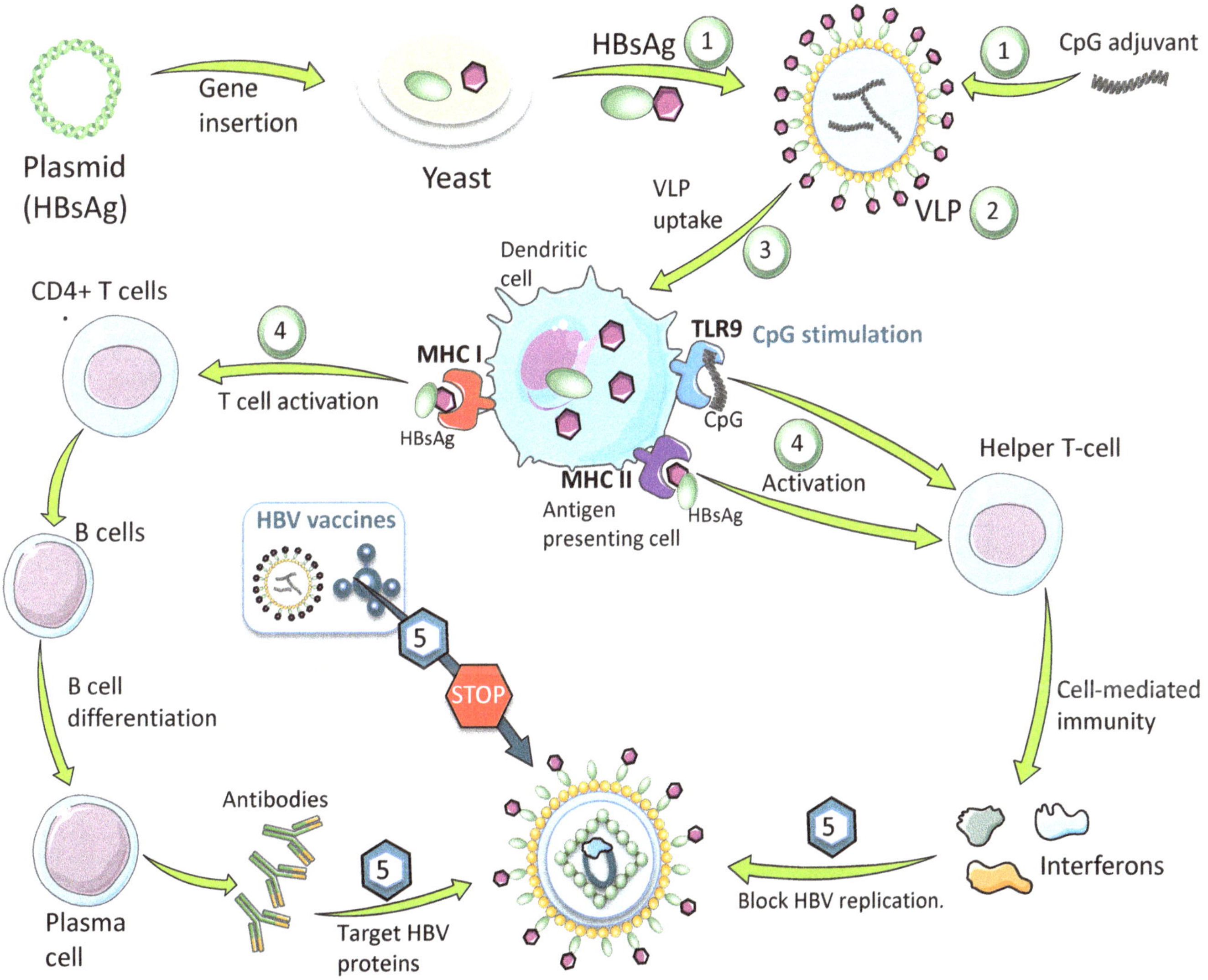

Plasmid (HBsAg)
Gene insertion
Yeast
HBsAg 1
CpG adjuvant 1
VLP 2
VLP uptake 3
Dendritic cell
CD4+ T cells
4 T cell activation
MHC I
HBsAg
TLR9 CpG stimulation
CpG
4 Activation
Helper T-cell
MHC II
HBsAg
Antigen presenting cell
B cells
HBV vaccines
5
STOP
B cell differentiation
Cell-mediated immunity
Antibodies
Plasma cell
5 Target HBV proteins
5 Block HBV replication.
Interferons

Human papillomavirus (HPV) virus

Human papillomavirus (HPV) is the most common sexually transmitted infection that **infects keratinocytes** and the basal layer of stratified squamous epithelial skin or mucosal cells.

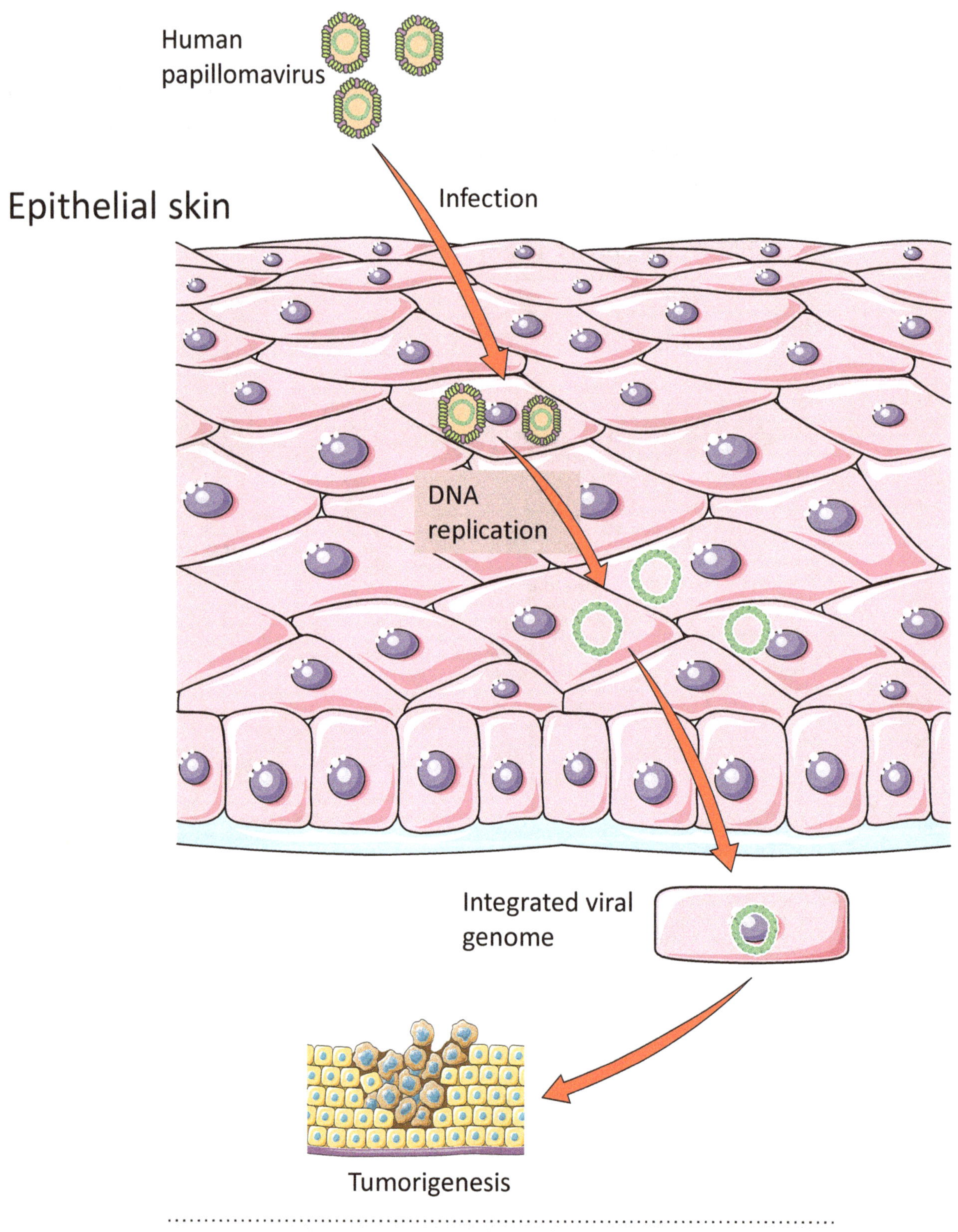

DNA viruses: Description of the human papillomavirus virus.

Human papillomavirus (HPV) virus

Human papillomavirus (HPV) is the most common sexually transmitted infection that **infects keratinocytes** and the basal layer of stratified squamous epithelia skin or mucosal cells.

Human papillomavirus (HPV) is a small, icosahedral, **nonenveloped deoxyribonucleic acid (DNA) virus** with a diameter of 55 nm and consists of a single double-stranded DNA molecule of 8 kB bound to host cell histones within a protein capsid. **The genome encodes for 6 early proteins** responsible for virus replication and **2 late proteins, L1 and L2**, which are the viral structural proteins.

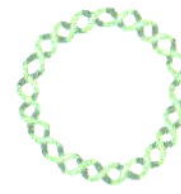

The genome has an early region which codes for **six regulatory proteins** (E1, E2, E4, E5, E6 and E7) that are expressed immediately on infection, plus a late region encoding the **capsid proteins L1 and 2**.

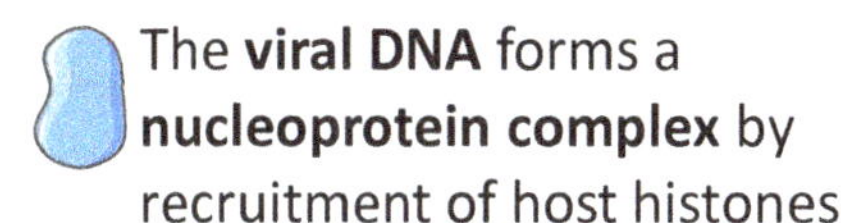

The **viral DNA** forms a **nucleoprotein complex** by recruitment of host histones.

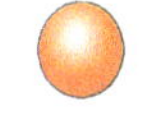

E1 and E2 proteins maintain the **circular viral DNA. structure and initiate replication.**

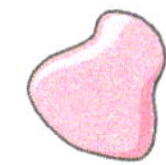

E4 promotes viral genome amplification and mature viral release by disrupting the host cell cytoskeleton.

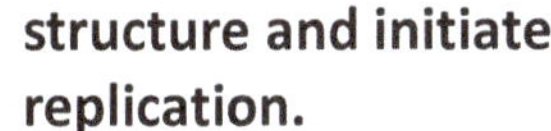

Vaccine, L1 protein antigen

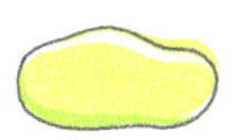

L1 protein

- Forms the capsid.
- Interacts with negatively charged sugars on the host cell surface for **initial attachment**.
- Interacts with a cell surface protein (integrin) **to promote viral entry.**

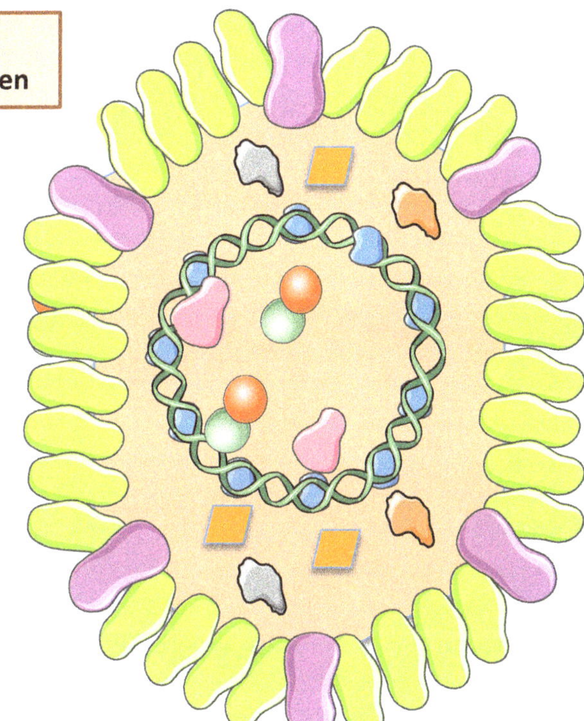

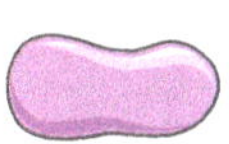

L2 protein

- Facilitates the **packaging of the viral genome** into nascent virions and **entry into the infected cell.**
- **Disrupts host cell membranes** through a negatively charged cell-penetrating peptide which allows escape of **viral DNA** with L2 to the **host cell nucleus.**

E5 **down regulates** HLA class I proteins on the host cell surface and action of $CD8^+$ **cytotoxic T cells.**

E6 and E7 promote **replication of viral DNA** and interfere with type 1 interferon responses blocking antiviral cascades in the host cell.

DNA viruses: Description of the human papillomavirus virus.

The disease: Human papillomavirus infection

Human papillomavirus (HPV) is a viral infection passed through skin-to-skin contact and commonly causes skin or mucous membrane growths (warts). There are **over 40 strains of HPV**, which are passed through sexual contact and can affect genitals, mouth, or throat and **can cause six types of cancers** later in life including **cervical cancer.**

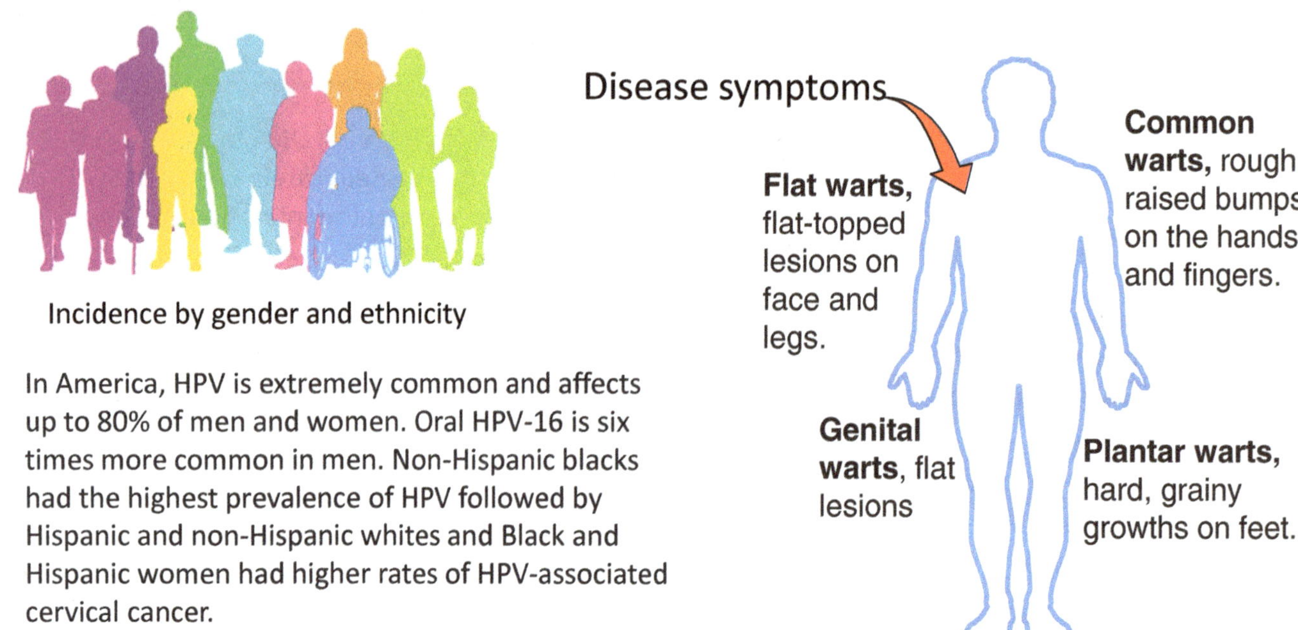
Disease symptoms
Flat warts, flat-topped lesions on face and legs.
Common warts, rough, raised bumps on the hands and fingers.
Genital warts, flat lesions
Plantar warts, hard, grainy growths on feet.

Incidence by gender and ethnicity

In America, HPV is extremely common and affects up to 80% of men and women. Oral HPV-16 is six times more common in men. Non-Hispanic blacks had the highest prevalence of HPV followed by Hispanic and non-Hispanic whites and Black and Hispanic women had higher rates of HPV-associated cervical cancer.

The medicine

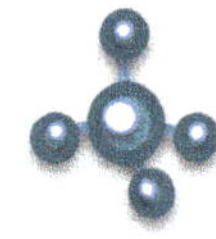
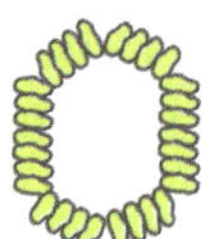

Human papillomavirus vaccine (Recombinant), Gardasil-9, 2014

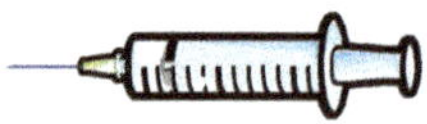

Vaccination by intramuscular injection into the deltoid muscle.

Gardasil-9 is a noninfectious **9-valent recombinant vaccine** prepared from the purified virus-like particles (VLPs) of the major capsid (L1) protein of 9 HPV types 6, 11, 16, 18, 31, 33, 45, 52, and 58. Vaccination of children (2 doses) at ages 11–12 years can prevent 90% of cervical cancers.

Human papillomavirus virus : Gardasil-9 vaccine

Action of Gardasil-9 vaccine on cell and disease biology

1 **Plasmid initiates yeast expression of HPV** L1 protein, which is purified and adsorbed on an aluminum-containing adjuvant.

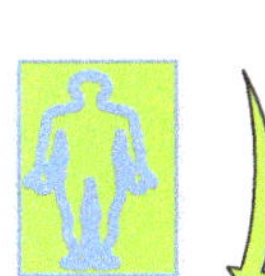

2 **Virus-like particles (VLPs) are assemblies of L1 proteins** without genetic material **and similar to viral structures and size.**

3 **VLPs strong activators of dendritic cells,** VLP peptides are loaded on major histocompatibility complex **(MHC) class I proteins** to **activate CD4+ T cell** with B cell differentiation into antibody producing cells.

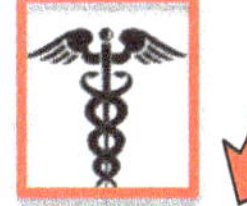

4 **HPV infection of injured epithelial cells promotes the** development of precancerous states.

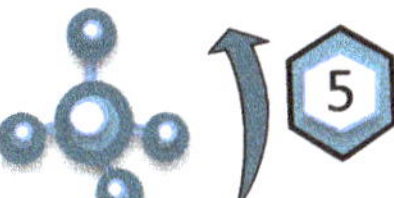

5 **Gardasil-9** induces **high serum levels of antibodies** specific to the targeted HPV types.

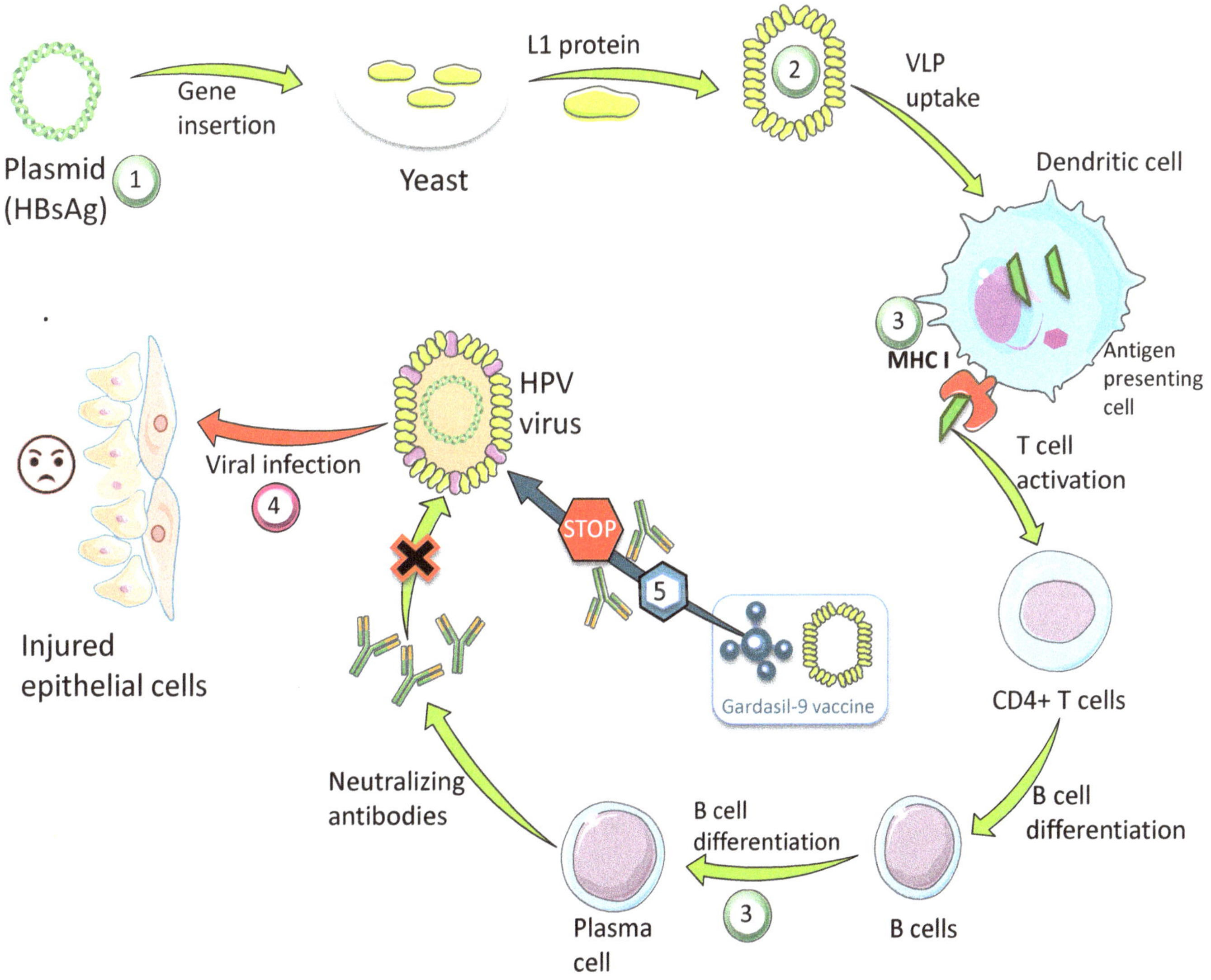

Plasmid (HBsAg) 1
Gene insertion
Yeast
L1 protein
2
VLP uptake
Dendritic cell
3
MHC I
Antigen presenting cell
T cell activation
CD4+ T cells
B cell differentiation
B cells
B cell differentiation
3
Plasma cell
Neutralizing antibodies
STOP
5
Gardasil-9 vaccine
HPV virus
Viral infection
4
Injured epithelial cells

Human papillomavirus virus : Gardasil-9 vaccine

Additional reading

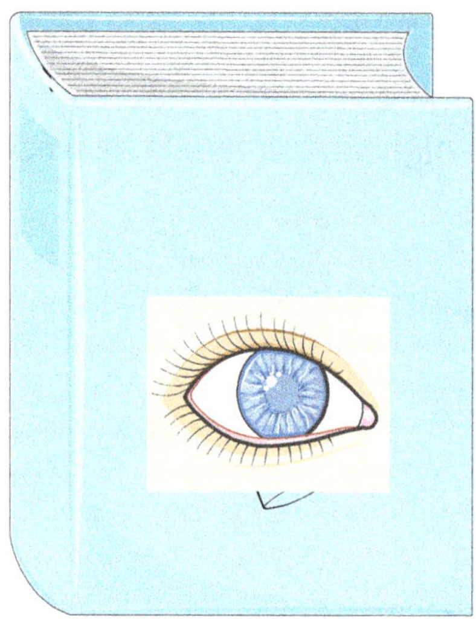

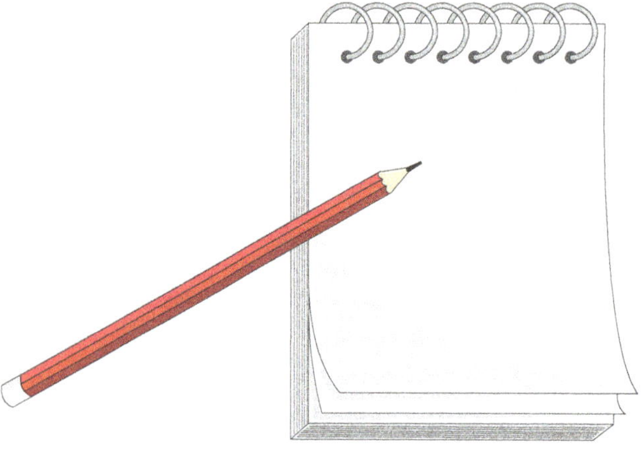

Chapter 1

Illustration: get your research the attention it deserves, Andy Tay, Nature, 586, 157–158 (2021)
https://www.nature.com/articles/d41586-020-02660-3
Three scientific artists explain how to create impact with attractive visuals.

Jargon shuts readers out, Chris Woolston, Nature, 579, 309–310 (2020)
https://media.nature.com/original/magazine-assets/d41586-020-00580-w/d41586-020-00580-w.pdf
Non-scientists feel confused by technical language — even if it's defined.

Family Medicine, James Marcus, New Yorker, March 11, 34-39 (2019)
https://www.newyorker.com/magazine/2019/03/11/family-medicine
At the end of his life, my father went from doctor to patient, from scientist to subject.

Chapter 2

The changing landscape of atherosclerosis, Peter Libby, Nature, 592, 524–533 (2021)
https://www.nature.com/articles/s41586-021-03392-8
Advances in our understanding of the biology of atherosclerosis have opened avenues to therapeutic interventions that promise to improve the prevention and treatment of now-ubiquitous atherosclerotic diseases.

Hepatocellular Carcinoma — Origins and Outcomes, Robin Kelley and Tim Greten, New England J of Medicine
https://www.nature.com/articles/s41572-020-00240-3
New trials are exploring combination therapies, including checkpoint inhibitors and tyrosine kinase inhibitors or anti-VEGF therapies, or even combinations of two immunotherapy regimens. The outcomes of these trials are expected to change the landscape of HCC management at all evolutionary stages.

Can Brain Science Help Us Break Bad Habits? Jerome Groopman, New Yorker, October 28, 83-85 (2019)
https://www.newyorker.com/magazine/2019/10/28/can-brain-science-help-us-break-bad-habits
Studies suggest that relying on will power is hopeless. Instead, we must find strategies that don't require us to be strong.

Chapter 3

Tissues, not blood, are where immune cells function, Donna Farber, Nature, 593, 507-509, 2021
https://www.nature.com/articles/d41586-021-01396-y
COVID has shown we must study immunity in the whole body — let's sort the logistics to acquire the right samples.

Age-Related Macular Degeneration, Rajendra Apte, New England J of Medicine, 385, 539-547, 2021.
https://www.nejm.org/doi/pdf/10.1056/NEJMcp2102061
Age-related macular degeneration is the leading cause of vision loss in older persons in industrialized nations. Micronutrient supplementation can reduce the risk of progression to advanced AMD. Treatment of neovascular AMD with anti–vascular endothelial growth factor pharmacotherapy reduces vision loss.

A deadly spread to the brain, Nature, Natalie Healey, 587, S14-15, 2020,
https://media.nature.com/original/magazine-assets/d41586-020-03155-x/d41586-020-03155-x.pdf
Lung cancer commonly advances to the brain, leading to distressing neurological symptoms and a poor chance of survival. Better treatments are emerging for the disease, but will they help people with brain tumours?

Seeds of cancer in normal skin, Inigo Martincorena, Nature News &Views, 586, 502-506, 2020
https://www.nature.com/articles/d41586-020-02749-9
Sequencing the genomes of individual skin cells called melanocytes has revealed a rich landscape of DNA changes. These insights shed light on the origins of melanoma, an aggressive type of cancer.

Red blood cells may be immune sentinels, Mitch Leslie, Science, 374, 583-584 (2021)
https://www.science.org/content/article/red-blood-cells-may-be-immune-sentinels
Oxygen-carrying cells also capture DNA from pathogens and damaged cells

Chapter 4

The history of blood, Jerome Groopman, New Yorker, January 14, 58-64 (2019)
https://www.newyorker.com/magazine/2019/01/14/the-history-of-blood
For centuries, curiosity about the mystical and biological functions of blood has fuelled both dangerous misunderstandings and revolutionary discoveries.

Insights into Salt Handling and Blood Pressure, David Ellison and Paul Welling, New England J of Medicine, 385, 1981-1990, 2021
https://www.nejm.org/doi/full/10.1056/NEJMra2030212
Salt intake is associated with blood pressure, but the relationship is complex. This review highlights the interplay among renal salt transport, salt storage in the skin and interstitium, vascular adaptation to changes in the salt concentration, and neurohormonal signaling.

Carbohydrates, insulin, and obesity, John Speakman and Kevin Hall, Science, 372, 577-588 (2021)
https://www.science.org/doi/10.1126/science.aav0448
Insulin plays a role in body fat regulation independent of dietary carbohydrates.

Obesity, Immunity, and Cancer, Jeffrey Rathmell, New England J of Medicine, 384, 1160-1162, 2021
https://www.nejm.org/doi/full/10.1056/NEJMcibr2035081
Obesity is linked to a risk of certain types of cancer, such as liver cancer and uterine cancer. A recent study provides some clues as to why.

Immune-cell shutdown harms old brains, Jonas Neher , Nature News &Views, 590, 2021
https://media.nature.com/original/magazine-assets/d41586-021-00063-6/d41586-021-00063-6.pdf
Immune cells called macrophages have been found to shut down major metabolic pathways during ageing. Restoring metabolism in these cells is sufficient to alleviate age- associated cognitive decline in mice.

Chapter 5

A sense of self, Emily Underwood, Science, 372, 1142-1145 (2021)
https://www.science.org/doi/abs/10.1126/science.372.6547.1142
Communication between the brain and other organs shapes how we think, remember and feel.

The simplest of slumbers, Elizabeth Pennesi, Science, 374, 526-529, 2021.
https://www.science.org/doi/epdf/10.1126/science.acx9444
"Evidence from evolutionary ancient creatures is revealing that sleep is just not for our brain".

Medicine and the Mind — The Consequences of Psychiatry's Identity Crisis, Caleb Gardner and Arthur Kleinman**,** New England J of Medicine, 381, 1697-1699, 2019.
https://www.nejm.org/doi/full/10.1056/NEJMp1910603
"Checklists of symptoms now take the place of thoughtful diagnosis, trial-and-error "medication management" dominates practice with less time to work with patients on difficult problems".

Schizophrenia, Stephen Marder and Tyrone Cannon, New England J of Medicine, 381, 1753-1761, 2019.
https://www.nejm.org/doi/full/10.1056/NEJMra1808803
"Schizophrenia involves multiple neurochemical pathways and brain circuits. Treatment is directed at ameliorating acute psychosis and reducing relapses.".

Multiple sclerosis enters a grey area, Jenna Pappalardo and David Hafler, Nature, 566, 465-466, 2019.
https://www.nature.com/articles/d41586-019-00563-6#:~:text=Studying%20a%20rat%20model%20of,is%20present%20in%20grey%20matter
Studies of multiple sclerosis have long focused on the white matter of the brain. Insights into how immune cells target the brain's grey matter now illuminate the stage of the disease at which neurodegeneration occurs.

Chapter 6

Overlooked and underfunded: neglected diseases exert a toll, Michael Eisenstein, Nature, 598, S20-22 (2021)
https://www.natureindex.com/news-blog/overlooked-and-underfunded-neglected-diseases-exert-a-toll
Solutions for overlooked and underfunded sicknesses demand committed advocates.

Personalized RNA drugs may soon be available for more rare genetic diseases, Jocelyn Kaiser, Science, 374, 672 (2021).
https://www.science.org/content/article/personalized-rna-drugs-may-soon-be-available-more-rare-genetic-diseases
Foundation aims to accelerate "n-of-1" approach being tested by academic teams in several countries.

The less-personal touch, Anthony King, Nature, 585, S4-S6 (2020)
https://media.nature.com/original/magazine-assets/d41586-020-02675-w/d41586-020-02675-w.pdf
CAR-T immunotherapy is a specialist and complex treatment for cancer. Now, researchers are looking to provide an off-the-shelf version to make the therapy available to more people.

Fix what's broken, Sarah DeWeerdt, Nature, 583, S2-S4 (2021).
https://media.nature.com/original/magazine-assets/d41586-020-02106-w/d41586-020-02106-w.pdf
Drugs that target specific mutations in the protein at the root of cystic fibrosis have supercharged treatments for the disease and spurred the search for further therapies.

.

Chapter 7

The incredible diversity of viruses, Amber Dance, Nature, 595, 22-25 (2021)
https://media.nature.com/original/magazine-assets/d41586-021-01749-7/d41586-021-01749-7.pdf
"They are everywhere virologists look, and they are not all bad. Scientists are beginning to identify and classify the nonillions of viruses on the planet and their contributions to global ecosystems".

The tangled history of mRNA vaccines, Elie Dolgin, Nature Nature, 597, 318-324 (2021)
https://www.nature.com/articles/d41586-021-02483-w
Hundreds of scientists had worked on mRNA vaccines for decades before the coronavirus pandemic brought a breakthrough.

The Message of Measles, Nick Paumgarten, New Yorker, September 2, 38-47 (2019)
https://www.newyorker.com/magazine/2019/09/02/the-message-of-measles
As public-health officials confront the largest outbreak in the U.S. in decades, they've been fighting as much against dangerous ideas as they have against the disease.

Infectious triggers, Anthony King, Nature, 595, S48-S50 (2021)
https://media.nature.com/original/magazine-assets/d41586-021-01835-w/d41586-021-01835-w.pdf
The body's response to viruses has long been proposed to spark autoimmune disease. Pandemics could clarify the connection.

Ebola virus may lurk in survivors for many years, Kai Kupferschmidt, Science, 371, 1188 (2021)
https://www.science.org/doi/10.1126/science.371.6535.1188
Genomic analysis of Guinea patients points to "new paradigm" for how outbreaks start.

Appendix 1: Diseases (organ involved)

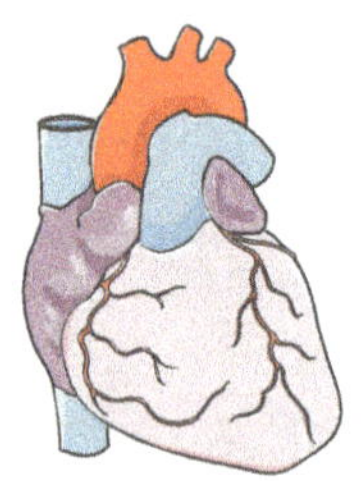

Heart

Amyloid cardiomyopathy (8)

Angina *(11)*

Coronary artery disease (20)

Hereditary transthyretin amyloidisis (36)

Hypercholesterolemia (40)

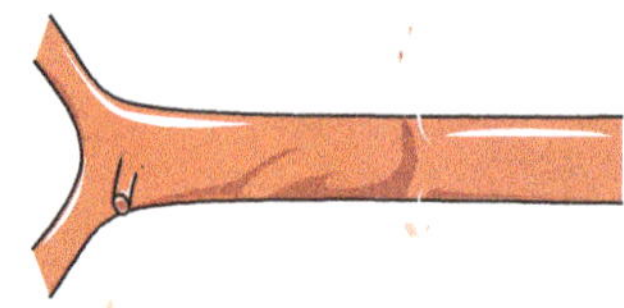

Blood and vessels

Anemia (10)

Acquired thrombotic thrombocytopenic purpura (3)

Fabry disease (29)

Hemophilia A (33)

Hypertension (41)

Non-Hodgkin lymphoma (54)

Thrombocytopenia (69)

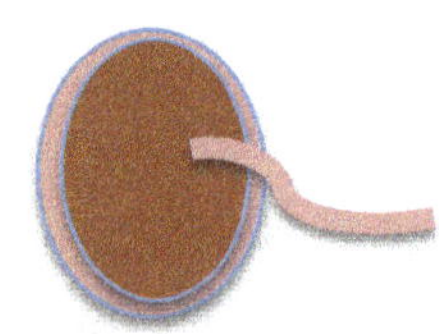

Prostate

Benign prostatic hyperplasia (15)

Prostate cancer *(62)*

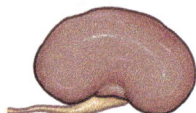

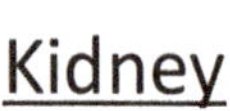

Kidney

Primary hyperoxaluria type 1 (61)

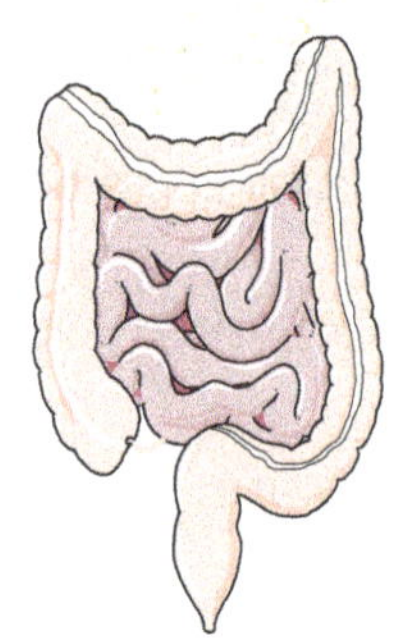

Stomach

Gastroesophageal reflux disease (30)

Gastrointestinal stromal tumors (31)

Hereditary angioedema (35)

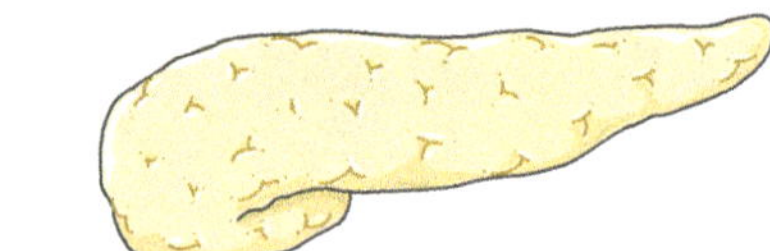

Pancreas

Severe early-onset obesity (66)

Type 1 diabetes (71)

Type 2 diabetes *(72)*

Liver

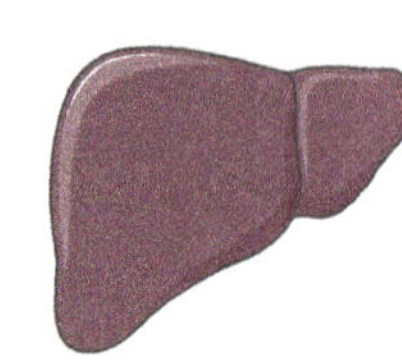

Acute hepatic porphyria (4)

Hepatitis B (34)

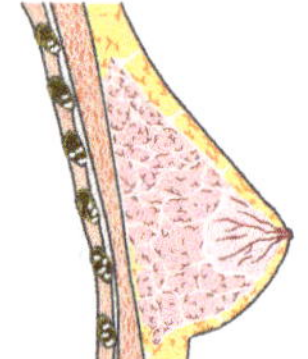

Breast

Breast cancer (18)

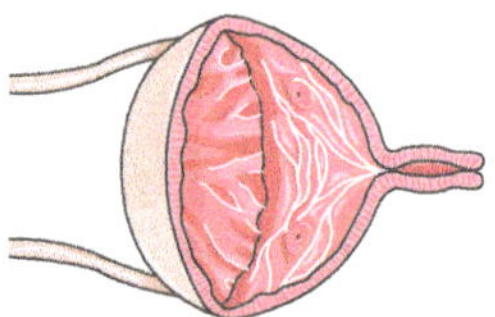

Bladder

Bladder cancer (16)

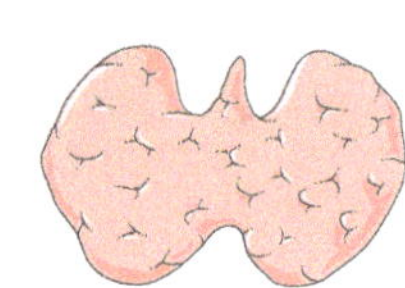

Thyroid

Hypothyroidism (42)

Appendix 1: Diseases (organ involved)

Eye
Neuromyelitis optica spectrum disorder (52)
Neurotropic keratitis (53)
Thyroid eye disease (70)
Wet macular degeneration (73)

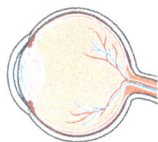

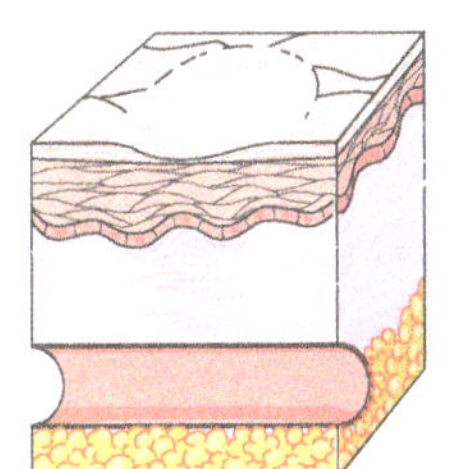

Skin
Acne vulgaris (1)
Epithelioid sarcoma (27)
Erythropoietic protoporphyria (28)
Psoriasis *(63)*

Bone
Gout (32)
Multiple myeloma (48)
Neuroblastoma (51)
Osteoporosis (56)
Rheumatoid arthritis (64)
X-linked hypophosphatemia (74)

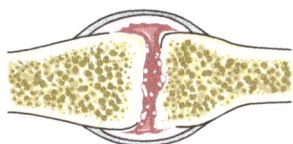

Muscle
Amyotrophic lateral sclerosis (9)
Duchenne muscular dystrophy (24)
Spinal muscle atrophy (68)

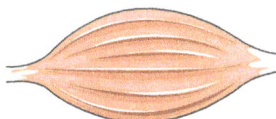

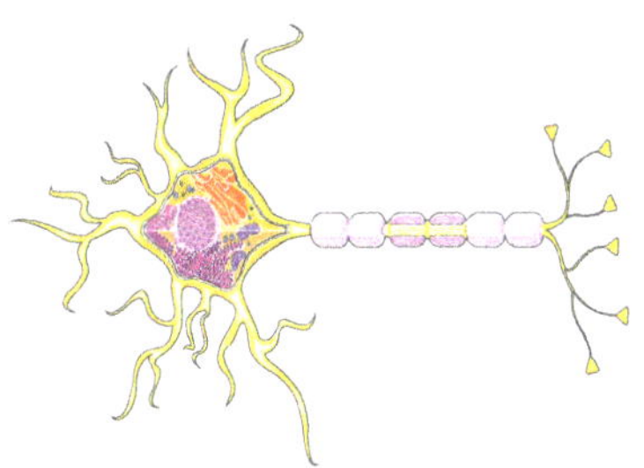

Neurological disorders
Acute pain (5)
Chronic inflammation (19)
Dravet syndrome (23)
Epilepsy (26)
Huntington's disease (38)
Hutchinson-Gilford (progeroid) syndrome (39)
Lennox-Gastaut syndrome (46)
Multiple sclerosis (49)
Parkinson's disease (57)

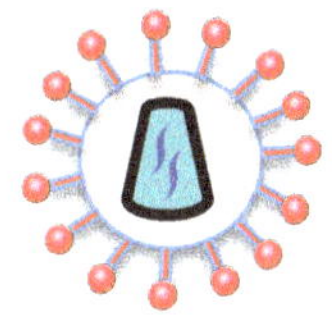

Virus
Acquired immunodeficiency syndrome (2)
Covid-19 (21,22)
Ebola (25)
Human papillomavirus (37)
Influenza (44)
Smallpox, *Tpoxx, ACAM2000 Vaccine (67)*

Appendix 1: Diseases (organ involved)

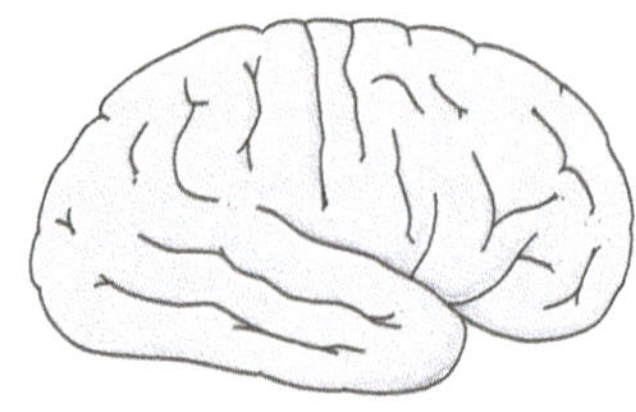

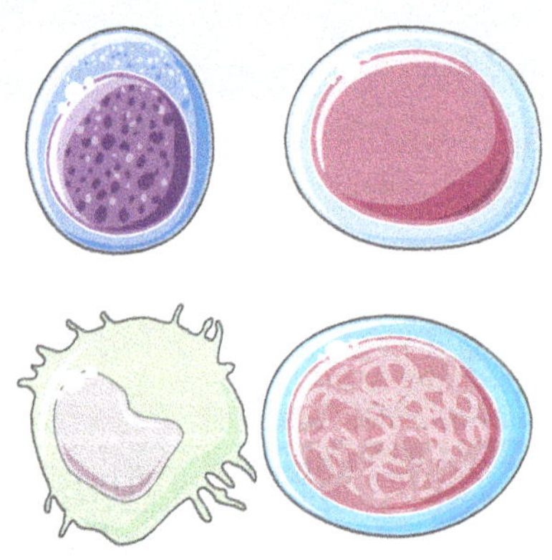

	Appendix 1 Diseases	Symptoms	Chapter	Page
	Disease, *medicine (generic name)*			
1	Acne vulgaris, *Trifarotene*	sebum secretions with inflammation of hair follicles	3	72
2	Acquired immunodeficiency syndrome, *Tenofovir, Darunavir, Dolutegravir, Enfuvirtide*	sexually transmitted infection of HIV virus	7	236, 238,240, 242
3	Acquired thrombotic thrombocytopenic purpura, *Caplacizumab*	unrestrained growth of microthrombi	3	76
4	Acute hepatic porphyria, *Givosiran*	abdominal neuropathic pain	6	210
5	Acute pain, *Hydrocodone*	derives from physical trauma	5	174
6	Adenosine deaminase deficiency, *Elapegademase*	severe combined immunodeficiency	1	10
7	Alzheimer's disease, *Donepezil*	progressive neurological disorder	5	176
8	Amyloid cardiomyopathy, *Tafamidis*	deposition of fibrils in the heart, heart failure	6	188
9	Amyotrophic lateral sclerosis, *Edaravone*	degeneration of motor neurons in spinal cord and brain	5	138
10	Anemia, *Epoetin alpha*	insufficient healthy red blood cells	4	92
11	Angina, *Nitroglycerin*	chest pain	1	16
12	Anxiety disorders, *Alprazolam*	extreme worry, panic disorders	5	160
13	B-cell lymphoma, *Axicabtagene ciloleucel*	blood cancer of B lymphocytes at lymph nodes	6	218
14	Bacterial meningitis, *Ceftriaxone*	inflammation of blood brain barrier, fever, headache	5	132
15	Benign prostatic hyperplasia, *Tamsulosin*	enlargement of the prostate gland	4	124
16	Bladder cancer, *Erdafitinib*	malignant cells in the lining of the bladder	4	122
17	Blastic plasmacytoid dendritic cell neoplasm, *Tagraxofusp*	blood cancer of the bone marrow	6	192
18	Breast cancer, *Raloxifene,Talazoparib, Alpelisib*	invasive ductal and metastatic cancer	1, 6	18,184, 186
19	Chronic inflammation, *Aspirin, Prednisone*	inflammatory process with destruction of tissue	4	114, 116
20	Coronary artery disease, *Colchicine*	reduction of blood flow to heart muscle	2, 4	50, 126
21	Covid-19, *Remdesivir, Molnupiravir, Nirmatrelvir, Bamlanivimab/Etesevimab,*	infection of upper and lower respiratory tract	7	252, 254, 256, 258
22	Covid-19, *Casirivimab/imdevimab, BNT162b2, mRNA-1273, Ad26.COV2*	infection of upper and lower respiratory tract	7	258, 260
23	Dravet syndrome, *Epidiolex*	epileptic syndrome	6	180
24	Duchenne muscular dystrophy, *Golodirsen*	muscle degeneration with progressive weakness	6	212

	Appendix 1 Diseases	Symptoms	Chapter	Page
25	Ebola, *Inmazeb, Ebola Zaire Vaccine*	lymph and blood system infected	7	246, 248
26	Epilepsy, *Lamotrigine*	recurrent seizures with convulsions	5	158
27	Epithelioid sarcoma, *Tazemetostat*	cancer of soft tissue under skin	3	68
28	Erythropoietic protoporphyria, *Afamelanotide*	intense skin pain, redness and thickening	3	74
29	Fabry disease, *Migalastat*	blood vessel narrowing, cardiac and kidney problems	6	182
30	Gastroesophageal reflux disease, *Omeprazole*	back up of acid and food into esophagus	2	28
31	Gastrointestinal stromal tumors, *Avapritinib*	connective tissue malignancies, stomach, small intestine	2	30
32	Gout, *Allopurinol*	acute arthritis, urate crystals in joints and bones	2	38
33	Hemophilia A, *Emicizumab*	excessive internal and external bleeding	6	204
34	Hepatitis B, *Entecavir, Recombivax, Engerix, Heplisav-B*	liver infection via transmission from infected bodily fluids	7	270, 272
35	Hereditary angioedema, *Lanadelumab*	severe swelling of stomach, limbs, face and throat	6	198
36	Hereditary transthyretin amylodsis, *Patisiran*	destruction of heart, GI tract, peripheral nervous system	6	214
37	Human papillomavirus, *vaccine Gardasil-9*	infection via skin to skin transmission	7	276
38	Huntington's disease, *Deutetrabenazine*	involuntary repetitive movements with chorea	5	150
39	Hutchinson-Gilford (progeroid) syndrome, Lonafarnib	premature aging	6	190
40	Hypercholesterolemia, *Bempedoic acid, Atorvastatin, Colchicine*	high levels of LDL cholesterol, cardiovascular disease	2	46,48, 50
41	Hypertension, *Lisinopril, Metoprolol, Amlodipine, Hydrochlorothiazide*	high blood pressure, chest pain, damage to arteries	4	96, 98,100, 102
42	Hypothyroidism, *Levothyroxine*	underactive thyroid, low levels of thyroid hormones T3 and T4	4	88
43	Immune system rejection, inflammatory skin conditions, *Mycophenolic acid*	psoriasis, connective tissue disorders and transplants	2	36
44	Influenza, *Zanamivir, Oseltamivir, Baloxavir, Fluzone*	infection of respiratory tract epithelial cells	7	228, 230, 232
45	Insomnia, *Eszopiclone, Lemborexant*	transient or chronic, inadequate sleep	5	162, 170

	Appendix 1 Diseases	Symptoms	Chapter	Page
46	Lennox-Gastaut syndrome, *Epidiolex*	epileptic syndrome	6	180
47	Migraine, *Galcanezumab, Lasmiditan, Ubrogepant*	throbbing/pulsing pain in one area of head	5	152, 168
48	Multiple myeloma, *Selinexor*	cancer of white blood cells in bone marrow	3	82
49	Multiple sclerosis, *Ocrelizumab, Mayzent*	inflammation of nervous system, impaired coordination	5	134, 136
50	Narcolepsy, *Solriamfetol, Pitolisant*	excessive daytime sleepiness, cataplexy	5	146, 154
51	Neuroblastoma, Naxitamab	cancer of bone and bone marrow	6	202
52	Neuromyelitis optica spectrum disorder, Satralizumab	vision loss due to inflammation of optic nerve	3	64
53	Neurotropic keratitis, *Cenegermin*	loss of corneal sensation with tissue breakdown	3	62
54	Non-Hodgkin lymphoma, *Polatuzumab, Vincristine*	cancer of lymphatic system	3	80
55	Non small lung cancer, *Lorlatinib*	group of lung cancers, effects both smokers and non smokers	3	66
56	Osteoporosis, *Romosozumab*	reduced quality of bone, increased fractures	6	200
57	Parkinson's disease, *Safinamide, Istradefylline*	progressive nervous system disorder, effects movement	5	148, 172
58	Phenylketonuria, *Pegvaliase*	cognitive, developmental and learning defects	1	12
59	Postpartum depression, *Brexanolone*	mood disorder occurring after childbirth	5	164
60	Primary hemophagocytic lymphohistiocytosis, *Emapalumab*	immune system disorder with autoimmune diseases	6	196
61	Primary hyperoxaluria type 1, *Lumasiran*	oxalate build up in kidney and urinary tract	6	216
62	Prostate cancer, *Apalutamide*	cancer of the gland cells of the prostate gland	4	120
63	Psoriasis, *Risankizumab*	chronic skin disease with raised patches of keratinocytes	3	70
64	Rheumatoid arthritis, *Upadacitinib*	inflammatory disease, effects lining of joints	4	118
65	Schizophrenia, *Lumateperone*	individual hears voices, becoming withdrawn and suspicious	5	144
66	Severe early-onset obesity, *Setmelanotide*	extreme hunger, obesity, adrenal insufficiency	6	208
67	Smallpox, *Tecovirimat, ACAM2000 Vaccine*	infection of respiratory mucosa, contact infected bodily fluids	7	264, 266

	Appendix 1 Diseases	Symptoms	Chapter	Page
68	Spinal muscle atrophy, *Onasemnogene abeparvovec*	lower limb and proximal muscle weakness with paralysis	6	220
69	Thrombocytopenia, *Lusutrombopag, Avatrombopag*	low platelet count with resulting deficiency in blood clotting	3	78
70	Thyroid eye disease, *Teprotumumab*	inflammation of orbital tissue	3	60
71	Type 1 diabetes, *Insulin glargine, Metformin*	low insulin production, high blood sugar levels	4	108
72	Type 2 diabetes, *Glimepiride, Empagliflozin, Semaglutide*	persistent hyperglycemia, insulin resistance	2, 4, 6	(42, 110), 106, 206
73	Wet macular degeneration, *Brolucizumab*	blurred vision due to damaged blood vessels	3	58
74	X-linked hypophosphatemia, *Burosumab*	rickets with impaired bone growth	6	194

Appendix 2: Medicines (site of action)

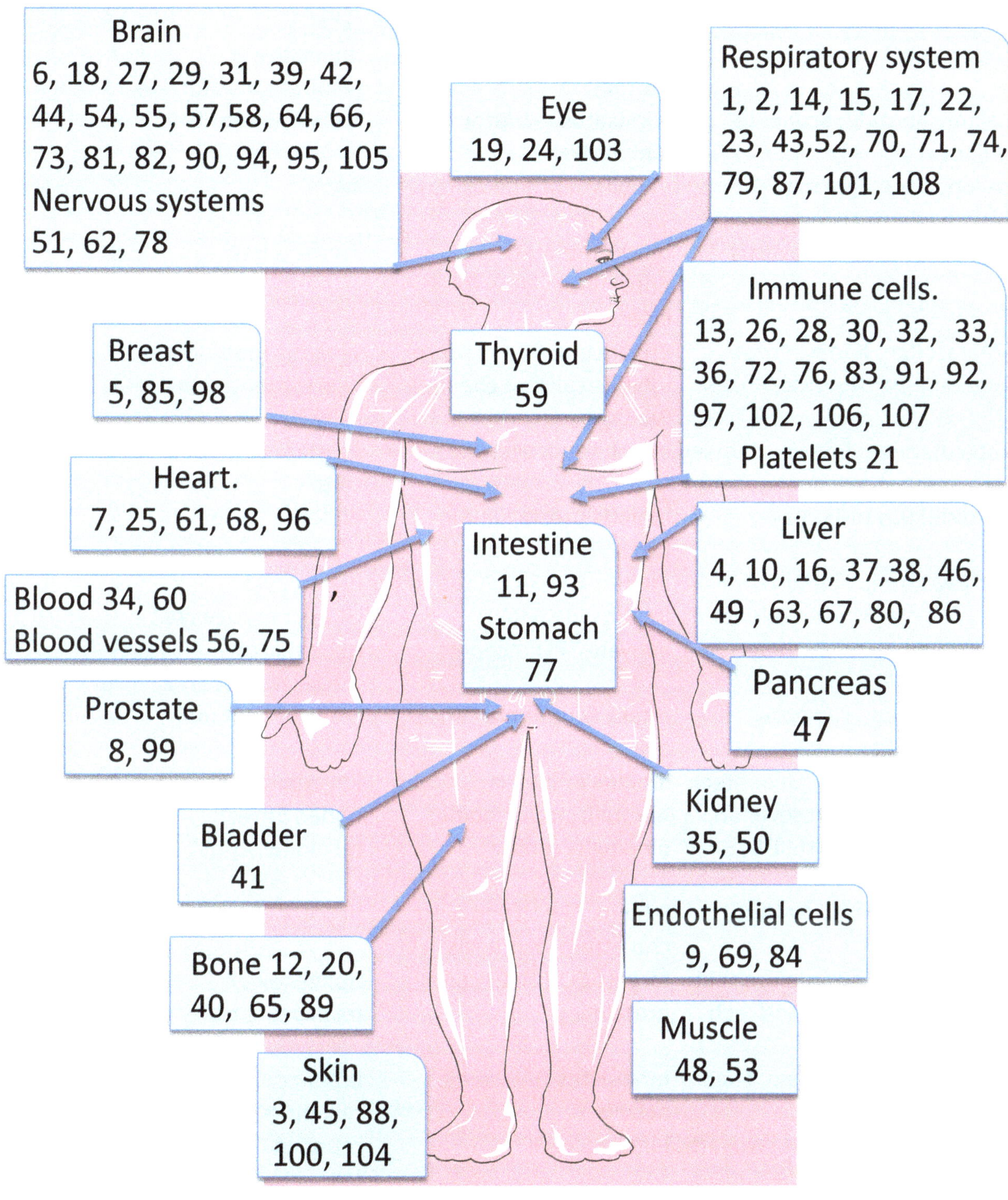
Brain
6, 18, 27, 29, 31, 39, 42,
44, 54, 55, 57,58, 64, 66,
73, 81, 82, 90, 94, 95, 105
Nervous systems
51, 62, 78
Eye
19, 24, 103
Respiratory system
1, 2, 14, 15, 17, 22,
23, 43,52, 70, 71, 74,
79, 87, 101, 108
Immune cells.
13, 26, 28, 30, 32, 33,
36, 72, 76, 83, 91, 92,
97, 102, 106, 107
Platelets 21
Breast
5, 85, 98
Thyroid
59
Heart.
7, 25, 61, 68, 96
Liver
4, 10, 16, 37,38, 46,
49 , 63, 67, 80, 86
Blood 34, 60
Blood vessels 56, 75
Intestine
11, 93
Stomach
77
Pancreas
47
Prostate
8, 99
Kidney
35, 50
Bladder
41
Endothelial cells
9, 69, 84
Bone 12, 20,
40, 65, 89
Muscle
48, 53
Skin
3, 45, 88,
100, 104

	Appendix 2 Medicines	mechanism	body organ	Chapter	Page
	Medicine (generic name, brand name & manufacturer)				
1	ACAM2000; Smallpox Vaccine, Sanofi Pasteur	targets smallpox virus	respiratory mucosa, skin	7	266
2	Ad26.COV2; Janssen	targets COVID-19 spike protein	upper, lower respiratory tract	7	260
3	Afamelanotide; Scenesse, Clinuvel	stimulates receptor for alpha-MSH	melanocytes, skin	3	74
4	Allopurinol; Zyloprim, Burroughs-Wellcome	inhibits xanthine oxidase	liver	2	38
5	Alpelisib: Piqray; Novartis	blocks mutated phosphatidylinositol-3 kinase	breast ducts	6	186
6	Alprazolam; Xanax, Pfizer	enhances GABA receptor	synaptic membranes	5	160
7	Amlodipine; Norvasc, Pfizer	inhibits calcium channel (voltage sensor)	heart smooth muscle cells	4	100
8	Apalutamide; Erleada, Janssen	inhibits androgen receptor	prostate epithelial cells	4	120
9	Aspirin; Bayer 81, Bayer	inhibits prostaglandins production	endothelial cells	4	114
10	Atorvastatin; Lipitor, Pfizer	inhibits HMG-CoA reductase	hepatocyte	2	48
11	Avapritinib; Ayvakit, Blueprint	inhibits PDGFRA	GI tract muscle cells	1	30
12	Avatrombopag; Doptelet, Dova	activate TPO receptor	bone marrow, megakaryocytes	3	78
13	Axicabtagene ciloleucel, Yescarta, Kite	attack lymphoma cancer cells	B-cell lymphoma	6	218
14	Baloxavir, Xofluza, Genentech	inhibits influenza	lung epithelial cells	7	230
15	Bamlanivimab, Etesevimab, LY-CoV555, LY-CoV016; Lilly	neutralizing antibodies, binding receptor	upper, lower respiratory tract	7	258
16	Bempedoic acid; Nexletol, Esperion	inhibits ATP citrate lyase, cholesterol synthesis	hepatocyte	2	46
17	BNT162b2; Comirnaty, Covid-19 vaccine, Pfizer-BioNTech	targets COVID-19 spike protein	upper, lower respiratory tract	7	260
18	Brexanolone; Zulresso, Sage	modulates GABAergic activity	brain neurosteroid receptors	5	164
19	Brolucizumab; Beovu, Novartis	binds to VEGF	retina in back layer of eye	3	58
20	Burosumab; Crysvita, Ultragenyx	inhibits fibroblast growth factor 23	osteoblasts, osteocytes	9	194
21	Caplacizumab; Cablivi, Sanofi	blocks von Willebrand factor	platlets	3	76

	Appendix 2 Medicines	mechanism	body organ	Chapter	Page
22	Casirivimab, imdevimab; REGEN-COV, Regeneron	neutralizing antibodies, binding receptor	upper, lower respiratory tract	7	258
23	Ceftriaxone; Rocephin, Roche	inhibits penicillin-binding protein	bacterial cell walls	5	132
24	Cenegermin; Oxervate, Dompe	replaces deficient nerve growth factor	front of eye	3	62
25	Colchicine; Colcrys, Mutual	inhibits NLRP3 inflammasome	arterial wall, macrophages	4	126
26	Darunavir; Prezista, Jannsen	inhibit HIV polyprotein cleavage	CD4+ T lymphocytes	7	238
27	Deutetrabenazine; Austedo, Teva	inhibits monoamine transporter 2	brain, dopamine circuitry	5	150
28	Dolutegravir; Tivicay, Viiv	inhibit HIV integrase	CD4+ T lymphocytes	7	240
29	Donepezil; Aricept, Eisai	inhibits acetylcholineesterase	basal forebrain, brain stem	5	176
30	Ebola Zaire Vaccine; Ervebo, Merck	targets ebola surface glycoprotein	macrophages, dendritic cells	7	248
31	Edaravone, Radicava, Mitsubishi Tanabe	free radical scavenger	brain motor neurons	5	138
32	Elapegademase,; Revcovi, Lediant	replace mutated adenosine deamidase	lymphoctes	1	10
33	Emapalumab; Gamifant, Novimmune	binds to interferon-gamma	natural killer T cells	6	196
34	Emicizumab; Hemlibra, Genentech	targets factor IXa and X	blood coagulation cascade	6	204
35	Empagliflozin; Jardiance, Lilly, Boehringer Ingelheim	inhibits glucose transport protein (SGLT2)	kidney proximal tubule	4	106
36	Enfuvirtide; Fuzeon, Roche	Inhibits HIV infusion into target cells	CD4+ T lymphocytes	7	242
37	Engerix; Hepatitis B virus vaccine, GSK	vaccine targets hepatitus surface antigen	liver inflammation	7	272
38	Entecavir; Baraclude, BMS	inhibits hepatitis virus reverse transcriptase	liver inflammation	7	270
39	Epidiolex; Cannabidiol, GW	increases serotonin action	postsynaptic neuron receptors	6	180
40	Epoetin alfa; Epogen, Amgen	supplements erythropoietin	bone marrow	4	92
41	Erdafitinib; Balversa, Janssen Eszopiclone	inhibits fibroblast growth factor receptors	bladder, urothelial cells	4	122
42	Eszopiclone; Lunesta, Sepracor	boosts the levels of GABA	pre-, post-synaptic membranes	5	162
43	Fluzone; Sanofi Pasteur	vaccine against influenza A and B	viral hemagglutinin (HA)	7	232

	Appendix 2 Medicines	mechanism	body organ	Chapter	Page
44	Galcanezumab; Emgality, Lilly	blocks calcitonin gene-related peptide	trigeminal ganglions neurons	5	168
45	Gardasil-9; Human papillomavirus vaccine, Merck	targets HPV major capsid protein	skin keratinocytes	7	276
46	Givosiran; Givlaari, Alnylam	reduces synthesis, delta-aminolevulinic acid	hepatocyte	6	210
47	Glimepiride; Amaryl, Sanofi Aventis	binds to SUR1 receptor	pancreatic beta cells	2,4	42, 110
48	Golodirsen; Vyondys, Sarepta	increases dystrophin synthesis	muscle fibers	6	212
49	Heplisav-B; Hepatitis B virus vaccine, Dynavax	vaccine targets hepatitus surface antigen	liver inflammation	7	272
50	Hydrochlorothiazide; Microzide, Merck	inhibits NaCl cotransporter	kidney nephron, distal tubule	4	102
51	Hydrocodone: Vicodin, Abbvie	activates mu-opiod receptor	neurons, pain inhibitory	5	174
52	Inmazeb; Regeneron	binds to viral surface glycoproteins	macrophages, dendritic cells	7	246
53	Insulin glargine; Lantus, Sanofi Aventis	stimulates insulin receptor	adipose, muscle, liver cells	4	108
54	Istradefylline; Nourianz, Kyowa Kirin	inhibits adenosine 2A receptor	forebrain, neuronal clusters	5	172
55	Lamotrigine; Lamictal, GSK	inhibits glutamate transporters	neurons and astrocytes	5	158
56	Lanadelumab; Takhzyro, Shire	inhibits plasma kallikrein	blood vessels	6	198
57	Lasmiditan; Reyvow, Lilly	stimulates serotonin-1F receptors	brain trigeminal system	5	152
58	Lemborexant; Dayvigo, Eisai	blocks orexin receptors	brain trigeminal system	5	170
59	Levothyroxine; Synthroid, Abbott	supplements thyroxine (T4)	thyroid gland	4	88
60	Lisinopril; Zestril, AstraZeneca	inhibits angiotensin converting enzyme	blood	4	96
61	Lonafarnib; Zokinvy, Merck	inhibits protein farnesyltransferase	heart muscle, adipose tissue	6	190
62	Lorlatinib; Lorbrena, Pfizer	inhibits ALK tyrosine kinase	lung nerve cells	3	66
63	Lumasiran; Oxlumo, Alnylam	reduces glycolate oxidase	hepatocyte	6	216
64	Lumateperone; Caplyta, Intra-cellular therapies, BMS	blocking action, dopamine, serotonin receptors	basal forebrain, limbic system	5	144
65	Lusutrombopag; Mulpleta, Shionogi	activate TPO receptor	bone marrow, megakaryocytes	3	78
66	Mayzent; Siponimod, Novartis	internalizes sphingosine-1-receptor	endothelial cells, astrocytes	5	136

	Appendix 2 Medicines	mechanism	body organ	Chapter	Page
67	Metformin; Glucophage, Merck	stimulates insulin receptor	adipose tissue, muscle, liver cells	4	108
68	Metoprolol;, Lopressor, AstraZeneca	blocks epinephrine binding to receptor	heart muscle cells	4	98
69	Migalastat; Galafold, Amicus	corrects misfolding, alpha-galactoside A enzyme	lysosomes in cells	6	182
70	Molnupiravir; Merck	corruption of RNA polymerase	upper, lower respiratory tract	7	254
71	mRNA-1273; Moderna	targets COVID-19 spike protein	upper, lower respiratory tract	7	260
72	Mycophenolic acid, Myfortic, Novartis	imhibits purine synthesis	B and T cells	2	36
73	Naxitamab; Danyleza, YmAbs therapeutics	binds disialoganglioside GB2	neuroblasts	6	202
74	Nirmatrelvir; Ritonavir, Paxlovid, Pfizer	inhibit viral protease	upper, lower respiratory tract	7	256
75	Nitroglycerin; Nitrostat, Parke-Davis	relaxes smooth muscle	small blood vessels	1	16
76	Ocrelizumab; Ocrevus, Genentech	binds to CD20 receptor on B cells	B lymphocytes	5	134
77	Omeprazole; Prilosec, AstraZeneca	inhibits stomach proton pump	stomach lining, bone marrow	2	28
78	Onasemnogene abeparvovec; Zolgensma, Novartis	repair survival of motor neuron complex	motor nerve cell	6	220
79	Oseltamivir, Tamiflu, Roche	inhibit influenza neuraminidase	lung epithelial cells	7	228
80	Patisiran; Onpattro, Alnylam	degrades mutant transthyretin	hepatocytes	6	214
81	Pegvaliase; Palynziq, Biomarin	replaces deficient phenylalanine hydroxlase	blood and brain tissue	1	12
82	Pitolisant; Wakix, Harmony	inhibits histamine H3 recepter	presynaptic histamine nerves	5	154
83	Polatuzumab; Polivy, Genentech	inhibition of CD79b B cells	lymphocytes	3	80
84	Prednisone; Rayos, Horizon	prednisone blocks glucocorticoid receptor	diverse distribution	4	116
85	Raloxifene; Evista, Lilly	inhibits estrogen receptor	breast tissue	1	18
86	Recombivax; Hepatitis B virus vaccine; Merck	vaccine targets hepatitus surface antigen	liver inflammation	7	272
87	Remdesivir; Veklury, Gilead	inhibits viral RNA polymerase	upper, lower respiratory tract	7	252
88	Risankizumab; Skyrizi, AbbVie	blocks interleukin 23, dendritic cells	keratinocyte, skin	3	70

	Appendix 2 Medicines	mechanism	body organ	Chapter	Page
89	Romosozumab; Evenity, Amgen	blocks sclerosin	bone osteocytes, osteoblasts	6	200
90	Safinamide; Xadago, Newron	inhibits monamine oxidase B	brain, synaptic cleft	5	148
91	Satralizumab; Enspryng, Genentech	inhibits IL-6 receptor	neutrophils	3	64
92	Selinexor; Xpovio, Karopharm	inhibits tumor supressor protein inactivation	plasma cells	3	82
93	Semaglutide; Rybelus, Novo Nordisk	activates glucagon-like peptide-1 receptor	intestine	6	206
94	Setmelanotide; Imcivree, Rhythm	activates melanocortin 4 receptors	hypothalamus	6	208
95	Solriamfetol; Sunosi, Jazz	block norepinephrine, dopamine transport	presynaptic neurons	5	146
96	Tafamidis; Vyndamax, Pfizer	stabilizes transthryetin	heart muscle	6	188
97	Tagraxofusp; Elzonris, Stemline	inhibits elongation factor 2	plasmacytoid dendritic cells	6	192
98	Talazoparib; Talzenna, Pfizer	inhibits PARP complex	breast ducts	6	184
99	Tamsulosin; Flomax, Boehringer Ingelheim	inhibits alpha-1A-adrenergic receptor	prostate smooth muscle cells	4	124
100	Tazemetostat; Tazverik, Epizyme	blocks EZH2 methyl transferase	skin, soft tissue	3	68
101	Tecovirimat, Tpoxx, Siga	inhibits envelope wrapping protein	respiratory mucosa, skin	7	264
102	Tenofovir disoproxil; Viread, Gilead	inhibition of HIV reverse transcription	CD4+ T lymphocytes	7	236
103	Teprotumumab; Tepezza, Horizon	binds to IGF receptor 1, inhibits IGF-1	orbital fibroblast	3	60
104	Trifarotene; Aklief, Galderma	stimulates retinoic acid receptor	skin epithelial cells, sebocytes,	3	72
105	Ubrogepant, Ubrelevy, Allergan	blocks calcitonin gene-related peptide	trigeminal ganglions, neurons	5	168
106	Upadacitinib; Rinvoq, AbbVie	inhibits Janus kinse-1	immune cells	4	118
107	Vincristine; Oncovin, Lilly	inhibits microtubule formation	lymphatic system	3	80
108	Zanamivir; Relenza, Glaxo Wellcome	inhibits influenza neuraminidase	lung epithelial cells	7	228

Target biochemistry for action of medicines

p=page number

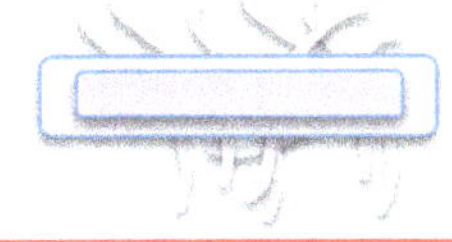

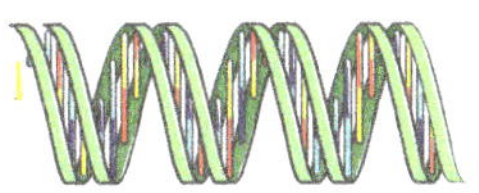

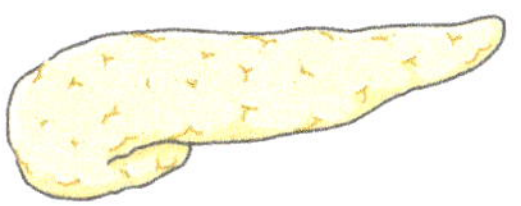

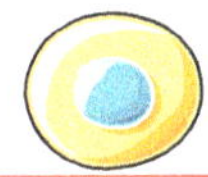

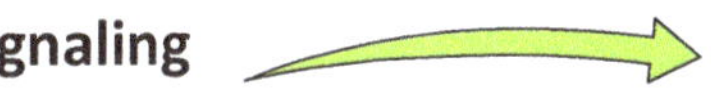

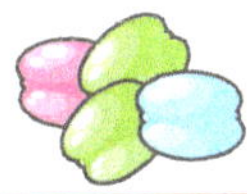

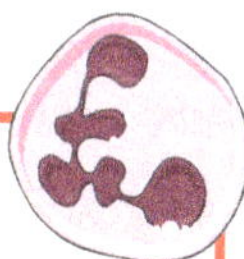

Target biochemistry for action of medicines

p=page number

Epithelial/ endothelial cells
Androgen receptor p121
Estrogen receptor p19
Glucose transport p107
NaCl transporter p103
Norepinephrine, alpha-1A receptor p125
Prostaglandin synthesis p115
SGLT2 transporter (sodium dependent
Sphingosine-1-phosphate receptor p137

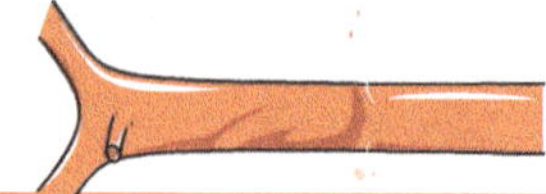

Blood
Glyoxalate metabolism p217
Hemostasis p77, 79, 205
Kallikrein p199
Red blood cells p93
Transthyretin p189, 215

Smooth Muscle
Calcium channel p101
Dystrophin p213
Epinephrine, andrenergic receptor p99
Nerve cell messages p31
Relaxation p17
Renin angiotensin system p97

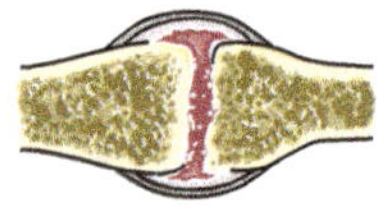

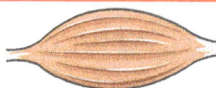

Bone
Fibroblast growth factor 23 (195)
Sclerostin p201
Xanthine oxidase p39

Neurons
Acetyl-choline esterase. p177
Adenosine A2A receptor p173
Calcitonin gene-related peptide, receptor p169
Dopamine receptors p145
Free radical scavenger p139
GABA-A receptor p161, 163, 165
Glutamate transporters p159
Histamine H3 receptor p155
Monoamine oxidase B p149
Monoamine transporters p147, 151
Mu-opioid receptor p175
Orexin 1,2 receptor p171
Serotonin receptors p153,181
Survival motor neuron protein 1 p221
Vesicular monoamine transporter 2 p151

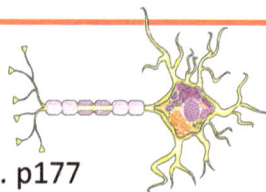

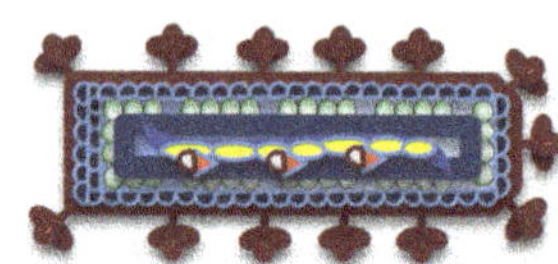

Virus
Capsid protein p275
Envelope wrapping protein VP37 p265
Hemagglutinin p233
Integrase p241
Neuraminidase p229
N-terminal fusion peptide p243
Reverse transcriptase p237, 271
RNA-dependent RNA polymerase p253, 255
RNA Endonuclease p231
Polyprotein protease 239, 257
Spike protein receptor binding domain p259, 261
Surface glycoprotein p247, 249
Viral particle p277

www.ingramcontent.com/pod-product-compliance
Lightning Source LLC
Chambersburg PA
CBHW081344190326
41458CB00018B/6084
9789811248191